IMMUNOLOGY FOR PHARMACY

evolve
learning system

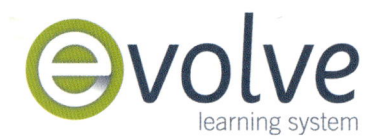

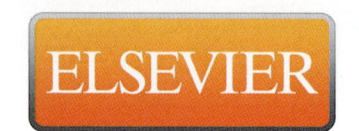

ELSEVIER

YOU'VE JUST PURCHASED
MORE THAN A TEXTBOOK

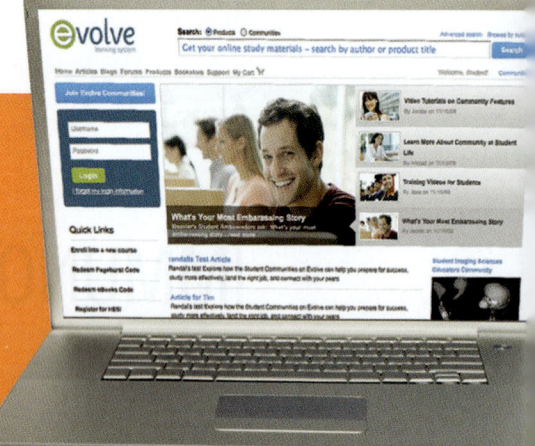

To access your online resources, visit

http://evolve.elsevier.com/Flaherty/immunology/

Register today and gain access to:

- Flashcards
- Animations
- For Instructors
    - Testbank with 300 questions and rationals
    - Image Collection

REGISTER TODAY!

IMMUNOLOGY FOR PHARMACY

Dennis K. Flaherty, PhD

Associate Professor
Department of Pharmaceutical Administrative Sciences
School of Pharmacy
University of Charleston
Charleston, West Virginia

ELSEVIER

ELSEVIER
MOSBY

3251 Riverport Lane
St. Louis, Missouri 63043

IMMUNOLOGY FOR PHARMACY   ISBN: 978-0-323-06947-2
Copyright © 2012 by Mosby, inc., an affiliate of Elsevier Inc.

No part of this publication may be reproduced or transmitted in any form or by any means, electronic or mechanical, including photocopying, recording, or any information storage and retrieval system, without permission in writing from the publisher. Details on how to seek permission, further information about the Publisher's permissions policies and our arrangements with organizations such as the Copyright Clearance Center and the Copyright Licensing Agency, can be found at our website: www.elsevier.com/permissions.

This book and the individual contributions contained in it are protected under copyright by the Publisher (other than as may be noted herein).

Notice

Knowledge and best practice in this field are constantly changing. As new research and experience broaden our understanding, changes in research methods, professional practices, or medical treatment may become necessary.

Practitioners and researchers must always rely on their own experience and knowledge in evaluating and using any information, methods, compounds, or experiments described herein. In using such information or methods they should be mindful of their own safety and the safety of others, including parties for whom they have a professional responsibility.

With respect to any drug or pharmaceutical products identified, readers are advised to check the most current information provided (i) on procedures featured or (ii) by the manufacturer of each product to be administered, to verify the recommended dose or formula, the method and duration of administration, and contraindications. It is the responsibility of practitioners, relying on their own experience and knowledge of their patients, to make diagnoses, to determine dosages and the best treatment for each individual patient, and to take all appropriate safety precautions.

To the fullest extent of the law, neither the Publisher nor the authors, contributors, or editors, assume any liability for any injury and/or damage to persons or property as a matter of products liability, negligence or otherwise, or from any use or operation of any methods, products, instructions, or ideas contained in the material herein.

ISBN: 978-0-323-06947-2

Vice President and Publisher: Linda Duncan
Executive Editor: Kellie White
Developmental Editors: Kelly Milford and Joe Gramlich
Publishing Services Manager: Catherine Jackson
Senior Project Manager: Mary Pohlman
Design Direction: Karen Pauls

Printed in China

Last digit is the print number: 9 8 7 6 5 4 3 2 1

To
Carol,
Wife and best friend

And
Dr. Robert G. Burrell,
Mentor, teacher, and scholar

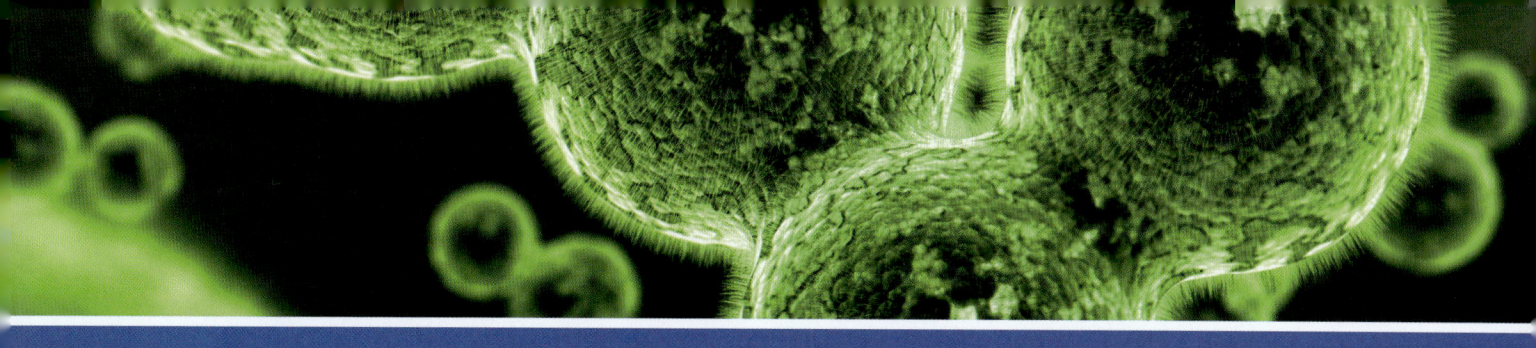

REVIEWERS

Ahmmed Ally, MD, PhD
Professor
Department of Pharmaceutical Sciences
South College School of Pharmacy
Knoxville, Tennessee

Vera C. Campbell, PhD
Assistant Professor
Department of Pharmaceutical Sciences
Hampton University School of Pharmacy
Hampton, Virginia

Deborah A. DeLuca, MS, JD
Assistant Professor
Health Law, Biomedical Ethics and Medical Sciences
School of Health and Medical Sciences
Seton Hall University
South Orange, New Jersey

Kristen Lehman Helms, PharmD
Associate Clinical Professor
Harrison School of Pharmacy
Auburn University
Auburn, Alabama

Paul Juang, PharmD, BCPS
Assistant Professor of Pharmacy Practice
St. Louis College of Pharmacy
St. Louis, Missouri

Brian J. Knoll, PhD
Associate Professor
Pharmacological and Pharmaceutical Sciences
College of Pharmacy
University of Houston
Houston, Texas

Donna Larson, EdD, MT(ASCP)DLM
Dean of Allied Health
Mt. Hood Community College
Gresham, Oregon

Puja Patel, PharmD
Ambulatory and Managed Care Resident
Kaiser Permanente of Georgia
Atlanta, Georgia

John R. Yannelli, PhD
Associate Professor of Microbiology, Immunology and Molecular Genetics
Markey Cancer Center
University of Kentucky
Lexington, Kentucky

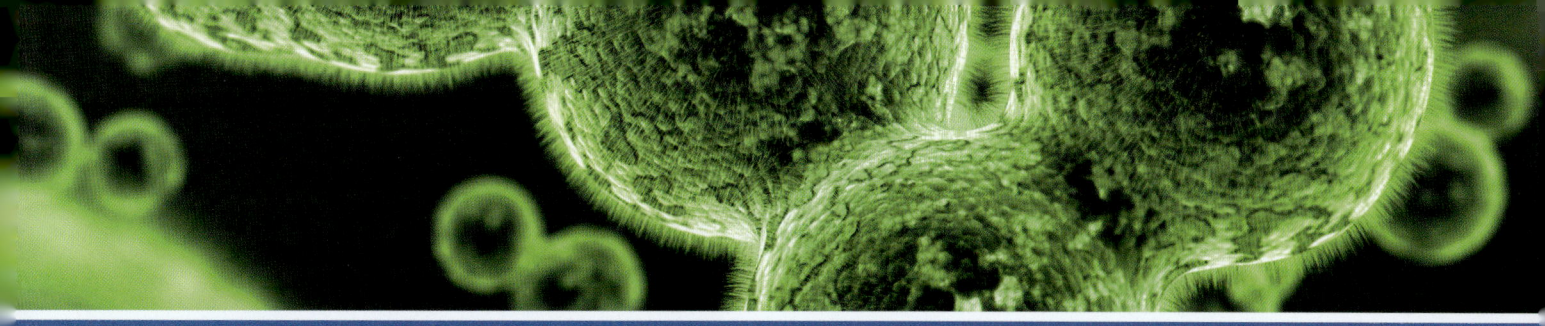

PREFACE

Immunology is discipline within the biomedical sciences that originally studied the host response to microbial infections and tumors. More recently, immunologists have discerned the role of the immune system in allergic reactions, autoimmune diseases and transplantation survival. This book presents basic immunological concepts and mechanisms while keeping the focus on the needs of student pharmacists in terms of pedagology, practical applications and therapy. Pedagogical features included in each chapter include:

- Objectives
- Key terms
- Assessment questions

This book is timely and unique for several reasons. Until now, there were no textbooks that meet the needs of both students and practicing pharmacists. Current textbooks are geared toward upper-level undergraduates or graduate students in immunology or microbiology. Moreover, this text discusses topics not found in current immunology textbooks, such as prophylaxis and vaccination (many states allow pharmacists to vaccinate patients); antibodies as therapeutic and diagnostic agents, biological modifiers and cancer vaccines. Treatment and therapeutics for various diseases and syndromes also are introduced in this text. Because this is an introductory text, dosing and specific treatment regimens are not discussed.

In many current immunology texts, chapters are arranged as independent silos with no apparent connections within the overall immune response. In this text, concepts and steps in an immune response are arranged sequentially as they would occur in nature. Other specialized topics (e.g., allergy, autoimmune disease, and immunodeficiencies) are logically arranged around antibody or cellular immune responses. This approach gives the reader a more logical approach to the study of immunology.

Dennis K. Flaherty, PhD

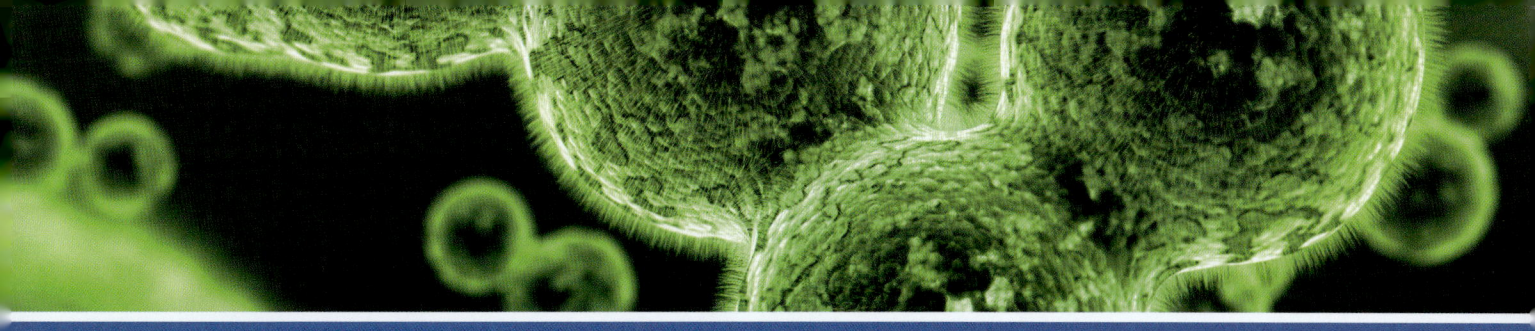

ACKNOWLEDGMENT

The author would like to thank the editorial team at Elsevier Publishing (Kellie White, Kelly Milford, Jennifer Watrous, Mary Pohlman, and Joe Gramlich) for their professionalism and dedication to this project.

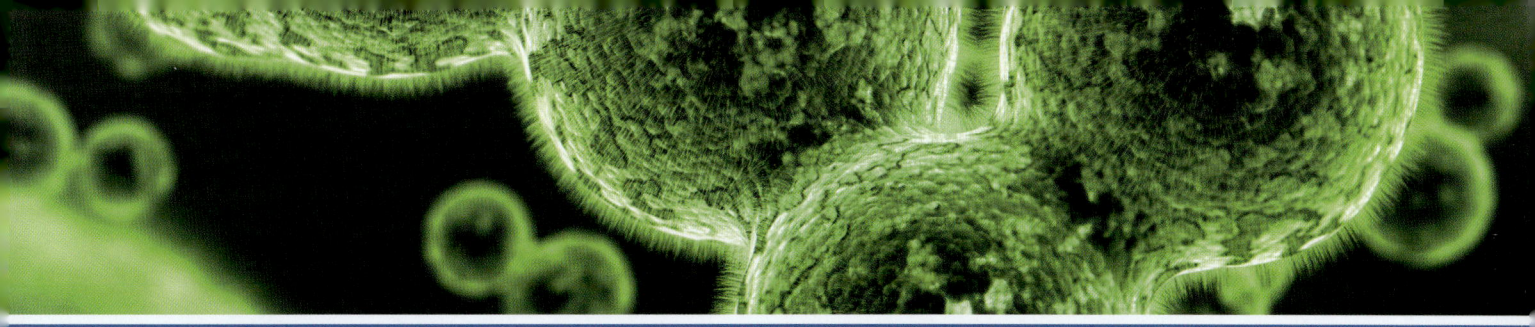

CONTENTS

1. CELLS AND ORGANS OF THE IMMUNE SYSTEM, 1
2. INNATE IMMUNITY, 15
3. IMMUNOGENICITY AND ANTIGENICITY, 23
4. ANTIGEN-PRESENTING MOLECULES, 31
5. ANTIGEN-PRESENTING CELLS, 37
6. SURFACE INTERACTIONS BETWEEN T CELLS AND ANTIGEN-PRESENTING CELLS, 45
7. INTRACELLULAR SIGNALING AND T CELL ACTIVATION, 55
8. B CELL ACTIVATION AND SIGNALING, 63
9. ANTIBODIES, 70
10. ANTIBODY DIVERSITY, 79
11. COMPLEMENT, 87
12. PHAGOCYTOSIS AND INTRACELLULAR KILLING, 97
13. ANTIBODIES AND IN VIVO THERAPY, 102
14. ANTIBODIES AND IN VITRO RESEARCH AND DIAGNOSTIC ASSAYS, 110
15. IMMEDIATE ALLERGIC REACTIONS, 118
16. AUTOIMMUNITY, 127
17. TRANSPLANTATION, 138
18. ANTIGEN PRESENTATION FOR CELL-MEDIATED RESPONSE, 147
19. DELAYED-TYPE HYPERSENSITIVITY REACTIONS, 152
20. CYTOTOXIC T CELLS, 162
21. NATURAL KILLER CELLS, 169
22. FACTORS THAT INFLUENCE THE IMMUNE RESPONSE, 175
23. CYTOKINES AND BIOLOGICAL MODIFIERS, 181
24. VACCINES IN THEORY AND PRACTICE, 189
25. VACCINE-PREVENTABLE DISEASES, 197
26. ACQUIRED IMMUNE DEFICIENCY SYNDROME, 214

ANSWERS TO ASSESSMENT QUESTIONS, 225

GLOSSARY, 227

INDEX, 239

CHAPTER 1

Cells and Organs of the Immune System

LEARNING OBJECTIVES

- Describe the structure and function of polymorphonuclear leukocytes or neutrophil
- Describe the structure and function of eosinophils
- Describe the structure and function of basophils
- Describe the structure and function of monocytes
- Compare and contrast monocytes and macrophages
- Describe the structure and function of large granular lymphocytes
- Identify the role of the T cell receptor (TCR) in an immune response
- Compare the pan-CD (cluster of differentiation) markers present on T and B cells
- Identify the function of T and B cell subsets
- Identify CD markers present on T and B cell subsets
- Describe the structure and function of natural killer (NK) cells
- Identify CD markers present on NK cells
- Describe the structure and function of the thymus
- Identify the roles of the thymic cortex and medulla in T cell maturation
- Understand positive and negative selection of T lymphocytes
- Identify anatomic sites responsible for B cell maturation
- Identify the role of the B cell receptor (BCR) in an immune response
- Compare and contrast the structure and function of peripheral blood and lymph systems
- Describe the structure of a lymph node
- Identify the cellular constituents of the cortical, paracortical, and medullary regions of the lymph node
- Describe the structure and function of the red and white splenic pulps
- Identify the roles of the cells localized in the splenic marginal zone
- Describe the role of Peyer's patches in immunity
- Identify the roles of intraepithelial lymphocytes (IELs) in mucosal immunity
- Describe the roles of microfold (M) cells in mucosal immunity
- Compare and contrast the advantage of mucosal versus peripheral blood immune responses
- Identify the location of three different tonsils
- Describe diapedesis of white blood cells
- Understand the roles of cell adhesion molecules, selectins, integrins, and chemokines in diapedesis
- Compare and contrast the symptoms, anatomic features, and immune defects present in DiGeorge and Nezelof syndromes
- Compare and contrast defects present in leukocyte adhesion deficiency types I and II

KEY TERMS

Antigen
B cell
B cell receptor (BCR)
CD4Th1 cell
CD4Th2 cell
CD8Tc1
CD8Tc2
Cluster of differentiation (CD) markers
Large granular lymphocyte (LGL)
Macrophage
Monocyte
Plasma cell
Small lymphocyte
T cell
T cell receptor (TCR)

INTRODUCTION

The immune system consists of a network of circulating blood cells, lymphoid tissues, and organs, which respond to foreign material by producing soluble antibodies (humoral response) or activated lymphocytes and macrophages (cellular response). Lymphoid tissue is composed of primary and secondary lymphoid organs. The bone marrow and thymus are considered primary lymphoid organs. The spleen, lymph nodes, and tonsils are regarded as secondary organs; the submucosa of the lung and intestine are also important secondary lymphoid organs. To accommodate these organs into a classification scheme, these organs are called the *bronchiole-associated lymphoid tissue (BALT)* and the *gut-associated lymphoid tissue (GALT)*. Together, these sites comprise the mucosal-associated lymphoid tissue (MALT). Lymphocytes and macrophages are the major effector cells in immunologic reactions.

HEMATOPOIESIS

Hematopoiesis refers to the development or maturation of red blood cells, white blood cells, and platelets. In the third month of gestation, hematopoietic stem cells migrate to the fetal liver. Later in gestation, stem cells localize in the spleen, where they undergo maturation. After birth, most stem cells are found in the bone marrow. Marrow is found in tubular, flat, and long bones and consists of a connective tissue framework, called *stroma*, which supports red or yellow pulp. Red pulp, which is the major source of hemopoietic stem cells, is found in flat bones such as the hip bone, breast bone, ribs, and vertebrae. The cancellous material at the epiphyseal plate of long bones contains red pulp. Yellow pulp is the major marrow constituent in long tubular bones and is comprised of aggregated fat cells.

Stem cells from red pulp produce four major cell lineages: (1) erythrocytes, (2) platelets, (3) myeloid cells (polymorphonuclear leukocytes, basophils, eosinophils, monocyte/macrophages), and (4) lymphocytes. These lineages undergo maturation in the bone marrow before being released into blood.

BLOOD

Blood contains red and white cells. Red cells are responsible for carrying oxygen to tissues, and white blood cells play a key role in fighting infections.

White Blood Cells

Peripheral blood contains red blood cells, white blood cells, and platelets. Based on the presence or absence of cytoplasmic granules, white blood cells can be defined as granulocytes and nongranulocytes. Granulocyte subsets include polymorphonuclear leukocytes, eosinophils, and basophils. Monocytes and small lymphocytes are generally considered nongranulocytic. However, a small subpopulation of lymphocytes, called *large granular lymphocytes (LGLs)*, does contain granules.

Polymorphonuclear Neutrophils

Polymorphonuclear neutrophils (PMN) (also referred to as polymorphonuclear leukocytes [PML]) constitute 50% to 70% of the white blood cells in peripheral blood. Their main function is to ingest and destroy foreign protein and bacteria. PMNs have a multi-lobed nucleus, which is usually divided into three or more segments (Figure 1-1).

The cytoplasm contains four distinct types of granules: (1) primary or azurophilic granules, (2) secondary granules, (3) gelatinase granules, and (4) secretory vesicles.

Primary Granules

These granules contain myeloperoxidase and lysozyme, which play major roles in the destruction of intracellular bacteria. Myeloperoxidase converts hydrogen peroxide into hypochlorous acid, which reduces pH and initiates the destruction of the bacterial cell wall. Lysozyme is an enzyme that disrupts the structural integrity of bacterial cell walls by breaking polymeric β 1-4 linkages.

Secondary Granules

Secondary granules contain additional enzymes such as apolactoferrin and collagenase, which prevent bacterial growth and increase PMN mobility. Apolactoferrin binds free iron and prevents the bacterial synthesis of heme-containing proteins such as cytochromes.

Tertiary Granules

Tertiary and secretory granules also play a role in immunity and host defense. Tertiary granules contain lysozyme and gelatinase. Gelatinase degrades ground substances between cells and increases PMN mobility. Secretory vesicles excrete N-formyl-1-methionyl-1-leucyl-1-phenylalanine (FMLP), which is a chemoattractant and activating agent for PMNs.

PMNs are produced in the bone marrow and undergo a 9-day to 2-week, seven-step maturation process from myeloblasts to mature cells. Mature cells entering the blood may remain in circulation (circulating pool) or marginate (marginating pool) by attaching to the endothelial lining of the vessels in capillary beds. Cells in capillary beds express certain molecules, called *selectins*, which preferentially attach PMNs to the vessel wall.

In response to infection or inflammation, PMNs "demarginate" and enter the blood circulation. At the same time, the bone marrow releases large numbers of immature neutrophils, called *neutrophilic "bands,"* into the circulation. The influx of immature band cells, commonly referred to by physicians as a

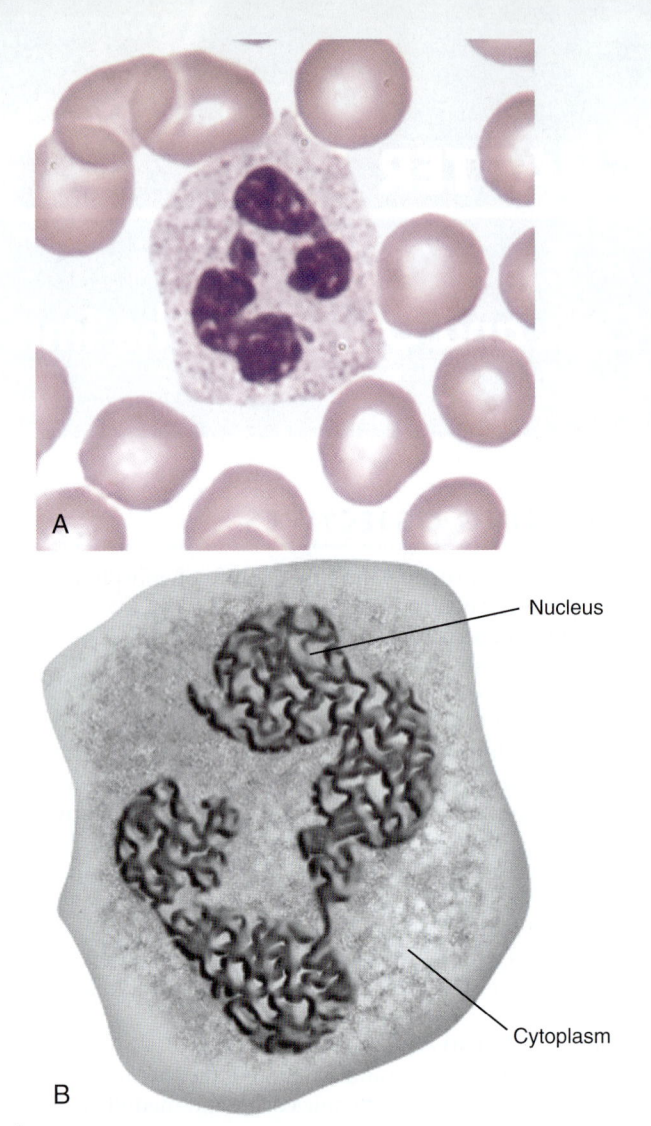

Figure 1-1

A, A polymorphonuclear neutrophils (PMN) in a blood smear also known as polymorphonuclear leukocyte (PML) (x1000). **B,** A schematic of a polymorphonuclear leukocyte. Note the multi-lobed nucleus. (From Carr J, Rodak B: Clinical hematology atlas, ed 3, St Louis, 2009, Saunders.)

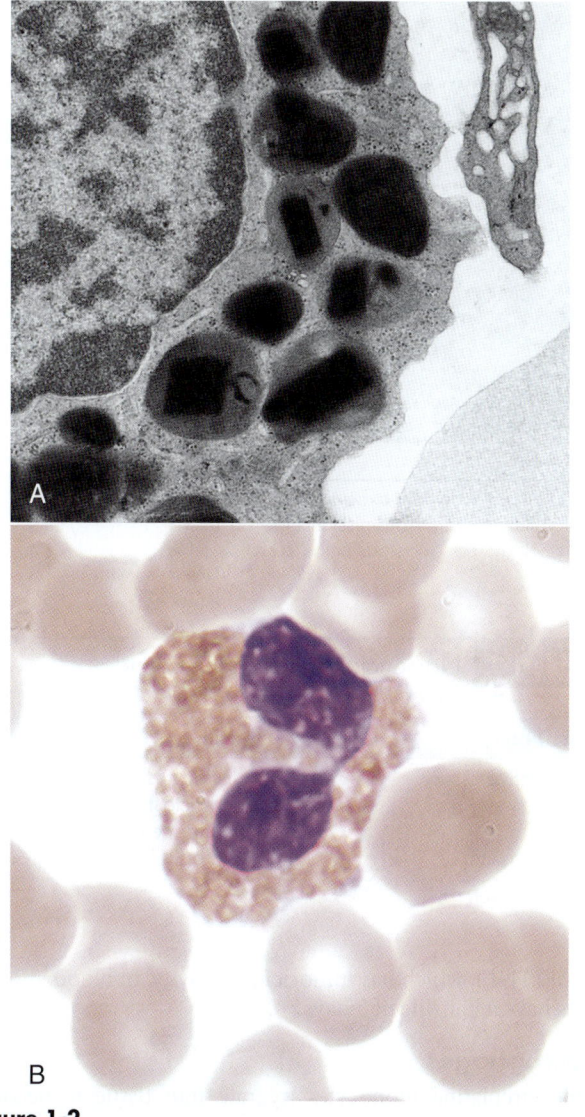

Figure 1-2

A, The internal structures of an eosinophilic granule are shown in this electron micrograph. **B,** An eosinophil in a blood smear (x1000). Note the reddish-orange granules. (From Carr J, Rodak B: Clinical hematology atlas, ed 3, St Louis, 2009, Saunders.)

left shift in blood cells, is indicative of an acute infection. The half-life of PMNs is 1 day in blood and 5 days in tissue.

Eosinophils

Eosinophils comprise 2% to 5 % of the circulating white blood cells. They are characterized by bi-lobed nuclei and the presence of large reddish-orange (eosin staining) granules and refractive crystals in the cytoplasm (Figure 1-2).

Eosinophils migrate to inflammatory sites and extrude granules into the external environment. The contents of these granules include major basic protein (MBP), eosinophilic cationic protein (ECP), eosinophil peroxidase (EPO), and eosinophil-derived neurotoxin (EDN). Extruded granules are a useful alternative for killing large extracellular pathogens that cannot be ingested by phagocytic cells. The proteins in granules have the following functions:

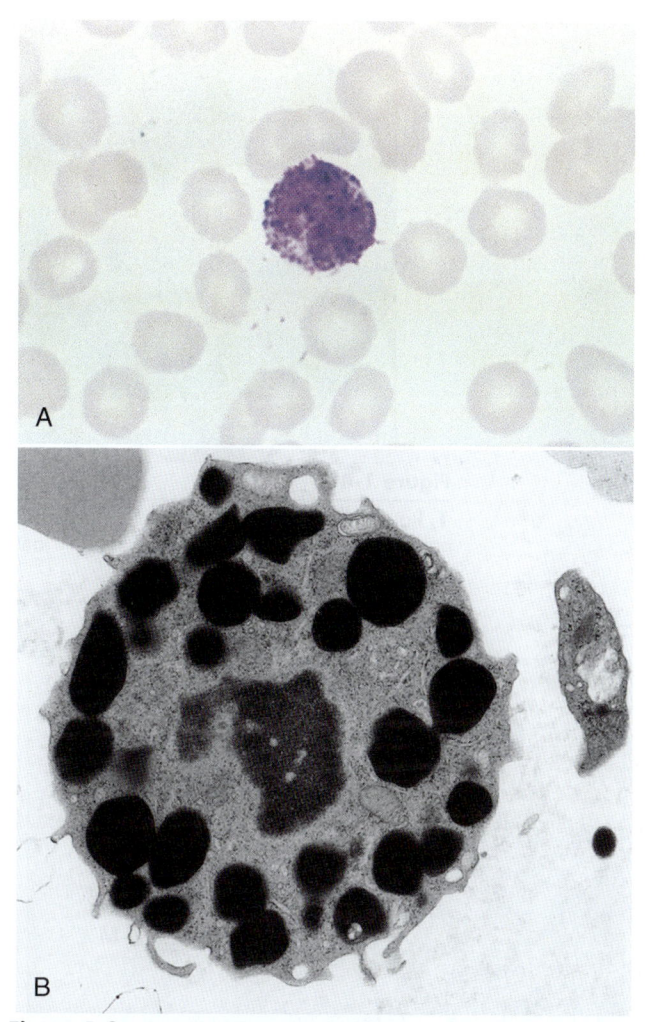

Figure 1-3

A, A basophil with an obscured nucleus. **B,** An electron micrograph of a basophil (x28,750). (A, from Rodak B, Fritsma G, Doig K: Hematology: Clinical principles and applications, ed 3, St Louis, 2007, Saunders. B, from Carr J, Rodak B: Clinical hematology atlas, ed 3, St Louis, 2009, Saunders.)

MBP	• Cytotoxic to helminth larvae • Releases histamine and other preformed mediators from basophils
ECP	• Cytotoxic by pore formation in cell walls
EPO	• Neuronal and axonal damage in the cerebellum and spinal cord

Basophils

Basophils constitute less than 1% of circulating leukocytes. They are small cells that have multi-lobed, heterochromatic nuclei and are easily stained with acidic or basophilic dyes (Figure 1-3). Basophils are one of the major effector cells in skin allergic reactions and termination of helminth infections. Cytoplasmic granules contain histamine, heparin, and tryptase.

Mast Cells

Mast cells are distributed beneath the epithelial linings of the skin and of the respiratory, intestinal, and genitourinary tracts. Although they have similar morphologies, mast cells are *not*

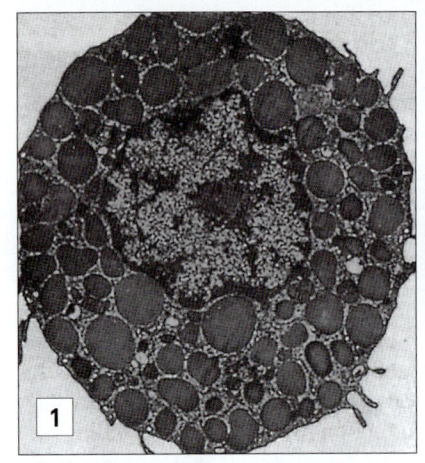

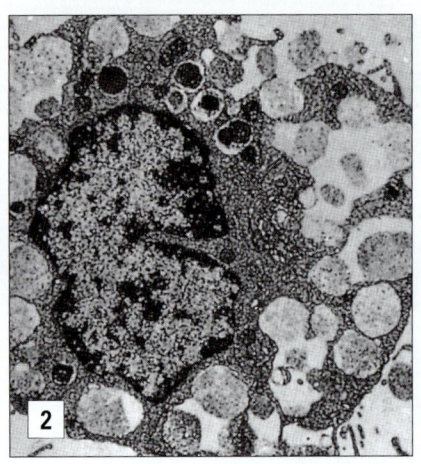

Figure 1-4

1, Rat peritoneal mast cells show electron-dense granules. **2,** Vacuolation with exocytosis of the granule contents has occurred after incubation with anti-immunoglobulin E (IgE). Transmission electron micrographs. (×2700.) (In Roitt I, Brostoff J, Male D, Roth D: Immunology, ed 7, Philadelphia, 2006, Mosby. Courtesy of Dr. D. Lawson.)

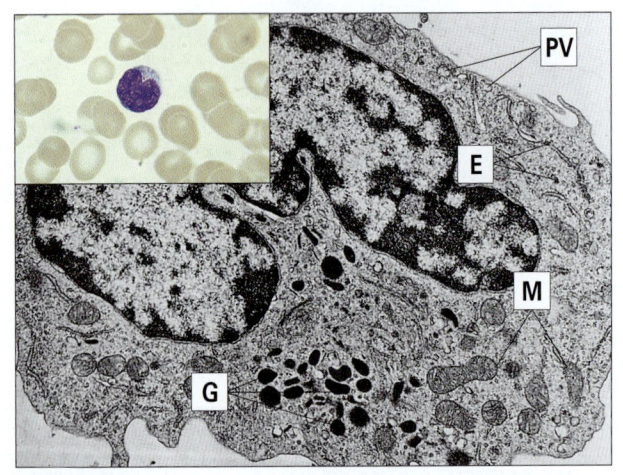

Figure 1-5

Ultrastructure of a monocyte showing the horseshoe-shaped nucleus, pinocytotic vesicles (*PV*), lysosomal granules (*G*), mitochondria (*M*), and isolated rough endoplasmic reticulum cisternae (*E*). (×8000.) *Inset:* Light microscope image of a monocyte from the blood. (×1200.) (In Roitt I, Brostoff J, Male D, Roth D: Immunology, ed 7, Philadelphia, 2006, Mosby. Courtesy of Dr. B. Nichols.)

Table 1-1	Nomenclature for Tissue-Bound Macrophages
Location	**Name**
Connective tissue	Histiocytes
Bone	Osteoclasts
Liver	Kupffer cells
Neural tissue	Microglial cells

basophils (Figure 1-4). They are derived from a different progenitor, have a different natural history, and express different cell surface markers.

Cytoplasmic granules are normal constituents of mast cells and contain the same inflammatory mediators as basophils. When released from mast cells, the inflammatory mediators facilitate allergic reactions in the respiratory tract and the intestine.

Monocytes

Monocytes comprise approximately 2% to 6% of the circulating white blood cells. They are the largest white blood cells in peripheral blood and contain large, indented nuclei, as well as abundant cytoplasm and azurophilic granules (Figure 1-5). As part of the immune response, monocytes degrade foreign material and present it to lymphocytes. Monocytes also produce reactive oxygen metabolites and the tumor necrosis factor (TNF), which has tumoricidal activity. In blood, monocytes have a half-life of 3 days.

Macrophages

Some circulating monocytes migrate into tissue to become fixed macrophages. Generally, these macrophages are located in certain anatomic areas, that is, bone, liver, brain, and connective tissue, where microbes are most likely to enter tissue. Tissue macrophages are usually named for their locations. For example, osteoclasts are found in bone, microglial cells are localized in the brain, and histiocytes are restricted to connective tissue.

The different types of tissue macrophages are presented in Table 1-1. Tissue macrophage populations are renewed every 6 to 16 days by an influx of monocytes or by the proliferation of tissue progenitor cells.

Lymphocytes

Between 20% and 45% of circulating white blood cells are lymphocytes. On the basis of size and staining patterns, lymphocytes are classified as small lymphocytes or large granular lymphocytes (Figure 1-6). Small lymphocytes have large, dark-staining nuclei, little cytoplasm, and no granules. Most small lymphocytes are localized in secondary lymphoid tissue (e.g., spleen or lymph nodes). Only 2% of these cells circulate in peripheral blood at any point in time. Large granular lymphocytes (LGLs), which arise in bone marrow, have large nuclei, plentiful cytoplasm, and multiple azurophilic granules. LGLs function as NK cells, which induce apoptosis in virus-infected cells and tumor cells. Lymphocytes have a half-life of several weeks to years.

CHAPTER 1   CELLS AND ORGANS OF THE IMMUNE SYSTEM

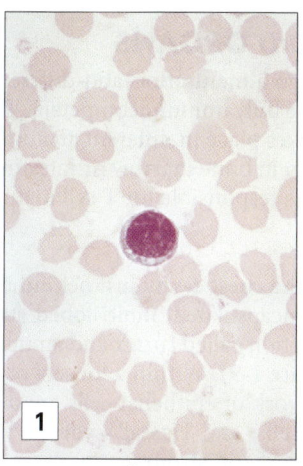

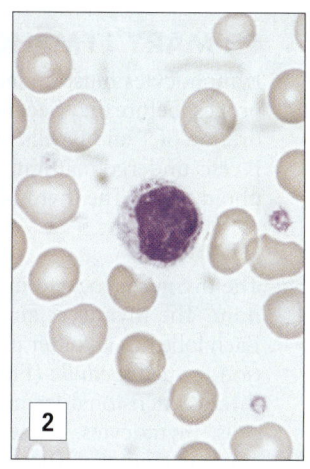

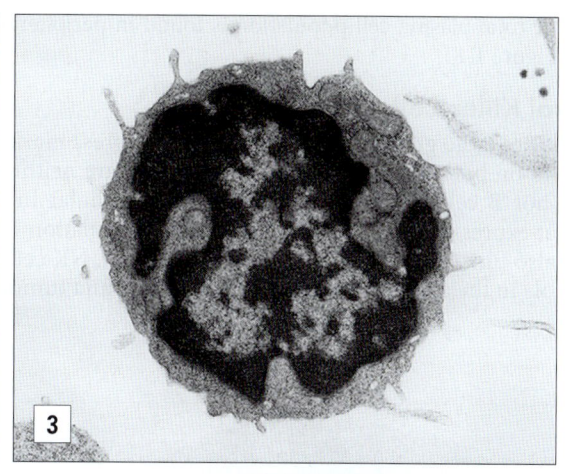

Figure 1-6

1, The small lymphocyte has no granules, a round nucleus, and a high N:C ratio. **2**, The large granular lymphocyte *(LGL)* has a lower N:C ratio, indented nucleus, and azurophilic granules in the cytoplasm. Giemsa stain (Courtesy of Dr. A. Stevens and Professor J. Lowe.). **3**, An electron micrograph of a lymphocyte (x30,000). In general, the distinction between what is a large granule lymphocyte and what is a small lymphocyte is determined by the amount of cytoplasm within the cell. (From Carr J, Rodak B: Clinical hematology atlas, ed 3, St Louis, 2009, Saunders.)

Subdivision of Small Lymphocytes

Small lymphocytes are divided into T and B cells on the basis of differentiation in the thymus (T cells) or in bone marrow (B cells). T cells are involved in the apoptosis of tumor cells, inflammatory responses to intracellular bacteria, and immuneregulation. B cells differentiate into plasma cells that produce soluble, protein antibodies directed toward foreign protein, carbohydrates, and extracellular microbial pathogens called antigens.

T and B cells cannot be distinguished by light microscopy, since all small lymphocytes have the same morphology. The presence of surface glycoproteins and glycolipids, called *cluster of differentiation (CD) markers*, is used to identify T and B cells. All T cells express CD3, which is part of a TCR that interacts with antigenic fragments. Each lymphocyte has only a single TCR type and recognizes only one antigen.

Within the T cell population are several subpopulations with different immunologic functions (Table 1-2). T cells are classified into helper/amplifier (CD4) cells and cytotoxic (CD8) cells. On the basis of cytokine production patterns, several CD4 subsets have been defined. For example, one population of CD4 T helper 2 (Th2) cells assists B cells in the production of antibodies. A second CD4 T cell amplifier (Th1) cell population generates inflammatory responses to foreign material.

Two subpopulations of CD8 cytotoxic T cells have been identified as well. Following stimulation, CD8 Tc1 induce apoptosis in tumor cells and virus-infected cells. The other population of CD8 Tc2 cells has limited cytolytic capacity but secretes proteins that inhibit cellular division or viral replication. When infection of critical, nonregenerative organs (e.g., brain) is present, Tc2 cells inhibit the replication of tumors or viruses without destroying infected cells and tissue.

All B cells express CD19-21 cell surface markers. B cells must differentiate into plasma cells before producing antibodies. Plasma cells contain more condensed, eccentrically placed nuclei and abundant cytoplasm. These cells also develop ribosomes and a large rough endoplasmic reticulum, as well as the Golgi apparatus, which is used for antibody secretion (Figure 1-7). Plasma cells are usually found in lymph nodes. Less than

Table 1-2 Cluster of Differentiation Markers on Lymphocytes

CD Marker	Lymphocyte Populations Expressing Specific CD Markers
CD3	All T cells
CD4	Helper/amplifier population
CD4, CD45RA, CD30	Th2 helper cells
CD4, CD45RO, CD30+	Th1 amplifier cells
CD8	Cytotoxic T cell population
CD8, CD28-	Tc1 cells
CD8, CD28+	Tc 2 cells
CD19-21	Most B cells
CD16, CD56	Natural killer cells

CD, Cluster of differentiation.

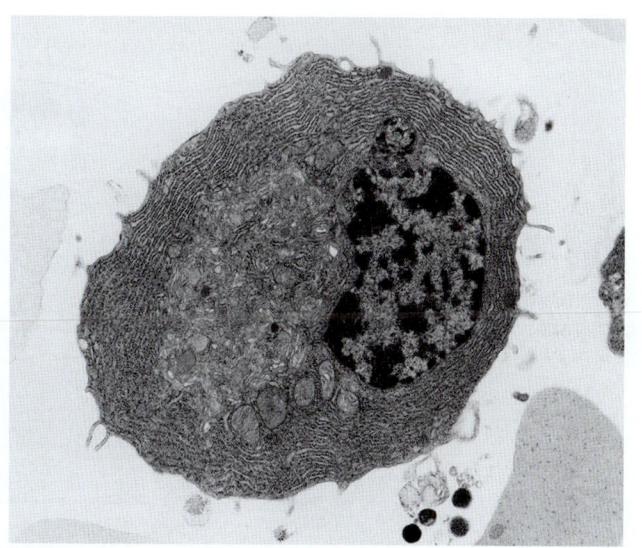

Figure 1-7

An electron micrograph of a plasma cell (x17,500). The cell is characterized by the parallel arrays of rough endoplasmic reticulum that are observed in its periphery. (From Carr J, Rodak B: Clinical hematology atlas, ed 3, St Louis, 2009, Saunders.)

1% of the total plasma cell population is found in peripheral blood (Figure 1-8).

Natural Killer Cells

NK cells are large granular lymphocytes that express markers found on both T and B cells. Most NK cells are neither T cells nor B cells and may represent a third cellular lineage that expresses CD16 and CD56. A small population of T cells also functions as NK cells (see Chapter 21). NK cells play a role in the apoptosis of virus-infected cells and tumor cells.

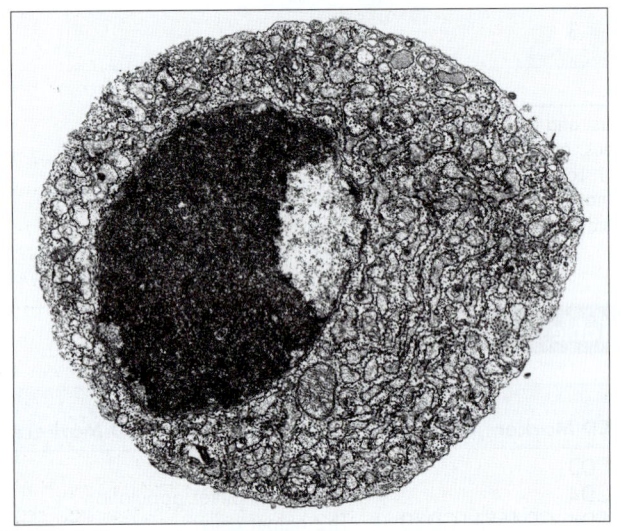

Figure 1-8
Plasma cells are short-lived and die by apoptosis (cell suicide). Note the nuclear chromatin changes, which are characteristic of apoptosis. (×5000.) (From Roitt I, Brostoff J, Male D, Roth D: Immunology, ed 7, Philadelphia, 2006, Mosby.)

PRIMARY LYMPHOID ORGANS

Lymphocytes must undergo a maturation-and-differentiation process before they become fully immunocompetent. The maturation of T and B cells takes place in different anatomic sites. B cells undergo maturation in bone marrow or intestinal lymphoid tissue. The thymus is responsible for T cell maturation.

Thymus

The thymus is located in the chest cavity just behind the sternum. The thymus is an encapsulated, multi-lobed structure. Each lobe has an outer portion called *cortex* and an inner portion termed *medulla* (Figure 1-9). Within a loosely organized three-dimensional framework of epithelial cells are dendritic cells, thymocytes, nurse cells, and Hassall's corpuscles. This cortical epithelial framework or stroma provides a unique environment for T cell maturation. Bone marrow lymphocytes entering the thymus are called *thymocytes*. These cells eventually become mature T cells.

At birth, the thymus is one of the largest organs in the body with a weight of 25 to 30 g, and it continues to grow and expand until puberty. During puberty, sex hormones cause the thymus to atrophy (involute), and its normal architecture is replaced by fat. After puberty, the hormones secreted by the epithelium are important in the maintenance of activated lymphocytes. By 30 years of age, only vestiges of the thymic epithelium remain.

Maturation of T Cells in the Thymus

In the cortex, immature T cells begin an initial round of proliferation during which the cortex becomes densely packed with lymphocytes. Cortical epithelial cells called *nurse cells* sustain proliferation by secreting interleukin 7 (IL-7). As they navigate the stromal network from the cortex to the medulla, thymocytes undergo a maturation-and-differentiation process (Figure 1-10). During maturation, a genetic rearrangement of TCRs

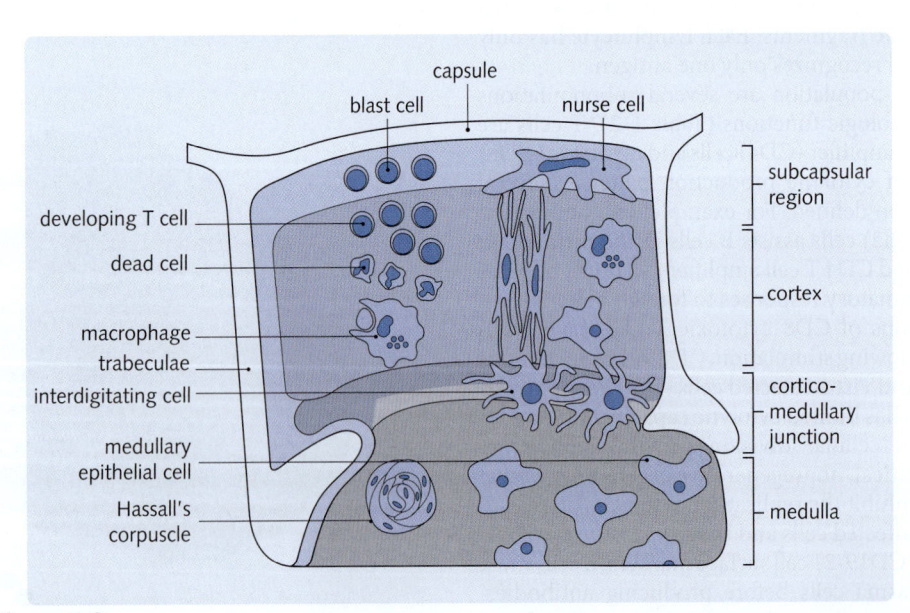

Figure 1-9
A schematic representation of the various cells found within the thymic lobule, including the T cells. T cells begin as thymocytes, which are lymphocytes originating from the bone marrow. Their maturation begins in the subcapsular region and ends in the medulla. (From Novak R: Crash course: Immunology, Philadelphia, Saunders, 2006.)

ensures that at least one lymphocyte that recognizes each of the 10^{13} possible antigens (protein or carbohydrate molecules recognized as foreign by the host) is present. Unfortunately, some of the maturing T cells now recognize antigens expressed by host cells as well. These auto-reactive cells must be destroyed before they can attack host tissue. Auto-reactive cells are removed by a two-step—positive and negative—selection process.

In positive selection, thymocytes react with major histocompatibility complex (MHC) molecules expressed on cortical epithelial cells. MHC molecules are present on all nucleated cells and serve two functions: (1) They are markers of "self" or host tissue, and (2) they present antigens to lymphocytes. The survival or death of thymocytes is dependent on their affinity for binding to the MHC molecules. Thymocytes that do not interact with MHC molecules undergo apoptosis and are phagocytosed in Hassell's corpuscles. Cells binding to the MHC markers with high affinity are considered auto-reactive; they undergo apoptosis or are prevented from maturation. Cells binding to the self-markers with low affinity are considered nonthreatening to the host, and they move deeper into the cortex.

Negative selection removes thymocytes that have auto-reactivity to the self-antigens that are unique to tissue such as the thyroid, muscle, intestinal, or neural tissue. In negative selection, tissue-specific antigens are presented in the context of MHC molecules expressed on dendritic cells, macrophages, and thymic epithelial cells. Again, thymocytes that bind with high affinity are considered auto-reactive, and they undergo apoptosis. T cells with little or no affinity for the self-antigens are allowed to enter peripheral blood.

Hormones and T Cell Maturation

T cell maturation is under the control of the hormones secreted by the thymic epithelium. These hormones include thymosin α1, thymopoietin, thymopentin, thymosin β4, and thymulin. On hormonal stimulation, most thymocytes express a CD8+ marker but quickly transition into dual positive (CD4+, CD8+) cells. Over 80% of the total cells in the adult thymic cortex are dual positive. After 12 to 19 days of maturation, only 20% of the original thymocyte population remains in the thymus. Mature CD4+, CD8-, and TCR+ cells (12%–15% of the total population) are released into peripheral blood as CD4 T helper/amplifier cells. CD4-, CD8+, and TCR+ cells (3% of total thymocytes) are also released into peripheral blood in high numbers to become CD8 cytotoxic cells. A small percentage of cells (2%) that have TCRs but no surface markers (CD4-, CD8-, TCR+) also are seeded into peripheral blood. These cells represent a small population of T cells that have escaped the selection process.

Bone Marrow and Peyer's Patches

The B cell maturation process in humans is still being debated. Some data suggest that intestinal Peyer's patches and other gut-associated lymphoid tissue play critical roles in the differentiation and maturation of B cells. Other evidence indicates that bone marrow is involved in B cell maturation. It is clear, however, that B cells undergo a gene rearrangement similar to that in T cells. Like T cells, B cells have a receptor (BCR) that reacts with antigens. Therefore, gene rearrangements result in B cells specific for each of the 10^{13} possible antigens.

THE LYMPH SYSTEM

The lymph system is a unique anatomic feature that allows the immune system to monitor tissue for infections and mutant cells (Figure 1-11). By using hydrostatic pressure and diapedesis, lymphocytes and monocytes exit the capillaries, move through the tissue layer, and are collected in small lymph vessels.

The presence of antigen in tissue activates immunocompetent macrophages, which process antigen for presentation to naïve lymphocytes. Activated macrophages are transferred to progressively larger vessels until they reach the lymph nodes. Antigen presentation activates and expands clones of lymphocytes that can react with the antigen. After exiting a lymph node, activated lymphocytes move into lymph vessels that eventually drain into the subclavian vein near the heart. Antigen-specific lymphocytes then circulate in the blood. On reaching the site

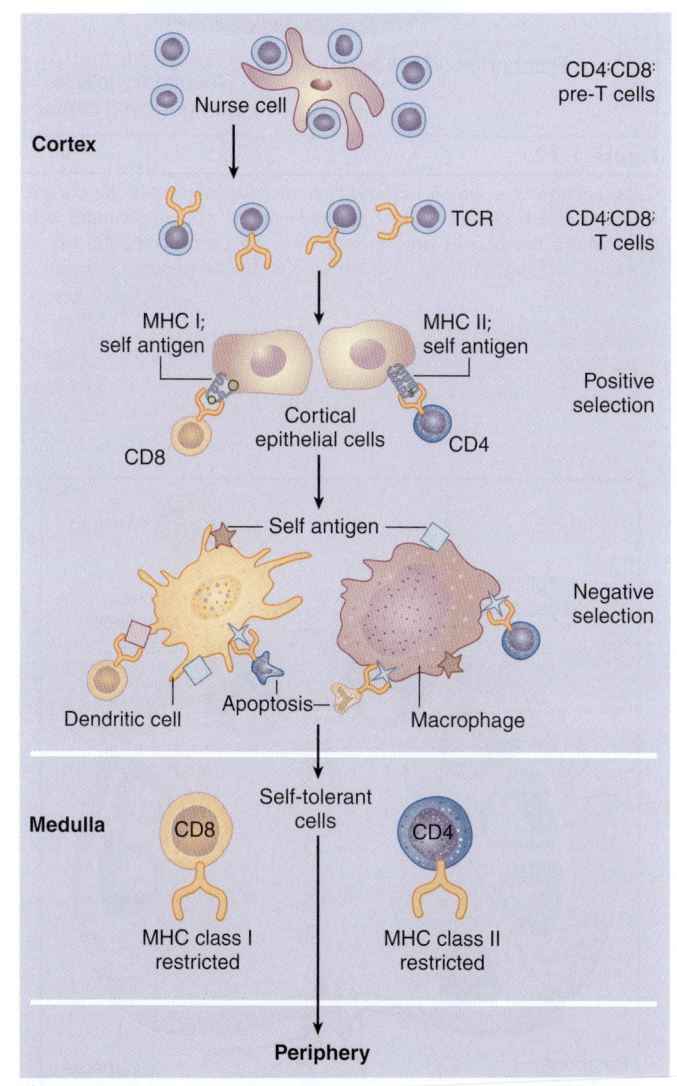

Figure 1-10

Development of the T cells in the thymus. Precursors committed to the T cell lineage arrive in the thymus and begin to rearrange their T cell receptor genes. Immature T cells with receptors binding to self–major histocompatibility complex (MHC) on cortical epithelial cells receive signals for survival (positive selection). At the corticomedullary junction, surviving T cells probe self-antigens presented by dendritic cells and macrophages. T cells reacting strongly to self-antigens are deleted by apoptosis (negative selection). T cells released into the periphery are tolerant toward self and recognize antigens in the context of self-MHC. (From Goldman L, Ausiello D: Cecil medicine, ed 22, Philadelphia, Saunders, 2008.)

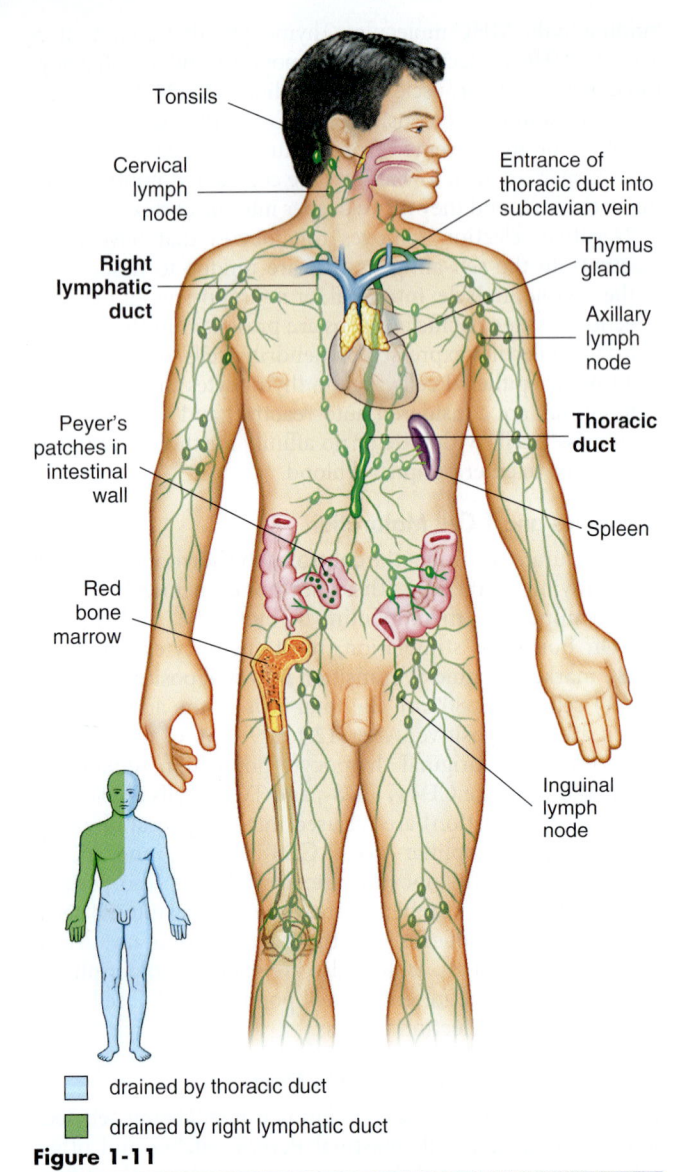

Figure 1-11
Lymph nodes are found at junctions of lymphatic vessels and form a network that drains and filters interstitial fluid from the tissue spaces. They are either subcutaneous or visceral, the latter draining the deep tissues and internal organs of the body. The lymph eventually reaches the thoracic duct, which opens into the left subclavian vein and thus back into the circulation. (From Salvo S: Mosby's pathology for massage therapists, ed 2, St Louis, 2009, Mosby.)

Figure 1-12
Cross-section of a lymph node with numerous follicles in the cortex, some of which contain lightly stained central areas (germinal centers, where the B cells proliferate), and the central medulla. (From Abbas A, Lichtman A: Basic immunology, ed 3, Philadelphia, Saunders, 2009.)

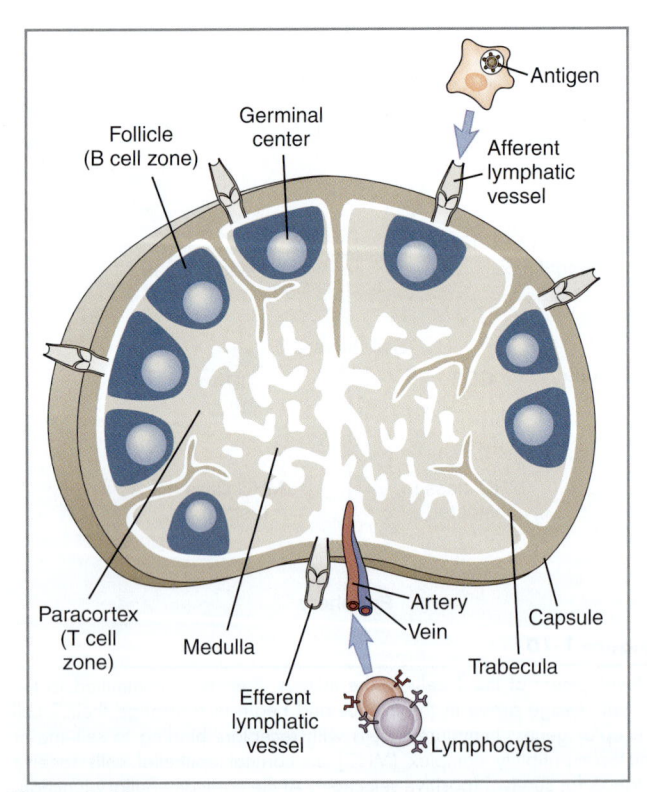

Figure 1-13
The morphology of lymph nodes. This schematic diagram shows the structural organization and blood flow in a lymph node. (From Abbas AK, Lichtman AH: Basic immunology: functions and disorders of the immune system, ed 2 [updated edition 2006-2007], Philadelphia, 2006, Saunders.)

of an infection or cancer, activated lymphocytes leave the capillary to mount an immune response in tissue.

SECONDARY LYMPHOID ORGANS

Lymph Node

The lymph node is a complex, kidney-shaped structure usually located at the junction of several lymph vessels. From an anatomic perspective, nodes consist of a cortex (outer portion), a paracortex, and a medulla (inner portion). The sections of lymph nodes are shown in Figure 1-12 and Figure 1-13.

The cortex is densely packed with lymphocytes and macrophages. Primary follicles of virgin or naïve B cells, interspersed in a framework of follicular dendritic cells, are prevalent

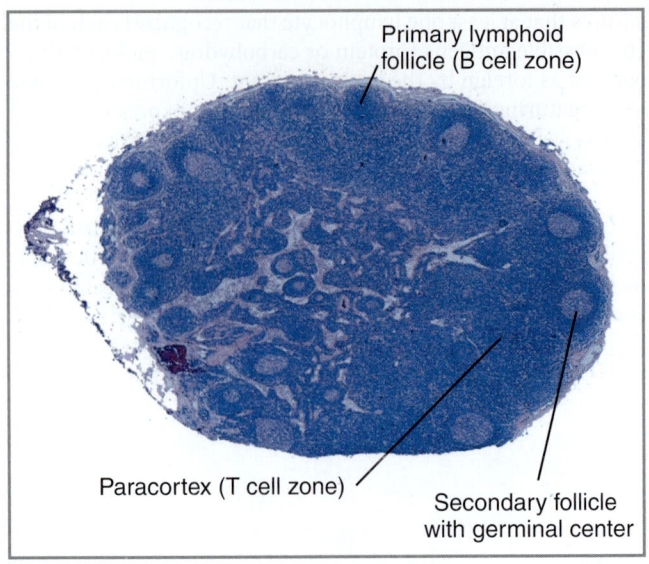

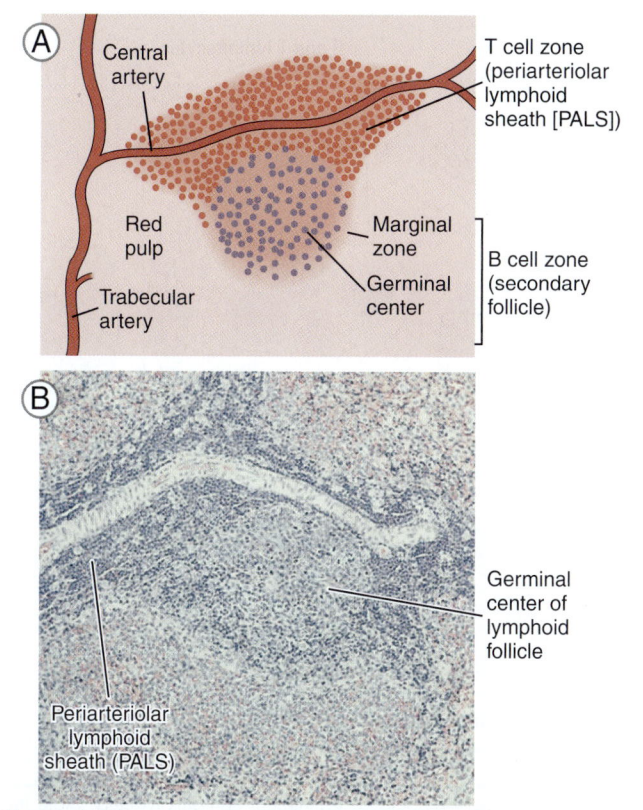

Figure 1-14

Morphology of the spleen. **A,** This schematic diagram shows a splenic arteriole surrounded by the periarteriolar lymphoid sheath (PALS) and attached follicle containing a prominent germinal center. The PALS and lymphoid follicles together constitute the white pulp. **B,** This light micrograph of a section of a spleen shows an arteriole with the PALS and a secondary follicle. These are surrounded by the red pulp, which is rich in vascular sinusoids. (From Abbas AK, Lichtman AH: Basic immunology: functions and disorders of the immune system, ed 2 [updated edition 2006-2007], Philadelphia, 2006, Saunders.)

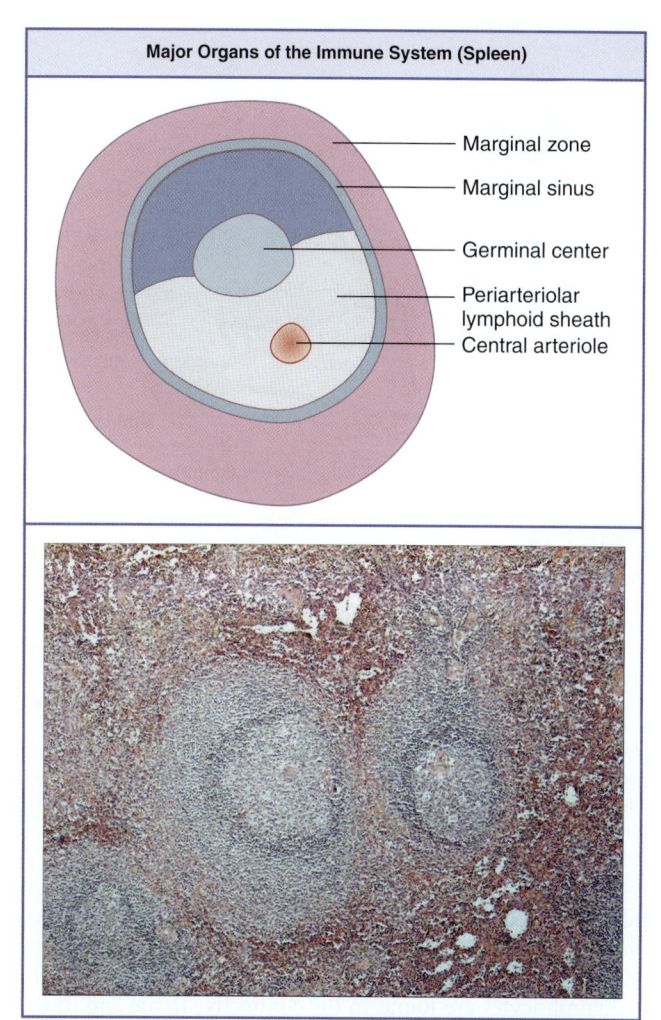

Figure 1-15

The spleen. The white pulp of the spleen contains a central artery and associated follicle (germinal center, marginal zone, and periarteriolar lymphoid sheath). (From Actor, JK: Elsevier's integrated immunology and microbiology, Philadelphia, 2007, Mosby.)

in the outer cortex. When B cells are actively proliferating within a follicle, the central area is referred to as the *germinal center*. Surrounding the germinal center is the mantle layer that contains B memory cells. Interspersed between the follicles is the paracortical region. The paracortex contains CD4 helper cells, a few cytotoxic CD8 cells, macrophages, granulocytes, and neutrophils.

The medulla, or the middle region of a lymph node, consists of a series of cavernous, cellular cords and connecting sinuses containing macrophages and plasma cells. Lymphoid tissue containing B cells and histiocytes is arranged in medullary cords between the connecting sinuses. Lymph fluid containing T cells and plasma cells flows into medullary sinuses and into efferent lymphatic vessels.

Spleen

The spleen, the largest lymphoid organ in the body, is located in the upper left quadrant of the abdomen and tucked under the diaphragm. The parenchyma or splenic bulk is divided into the red and white pulp (Figure 1-14).

Red pulp contains splenic sinuses with numerous thin-walled blood vessels interspersed between strands of connective tissue. Sinuses filter foreign material and purify blood. Old or damaged red blood cells are concentrated and destroyed by macrophages within venous sinuses. Sinuses also serve as storage facilities for platelets and red blood cells. Over 30% of platelets are sequestered in the spleen. On demand, platelets are expelled by the simple contraction of the organ.

White pulp is composed of lymphocytes that are clustered around and along the length of small, central splenic arteries to form a periarteriolar lymphoid sheath (PALS). Two thirds of the PALS are made up of CD4+ cells. B cells are also found in the PALS in the form of primary follicles and germinal centers. Along the rim of each splenic follicle is the marginal zone, which contains a mixed population of virgin and memory B cells (Figure 1-15). Marginal zone B cells are unique in that they produce antibodies directed toward carbohydrate antigens.

LYMPHOID TISSUE ORGANIZED INTO ANATOMIC UNITS

Mucosal-Associated Lymphoid Tissue

Lymphocytes are scattered beneath the epithelium along the entire gastrointestinal tract. Organized lymphocyte clusters, called *Peyer's patches*, are found in the ileum (Figure 1-16). Under light microscopy, Peyer's patches appear as lymphoid

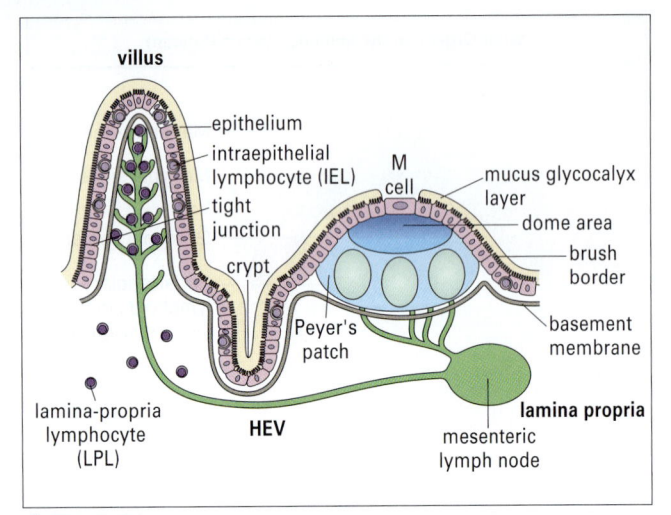

Figure 1-16
Peyer's patches, as well as tonsils and other lymphoid areas of mucosal-associated lymphoid tissue (MALT), are sites of lymphocyte priming by antigens, which are internalized by M cells in the follicle-associated epithelium (FAE). The subepithelial region, the dome, is rich in antigen-presenting cells (APCs) and also contains a subset of B cells similar to those found in the splenic marginal zone. Lymphoid follicles and intervening T-dependent zones are localized under the dome region. Lymphocytes primed by antigens in these initiation sites of the gut mucosa migrate to the mesenteric lymph nodes and then to the effector sites (the intestinal villi), where they are found both in the lamina propria (LPLs) and within the surface epithelium (IELs). (From Roitt I, Brostoff J, Male D, Roth D: Immunology, ed 7, Philadelphia, 2006, Mosby.)

follicles that contain CD4+ T helper cells, mature B cells, macrophages, and dendritic cells. Surrounding the follicle is a mantle of B cells that are analogous to the splenic marginal zone B cells.

Lymphocytes are found in the connective tissue and in the epithelial layer of the mucosa. Intraepithelial Lymphocytes (IELs) are found in the surface epithelium and have the closest contact with bacteria and parasites. These lymphocytes express CD8 and are constitutively cytotoxic. The exact function of IELs is difficult to determine because both the phenotype and the function differ depending on anatomic location. Lamina propria lymphocytes (LPLs) are T cells and activated B cells and plasma cells that produce specialized antibodies released into the intestinal lumen.

In the intestine, antigens are recognized by intestinal microfold (M) cells present in the dome epithelium of Peyer's patches (Figure 1-17). These cells lack the villi normally present on intestinal cells and have deeply invaginated basal surfaces that trap antigens. Antigens are endocytosed by M cells, transported in vesicles to the submucosa, and exocytosed to lymphocytes in the intraepithelial spaces.

After antigenic stimulation in the intestinal mucosa, T cells and antigen-presenting macrophages travel to the mesenteric lymph node where the immune response is amplified. Lymphocytes activated in the node enter the thoracic duct, which empties into bloodstream (Figure 1-18). After entering the peripheral circulation, activated lymphocytes are evenly distributed to mucosal tissues in the genitourinary tract, lung, salivary and lacrimal glands, lactating mammary glands, and the gut intestinal mucosa. Therefore, antigenic stimulation of one mucosal surface provides protection to all mucosal surfaces. After localization in mucosal tissue activated B cells initiate the production of specialized secretory antibodies.

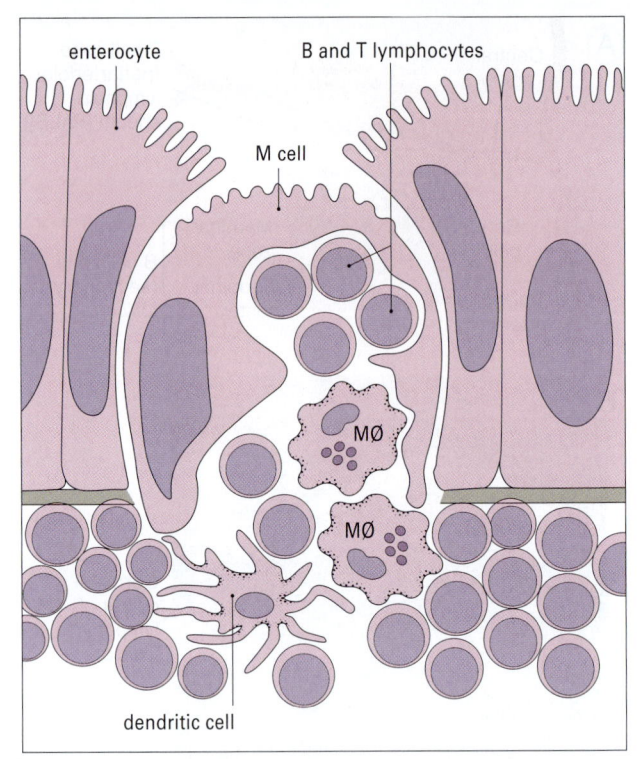

Figure 1-17
The intestinal follicle–associated epithelium contains M cells. Note the lymphocytes and occasional macrophages (MØ) in the pocket formed by invagination of the basolateral membrane of the M cell. Antigens endocytosed by the M cell are passed via this pocket into the subepithelial tissues (*not shown*). (From Roitt I, Brostoff J, Male D, Roth D: Immunology, ed 7, Philadelphia, 2006, Mosby.)

Tonsils

The entrance to the respiratory tract is guarded by tonsils, which are localized in three areas of the oral pharynx. (1) *Palatine* tonsils are found on the lateral wall of the oral pharynx. They are covered with respiratory squamous epithelium and surrounded by a capsule of connective tissue. (2) *Lingual* tonsils are found at the root of the tongue. Both the palatine and lingual tonsils have deep crypts that increase the surface area available to trap bacteria and other antigens. (3) A third tonsillar tissue is the *pharyngeal* tonsil or adenoid that is located in the roof of the pharynx behind the soft palate.

Tonsils are lymphoid organs. All three tonsils are densely packed with subepithelial and intraepithelial lymphocytes. Subsets of CD4 and B cells, along with macrophages, are the major constituents of tonsils. Tonsils produce secretory antibodies aimed at diphtheria, *Streptococcus*, and a number of respiratory viruses including polio and rubella viruses. The removal of tonsils (tonsillectomy) severely reduces the production of secretory antibodies and may increase the risk for repeated infections of the oropharynx.

LYMPHOCYTE DIAPEDESIS

Tissue damage, infection, or inflammation cause the migration of white blood cells from the blood vessel to tissue through a process called *diapedesis*. Within 2 hours of the initiation of an inflammatory response, small-molecular-weight proteins, called *cytokines*, are released by monocytes. Cytokines upregulate adhesion molecules, called *E-selectin* and *P-selectin*,

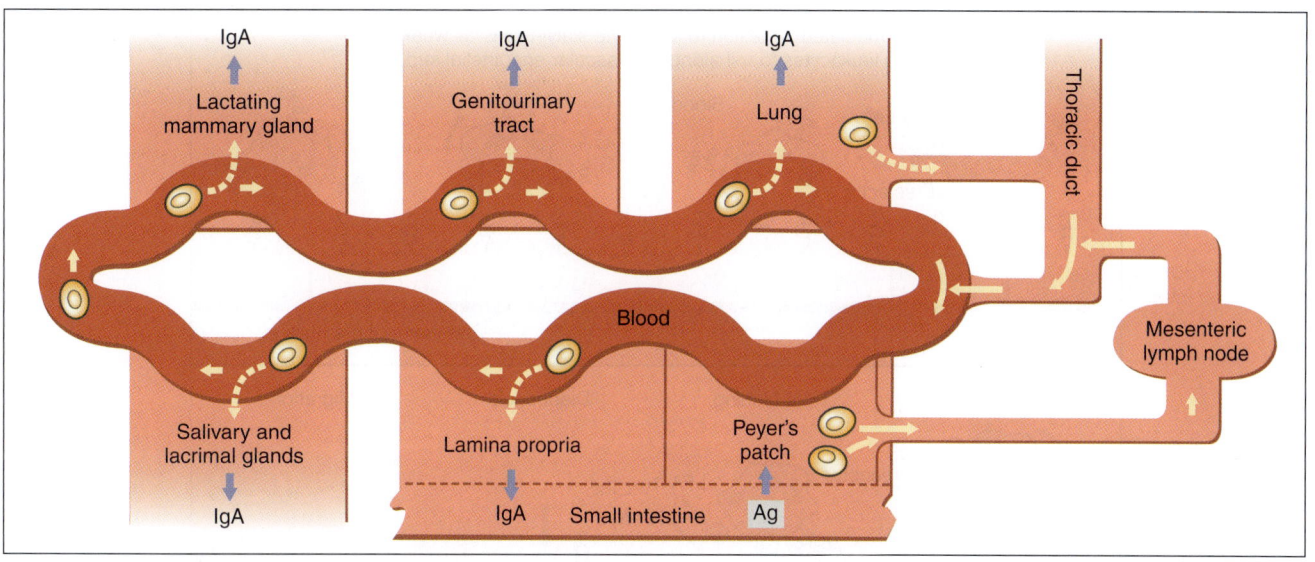

Figure 1-18

Lymphocyte circulation with the mucosal lymphoid system. (From Roitt, I: Essential immunology, ed 6, Philadelphia, 2001, Mosby.)

Table 1-3 Selectins, Integrins, and Adhesion Factors Used in Diapedesis

Factor	Cellular Location
Selectins	
E-selectin	Endothelial cells
L-selectin	Leukocytes
P-selectin	Platelets and endothelial cells
Integrins	
CD11a/CD18 (LFA-1)	Leukocytes
CD11b/CD18 (Mac-1, CR3)	Leukocytes
CD11c/CD18 (CR4)	Leukocytes
Cell Adhesion Factors	
EP-CAM	Epithelial cells
GlyCAM	Endothelial cells
ICAM-1	Endothelial cells
VCAM	Endothelial cell
VLA	Lymphocytes

CD, Cluster of differentiation; *EP-CAM*, epithelial cell adhesion molecule; *GlyCAM*, glycosylation-dependent cell adhesion molecule 1; *ICAM*, intercellular adhesion molecule-1; *VCAM*, vascular cell adhesion molecule 1; *VLA*, very late antigen.

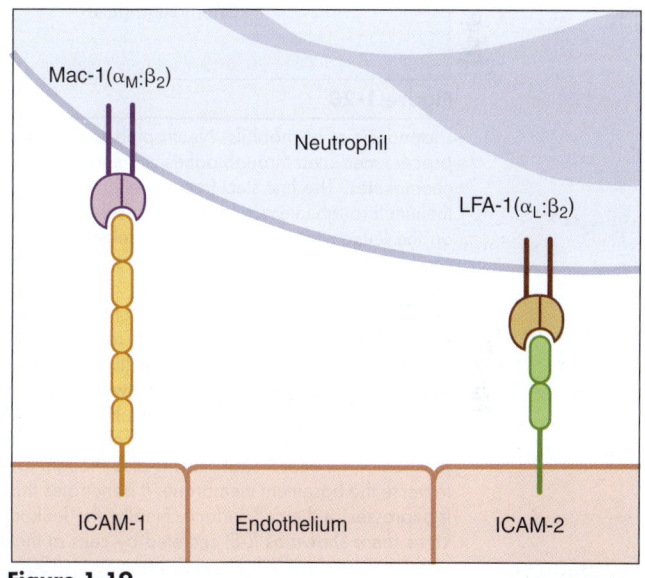

Figure 1-19

Phagocyte adhesion to vascular endothelium is mediated by integrins. The vascular endothelium, when it is activated by inflammatory mediators, expresses two adhesion molecules—ICAM-1 and ICAM-2. These are ligands for integrins expressed by phagocytes—$\alpha_L:\beta_2$ (also called LFA-1 or CD11a:CD18) and $\alpha_M:\beta_2$ (also called Mac-1, CR3, or CD11b:CD18). (From Murphy K, Travers P, Walport M: Janeway's immunobiology, ed 7, New York, 2008, Garland Science, Taylor & Francis Group, LLC.)

on vessel walls. Other molecules, called *chemokines*, also are released by endothelial cells.

Chemokines attach to endothelial cells along a concentration gradient that is counter to blood flow (the highest concentration is at the site of diapedesis). In essence, chemokines attract leukocytes to the site of infection or tissue damage. However, leukocytes move through blood vessels at great speed and must be slowed and tethered to the vessel walls before they exit the vessel and enter tissue.

To slow the speed of leukocytes, E-selectins and chemokines interact with carbohydrate ligands on leukocytes (Table 1-3). Different selectin–ligand interactions help slow rolling PMNs and lymphocytes. PMNs are slowed by interactions between a tetrasaccharide carbohydrate present on PMNs and monocytes called *sialyl-Lewis^x* and E-selectins. Lymphocytes roll faster than monocytes or PMNs and require interactions among E-selectin, P-selectin, and lymphocyte VLA-4 (very late antigen 4) in the deceleration process.

To tether leukocytes to the vessel walls, additional interactions between endothelial intercellular adhesion molecules (ICAM-1 and ICAM-2) and lymphocyte function associated antigen -1 (LFA-1) are required (Figure 1-19). Once the cells are tethered to the endothelium, they flatten out and

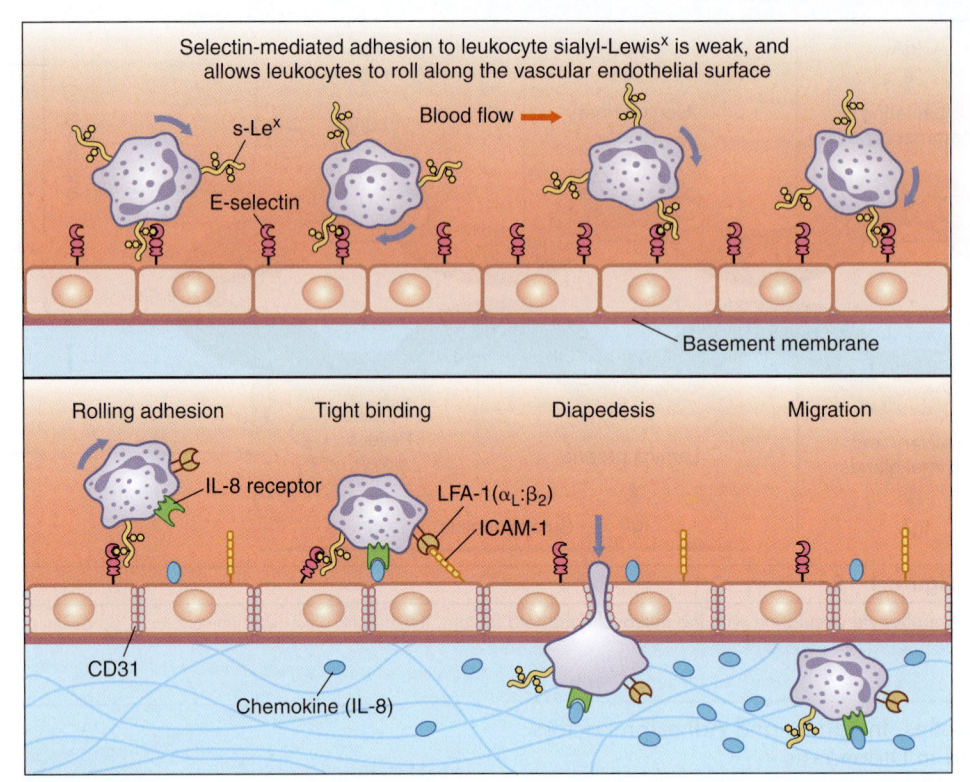

Figure 1-20

Diapedesis of neutrophils. Neutrophils leave the blood and migrate to sites of infection in a multiple-step process mediated through adhesive interactions that are regulated by macrophage-derived cytokines and chemokines. The first step (*top panel*) involves the reversible binding of leukocytes to the vascular endothelium through interactions between selectins induced on the endothelium and their carbohydrate ligands on the leukocyte, shown here for E-selectin and its ligand the sialyl-Lewis^x moiety (s-Le^x). This interaction cannot anchor the cells against the shearing force of the flow of blood; and, instead, they roll along the endothelium, continually making and breaking contact. The binding does, however, allow stronger interactions, which occur as a result of the induction of intracellular adhesion molecule 1 (ICAM-1) on the endothelium and the activation of its receptors LFA-1 and Mac-1 (*not shown*) on the leukocyte by contact with a chemokine like interleukin 8 (IL-8). Tight binding between these molecules arrests the rolling and allows the leukocyte to squeeze between the endothelial cells forming the wall of the blood vessel (to extravasate). The leukocyte integrins LFA-1 and Mac-1 are required for extravasation and for migration toward chemoattractants. Adhesion between molecules of CD31, expressed on both the leukocyte and the junction of the endothelial cells, is also thought to contribute to extravasation. The leukocyte also needs to traverse the basement membrane; it penetrates this with the aid of a matrix metallo-proteinase enzyme that it expresses at the cell surface. Finally, the leukocyte migrates along a concentration gradient of chemokines (*here shown as IL-8*) secreted by cells at the site of infection. (From Murphy K, Travers P, Walport M: Janeway's immunobiology, ed 7, New York, 2008, Garland Science, Taylor & Francis Group, LLC.)

transmigrate through the endothelial layer and the underlying matrix. A schematic of diapedesis is shown in Figure 1-20.

The tethering or adherence process may take only seconds, but the transmigration of leukocytes may take 10 to 20 minutes. During transmigration, immunocompetent cells change from a round structure to a flat structure and crawl to the exit site. Cells can exit the vasculature by passing between or through endothelial cells. Passage between cells is facilitated by the production of *hevin*, which temporarily disrupts cell junctions and allows cell movement between cell junctions. Migration through cells is a more complex process. Following attachment, the lymphoid cells are concentrated in the caveolin-rich areas on the cell surface, which are called *transmigratory cups*. Caveolins are a family of proteins that mediate the endocytosis of receptor-bound molecules. Following the endocytosis of leukocytes, ICAMs and caveolins form a protective channel that allows the leukocyte passage through the cell. The formation of another transmigratory cup allows the leukocyte to exit both the vascular endothelial cell and the underlying matrix.

ANATOMIC DEFECTS AND IMMUNODEFICIENCIES

DiGeorge Syndrome

DiGeorge syndrome is caused by abnormal migration of cells to select tissues during development. The major defect is a 30-gene deletion on chromosome 22 at position 22q11.2. This deletion prevents the development of the third and fourth pharyngeal pouches during the twelfth week of gestation. Major organs affected by the defect are the thymus, the parathyroid, and the heart. In addition, facial abnormalities, including underdeveloped chins, droopy eyelids, and upper ears that are rotated backward, occur. Children with this syndrome have a nonfunctioning, rudimentary thymus and lack mature T cells in the circulation and in secondary lymphoid tissue. Because the underdeveloped parathyroid cannot control calcium levels, muscular tetany and seizures are common. Most of the deaths are associated with infection or cardiac problems.

Nezelof Syndrome

Nezelof syndrome is a very rare disease that has affected less than 200,000 children in the United States. Affected children have a rudimentary thymus, but their parathyroid function is normal.

Although classified as a primary T cell deficiency, Nezelof syndrome has associated defects in B cell development and maturation. Some classifications place the syndrome in the severe combined immunodeficiency category. Evidence indicates that children exhibiting only a T cell deficiency have a purine nucleoside phosphorylase (PNP) deficiency in the purine salvage pathway. Metabolites are toxic to developing T cells. In some instances, adenosine deaminase (ADA) enzymes also are nonfunctional. Toxic metabolites that are generated as a consequence of the ADA deficiency block the development of T cells, B cells, and NK cells.

Leukocyte Adhesion Deficiency

Defective diapedesis is reflected in two immunodeficiencies called *leukocyte adhesion deficiency (LAD) I* and *II*. LAD I is an autosomal recessive disease, in which expression of CD18 on macrophages, neutrophils, and lymphocytes fails to occur. CD18 consists of LFA-1, macrophage-antigen-1 (MAC-1), and receptors that bind leukocytes to the molecules expressed on the endothelium of the blood vessel.

LAD II is the result of defective fucose transport and fucosylation, which are necessary for the synthesis of sialyl-Lewis^x (s-Le^x) on PMNs and monocytes. As a consequence, monocytes and PMNs cannot exit the vasculature in response to infections or tissue damage. The disease is extremely rare, with only 200 cases reported in the last 20 years. Unfortunately, most individuals with this disease die of overwhelming infections within the first 2 years of life.

SUMMARY

- White blood cells are involved in the body's response to infections and tumors.
- Lymphocytes and monocytes/macrophages are the major effector cells in an immune response.
- Bone marrow and the thymus are the primary lymphoid organs.
- The spleen, lymph nodes, and tonsils are the secondary lymphoid organs.
- Lymphocytes are classified into T cells and B cells on the basis of function and site of maturation.
- Subsets of T cells and B cells have different immunologic functions.
- The secondary lymphoid organs and tissue are organized into anatomic units.
- Lymphocytes and other immunocompetent cells exit blood vessels and enter tissue by diapedesis.
- Developmental and genetic abnormalities can cause abnormal thymus function or diapedesis of white blood cells.

REFERENCES

Anderson SJ, Perlmutter RM: A signaling pathway governing early thymocyte maturation, Immunol Today 16:99, 1995.

Craig SW, Cebra JJ: Peyer's patches: An enriched source of precursors for IgA producing immunocytes in the rat, J Exp Med 134:188, 1971.

Geissmann F, Manz MG, Jung S, et al: Evolving views on the genealogy of B cells, Nat Rev Immunol 8(2):95, 2008.

Girard JP, Springer TA: High endothelial venules (HEVs): Specialized endothelium for lymphocyte migration, Immunol Today 16:449, 1995.

Kroese FGM, Timens W, Nieuwenhuis P: Germinal center reaction and B lymphocytes: Morphology and function, Berlin, 1990, Springer Verlag.

Laman JD, Van den Eertwegh AJM, Claassen E, et al: Cell-cell interactions: In situ studies of splenic humoral responses. In Fornusek L, Veivicka V, editors: Immune system accessory cells, Boca Raton, 1992, CRC Press.

Pawlowski TJ, Staerz UE: Thymic education—T cells do it for themselves, Immunol Today 15:205–208, 1994.

Szakal AK, Kosco MH, Tew JG: Microanatomy of lymphoid tissue during a humoral immune response: Structure function relationships, Annu Rev Immunol 7:91–109, 1989.

Webster ADB: Laboratory investigations of primary deficiencies of the lymphoid system, Clin Allergy Immunol 5:447–467, 1985.

ASSESSMENT QUESTIONS

1. Which of the following cells are involved in allergic reactions?
   I. Mast cells
   II. Basophils
   III. Eosinophils
   A. I and II
   B. I and III
   C. II and III
   D. I, II, and III

2. Which of the following cells are the major effector cells in an immune response?
   I. Lymphocytes
   II. Monocytes
   III. Basophils
   A. I and II
   B. I and III
   C. II and III
   D. I, II, and III

3. In positive selection in the thymus, immature thymocytes react with:
   A. MHC molecules on cortical epithelial cells
   B. T cell receptors (TCRs)
   C. B cell receptors
   D. Thymic epithelium

4. Leukocyte adhesion deficiency II is caused by a:
   A. Deficiency in CD3
   B. Deficiency in TCRs
   C. Deficiency in fucose transport
   D. Deficiency in CD18

5. Cells that actually produce antibodies are:
   A. Plasma cells
   B. B cells
   C. Monocytes
   D. T cells

6. The subpopulation of T cells that assist in the production of antibodies is:
   A. CD4 Th1 cells
   B. CD4 Th2 cells
   C. CD8 Tc1 cells
   D. CD8 Tc2 cells

7. In mammals, B cell maturation is believed to occur in:
   I. Bone marrow
   II. Peyer's patches
   III. Bursa of Fabricus
   A. I and II
   B. I and III
   C. II and III
   D. I, II, and III

8. Which of the following cells reside in tissue?
   I. Macrophages
   II. Mast cells
   III. Basophils
   A. I and II
   B. I and III
   C. II and III
   D. I, II, and III

9. Large granular lymphocytes have the following characteristics:
   I. CD 16 expressed on the cell membrane
   II. Ability to lyse virus-infected cells and tumor cells
   III. Representative of a third lymphocyte lineage
   A. I and II
   B. I and III
   C. II and III
   D. I, II, and III

CHAPTER 2

Innate Immunity

LEARNING OBJECTIVES

- Describe the barriers that prevent microbial infection of the skin
- Describe the respiratory tract barriers that prevent microbial infection
- Define pathogen-associated microbial patterns (PAMPs)
- Define Toll-like receptors on leukocytes and describe their function
- List 11 different Toll-like receptor ligands
- Compare and contrast the roles of Toll-like receptors in innate and adaptive immunologic responses
- Explain the immunologic mechanisms involved in endotoxins or septic shock
- Describe the components of an acute phase response
- List five acute-phase proteins synthesized by the liver and their function
- Identify antimicrobial agents produced by cells and tissue

KEY TERMS

Acute-phase proteins
Acute-phase response
Adaptive immune response
Complement
Innate immune response
Opsonin
Pyrogen
Toll-like receptor

INTRODUCTION

The body is protected from infection by anatomic and physiologic barriers in the skin and in the respiratory, intestinal, and urogenital tracts. If these barriers are breached an innate immune response is generated. In the response, phagocytic cells, antimicrobial proteins and serum enzymes are activated by molecules common to most bacteria. The innate immune response functions to contain an infection until an adaptive response can be mounted against the infective agent. An adaptive response begins 7 to 10 days after infection and consists of antibodies, CD4Th1 inflammatory response or CD8 cytotoxic cells.

ANATOMIC AND PHYSIOLOGIC BARRIERS

Skin

The skin is an inhospitable environment for bacterial colonization and growth with the exception of staphylococcus epidermidis, bacteria cannot attach to the outer layer of skin or stratum corneum because it is composed of dead keratinocytes, keratin, ceramides, free fatty acid, and cholesterol. Moreover, the stratum corneum is continually shed and renewed by younger keratinocytes pushing up from below. Bacterial colonization is prevented by other factors as well. Perspiration deposits salt on the skin. High salt concentrations create a hypertonic environment that inhibits bacterial growth. Sebaceous glands also produce a waxlike substance called *sebum*, which contains lactic acid and propionic acid produced by *Propionibacterium acnes*—a commensal organism found in the sebaceous gland. Sebum reduces the skin pH to between 3.0 and 5.0, and this acidic environment inhibits bacterial growth.

Respiratory Tract

The respiratory tract is protected from infection by ciliated epithelial cells and a mucous layer. Glycosylated mucous proteins cover the entire respiratory tract and trap particulate matter. The coordinated beating of the cilia on respiratory epithelial cilia moves the mucus upward to the glottis, where it is expelled from the airways or swallowed. This mechanism is referred to as the *mucociliary escalator*. The mucous covering is replaced several times each day, leading to the production of a pint to a quart of mucus per day. Defective escalator function increases the risk of developing respiratory tract infections, sinusitis, and otitis media.

Mucociliary escalator dysfunction can be inherited or can be the result of environmental insults. For example, primary ciliary dyskinesia (PCD) is an inherited syndrome characterized by impaired transport and the abnormal structure of cilia. In this syndrome, lungs and sinuses are prone to repeated infections.

Environmental insults and drugs often affect the function of the mucociliary escalator. For example, halothane, cocaine, and sulfur dioxide are toxic to epithelial cells. Smoking or inhalation of toxic fumes also injures the epithelium causing loss of ciliated cells. Escalator function can be compromised by cold or dry air that often creates a highly viscous mucus that cannot be moved upward by ciliated cells.

Stomach and Intestine

Stomach acid forms a passive barrier to prevent infection of the intestinal tract. With the exception of *Helicobacter pylori* (the etiologic agent of gastric and duodenal ulcers), most ingested pathogenic bacteria cannot survive in stomach acid. Bile salts found in the intestine also are toxic to bacteria.

Urogenital Tract

The components of the urogenital tract that actively participate in the innate immune response are the urethra and the vaginal mucosa. The urethra is usually sterile because the persistent flushing of urine prevents bacterial attachment to urethral epithelial cells. The acidity of urine also prevents bacterial colonization. In females, the normal flora of the vaginal mucosa prevents colonization by pathogenic microbes. Acids produced by lactobacilli create a slightly acidic mucosal environment that inhibits bacterial growth. The risk of infection increases when the lactobacillus population is reduced, the pH of urine is increased, or both.

PATHOGEN-ASSOCIATED MOLECULAR PATTERNS

Pathogen-associated molecular patterns (PAMPs) are molecular structures or molecules that are shared by most pathogenic bacteria and some viruses. Most components are constituents of microbial cell walls, single-stranded and double-stranded nucleic acids, or unmethylated deoxyribonucleic acid (DNA). Common PAMPs are presented in Table 2-1. In an innate immune response, PAMPs are recognized by several different mechanisms, including the following:
- Serum complement components
- Receptors on leukocytes and tissue cells
- Acute phase proteins

SERUM COMPLEMENT COMPONENTS AND PATHOGEN-ASSOCIATED MOLECULAR PATTERNS

Complement comprises nine serum proteins (Figure 2-1) and produces proinflammatory factors that are chemotactic for phagocytic cells (see Chapter 11). Complement fragments coat bacteria to create opsonins, which are, by definition, molecules that attach to microbes and promote phagocytosis.

Complement can be activated by different mechanisms. In an adaptive response, complement is activated by antigen–antibody complexes (see Chapter 11). Three other mechanisms do not require the presence of antibody and are activated during an innate immune response. Complement can be activated by interaction with select molecules (e.g., zymozan) on microbial surfaces in an alternative complement activation pathway. Lectins (proteins that bind to sugars) also activate the complement cascade in the mannose-binding lectin (MBL) pathway. Some acute phase proteins produced by the liver during inflammation activate the complement cascade (see Acute Phase Response).

Mannose-Binding Lectin Complement Activation Pathway

Collectins are a family of lectins that react with terminal mannose or fructose molecules on microbes and activate complement. The collectin family includes Mannose-binding lectin (MBL), bovine conglutinin, lung surfactants A and D, and bovine collectin 43. Structurally, collectins are multi-meric proteins with a "flower bouquet" or an "X-like" structure (Figure 2-2).

MBL is the most studied of the collectins. MBL circulates in a complex with MBL-associated serine protease 1 and 2 (MASP1 and MASP2). In the presence of calcium, MBL or MASP binds to PAMPs such as N-acetylglucosamine, mannose, and N-acetylmannosamine residues expressed on bacteria, fungi, human immunodeficiency virus (HIV) and influenza virus. Following an initial interaction with target molecules, the serum complement cascade is activated. MBL or MASP activates the C2 and C4 complement component to create a C3 convertase (Figure 2-3).

Cascade fragment C3b binds to bacterial PAMPs and acts as an opsonin. Other complement fragments such C3a and C5a induce the release of histamine and pharmacologic mediators from mast cells and basophiles. These fragments are called *anaphylatoxins*. Histamine increases capillary permeability and fluid leaks into tissue. Fluid leaking from capillaries reduces fluid levels in the vessels and precipitates bacteria, rendering them more susceptible to phagocytosis. In addition to their role as anaphylatoxins, C3a and C5a are chemoattractants for phagocytic cells. Complexes of C5b, C6, and C7-C9 create a membrane attack complex that inserts a "tube-like" structure through the bacterial membrane, which results in the death of the bacterium.

Receptor Recognition of Pathogen-Associated Molecular Patterns

Phagocytic cells have a number of receptors that recognize PAMPs on pathogenic microbes. Scavenger, carbohydrate, and Toll-like receptors are important in the recognition of PAMPs. Scavenger receptors bind lipoteichoic acids, endotoxins from gram-negative bacteria, and peptidoglycans from gram-positive bacteria. Carbohydrate receptors recognize mannose or fructose in the terminal sugars of bacterial glycoproteins (Figure 2-4).

Toll-like receptors (TLRs) present on lymphocytes, macrophages, and dendritic cells play a more important role in innate immunity. The 11 different TLRs in mammals usually recognize only one type of PAMP (Table 2-2). For example, TLR-2 binds to the peptidoglycans of *Streptococcus* and *Staphylococcus*, whereas TLR-5 only binds the proteins of bacterial flagellae. The ligands for TLR receptors are listed in Table 2-3. Interactions between the PAMP and its receptor activate intracellular

Table 2-1	Common Pathogen-Associated Microbial Patterns in Bacteria, Fungi, and Viruses
Peptidoglycan	Gram-positive bacteria
Lipopolysaccharide	Gram-negative bacteria
Lipoteichoic acids	Gram-positive bacteria
Flagellin	Bacteria
Lipoarabinomannan	Mycobacteria
Beta 1,3 glycan	Fungi
Respiratory syncytial virus (RSV) protein	Viruses
Double-stranded ribonucleic acid (RNA)	Viruses
Lipopeptides	Mycoplasma
Unmethylated CpGDNA*	Bacteria
Profilin-like molecules	Toxoplasma

*Unmethylated bacterial deoxyribonucleic acid (DNA) containing cytosine phosphate guanine motifs.

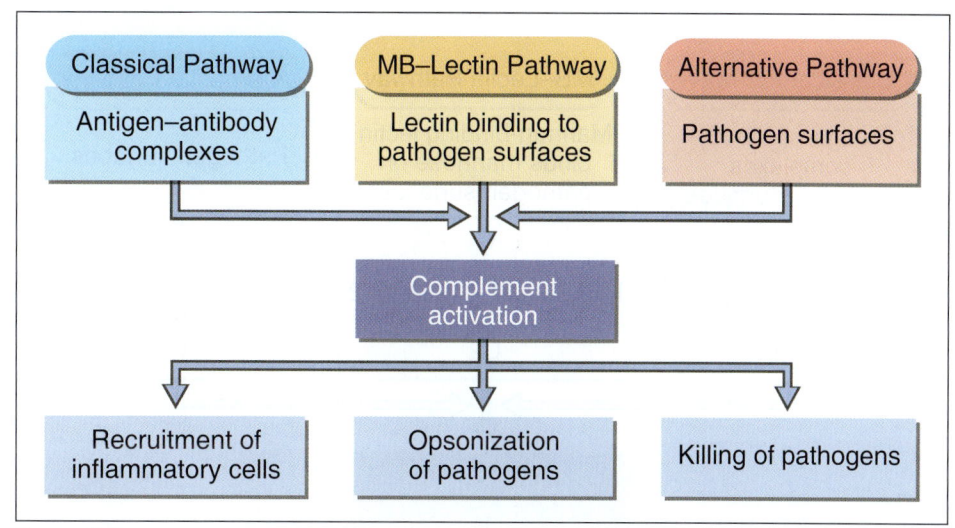

Figure 2-1

Schematic overview of the complement cascade. The three pathways of complement activation are (1) the classic pathway, which is triggered by antibody or by direct binding of complement component C1q to the pathogen surface; (2) the mannan (MB)-binding–lectin pathway, which is triggered by mannan-binding lectin, a normal serum constituent that binds some encapsulated bacteria; and (3) the alternative pathway, which is triggered directly on pathogen surfaces. All of these pathways generate a crucial enzymatic activity that, in turn, generates the effector molecules of complement. The three main consequences of complement activation are opsonization of pathogens, the recruitment of inflammatory cells, and direct killing of pathogens. (From Murphy K, Travers P, Walport M: Janeway's immunobiology ed 7, New York, 2008, Garland Science, Taylor & Francis Group, LLC.)

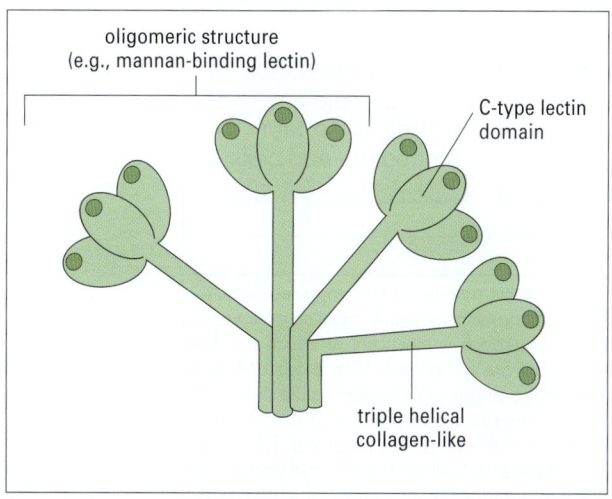

Figure 2-2

Collectins are oligomers of triple-helical molecules with C-type lectin domains. They recognize a variety of microbial pathogen-associated microbial patterns (PAMPs). (From Roitt I, Brostoff J, Male D, et al: Immunology, ed 7, Philadelphia, 2006, Mosby.)

signaling and the synthesis of specific small-molecular-weight messengers called *cytokines* that activate both the innate immune system and the adaptive immune system.

RECEPTOR ACTIVATION AND FUNCTIONAL RESPONSES IN INNATE IMMUNITY

The ligation of PAMPs with Toll-like receptors accelerates the phagocytosis of microbes. During phagocytosis, the cell membrane envelopes bacteria and creates an intracellular vacuole called *phagosome*. Primary granules fuse with the phagosome to create a *phagolysosome*. Enzymes in the granule kill the microbes by breaking their cell walls and disrupting membrane function (Figure 2-5). At the same time, the oxygen-dependent killing mechanism produces singlet oxygen, hydrogen peroxide, and hypochlorous acid. These substances, along with nitric oxide, are released into the phagolysosone to kill bacteria.

Interactions between PAMPs and Toll-like receptors on macrophages cause the release of interleukin 6 and interleukin 12 (IL-6 and IL-12) from phagocytic cells. IL-6 plays a role in the proliferation of CD8 cytotoxic T cells. It also upregulates adhesion factors on endothelial cells, which allows the egress of phagocytic cells and lymphocytes from the vasculature. IL-6 may also play a role in autoimmune reactions.

Toll-Like Receptors and Autoimmunity

The ligation of Toll-like receptors and the production of IL-6 result in the inactivation of regulatory cells that control the autoimmune B cells in peripheral blood. The disruption of the regulatory network allows B cells to produce autoantibodies directed at host tissue. For example, systemic lupus erythematosus (SLE) is an autoimmune response that is characterized by autoantibodies directed at DNA. The disease is exacerbated by the recognition of cytosine- and guanosine-containing unmethylated DNA by TLR-9 receptors on leukocytes and the release of IL-6.

Toll-Like Receptors, Endotoxins, and Septic Shock

Lipopolysaccharide endotoxins are biologically important PAMPs. Endotoxins, which are an integral part of the gram-negative cell wall, are released on the death of the bacterium and react with CD14 and TLR-4 receptors on the macrophage surface. Intracellular signaling induces the synthesis and

CHAPTER 2 INNATE IMMUNITY

Classical Pathway	MB–Lectin Pathway	Alternative Pathway
Antigen:antibody complexes (pathogen surfaces)	Mannan-binding lectin binds mannose on pathogen surfaces	Pathogen surfaces
C1q, C1r, C1s C4 C2	MBL, MASP-1, MASP-2 C4 C2	C3 B D

↓ ↓ ↓

C3 convertase

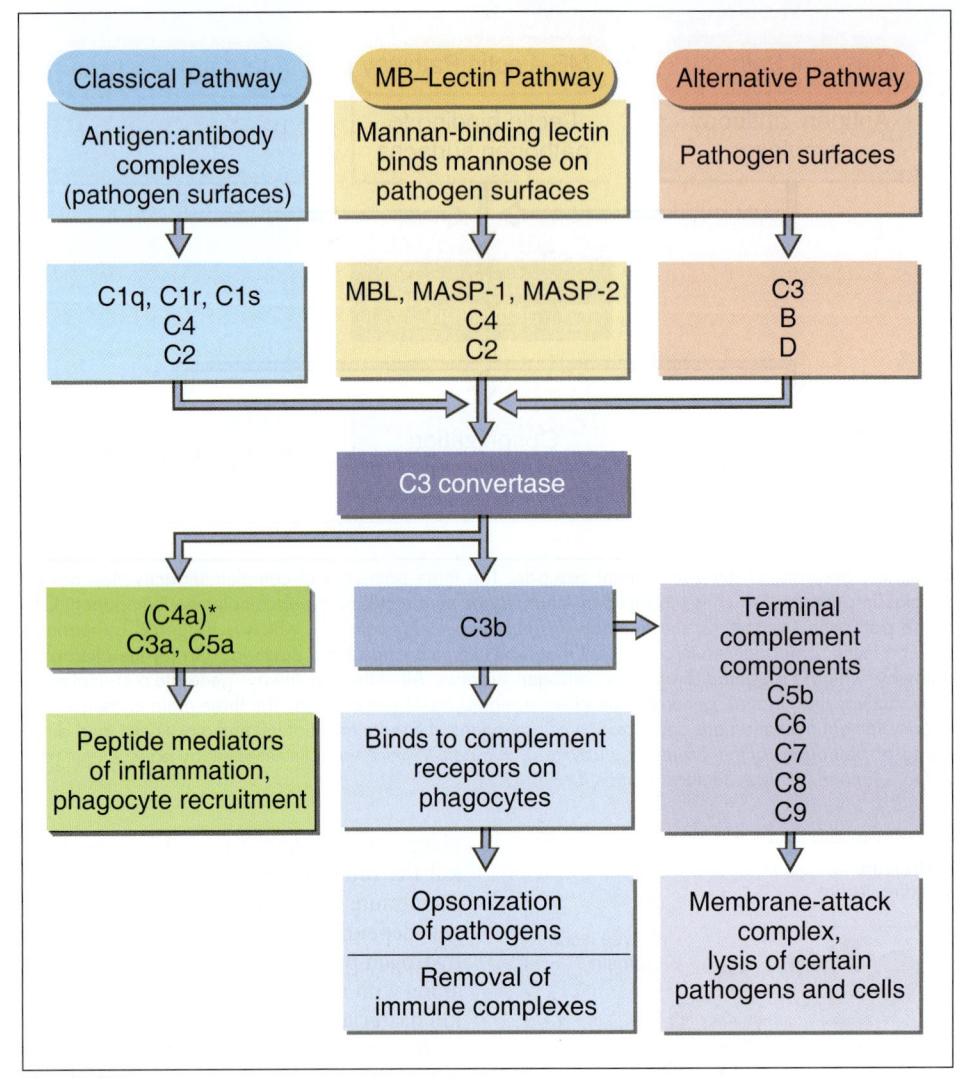

(C4a)* C3a, C5a	C3b	Terminal complement components C5b C6 C7 C8 C9
Peptide mediators of inflammation, phagocyte recruitment	Binds to complement receptors on phagocytes	Membrane-attack complex, lysis of certain pathogens and cells
	Opsonization of pathogens Removal of immune complexes	

Figure 2-3

The early events of all three pathways of complement activation involve a series of cleavage reactions that culminate in the formation of an enzymatic activity called a *C3 convertase*, which cleaves complement component C3 into C3b and C3a. The production of the C3 convertase is the point at which the three pathways converge and the main effector functions of complement are generated. C3b binds covalently to the bacterial cell membrane and opsonizes the bacteria, enabling phagocytes to internalize them. C3a is a peptide mediator of local inflammation. C5a and C5b are generated by cleavage of C5b by a C5 convertase formed by C3b bound to the C3 convertase *(not shown in this simplified diagram)*. C5a is also a powerful peptide mediator of inflammation. C5b triggers the late events in which the terminal components of complement assemble into a membrane-attack complex that can damage the membrane of certain pathogens. C4a is generated by the cleavage of C4 during the early events of the classic pathway and not by the action of C3 convertase, hence the *; it is also a peptide mediator of inflammation but its effects are relatively weak. Similarly, C4b, the large cleavage fragment of C4 *(not shown)*, is a weak opsonin. Although the classic complement activation pathway was first discovered as an antibody-triggered pathway, it is now known that C1q can activate this pathway by binding directly to pathogen surfaces, as well as paralleling the mannan-binding (MB)–lectin activation pathway by binding to antibody that is itself bound to the pathogen surface. In the MB-lectin pathway, MASP stands for mannan-binding lectin-associated serine protease. (From Murphy K, Travers P, Walport M: Janeway's immunobiology, ed 7, New York, 2008, Garland Science, Taylor & Francis Group, LLC.)

release of proinflammatory cytokines (IL-1, IL-2, IL-6, IL-8, and TNF-α [tumor necrosis factor–alpha]). TNF-α is the central cytokine involved in *septic shock syndrome*. Manifestations of septic shock include tachycardia, tachypenia, alterations in temperature, and activation of the coagulation cascade. Arterial and venous dilation results in septic shock. As a consequence of hypovolemia, tissue perfusion becomes inadequate, which results in cellular dysfunction. Mortality rate among patients with septic shock ranges from 20% to 80%.

ACUTE PHASE RESPONSE

In innate immunity, mammals respond to tissue injury or infection by initiating an acute phase response. The response is characterized by fever, demargination of

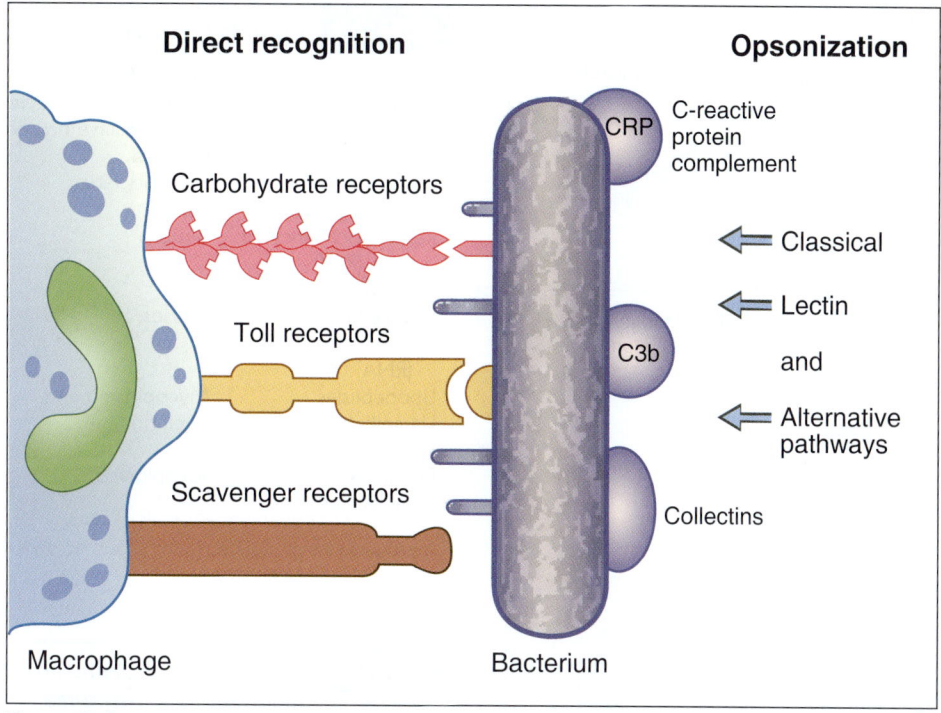

Figure 2-4
Macrophages can recognize pathogen-associated microbial patterns (PAMPs) either directly or following opsonization with serum molecules. (Adapted from Roitt I, Brostoff J, Male D, et al: Immunology, ed 7, Philadelphia, 2006, Mosby.)

polymorphonuclear leukocytes (PMNs) and the synthesis of acute-phase proteins by the liver. Acute-phase proteins inhibit bacterial growth or activate the complement cascade. The most common acute-phase proteins are listed in Table 2-3. During the response, white blood cells also produce a wide variety of antimicrobial agents such as cathelicins, defensins, and nitric oxide.

Temperature

Most pathogenic bacteria have a narrow growth range at temperatures between 96°F and 100°F. An elevation in body temperature or fever slows bacterial replication until an adaptive immune response can be generated. Fever is induced by IL-1 and Interferon-gamma (IFN-γ) released by monocytes. The interleukins travel to the hypothalamus and increase the temperature set point. Since these cytokines can regulate temperature, they are termed *endogenous pyrogens*. Other cytokines (anti-pyretic) such as IL-10 and TNF-α modulate and maintain the temperature response.

Acute Phase Proteins

C-reactive protein (CRP), the most studied acute-phase protein (see Table 2-3), activates the complement cascade. Cleavage of other complement components creates opsonins that bind to microbial PAMPs and promotes phagocytosis. Others acute-phase proteins such as ferritin, haptoglobin, and ceruloplasmin bind or oxidize free iron in serum to prevent microbial growth. Iron is necessary for the synthesis of cytochromes and the production of adenosine triphosphate (ATP).

Antimicrobial Agents Produced by Cells and Tissues

Cathelicidins

Cathelicidins are proteins produced by the PMNs, keratinocytes, and epithelial cells of the respiratory and gastrointestinal tracts. Cathelicidin subsets have different biologic functions. PMN-produced cathelicidins have broad-spectrum microbial toxicity. Other cathelicidins synthesized by epithelial cells bind and neutralize lipopolysaccharide endotoxins. In the skin, keratinocyte cathelicidins are chemotactic for phagocytes and T cells. Animal studies show that cathelicidins are important in host defense against Group A streptococci that cause necrotic skin lesions.

Defensins

Defensins are small (29–35 amino acids) proteins produced by circulating white blood cells and tissue cells. Defensins can be classified into alpha and beta families. Alpha-defensins (α-defensins) are found in neutrophils, macrophages, and Paneth cells in the intestine. Paneth cell defensins are called *crypticidins* and serve to reduce the number of bacteria in the intestinal lumen. Beta-defensins (β-defensins) are secreted by most leukocytes and epithelial cells.

Defensins have broad-spectrum activity against gram-positive and gram-negative bacteria and kill bacteria in a number of ways. Some defensins create voltage-dependent channels in bacterial membranes that allow the influx of water. Increased osmotic pressure ruptures the bacterial membranes. Other defensins move through bacterial cell walls, bind to target cells, and disrupt normal metabolism.

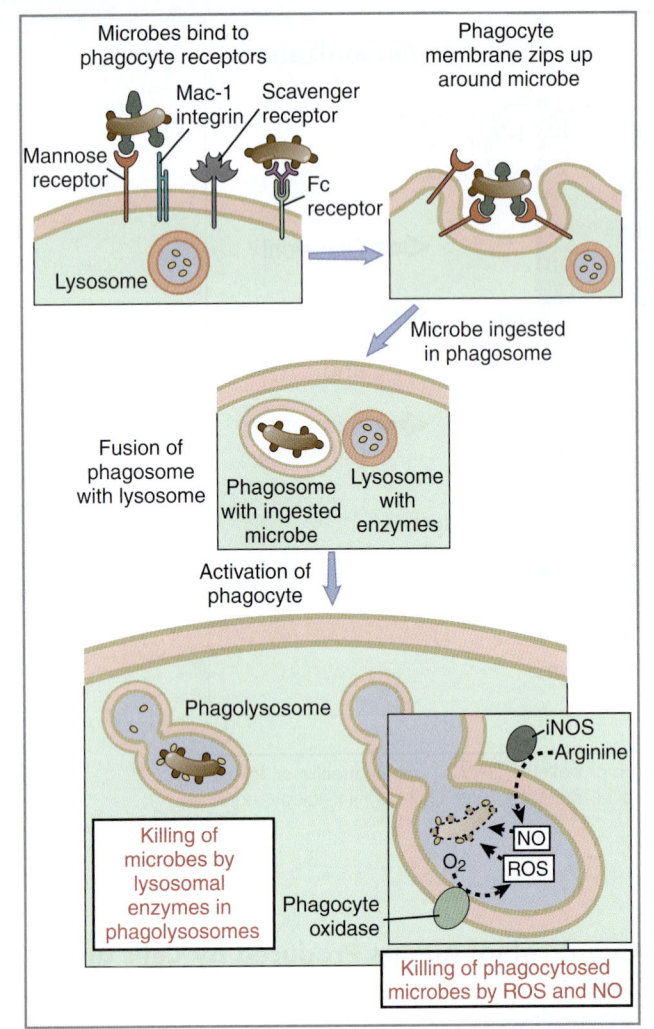

Table 2-2 Ligands for Toll-Like Receptors

Peptidoglycan	Gram-positive bacteria	TLR-2, TLR-6
Lipopolysaccharide	Gram-negative bacteria	TLR-4
Lipoteichoic acids	Gram-positive bacteria	TLR-1, TLR-6
Flagellin	Bacteria	TLR-5
Lipoarabinomannan	Mycobacteria	TLR-2, TLR-6
Beta 1,3 glucan	Fungi	TLR-1, TLR-6
Respiratory syncytial virus (RSV) protein	Viruses	TLR-4
Double-stranded ribonucleic acid (RNA)	Viruses	TLR-3
Lipopeptides	Mycoplasma	TLR-7
Unmethylated CpGDNA*	Bacteria	TLR-9
Profilin-like molecules	Toxoplasma	TLR-11

*Unmethylated bacterial deoxyribonucleic acid (DNA) containing cytosine phosphate guanine motifs.

Table 2-3 Acute Phase Proteins Produced during an Inflammatory Response

Acute Phase Proteins	Biologic Effects
C-reactive protein (CRP)	Activates complement and forms opsonins
Ferritin	Binds iron
Haptoglobin	Binds hemoglobin and prevents iron uptake
Ceruloplasmin	Oxidizes iron
Serum amyloid protein	Recruits inflammatory cells

Figure 2-5
Phagocytosis and intracellular killing of microbes. Macrophages and neutrophils express many surface receptors that may bind microbes for subsequent phagocytosis; selected examples of such receptors are shown. (*iNOS*, inducible nitric oxide synthase; *NO*, nitric oxide; *ROI*, reactive oxygen intermediate.) (From Abbas AK, Lichtman AH: Basic immunology: Functions and disorders of the immune system, ed 3, Philadelphia, 2009, Saunders.)

A specific β-defensin called *tracheal antimicrobial peptide (TAP)* is found along the entire length of conducting airways. In the lung, the β-1 TAP defensin prevents infection by virulent or opportunistic pathogens. In patients with cystic fibrosis (CF), the TAP is inactivated by high salt concentrations in the respiratory mucosa. This allows development of respiratory tract infections with opportunistic pathogens such as *Pseudomonas aeruginosa*.

Defensins also prevent the influenza virus from entering target cells. Influenza hemagglutinins are necessary for binding the virus to the target cell. Defensins render the virus noninfectious by cross-linking hemagglutinins, which prevents the normal interaction between the virus and the host cell membrane.

Nitric Oxide

Nitric oxide is a highly reactive molecule produced by macrophages following interactions between Toll-like receptors and PAMPs. In a chemical reaction, nitric oxide synthase oxidizes L-arginine to L-citrulline and nitric oxide (NO). Exposure to NO is cytotoxic to bacteria, fungi, parasites, and tumor cells. Toxicity is related to NO's ability to inhibit DNA synthesis and mitochondrial respiration. Prolonged NO generation can be detrimental to the body. Chemical reactions between NO and oxygen (O_2) forms dinitrogen trioxide in mammalian cell membranes and disrupts normal cellular function.

PATHOGEN-ASSOCIATED MICROBIAL PATTERNS AND VACCINES

PAMPs are being considered as additional components of vaccines because they stimulate both the innate and the adaptive immune systems. When added to vaccines, compounds that stimulate and direct the immune response are termed *adjuvants* (see Chapter 24). Adjuvants work by reducing antigen solubility and releasing small amounts of antigens over an extended period. PAMPs are used adjuvants. A purified PAMP from the tuberculosis bacterium called *muramyl dipeptide* is used in Freunds complete adjuvant to induce cell-mediated immune response to antigens.

IMMUNODEFICIENCY AND INNATE IMMUNITY

Most individuals with an MBL deficiency are healthy, but an increased incidence of otitis media, chronic upper respiratory tract infections, chronic diarrhea, and autoimmunity is seen among them. In infants, MBL may play an important role in the transition from passive immunity from the mother to mature adaptive immune responses.

SUMMARY

- The innate immune response involves the recognition of highly conserved microbial molecular structures called *pathogen-associated molecular patterns (PAMPs)*.
- PAMPs are recognized by serum proteins and phagocytic cell receptors.
- Additional antimicrobial agents are synthesized during an acute-phase response, which is characterized by physiologic changes in the host.
- The innate response controls pathogenic microbes until an adaptive immune response is generated.

REFERENCES

Baumann H, Gauldie J: The acute phase response, Immunol Today 15(2):74, 1994.

Hoppe HJ, Reid KB: Collectins-soluble proteins containing collagenous regions and lectin domains and their roles in innate immunity, Protein Sci 3:1143, 1994.

Kagan BL, Ganz T, Lehrer RI: Defensins: A family of antimicrobial and cytotoxic peptides, Toxicology 87:131, 1994.

Malhotra R, Merry T, Ray KP: Innate immunity: A primitive system in humans, Immunol Today 21(11):534, 2000.

Turner MW: Mannose-binding lectin: The pluripotent molecule of the innate immune system, Immunol Today 17(11):532, 1996.

ASSESSMENT QUESTIONS

1. Which of the following is found on skin?
   I. Perspiration
   II. Sebum
   III. Lactic acid
   A. I
   B. III
   C. I and II
   D. II and III
   E. I, II, and III

2. In which of the following is the mucociliary escalator found?
   A. Skin
   B. Respiratory tract
   C. Intestinal tract
   D. Urogenital tract

3. Pathogen-associated molecular patterns (PAMPs) are:
   I. Highly conserved molecular structures
   II. Common to most pathogenic bacteria
   III. Found on the surface of phagocytic cells
   A. I
   B. III
   C. I and II
   D. II and III
   E. I, II, and III

4. Which of the following are characteristics of serum complement?
   I. Nine serum proteins are present
   II. Fragments are opsonins
   III. Fragments are chemotactic
   A. I
   B. III
   C. I and II
   D. II and III
   E. I, II, and III

5. Which of the following is *not* considered a collectin?
   A. Zymosan
   B. Mannose-binding lectin (MBL)
   C. Bovine conglutinin
   D. Bovine collectin 43

6. Which of the following are functional responses of Toll-like receptor ligation?
   A. Phagocytosis and intracellular killing
   B. Proliferation of CD8 cells
   C. Synthesis of nitric oxide
   D. All of the above

7. Which of following are associated with toxic shock caused by endotoxins?
   I. Lipopolysaccharide
   II. Toll-like receptor 4 (TLR-4)
   III. Tumor necrosis factor–alpha (TNF-α)
   A. I
   B. III
   C. I and II
   D. II and III
   E. I, II, and III

8. Which of the following is associated with the acute-phase response?
   I. Fever
   II. Synthesis of acute-phase proteins
   III. Demargination of lymphocytes
   A. I
   B. III
   C. I and II
   D. II and III
   E. I, II, and III

9. Which of the following are small -(29–35 amino acids)- molecular-weight proteins produced by white blood and tissue cells?
   A. Cathelicidins
   B. Ferritin
   C. Defensins
   D. Haptoglobin

CHAPTER 3

Immunogenicity and Antigenicity

LEARNING OBJECTIVES

- Compare and contrast immunogens and antigens
- List the four major characteristics of an immunogen
- Identify the four biological factors that influence immunogenicity
- Define what an epitope is
- Compare and contrast linear and conformational epitopes
- Explain the relationship between epitopes and T and B cells
- Compare and contrast isoantigens and alloantigens
- Illustrate the differences between the hemolytic transfusion reactions of isoantigens and alloantigens
- Explain the role of RhoGam in preventing an immune response to Rh-positive fetal red blood cells
- Recognize the differences between exogenous and endogenous antigens
- Define what a hapten is
- List the metabolites of penicillin
- Recognize the pharmaceuticals that create neoantigens on red blood cells
- Identify the drugs that cause delayed cutaneous drug reactions

KEY TERMS

Alloantigens
Conformational epitope
Endogenous antigen
Epitope
Exogenous antigen
Hapten
Isoantigen
Neoantigen
Linear epitope

INTRODUCTION

This chapter begins the exploration of an adaptive immune response. Unlike innate immunity, which recognizes highly conserved microbial structures, the adaptive response is designed to protect the host against microbial antigens that constantly change and evolve. As the microbe changes its tactics for infection, the immune system adapts to counter the tactic and destroy the microbe. Adaptive immunity requires the stimulation of the immune system, the proliferation of effector cells, and the synthesis of cytokines and antibodies.

The concepts of immunogenicity and antigenicity are critical to the understanding of adaptive immunity. By definition, an *immunogen* is a molecule that stimulates the immune system to produce a response. An *antigen* is the part of the immunogen that reacts with immune effector cells or soluble antibodies. The term *allergen* is used to denote an immunogen that elicits the production of allergic antibody.

CHARACTERISTICS OF AN IMMUNOGEN

Foreignness

Immunogens that are considered "self" do not evoke an immune response; thus, foreignness is a critical attribute of immunogens. Phylogenetic differences between the host and the immunogen determine foreignness. For example, a vigorous response is generated when human serum albumin is injected into a mouse. In contrast, when mouse albumin is injected into a rat, only a minimal immune response is observed.

Internal Rigidity and Tertiary Structure

Most immunogens are proteins, which are complex rigid structures with a conformation defined by primary, secondary, and tertiary structures. Carbohydrates are composed of linear, repeating carbohydrate units with minimal structural rigidity. Therefore, carbohydrates are generally poor immunogens. The immunogenicity of deoxyribonucleic acid (DNA) depends on molecular weight and the extent of methylation. High-molecular-weight hypomethylated DNA is immunogenic. Other forms of DNA do not evoke an immune response.

Lipids, which are linear carbon chains with no defined tertiary structure, are rarely immunogenic because they lack structural rigidity. The exception is cardiolipin which is used as an antigen in the Wassermann test for syphilis.

Size

Size is an important determinant for antigenicity. Molecular structures less than 3000 MW (molecular weight) do not elicit an immune response, whereas maximum stimulation of the immune system is achieved with large antigens (e.g., 100,000 MW). Large macromolecules are better immunogens because they are insoluble and more easily ingested and processed by macrophages for presentation to lymphocytes.

Degradability

Immunogens must be degradable by macrophages to stimulate an immune response, antigen presenting cells must process the immunogen to yield small polypeptides between 7 and 30 amino acids. The small polypeptides are presented to lymphocytes.

BIOLOGIC FACTORS INFLUENCING IMMUNOGENICITY

Genetics

Genetics influences a person's ability to respond to specific immunogens. Genetic nonresponsiveness is the result of two defects. Some individuals lack a lymphocyte clone with a T cell receptor (TCR) directed at the antigen. Other individuals have a defect in antigen processing and cannot present the antigen to T cells.

Age

The immune response is influenced by a person's age. Infants are born with a still-developing immune system and cannot mount an immune response to some antigens. Infants are protected by maternal antibodies that cross the placenta before birth and by antibodies in breast milk after birth. An infant's immune system becomes fully functional between 6 and 12 months of age.

On the other end of the spectrum, the functional capacity of the immune system wanes with age, and older adults have a reduced ability to mount an effective immune response.

ANCILLARY FACTORS INFLUENCING IMMUNOGENICITY

Concentration

The immune response is a reflection of immunogen concentration and follows a bell-shaped curve, referred to as *gaussian distribution*. Small amounts of antigen fail to stimulate the immune system and induce an irreversible tolerance to the antigen. Excessively large concentrations paralyze the antigen-presenting cells. Only optimal concentrations on the bell-shaped curve generate an immune response.

Route of Administration

The magnitude and the nature of the immune response are determined by the route of administration. Subcutaneous or intramuscular administration stimulates the systemic immune system and protects the host from dying of the disease. Slow release of the antigen from the subcutaneous depot stimulates the immune system maximally. When the antigen is administered by the mucosal route, the host is protected from infection and mortality from the infection. Oral administration is less effective because of rapid clearance of the antigen from the circulation or inactivation of the antigen by gastric fluids.

EPITOPES

The molecular fragment of an antigen that interacts with effector cells or antibodies is called an *epitope*, or *antigenic determinant*. Proteins are usually large, complex structures that have multiple and different epitopes. One epitope, however, is dominant in the elicitation of an immune response.

Epitopes are either linear or conformational. Proteins have both linear and conformational epitopes. Linear epitopes comprise six to eight contiguous amino acids in the primary amino acid sequence of a polypeptide (Figure 3-1). Lymphocyte receptors or antibodies recognize linear epitopes in the native, fragmented, or extended conformations of the polypeptide. In contrast, conformational epitopes are created when protein segments are folded into a tertiary structure. The immune system recognizes the native conformational epitopes or the isolated fragments that retain the appropriate conformational tertiary structure.

T CELL AND B CELL RECOGNITION OF EPITOPES

Linear epitopes are recognized by T cells. Often, these epitopes are internal hydrophobic amino acid sequences processed by macrophages and presented to T cells in the context of human leukocyte antigen (HLA) class I and class II molecules. Processed epitopes containing 7 to 17 amino acids are presented to T lymphocytes by antigen-presenting cells. B cell epitopes from globular proteins, which range from 5 to 30 amino acids, are usually conformational. The length and flexibility of the epitope ensures high-affinity bonding to B cell receptors or circulating antibodies.

TYPES OF ANTIGENS

White Blood Cell Alloantigens

White blood cells express alloantigens, which are part of the body's self-recognition system. Alloantigens are found in some, but not all, members of a species. In mice, the genes for white cell alloantigens are localized in the MHC on chromosome 17. Humans have a similar locus called the *human leukocyte antigen (HLA)* complex located on chromosome 6. These glycoproteins are subdivided into class I and class II antigens. These antigens are involved in the presentation of antigen (see Chapter 4), the rejection or acceptance of grafts (see Chapter 17) between members of the same species (e.g., allografts), or both. Class I HLA antigens are constitutive and are expressed on all nucleated cells. Class II antigens are inducible and are only expressed on macrophages and monocytes. Multi-parous women and transplant recipients often develop antibodies directed at alloantigens.

Transfusion-Related Acute Lung Injury

Transfusion-related acute lung injury (TRALI) is caused by the transfusion of blood products containing anti-HLA antibodies. The antibodies react with HLA molecules on circulating neutrophils, which pool in the lung capillaries and move into extravascular spaces. Antibody-coated neutrophils release free oxygen radicals, enzymes, and arachidonic acid metabolites, which damage the alveolar epithelium. Leakage of fluid into alveoli from capillaries causes pulmonary edema. Patients present with shortness of breath, hypoxia, and fever.

Red Blood Cell Antigens

The best-studied antigens in humans are found on red blood cells. Red blood cell antigens are water-soluble glycopeptides consisting of heterosaccharides attached by a glycosidic linkage at the reducing ends. The common core structure consists of a galactose and N-acetyl glucosamine attached to a glycoprotein core and is called the *H-antigen*. Most individuals have a fucosyltransferase enzyme that attaches a fucose to the terminal end of the H antigen. Two variants of a glycosyltransferase enzyme add additional sugars to the H antigen.

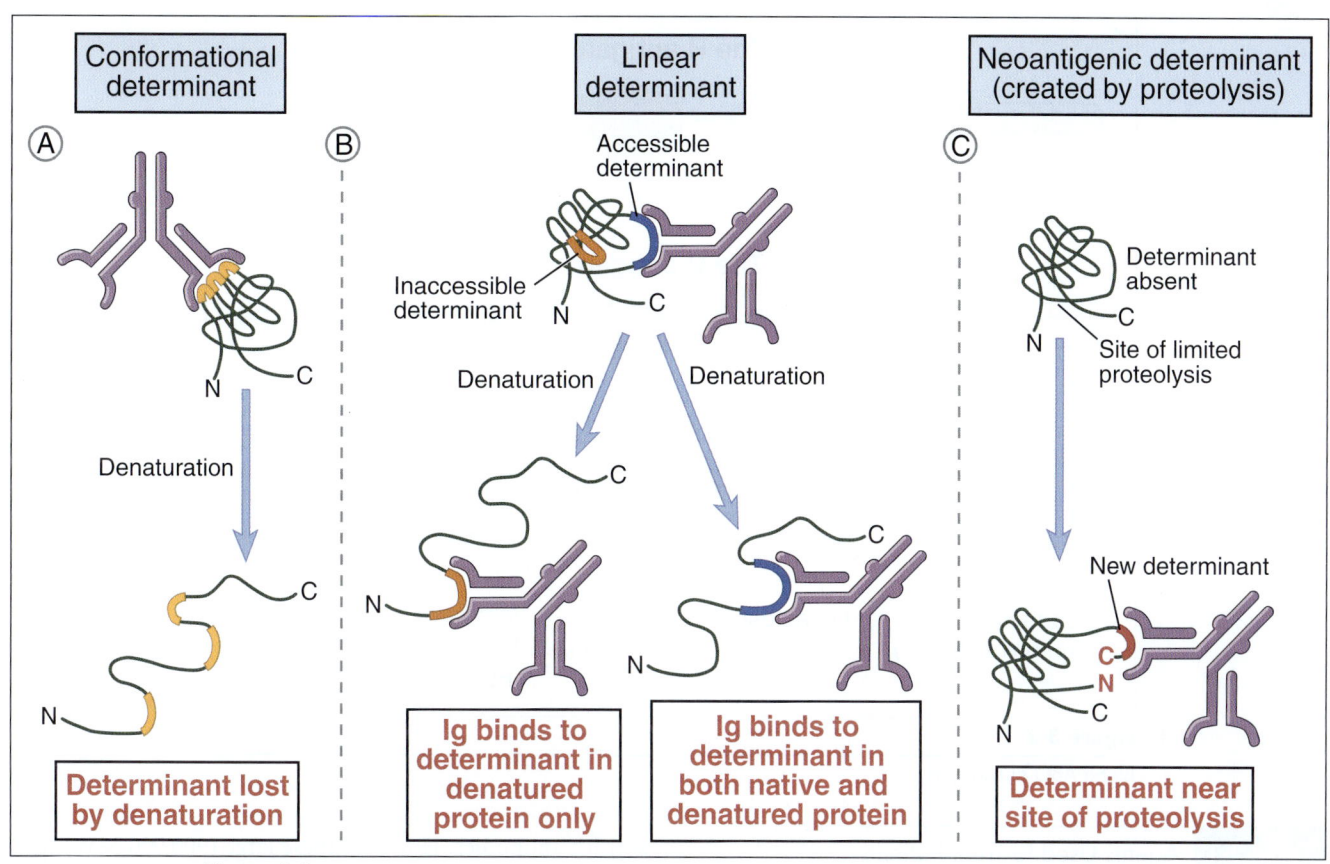

Figure 3-1

The nature of antigenic determinants. Antigenic determinants (*shown in orange, red, and blue*) may depend on protein folding (conformation) as well as on primary structure. Some determinants are accessible in native proteins and are lost on denaturation (**A**), whereas others are exposed only on protein unfolding (**B**). Neodeterminants arise from postsynthetic modifications such as peptide bond cleavage (**C**). (From Abbas AK, Lichtman AH, Pillai S: Cellular and molecular immunology, ed 6 [updated edition], Philadelphia, 2010, Saunders.)

The type A antigen is created when *N*-acetylgalactosamine is added to the terminal galactose. When an additional galactose is added to the terminal sugar, it produces a type B red cell antigen. In individuals who are heterozygous for blood group antigens, a galactosamine and N-acetylglucosamine are added to the core H antigen, which creates the AB blood type (Figure 3-2).

Using the ABO isoantigens, it is possible to classify red blood cell types into populations of universal donors or universal recipients. Since the O type contains an epitope that is common to all red blood cells (H antigen) and is non-immunogenic, individuals are universal donors. Conversely, persons with type AB blood are considered universal recipients because they express both A and B antigens. When transfused with type O, A, or B blood, persons with type AB blood do not mount an immune response because neither the A antigen nor the B antigen is foreign.

Antibodies directed at non-self blood group antigens are often present in serum. These natural antibodies are formed because A and B antigens are found in a wide variety of unrelated plant and animal tissues. Ingestion of these heterologous antigens stimulates the production of antibodies directed at non-self red cell antigens. For example, antibodies directed at blood group A are present in the serum of people with type B red blood cells. Conversely, persons with blood group A have anti-B antibodies in the serum. Antibodies directed at ABO blood group antigens can also be generated as a consequence of previous pregnancies, transfusions, or organ transplantations.

Hemolytic Transfusion Reactions

Hemolytic transfusion reactions occur when a patient receives red blood cells with major or minor antigens to which they have antibodies. An ABO mismatch typically occurs when a patient with group O blood type is transfused with group A, B, or AB blood cells. Antibodies in the recipient's blood react with red cell isoantigens and activate complement that lyses the recipient's red blood cells. As a result, hemoglobin is found in blood and urine, and microthrombi are formed. These small thrombi localize in the capillaries of the hands and feet. Obstruction of blood flow in the capillaries causes tissue necrosis and gangrene. Renal failure and cardiovascular collapse are other dangerous sequelae in these patients.

Treatment of Hemolytic Transfusion Reactions

Patients undergoing hemolytic transfusion reactions may experience mild or severe reactions. Mild symptoms include rashes, fever, and back pain. Acute kidney failure is a significant and severe problem in some patients. Treatment is directed at reducing the mild symptoms, increasing renal blood flow, and preserving urinary output (Table 3-1).

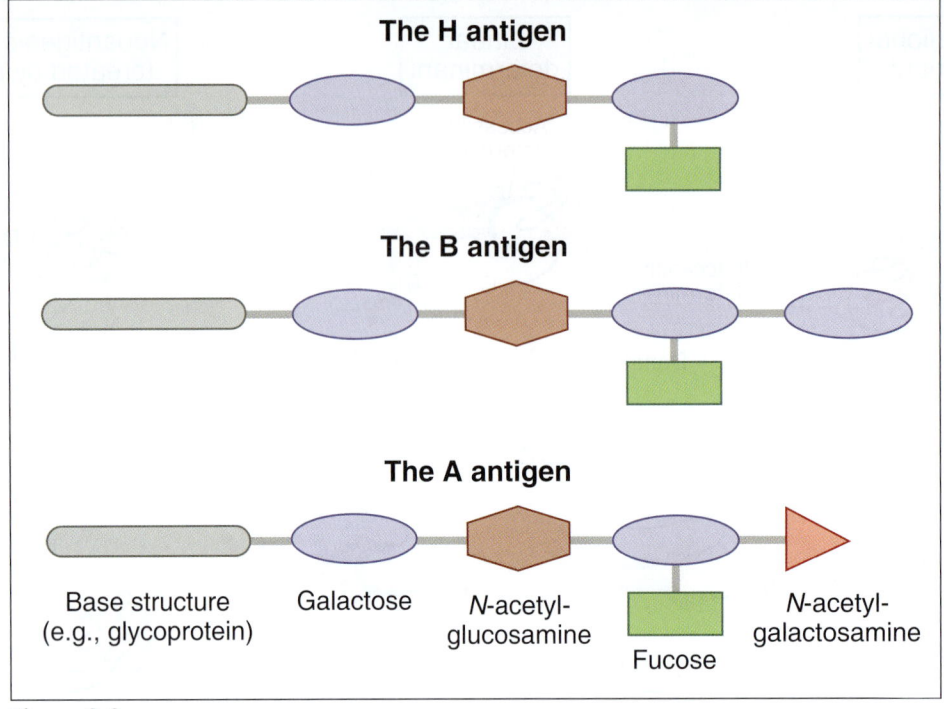

Figure 3-2
Blood ABO phenotypes.

Table 3-1	Agents Used to Treat Patients Experiencing Mild or Severe Hemolytic Transfusion Reactions
Agent	**Reaction**
Furosemide	Increases renal blood flow and preserves urinary output
Epinephrine	Increases bronchodilatation and peripheral vascular resistance
Antihistamines	Decreases the histamine response in nerve endings and blood vessels
Methylprednisolone	Decreases inflammation

Rhesus Factor Isoantigens

Rhesus factor (Rh or RhD), or *Rhesus antigen*, is another isoantigen found on red blood cells. The name is derived from the fact that the blood antigen was first described in the Rhesus monkey. Rh antigens are nonglycosylated, hydrophobic cell membrane antigens expressed in 85% of the human population (Rh positive, or Rh+). Individuals with alterations or a deletion of the Rh protein are considered Rh negative (Rh−). If individuals with Rh− blood are exposed to Rh+ antigens, a vigorous antibody response is evoked. An Rh mismatch during transfusion causes a unique extravascular hemolytic anemia. Antibodies directed at the Rh factor do not activate complement. Hence, no intravascular hemolysis occurs. Rather, red cells are coated with antibody and removed by splenic macrophages.

Rh antigens play a significant role in transfusion reactions; however, Rh compatibility takes on an even more significant and crucial role in pregnancy. Serious problems arise when the Rh− mother is exposed to Rh+ cells. Exposure can occur as a consequence of normal delivery, trauma, or blood transfusions. Within 30 days of exposure, the mother will develop anti-Rh antibodies. However, these large (900,000 MW) IgM antibodies cannot cross the placenta. Therefore, the first child will be unaffected. If the mother is exposed to Rh T cells during a second pregnancy, small (150,000 MW) IgG antibodies are produced. These antibodies can cross the placenta and attack the fetal red blood cells, causing an autoimmune hemolytic anemia, called *erythroblastosis fetalis*, with severe consequences. The lysis of red cells liberates hemoglobin, which is converted to bilirubin. Accumulation of bilirubin damages the central nervous system, and the infants develop hypotonia, hearing loss, and intellectual disabilities.

Severe forms of erythroblastosis fetalis are characterized by cardiac failure, pericardial effusions, and edema (hydrops fetalis).

Treatment of Rh Incompatibility

Pooled human anti-D immune globulin (Rh IgG or RhoGAM) treatment is indicated at 28 weeks and within 72 hours after delivery if the baby is Rh+. It is also indicated following spontaneous or induced termination and any event that could lead to transplacental hemorrhage. A single dose (50 micrograms [μg]), which is administered following first-trimester pregnancy termination, is enough to neutralize 2.5 mL of fetal blood. A 300-μg dose, which can neutralize 15 mL of fetal blood, is administered for all other indications. When properly administered, the incidence of adverse effects is less than 0.5%.

EXOGENOUS AND ENDOGENOUS ANTIGENS

Exogenous Antigens

Exogenous antigens enter the body via the oral, respiratory, and parenteral routes. In general, exogenous antigens are immunogenic structures expressed on extracellular bacteria, fungi, viruses, and pollens. Exogenous antigens are ingested

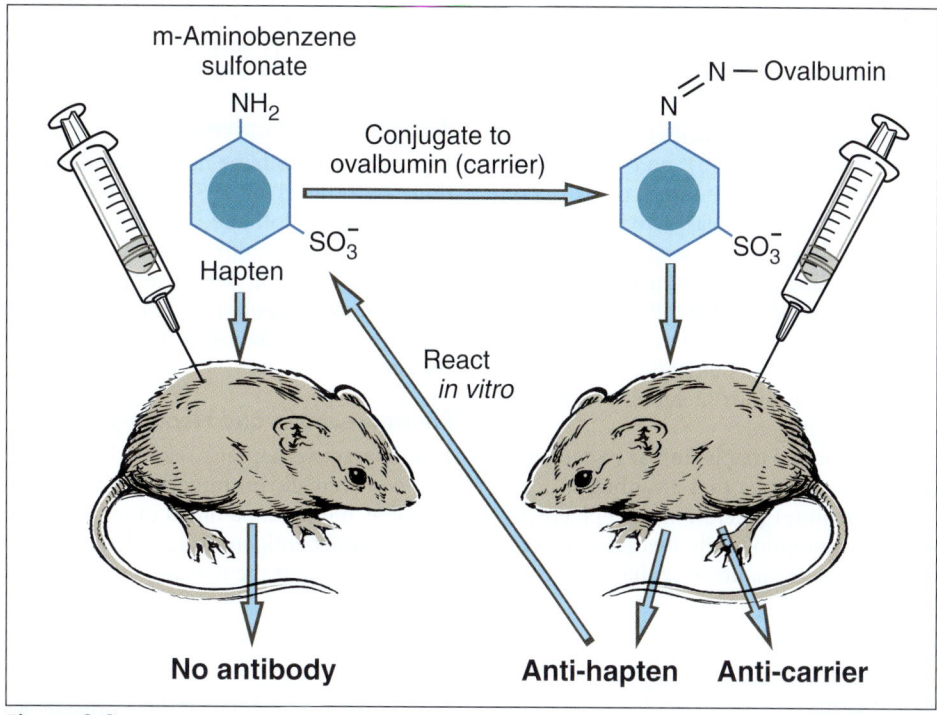

Figure 3-3
Hapten conjugation to ovalbumin.

by macrophages, and epitopes are presented in the context of class II molecules to Th2 cells. In some cases, exogenous antigens may be secretory products of bacteria or liberated on the death of the bacterium. For example, secreted protein exotoxins are both immunogenic and toxic to mammalian tissue. Lipopolysaccharide endotoxins are an integral part of the gram-negative cell wall and are released into the circulation following bacterial death.

Endogenous Antigens
Endogenous antigens are generated by cells infected by viruses, intracellular parasites, or tumor cells. These antigens are produced internally, processed in the cytosol, and loaded onto HLA class I molecules for presentation to CD8 cells. Antigen-specific CD8 cells then destroy the tumor cells.

Autoantigens
Autoantigens are the result of mutation, neoantigen formation, or exposure of previously hidden self-antigens. Genes producing self-proteins can mutate and create a new immunogenic protein called *neoantigen*. Viral infections and drugs can create neoantigens that stimulate an immune response. In some cases, auto-reactive proteins found in organs that develop late in gestation (e.g., eyes, testes) are not present when lymphocytes undergo positive and negative selection in the thymus. Therefore, auto-reactive T cells are not selected for destruction in the thymus and enter peripheral blood. Under normal circumstances, autoantigens are protected from the immune system by anatomic barriers (e.g., testes), a lack of blood vessels, or cellular structures that force immunocompetent cells to undergo apoptosis (e.g., eyes). Trauma or infection can expose autoantigens, and the resulting immune response damages the tissue.

HAPTENS
Haptens are small-molecular-weight compounds that evoke an immune response only when they are attached to carrier proteins. In vivo, haptens readily bind to serum proteins such as albumin. The combined molecular weights of albumin and the hapten need to exceed 3000 MW to stimulate the immune system. The immune response is directed at both the hapten and the carrier protein. The carrier protein has a different and unique antigenic structure after binding to the hapten.

The concept of haptens was introduced by Landsteiner. Subsequently, experiments with murine models demonstrated that immunization with m-aminobenzene sulfonate failed to elicit an immune response (Figure 3-3).

However, a vigorous antibody response was observed when m-aminobenzene sulfonate was linked to carrier protein (ovalbumin). Antibodies were directed to both the aminobenzene and the carrier protein. The phenomenon was termed *haptenic response*, from the Greek *haptein*, which means "to fasten."

Pharmaceuticals as Haptens
Most pharmaceuticals and antibiotics are small (at or less than 3000 MW) compounds. The native drug or metabolites are often haptens that bind to serum proteins or molecules expressed on cells and elicit either an antibody response or a cellular response. An immune response to the hapten carrier complex can result in skin eruptions, asthma, anaphylaxis, and autoimmune reactions. Antibiotics and anesthetics are common biologically active haptens.

Antibiotics as Haptens
Penicillin is the leading cause of immunologically mediated adverse health effects. Approximately 2% of patients receiving penicillin therapy develop urticaria, asthma, or angioedema.

Anaphylaxis, which is a serious and often fatal reaction to penicillin, results in 500 to 1000 deaths each year in the United States. Penicillin is composed of an acyl side chain linked to a β-lactam ring combined with a thiazolidine ring. Natural penicillin (PenG), penicillinase-resistant penicillin (methicillin), extended-spectrum penicillin (amoxicillin), and broad-spectrum penicillin (carbenicillin) all have the same core β-lactam ring, which is essential for antimicrobial activity. Bacteria secrete a β-lactamase that breaks the lactam ring, rendering the antibiotic ineffective and creating highly charged metabolites (Figure 3-4). The major antigenic determinant (90%–95% of the breakdown products) is a benzylpenicilloyl derivative (BPO).

Minor metabolites include parental penicillin, penicilloate, and penicilloylamine. Major and minor metabolites combine with proteins to become immunogenic.

Cephalosporins have a structure that is similar to penicillin and are reactive haptens. For reasons that are unclear, third (ceftriaxone) and fourth (cefepime) generations of cephalosporins are more involved in immunologically mediated adverse health effects. The haptenic determinants of cephalosporin are not fully delineated. It has been suggested that serologic reactivity is directed at both the acyl side chains and the β-lactam ring linked to the carriers.

Anesthetics as Haptens
Exposure to halothane may also induce an autoimmune reaction. Introduced in 1951 as a potent, nonflammable anesthetic agent, halothane is metabolized in oxidative pathways to trifluoroacetyl chloride (TFAC). In a subsequent chemical reaction, TFAC acetylates liver proteins to form a neoantigen. An immune response to the neoantigen causes halothane hepatitis. Inflammation of the liver abates when the drug is discontinued.

Pharmaceuticals and Neoantigens
Highly reactive haptens readily bind to red blood cell membranes to create immunogenic neoantigens (Box 3-1). For example, methyldopa binds to red blood cell membrane, thus creating a neoantigen. A hemolytic anemia results when antibodies react with the neoantigen and lyse the red cells.

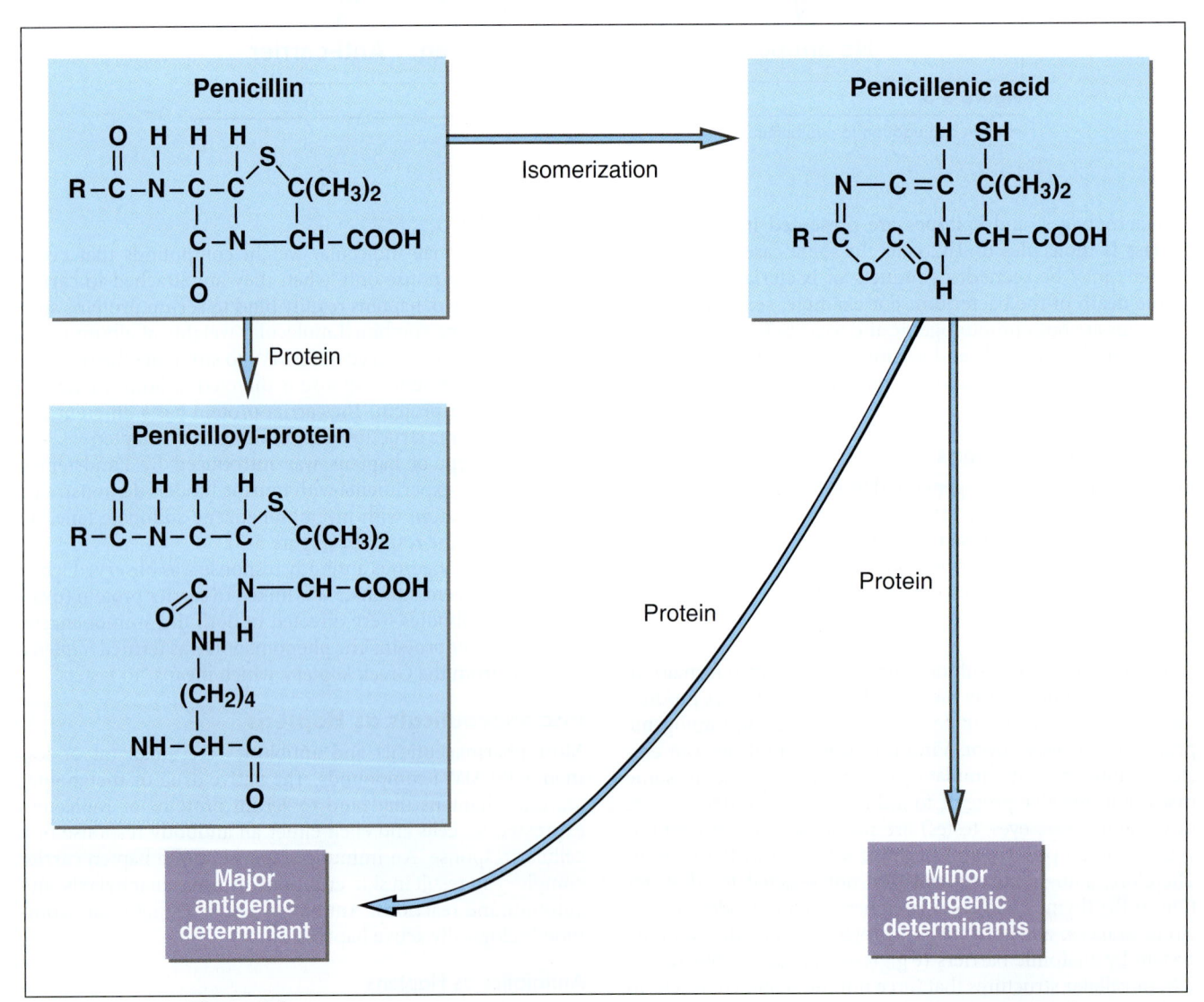

Figure 3-4

Penicillin haptenic metabolites. The conjugation of penicilloyl derivatives to protein via an amide linkage is shown in the lower left.

> **BOX 3-1**
> **Drugs or Their Metabolites That React with Red Blood Cells or Serum Proteins**
>
> **Drugs Reacting with Red Blood cells**
> Diclofenac
> Ibuprofen
> Levodopa
> Mefenamic acid
> Methyldopa
> Procainamide
>
> **Drugs Reacting with Serum Proteins**
> Penicillins
> Cephalosporins
> Tetracycline
> Tolbutamide

Haptens and Cell-Mediated Reactions

Some responses to pharmaceuticals are mediated by inflammatory cells rather than by antibodies. Skin lesions, which are characterized by redness, induration, or blistering, occur 24 to 48 hours after exposure and are mediated by CD4Th1 cells and inflammatory macrophages. Inflammatory responses in the liver and kidney have also been reported. Clinical symptoms may persist after discontinuation of the drug.

Delayed hypersensitivity reactions in the skin or cutaneous drug reactions (CDRs) occur following systemic administration of a wide variety of drugs. Antimicrobial agents (sulfonamides), anticonvulsants (carbamazepine), anesthetics (lidocaine), anti-psychotics (clozapine), cardiovascular agents (procainamide, hydrazaline) and nonsteroidal anti-inflammatory drugs (diclofenac) are metabolized by the liver with the creation of reactive haptens, which bind to skin cells. An inflammatory response in the skin is characterized by widespread rashes and eruptions. Reactions in the skin usually occur 7 to 10 days after drug administration.

SUMMARY

- The adaptive immune response is affected by changing and evolving microbial immunogens rather than by the highly conserved molecules recognized by the innate response.
- Immunogens are large-molecular-weight molecules that have defined structural and biologic characteristics.
- Haptens are small-molecular-weight compounds that require protein binding to stimulate an immune response.
- Immunogens can be molecules expressed on cells, bacterial proteins and lipopolysaccharides, viral and fungal proteins, and tumor cells.

REFERENCES

Benacerraf B, Paul WE, Green I: Hapten-carrier relationships, Ann N Y Acad Sci 169(1):93, 1970.

Benjamin D, Berzofsky J, East I: The antigenic structure of proteins: A reappraisal, Annu Rev Immunol 2:67, 1984.

Smerdou C, Anton IM, Plana J, et al: A continuous epitope from transmissible gastroenteritis virus S protein fused to *E. coli* heat-labile toxin B subunit expressed by attenuated Salmonella induces serum and secretory immunity, Virus Res 41:1, 1996.

ASSESSMENT QUESTIONS

1. Which of the following is *not* a characteristic of an immunogen?
   A. Foreignness
   B. Tertiary structure
   C. Molecular weight less than 3000
   D. Degradability

2. Which of the following describes an epitope?
   I. Is a fragment of an immunogen
   II. Reacts with effector cells or antibodies
   III. Is a part of the T cell receptor (TCR)
   A. I
   B. III
   C. I and II
   D. II and III
   E. I, II, and III

3. On which of the following do linear epitopes usually react with receptors?
   A. B cells
   B. T cells
   C. Dendritic cells
   D. Macrophages

4. Which of the following describes alloantigens?
   I. Are present on white blood cells
   II. Are present on cells from some but not all members of a species
   III. Are part of the body's self-recognition system
   A. I
   B. III
   C. I and II
   D. II and III
   E. I, II, and III

5. Which of the following usually precipitates transfusion-related acute lung injury (TRALI)?
   A. Presence of antibodies to isoantigens on red blood cells
   B. Presence of antibodies to alloantigens on white blood cells
   C. Presence of antibodies to Rh+ red blood cells
   D. Extravascular destruction of red blood cells

6. Which of the following are characteristics of a hapten?
   I. Has a molecular weight of less than 3000
   II. Does not evoke an immune response
   III. Cannot bind to serum proteins
   A. I
   B. III
   C. I and II
   D. II and III
   E. I, II, and III

7. Which of the following is the major haptenic metabolite of penicillin?
   A. Penicillin
   B. Penicilloylamine
   C. Penicillioate
   D. Benzylpenicilloyl derivatives

8. Which of the following is the reason for proteins being excellent immunogens?
   I. A rigid tertiary structure
   II. Multiple epitopes
   III. A linear repeating epitope
   A. I
   B. III
   C. I and II
   D. II and III
   E. I, II, and III

9. Which of the following causes an antibody-mediated hemolytic anemia?
   A. Methyldopa
   B. Procainamide
   C. Lidocaine
   D. Hydralazine

CHAPTER 4

Antigen-Presenting Molecules

LEARNING OBJECTIVES

- Differentiate between major histocompatibility complex (MHC) and human leukocyte antigen (HLA) glycoproteins
- Explain the functions of HLAs
- Identify the major class I loci
- Identify the major class II loci
- Compare and contrast the structures of class I and II molecules
- Discuss the relationships between class I and class II molecules and CD4 and CD8 cells
- Identify the genes located in HLA class III loci
- Compare and contrast antigens binding to class I and class II molecules
- Define haplotype
- Understand the value of heterozygosity in species survival
- Explain how recombinant HLA molecules are generated
- Understand the value of allelic polymorphism in species survival
- Define a single nucleotide polymorphism (SNP)
- Restate the structural features of CD1 molecules
- Recognize the biologic function of CD1 molecules
- Define bare lymphocyte syndrome
- Explain the molecular defects associated with bare lymphocyte syndrome

KEY TERMS

Human leukocyte antigen (HLA) complex
Class I region
Class II region
Class III region
Haplotype
Heterozygosity
Allelic polymorphism
Single nucleotide polymorphism

INTRODUCTION

The immune system defends the host against microbial infections and mutant cells. In defense of the host, the immune system must differentiate between foreign proteins and "self-proteins." Surface display proteins are used as markers of "self." Early animal skin transplantation studies demonstrated that rejection or acceptance of grafts was dependent on "self" markers mapped to a gene cluster on chromosome 17. This gene cluster was called the *major histocompatibility complex (MHC)*. In humans, the MHC is called the *human leukocyte antigen (HLA) complex*. The term is derived from the use of white blood cell alloantigens in tissue typing of donors and recipients prior to organ transplantation. Although HLAs are important in transfusion reactions, organ transplantation, and autoimmunity, their most important role is antigen presentation to T cells. In this role, HLA molecules control susceptibility or resistance to infection, the generation of autoimmune responses, and antibody-mediated and cell-mediated responses.

THE HUMAN LEUKOCYTE ANTIGEN COMPLEX

The HLA complex is a gene cluster containing 128 functional genes and 96 partial genes or gene fragments called *pseudogenes*. Most gene products are expressed on nucleated cells in the body, but some are secreted proteins that augment an inflammatory response. On the basis of gene product structure and function, the HLA gene complex is subdivided into class I, II, and III regions. The function of pseudogenes is unclear, but evidence suggests that pseudogenes are coding sequences that contribute to the genetic diversity of HLA molecules. A map of the human MHC or HLA complex is shown in Figure 4-1.

Class I Region

The class I region is subdivided into three major loci, termed *HLA-A*, *HLA-B*, and *HLA-C*, and minor loci consisting of *HLA-G*, *HLA-E*, *HLA-F*, *HLA-H*, and *HLA-J* and MHC class I chain–related genes (MIC). The major class I loci (A, B, and C) present antigens to CD8 T cells.

Minor loci have various immunologic functions. HLA-E interacts with CD94 and NKG2 receptors on natural killer (NK) cells to augment or inhibit NK cell function. HLA-F has an unknown function. HLA-G presents a broad range of self-polypeptides with similar molecular structure and is found in high concentrations on the surface of extravillous cytotrophoblast and the placenta. The role of HLA-G in pregnancy is unclear, but it may shift immune responses from Th1 to Th2. The functions of HLA-H and J are unclear.

The MIC family represents a nonclassic HLA gene complex. Gene products are expressed as a stress response to virus infection or cellular damage in the intestine and synovia. Their structure resembles a class I molecule, but MIC gene products cannot present antigens. Expression of MIC marks the cell for destruction by CD8 and NK cells.

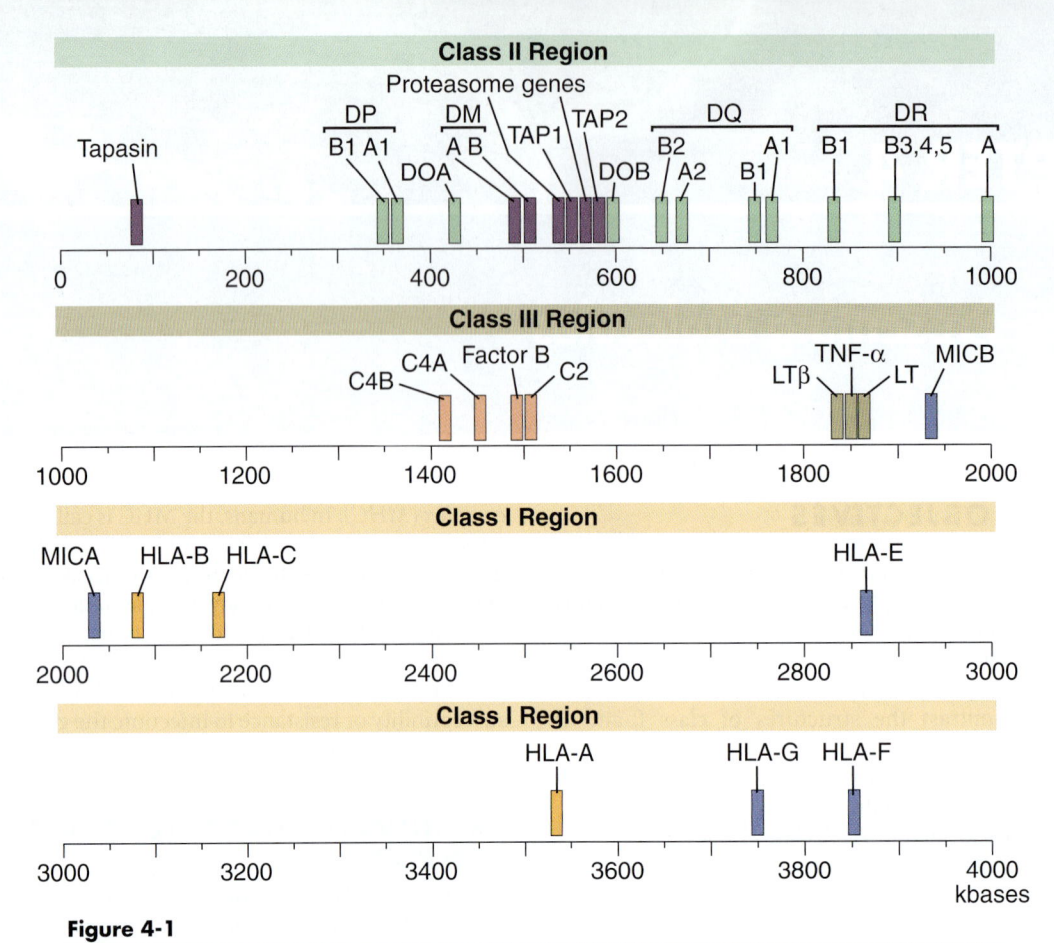

Figure 4-1
Map of the human leukocyte antigen complex (HLA). This map is simplified to exclude many genes that are of unknown function. HLA-E, HLA-F, HLA-G, and the MIC genes are class I–like molecules, many of whose products are recognized by natural killer (NK) cells; C4, C2, and factor B genes encode complement proteins; tapasin, HLA-DM, HLA-DO, transporter-associated antigen processing (TAP), and proteasome encode proteins involved in antigen processing; lymphotoxin A (LTA), lymphotoxin B (LTB) and tumor necrosis factor (TNF) encode cytokines. Many pseudogenes and genes whose roles in immune responses are not established are located in the HLA complex but are not shown. (From Abbas AK, Lichtman AH, Pillai S: Cellular and molecular immunology, ed 6 [updated edition], Philadelphia, 2010, Saunders.)

STRUCTURE OF CLASS I MOLECULES

Class I molecules comprise a single glycosylated α-chain (394 amino acids), which is noncovalently bound to β2-microglobulin (94 amino acids). The class I protein consists of two intracellular and three extracellular domains. The two intracellular domains attach the molecules to the cell membrane and extend into the cytoplasm. The three extracellular domains—designated $α_1$, $α_2$, and $α_3$—are each composed of 90 amino acids. The $α_1$- and $α_2$- domains have unique helical structures that form an antigen-binding cleft used to present antigens to T cells (Figure 4-2).

Peptides are tethered to the ends of the binding groove usually at positions 2 and 9. Thus, the binding cleft accommodates only small peptides containing 8 to 12 amino acids. Flexing of unbound peptides and side chains within the binding cleft creates a three-dimensional epitope structure that is recognized by T cells. The $α_3$-domain stabilizes the interaction between class I molecules and the lymphocyte T cell receptor.

Class II Region

Class II gene products are induced and expressed on monocytes, macrophages, dendritic cells, and B cells. Within the class II region are three loci (DP, DR, and DQ) involved in antigen presentation. Class II molecules present antigens to CD4Th1 and CD4Th2 cells. Other genes in the class II region code for proteins that are important in antigen processing.

STRUCTURE OF CLASS II MOLECULES

The class II region has three major loci (DP, DQ, and DR). Class II molecules consist of heavily glycosylated α- and β-chains. Although both chains have similar structure, the α-chain is larger (30–34 kiloDaltons [kDa]) compared with the β-chain (26–29 kDa). An antigen-binding cleft comprises the $α_1$- and $β_1$-domains (Figure 4-3). The peptide binding to the class II molecule occurs in the middle of the binding cleft at positions 1, 4, 6, and 9. Peptides are bound in a manner analogous to a long pipe being held in a centrally located vise. Peptides are held in place by hydrogen bonding and van der Waals forces. All class II antigens bind at the same anchor positions. However, they are much larger than class I antigens (10–30 amino acids) and protrude from either end of the cleft.

Class III Region

The class III region has 62 genes, which have diverse functions. Most class III gene products are not membrane proteins but are secreted into the environment. Products include

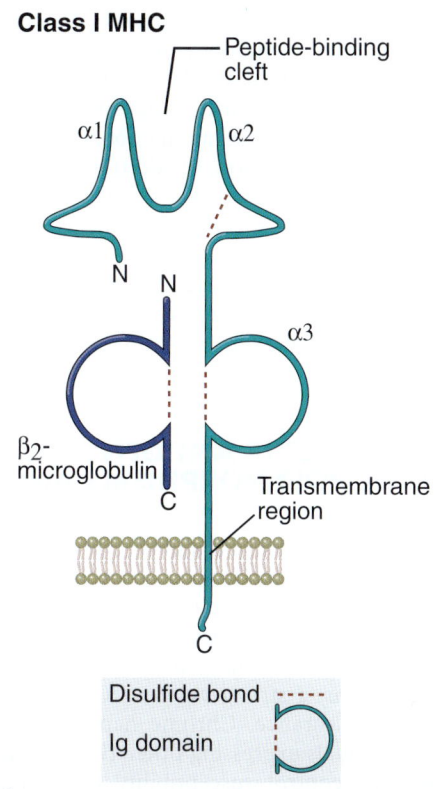

Figure 4-2
Structure of a class I MHC or HLA molecule. The schematic diagram illustrates the different regions of the HLA molecule (*not drawn to scale*). Class I molecules are composed of a polymorphic α-chain noncovalently attached to the nonpolymorphic β2-microglobulin (β2m). The α-chain is glycosylated; carbohydrate residues are not shown. (From Abbas AK, Lichtman AH, Pillai S: Cellular and molecular immunology, ed 6 [updated edition], Philadelphia, 2010, Saunders. Courtesy of Dr. P. Bjorkman, California Institute of Technology, Pasadena, Calif.)

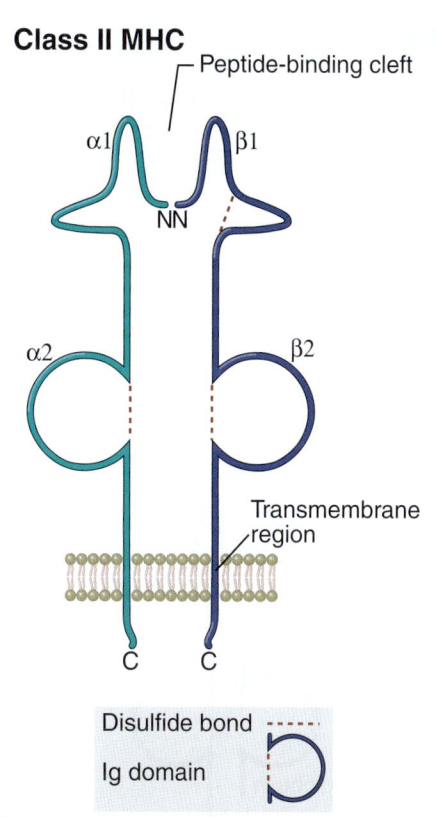

Figure 4-3
Structure of a class II MHC or HLA molecule. The schematic diagram illustrates the different regions of the HLA molecule (*not drawn to scale*). Class II molecules are composed of a polymorphic α-chain noncovalently attached to a polymorphic β-chain. Both chains are glycosylated; carbohydrate residues are not shown. (From Abbas AK, Lichtman AH, Pillai S: Cellular and molecular immunology, ed 6 [updated edition], Philadelphia, 2010, Saunders. Courtesy of Dr. P. Bjorkman, California Institute of Technology, Pasadena, Calif.)

three complement components and the tumor necrosis factor (TNF).

INHERITANCE OF HUMAN LEUKOCYTE ANTIGENS

A set of HLAs (HLA A, B, C, DP, DQ, and DR) on the same chromosome is called a *haplotype*. The genotype of each individual consists of two haplotypes. One set of HLA genes (N=6) is inherited from the father, and the other haplotype (N=6) is inherited from the mother. Both haplotypes are co-dominant and expressed on cells. HLA genes usually are inherited in blocks as haplotypes. Occasionally, deoxyribonucleic acid (DNA) segments are exchanged in a process called *gene conversion*. During meiosis, two homologous chromosomes with multiple genes arranged in tandem are misaligned. Crossing over of parental haplotypes and DNA recombination allows individual genes or parts of genes to transfer from one chromosome to another without any loss of function. Exchange of DNA causes multiple amino acid changes in the original gene and the formation of a recombinant HLA molecule.

HETEROZYGOSITY

The inheritance of duplicate genes at the same locus may be the result of a population balancing selection process, which, in theory, provides a survival advantage to heterozygotes. All HLA molecules can present antigens to T cells, but each HLA molecule binds a different range of antigens. In effect, the inheritance of paternal and maternal haplotypes doubles the antigen-presenting capability of the host and increases the probability that most individuals within a species will be heterozygotes. Heterozygotes at an HLA locus are more resistant to disease than are homozygotes because they have a more varied repertoire of antigen-presenting HLA molecules.

ALLELIC POLYMORPHISM

Additional genetic diversity critical to the disease resistance is provided by allelic and single nucleotide polymorphisms (SNPs). When several alternate forms of the same gene are present, the gene is termed *polymorphic*. Each variant of a polymorphic gene is called an *allele*. Over 3000 different alleles are present within the HLA complex. Two thousand polymorphic alleles have been reported in class I loci alone. Over 900 different alleles also are found in class II DR, DQ, and DP loci. Nonclassic, minor loci such as HLA-F, HLA-G, HLA-H, and HLA-J are less polymorphic compared with antigen-presenting loci and have restricted tissue distribution. The different alleles present in major loci are shown in Table 4-1. SNPs are single base pair changes in genes coding for each HLA allele. In effect, SNPs create additional alternative forms of each allele.

Allelic polymorphism and SNPs are associated with nonsynchronous amino acid substitutions in the α-helical sides of the binding cleft or alterations in the peptide anchoring β-strands forming the floor of the cleft. A change in the binding cleft alters the pattern of antigens binding to the allele (Figure 4-4).

CHAPTER 4 ANTIGEN-PRESENTING MOLECULES

Table 4-1 HLA Allelic Polymorphism

Class I Loci	No. of Alleles	Class II Loci	No. of Alleles
HLA-A	649	HLA-DR	643
HLA-B	1029	HLA-DQ	125
HLA-C	350	HLA-DP	154
HLA-E	9		
HLA-F	21		
HLA-G	31		

HLA, human leukocyte antigen.

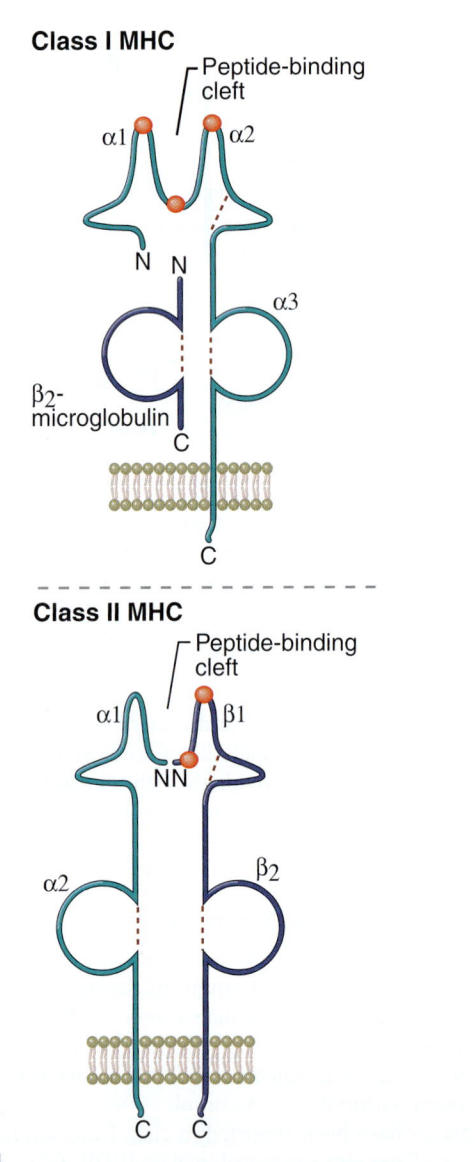

Figure 4-4
Polymorphic residues of human HLA molecules. The polymorphic residues of class I and class II HLA molecules (*shown as red circles*) are located in the peptide-binding clefts and the α-helices around the clefts. In the class II molecule shown (HLA-DR), essentially all the polymorphism is in the β-chain. (From Abbas AK, Lichtman AH, Pillai S: Cellular and molecular immunology, ed 6 [updated edition], Philadelphia, 2010, Saunders. Courtesy of Dr. J. McCluskey, University of Melbourne, Parkville, Australia.)

Allelic polymorphism is a response to the constant and continuing evolution of microbes and is essential to the survival of the species. Within an HLA locus, the presence of different alleles presenting a wide range of antigens from the same microbe ensures that some members of a species will survive the microbial infection. In addition, allelic polymorphism protects some members of a species when a microbe inadvertently expresses a specific HLA allele. Microbes that express an HLA allele would be considered "self" and evade immune detection. As a consequence of infection, significant population mortality may occur among individuals carrying the allele. However, individuals expressing other HLA polymorphic alleles within the same loci would be unaffected.

HUMAN LEUCOCYTE ANTIGEN SINGLE NUCLEOTIDE POLYMORPHISMS AND DISEASE

The HLA molecule's ability or inability to present antigens to T cells determines an individual's resistance or susceptibility to microbial infections. For example, self-limiting hepatitis B is associated with the expression of HLA-DR13. Individuals homozygous for DR13 have more efficient presentation of hepatitis antigens, a strong vigorous CD4 response, and accelerated viral clearance. Chronic hepatitis B infections develop in individuals expressing other HLA DR molecules. HLA alleles also control susceptibility to infections. The strongest relationship between HLA and disease is found in HLA alleles containing SNPs. For example, individuals expressing (DRB1*1501) molecules have a high risk for developing pulmonary tuberculosis. It is assumed that these class II molecules cannot present mycobacterium antigens to CD4Th1 cells.

ANTIGEN-PRESENTING MOLECULES OUTSIDE THE HUMAN LEUCOCYTE ANTIGEN COMPLEX

The CD1 family of genes is involved in antigen presentation. Unlike HLA molecules, they are encoded by a gene cluster on chromosome 1. The configuration of the CD1 molecule is similar to a class I protein with respect to subunit organization and the presence of B_2-microglobulin. CD1 molecules present highly conserved glycolipids to CD4Th1 cells. Glycolipids include mycolic acid, glucose monomycolate, phosphoinositol mannosides, and lipoarabinomannan derived from the *Mycobacterium* species that cause tuberculosis and leprosy.

Two families of CD1 molecules exist: (1) Group I consists of CD1a, CD1b, and CD1c. (2) CD1d is the only member of group II (Table 4-2). CD1a is expressed on thymocytes, dendritic cells, and Langerhans cells. CD1b is expressed on monocytes and macrophages. CD1c is found on circulating B cells, the splenic mantle zone, and tonsillar B cells. Monocytes, macrophages, dendritic cells, B cells, and some nonlymphoid cells express CD1d.

It is unclear whether the five members of the CD1 family present the same antigens or different antigens. It is conceivable that each represents a redundant system for the identification of conserved molecules. Some evidence suggests that group I CD1 is promiscuous and presents an overlapping set of glycopeptides. Other CD1 molecules may have individual binding properties.

Table 4-2: Tissue Distribution of Group I CD1 Molecules

CD1 Family Member	Tissue Distribution
CD1a	Thymocytes, dendritic cells, Langerhans cells
CD1b	Macrophages
CD1c	Circulating B cells, splenic mantle zone and tonsillar B cells
CD1d	Monocytes, macrophages, dendritic cells, B cells

Table 4-3: Therapeutic Agents Indicated for Suspected Viral or Microbial Infections in Children with Bare Lymphocyte Syndrome

Agent	Infection
Acyclovir	Herpes simplex, cytomegalovirus, varicella zoster
Fluconazole	Mucosal *Candida albicans*
Amphotericin B	Invasive *Candida albicans* and *Aspergillus*
Itraconazole	*Aspergillus*

ANTIGEN-PRESENTING MOLECULES AND IMMUNODEFICIENCY

Bare Lymphocyte Syndrome

The bare lymphocyte syndrome (BLS) is a form of severe combined immunodeficiency (SCID). In this syndrome, individuals lack class II molecules on the surface of B cells and monocytes. Class II molecules are not produced because of mutations in the consensus sequences of gene promoters that regulate HLA class II structural genes. Mutations prevent the docking of regulator factor X (RFX) and class II transactivator (CIIT) with the promoter genes. CIIT regulates the expression of the class II molecule.

Children with BLS have repeated infections with *Candida albicans* or *Pneumocystis jiroveci*. Common childhood viral infections with respiratory syncytial virus (RSV) or cytomegalovirus (CMV) are invariably fatal.

Treatment of Bare Lymphocyte Syndrome

Without hematopoietic stem cell transplantation, infants with this syndrome die within the first year of life. Aggressive antibiotic therapy is indicated for suspected microbial and viral infections. Agents used in the treatment of BLS are shown in Table 4-3.

SUMMARY

- The human leukocyte antigen (HLA) complex on chromosome 6 has three regions that code for antigen-presenting molecules.
- Three major class I and class II loci are present within the coding regions.
- Major loci within the class I region produce glycoproteins that present antigens to CD8 cells.
- Major loci within the class II region produce glycoproteins that present antigens to CD4 cells.
- Regions outside the HLA complex code for molecules that present highly conserved molecules.
- Each individual has two sets of HLA molecules. One is inherited from the mother and the other from the father.
- Heterozygosity, allelic polymorphism, and single nucleopeptide polymorphisms (SNPs) ensure that some members of the species will survive microbial infections.

REFERENCES

Bjorkman PJ, Parham P: Structure, function, and diversity of class I major histocompatibility complex molecules, Annu Rev Biochem 59:253, 1990.

Bjorkman PJ, Saper MA, Samraoui B, et al: The foreign antigen binding site and T cell recognition regions of class I histocompatibility antigens, Nature 329(6139):512, 1987.

Brown JH, Jardetzky T, Saper MA, et al: A hypothetical model of the foreign antigen binding site of class II histocompatibility molecules, Nature 332(6167):845, 1988.

Brown JH, Jardetzky TS, Gorga JC, et al: Three-dimensional structure of the human class II histocompatibility antigen HLA-DR1, Nature 364(6432):33, 1988.

Diepolder HM, Jung MC, Keller E, et al: A vigorous virus-specific CD4+ T cell response may contribute to the association of HLA-DR13 with viral clearance in hepatitis B, Clin Exp Immunol 113(2):244, 1998.

Fairhurst RM, Wang CX, Sieling PA, et al: CD1-restricted T cells and resistance to polysaccharide-encapsulated bacteria, Immunol Today 19(6):257, 1998.

Mehra NK, Rajalingam R, Mitra DK, et al: Variants of HLA-DR2/DR51 group haplotypes and susceptibility to tuberculoid leprosy and pulmonary tuberculosis in Asian Indians, Int J Lepr Other Mycobact Dis 63(2):241, 1995.

Porcelli SA, Segelke BW, Sugita M, et al: The CD1 family of lipid antigen-presenting molecules, Immunol Today 19(8):362, 1998.

Stern LJ, Brown JH, Jardetzky TS, et al: Crystal structure of the human class II MHC protein HLA-DR1 complexed with an influenza virus peptide, Nature 368(6468):215, 1994.

Touraine JL: The bare lymphocyte syndrome. Combined immune deficiency by absence of HLA antigen expression, Presse Med 13(11):671, 1984.

Wang JH, Meijers R, Xiong Y, et al: Crystal structure of the human CD4 N-terminal two-domain fragment complexed to a class II MHC molecule, Proc Natl Acad Sci U S A 98(19):10799, 2001.

Zeng Z, Castaño AR, Segelke BW, et al: Crystal structure of mouse CD1: An MHC-like fold with a large hydrophobic binding groove, Science 277(5324):339, 1997.

ASSESSMENT QUESTIONS

1. In which of the following are HLAs involved?
   I. Antigen presentation
   II. Transplantation
   III. Autoimmunity
   A. I
   B. III
   C. I and II
   D. II and III
   E. I, II, and III

2. Which of the following is a dual-chain class II molecule?
   A. MIC
   B. HLA-A
   C. HLA-DR
   D. HLA-C

3. HLA class I molecules present antigen to:
   A. CD8 cells
   B. CD4Th1 cells
   C. CD4Th2 cells
   D. B cells

4. HLA class II molecules can bind longer antigenic epitopes because:
   A. Antigens bind at the ends of the binding groove
   B. Antigens bind in the middle of the binding groove
   C. Antigens bind in both the middle and ends of the binding groove
   D. Antigens bind to β_2-microglobulin

5. By definition, allelic polymorphism is:
   I. A locus within the HLA complex
   II. Different forms of a gene within a loci
   III. SNPs within a polymorphic allele
   A. I
   B. III
   C. I and II
   D. II and III
   E. I, II, and III

6. Which of the following is an immunologically important gene cluster located outside the HLA complex on chromosome 6?
   A. MIC
   B. CD1
   C. BLS
   D. Class II

7. A set of HLA genes on the same chromosome is called a:
   A. Haplotype
   B. Genotype
   C. Heterozygote
   D. Cross-over

8. A class II molecule consists of:
   I. A single glycoprotein chain
   II. A single glycoprotein chain plus a β_2-microglobulin molecule
   III. Two glycoprotein chains
   A. I
   B. III
   C. I and II
   D. II and III
   E. I, II, and III

9. A DNA base pair change in a gene within the HLA complex is called a:
   A. Single nucleotide polymorphism
   B. Haplotype
   C. Genotype
   D. Gene conversion

CHAPTER 5

Antigen-Presenting Cells

LEARNING OBJECTIVES

- Differentiate between professional and amateur antigen-presenting cells
- Compare and contrast monocytes and macrophages
- Recognize dendritic cell subpopulations
- Compare and contrast the roles of follicular dendritic cells and interdigitating dendritic cells in antigen presentation
- Explain the roles of plasmacytoid dendritic cells in innate immunity and adaptive immunity
- Recognize the differences between a phagosome and an endosome
- Explain the roles of the invariant chain protein in antigen presentation
- Define class II-associated invariant chain peptide (CLIP)
- Recognize the biological roles of HLA-DM and HLA-DO in antigen presentation
- Identify the differences between phagocytosis and receptor-mediated endocytosis
- Discuss the concept of dendritic cell cross-priming and its usefulness in developing cancer vaccines

KEY TERMS

Class II-associated invariant chain peptide (CLIP)
Cross-priming
Dendritic cell
Endosome
Follicular dendritic cell
Iccosomes
Interstitial dendritic cell
Invariant chain
Langerhans cell
Macrophage
Monocyte
Phagosome
Plasmacytoid dendritic cell
Receptor-mediated endocytosis

INTRODUCTION

The previous chapter discussed molecules that present antigens to T cells. Prior to loading class I and II molecules with antigens, large-molecular-weight proteins must be degraded to a length of 8 to 30 amino acids. This chapter discusses the cells involved in antigen recognition and the processing of exogenous antigens. The processing of endogenous antigens is discussed later in Chapter 18.

To generate the small peptides, inhaled, ingested, or injected antigens are internalized by specialized antigen-presenting cells (APCs) and processed in an endocytic pathway.

APCs can be divided into "professional" and "amateur" subsets. Professional APCs such as monocytes, macrophages, dendritic cells, and B cells are fully committed to antigen presentation as an integral part of their function in the generation of the immune response. Other cells such as endothelial cells, fibroblasts, glial cells, pancreatic β- cells, keratinocytes, and thyroid cells present antigens only under select conditions. These cells are considered "amateur" APCs.

PROFESSIONAL ANTIGEN-PRESENTING CELLS

Monocytes and Macrophages

Monocytes and macrophages are responsible for the digestion of foreign material and for the presentation of antigenic epitopes to immunocompetent cells. Monocytes circulate in the blood, whereas macrophages are found in most tissues, for example, the brain (microglia), bone (osteoclasts), and connective tissue (histiocytes). Kupffer cells in the liver are the largest concentration of macrophages in the body.

Macrophages participate in both innate and adaptive immune responses. As part of innate immunity, macrophages are activated by antigens that are bound to PAMP, Toll-like, scavenger, and mannose receptors. In an adaptive response, antigens are recognized using receptors for intermediary molecules, such as antibody and complement fragments.

Dendritic Cells

In 1973, Steinman described a rare peripheral blood cell with membrane dendrites similar to a neuron. Other studies demonstrated that the dendritic cell (DC) is a "professional" antigen-producing cell present in lymphoid and nonlymphoid tissues. Dendritic cell precursors arise in bone marrow from committed CD34+ stem cells; differentiate into immature myeloid, monocytic, and lymphoid DCs; and are seeded into blood. Because of heterogeneity in cell surface markers, populations of DCs are difficult to identify. However, a putative hematopoietic differentiation pathway for DCs is shown in Figure 5-1.

Several DC subsets localize in tissues or circulate in peripheral blood. Two populations of dendritic cells are derived from

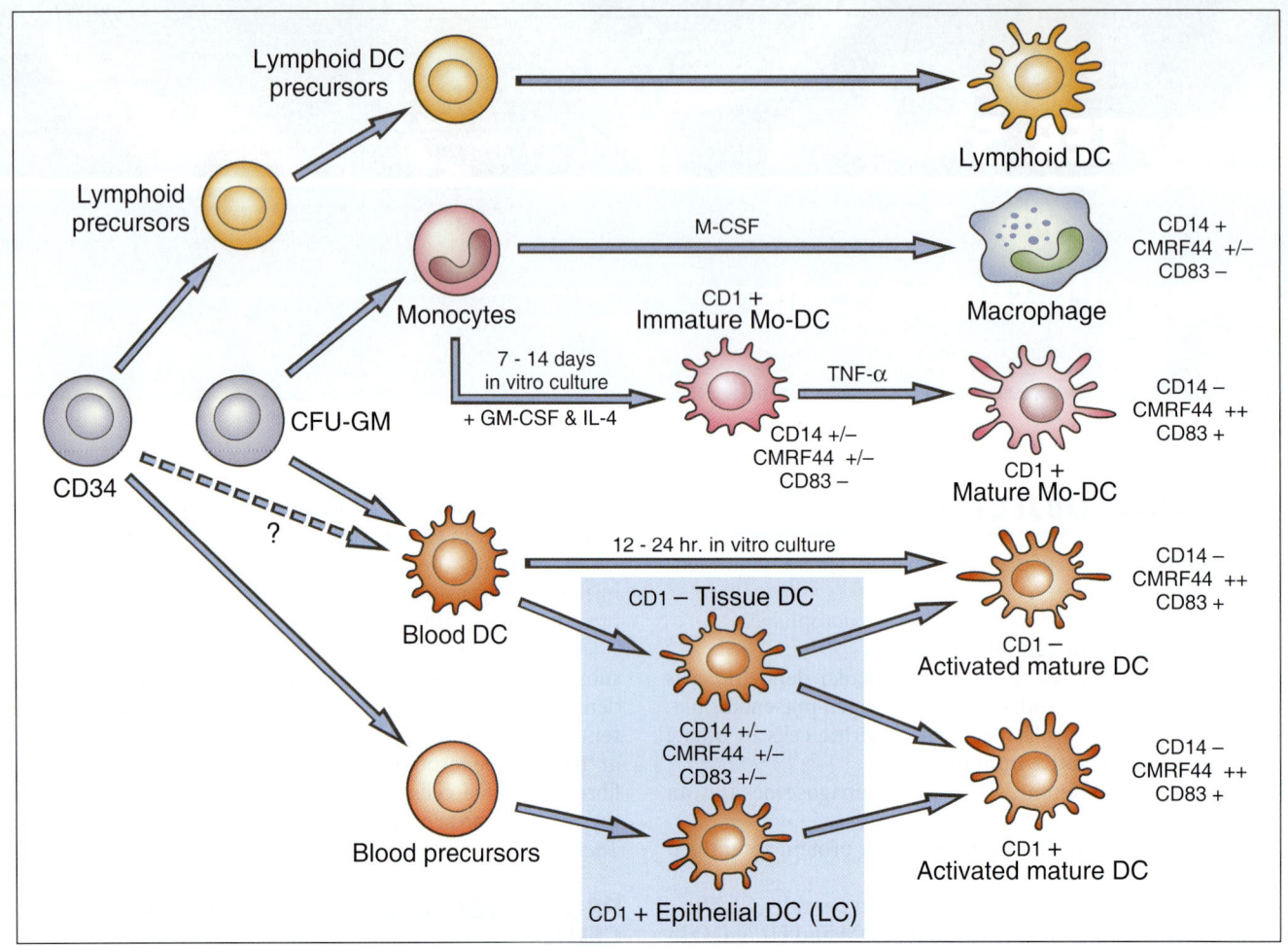

Figure 5-1

A putative hematopoietic differentiation pathway for myeloid and lymphoid dendritic cells (DCs). Lymphoid DCs have different properties (tolerizing) from myeloid DCs, which are immunostimulatory in most circumstances. The surveillance tissue-based DC–Langerhans cells (LCs) in the skin, DCs in the respiratory tract, gut, or other nonlymphoid tissues, migrate to the T-lymphocyte–dependent areas of the draining lymph node (LN). It is possible that epithelial based CD1+ DCs have an independent derivation from the stem cell. The ability of monocytes and macrophages to convert to DC in vivo has yet to be established. (From Hart, DN: Dendritic cells: Unique leukocyte populations which control the primary immune response, Blood 90(9):3245, 1997.)

a myeloid stem cell: (1) One population migrates to the lymph node where it becomes follicular dendritic cells. (2) A second population is found in nonlymphoid tissue and is referred to as *interstitial dendritic cells*. Lymphoid or plasmacytoid dendritic cells localize in the T cell compartment within the lymph node. Monocyte precursors may remain in peripheral blood as monocytic dendritic cells, although this concept is still being debated.

Dendritic cells are uniquely suited for antigen presentation. High numbers are concentrated at likely sites of microbial entry into the body (e.g., intestine and respiratory tract). Most DCs can efficiently capture and process antigen for presentation to T cells. Moreover, they are mobile and can migrate through tissue or stimulate immune responses in the regional lymph nodes.

Follicular Dendritic Cells

Follicular dendritic cells (FDCs) are found in the lymph node germinal follicles (Figure 5-2) and have several different functions, including activation of B cells and maintenance of immunologic memory.

Unlike other DCs, FDCs do not process antigen for presentation to T cells. Rather, they stimulate a CD4Th2 response and maintain memory by a unique mechanism. Using a repertoire of receptors, FDCs bind processed and unprocessed antigens onto beaded, three-dimensional structures called *iccosomes* (Figure 5-3).

Antigens may be retained in iccosomes for months and perhaps years. To stimulate antibody production, an antigen is slowly released, processed by B cells, and presented to T cells in the context of class II molecules. Cytokines produced from FDCs also contribute to the activation and differentiation of B cells into plasma cells. As a consequence of the continual stimulation of B cells, antibodies and memory cells are continually produced.

Interstitial Dendritic Cells

Interstitial dendritic cells are found in most tissue, with the exception of the brain and the eye. These cells serve as a sentinel for detecting foreign or antigenic molecules. The largest

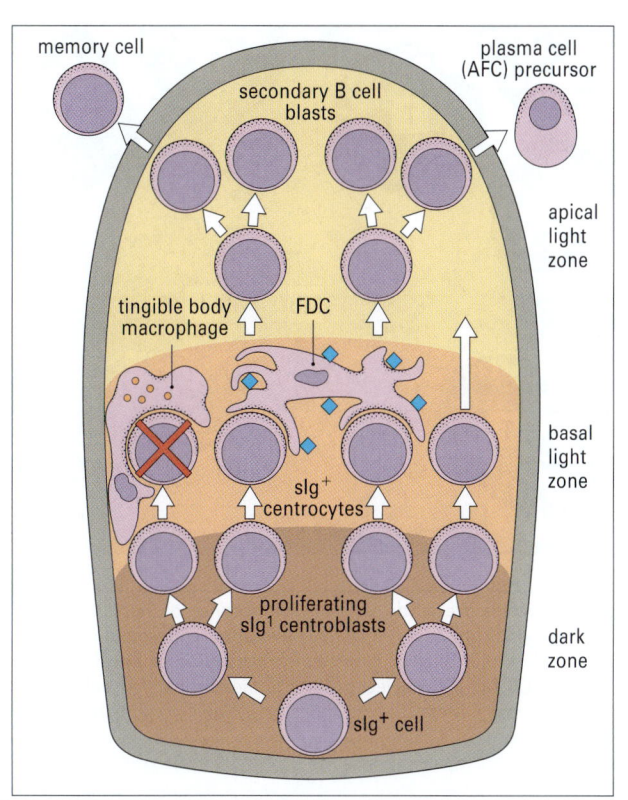

Figure 5-2

The functions of the germinal center are clonal proliferation, somatic hypermutation of immunoglobulin receptors, receptor editing, isotype class switching, affinity maturation, and selection by antigen. In this model, the germinal center is composed of three major zones: (1) a dark zone, (2) a basal light zone, and (3) an apical light zone. These zones are predominantly occupied by centroblasts, centrocytes, and secondary blasts, respectively. Primary B cell blasts carrying surface immunoglobulin receptors (sIg+) enter the follicle and leave as memory B cells or antibody forming cells (AFCs). Antigen-presenting follicular dendritic cells (FDCs) are mainly found in the two deeper zones, and cell death by apoptosis occurs primarily in the basal light zone, where tingible body macrophages are also located. Blue squares are iccosomes on the FDC. (Adapted from Delves PJ, et al: Roitt's essential immunology, ed 11, 2006, Blackwell Publishing.)

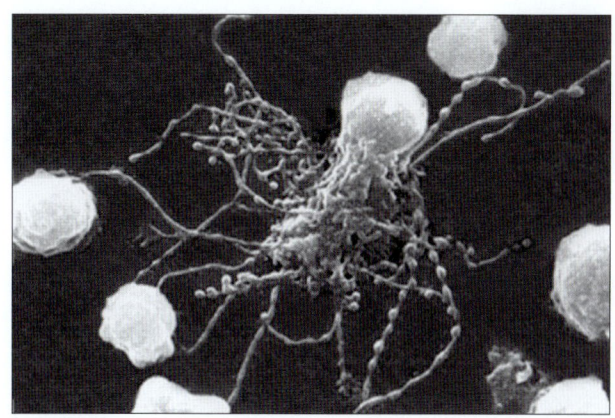

Figure 5-3

An isolated follicular dendritic cell (FDC) from the lymph node of an immunized mouse 24 hours after injection of antigen. The FDC is of intermediate maturity with smooth filiform dendrites typical of young FDCs, and beaded dendrites, which participate in the formation of iccosomes (antigen antibody complexes) in mature FDCs. The adjacent small white cells are lymphocytes. (In Roitt I, Brostoff J, Male D, et al: Immunology, ed 7, Philadelphia, 2006, Mosby. Electron micrograph kindly provided by Dr. Andras Szakal; reproduced by permission of the Journal of Immunology.)

reservoir of IDCs resides in the skin, where resident Langerhans cells (LC) occupy 25% of the skin surface area, but only 2% to 3% of skin cells. Resting or immature LCs reside in the suprabasilar epidermis and are identified by the presence of cytoplasmic Birbeck granules and by the expression of CD1, class I, class II molecules, and abundant receptors for pathogen-associated microbial patterns (PAMPs) and mannose. When antigens are captured, the immature LCs disengage from the epithelium and migrate to the paracortex or T cell zones of the regional lymph nodes. During migration, LCs undergo a transformation into "veiled cells." After entering the lymph node, the "veiled cells" assume the role of resident interdigitating dendritic cells that present antigen to naïve CD4 cells (Figure 5-4).

Resident lymph node IDCs can also process soluble antigens entering the lymph node via the lymph fluid. Lymph-borne soluble antigens percolate through the node in a manner that ensures contact with IDCs. Following internalization and processing, antigen is presented to naïve and effector CD4 T cells, which have close contact with the IDCs (Figure 5-5).

Plasmacytoid Dendritic Cells

Plasmacytoid dendritic cells (pDCs) resemble antibody-secreting plasma cells and are believed to arise from a lymphoid progenitor. pDCs are found in blood and in lymphoid tissues such as lymph nodes, tonsils, spleen, thymus, and Peyer's patches. Activated pDCs link innate immunity and adaptive immunity to viruses. In the innate response, Toll-like receptors 7 and 9 bind viral deoxyribonucleic acid (DNA) and ribonucleic acid (RNA) from herpes simplex virus (HSV), Sendai virus, human immunodeficiency virus type 1 (HIV-1), and influenza virus. Receptor activation of pDCs initiates synthesis of α-interferon and β-interferon. Interferon prevents the spread of the virus to uninfected cells and also activates natural killer cells. In the adaptive response, pDCs process and present antigens to T cells. Cytokines produced by pDCs also induce the expansion of antigen-specific CD8 memory cells and unique CD4Th1 cells responding to endogenous antigens.

B Cells

Under certain circumstances, B cells are able to present antigens to T cells. Antigens bind to an antigen-specific B cell receptor (BCR) which is a modified antibody. Cross-linking of BCRs internalizes antigens, which are degraded in the cytoplasm and presented to T cells in context with class II markers. B cells present antigens at 100 to 10,000 times lower concentration than that required for macrophage presentation.

PRESENTATION OF EXOGENOUS ANTIGENS

Exogenous antigens are degraded in the endocytic pathway and loaded onto class II molecules. The mechanism for class II molecule delivery differs with macrophages and B cells. Macrophages and dendritic cells bind antigens using a number of different receptors for PAMPs, complement fragments, or

CHAPTER 5 ANTIGEN-PRESENTING CELLS

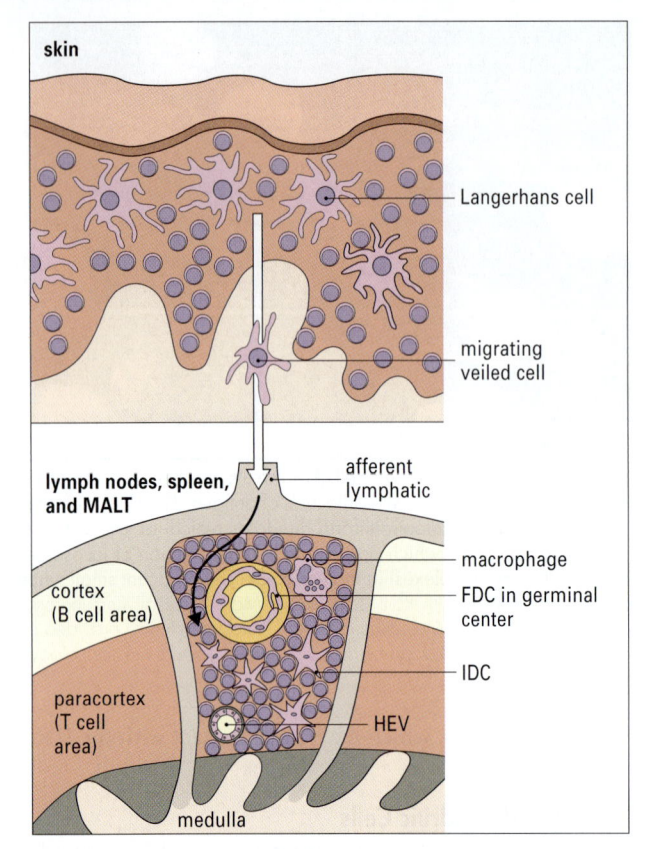

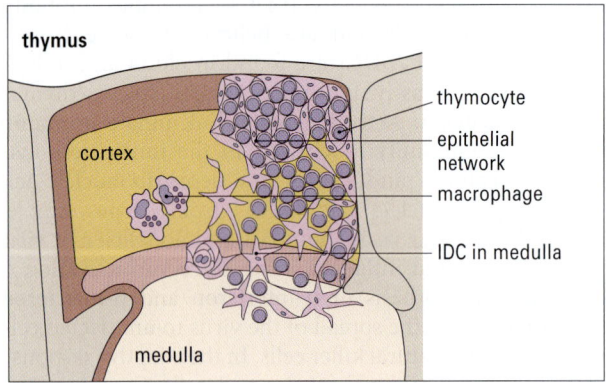

Figure 5-4

Bone marrow-derived antigen-presenting cells (APCs) are found especially in lymphoid tissues, in the skin, and in mucosa. APCs in the form of Langerhans cells are found in the epidermis and are characterized by special granules (the tennis racquet–shaped Birbeck granules; *not shown here*). Langerhans cells are rich in major histocompatibility complex (MHC) class II molecules and carry processed antigens. They migrate via the afferent lymphatics (where they appear as "veiled" cells) into the paracortex of the draining lymph nodes. Here they make contact with T cells. These interdigitating dendritic cells (IDCs), localized in the T cell areas of the lymph node, present antigens to T helper cells. Antigens are exposed to B cells on the follicular dendritic cells (FDCs) in the germinal centers of B cell follicles. Some macrophages located in the outer cortex and marginal sinus may also act as APCs. In the thymus, APCs occur as IDCs in the medulla. (*HEV*, high endothelial venule.) (From Roitt I, Brostoff J, Male D, et al: Immunology, ed 7, Philadelphia, 2006, Mosby.)

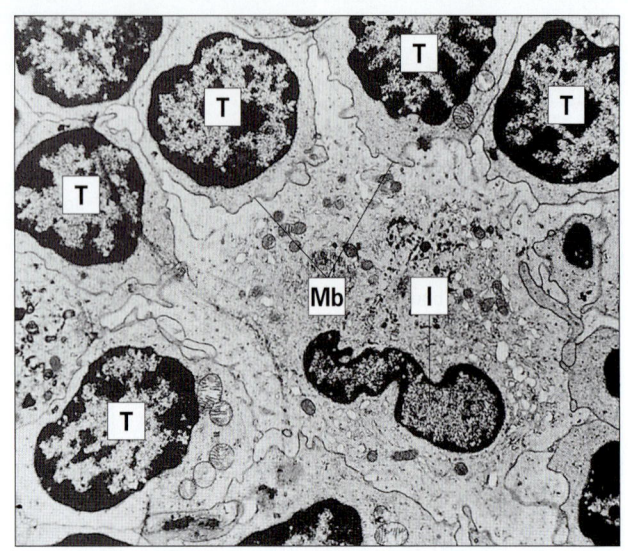

Figure 5-5

Intimate contacts are made with the membranes of the surrounding T cells. The cytoplasm contains a well-developed endosomal system and does not show the Birbeck granules characteristic of skin Langerhans cells. (× 2000.) (*I*, IDC nucleus; *Mb*, IDC membrane; *T*, T cell nucleus.) (In Roitt I, Brostoff J, Male D, et al: Immunology, ed 7, Philadelphia, 2006, Mosby. Courtesy of Dr. B.H. Balfour.)

B cells use receptor-mediated endocytosis to ingest foreign material. B cell receptors are localized in areas containing membrane clathrin. Receptor binding activates the clathrin and facilitates an inward folding of the cell membrane to form a vesicle. After recycling the clathrin molecules and the B cell receptors to the cell surface, the vesicle becomes a membrane-bound vacuole (Figure 5-6).

Different terms are used to describe the vacuoles in macrophages and B cells. In monocytes and macrophages, the vacuole is called a *phagosome*. Cytoplasmic lysosomal vesicles containing hydrolytic enzymes fuse with the phagosome membrane and empty their contents into the phagosome, which is now termed a *phagolysosome*. In B cells, endocytosis forms a vacuole called *early endosome*. In the endocytic pathway, early endosomes travel through a series of tubes and vesicles from the periphery to deep inside the cell (late endosome).

Class II molecules synthesized in the endoplasmic reticulum rapidly associate with a 30-kilodalton (kDal) invariant peptide chain (Ii). Homotrimers of Ii chain associate with three α-heterodimers or β-heterodimers of class II molecules. The Ii has two roles in antigen presentation: (1) It contains a signaling sequence that directs the class II molecule—into the endosome or the phagolysosome. (2) The Ii also prevents the loading of peptides into the binding groove until the class II molecule enters the endosome or the phagolysosome. The Ii may also contribute to the formation of the binding cleft and the overall structure of the class II molecule recognized by T cells. After entry into antigen-containing endosome or phagolysosome, the Ii is removed in an orderly proteolytic reaction (Figure 5-7).

In the endosome or phagolysosome, the invariant chain is truncated to a 3-kDal peptide called the class II-associated invariant chain peptide, or CLIP. In humans, the disassociation of the CLIP is facilitated by the HLA-DM (monocytes)

antibodies. Opsonized bacteria and antigens are ingested by a process called *phagocytosis*. During phagocytosis, a re-arrangement of cytoskeleton generates long membrane evaginations called *pseudopodia*, which surround and engulf membrane-bound material to form an internal vacuole.

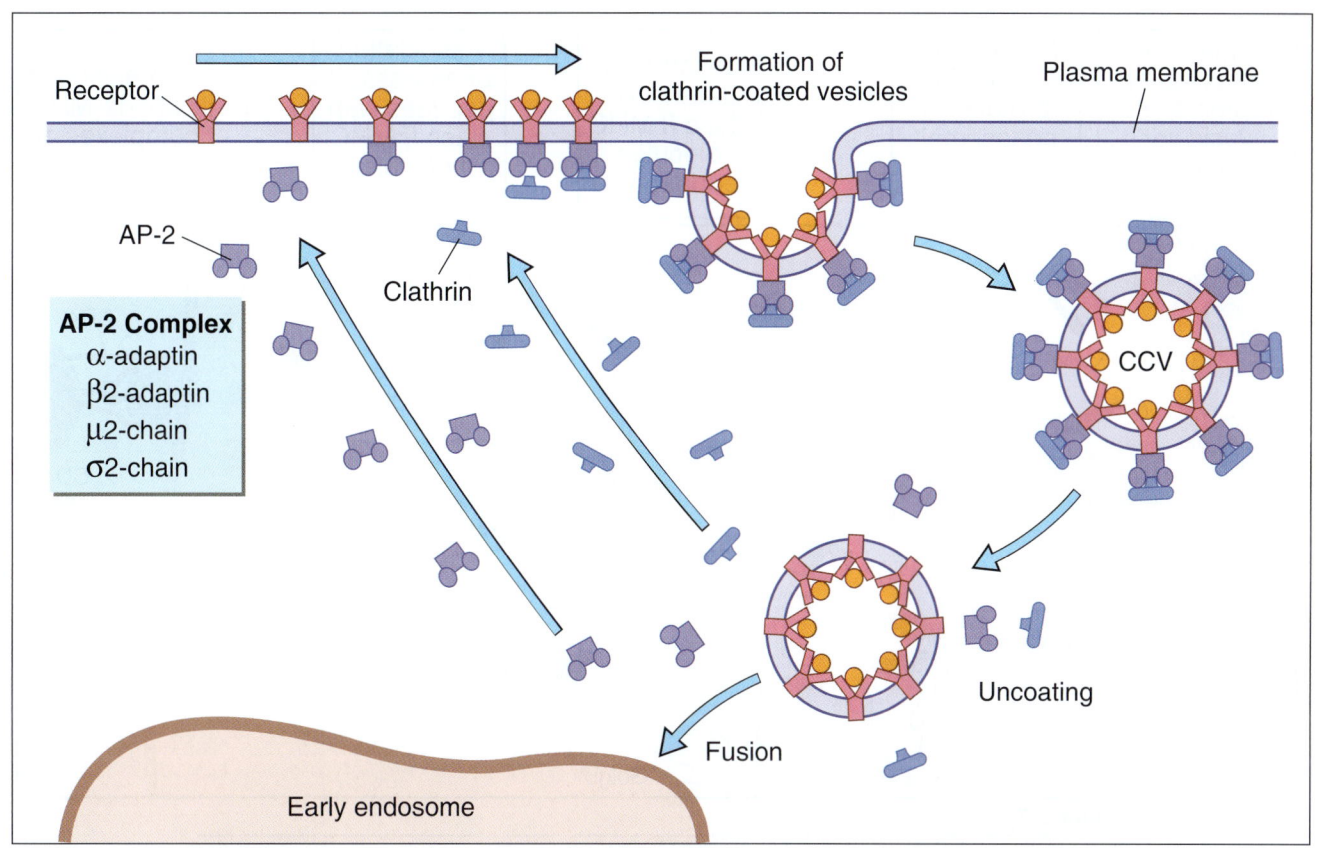

Figure 5-6

Mechanism of clathrin-dependent endocytosis. Clathrin and cargo molecules are assembled into clathrin-coated pits on the plasma membrane together with an adaptor complex called *AP-2*, which links clathrin with transmembrane receptors, concluding in the formation of mature clathrin-coated vesicles (CCVs). CCVs are then actively uncoated and transported to early, or sorting, endosomes. (From Barth D, Sato G, Sato M: Available from http://www.wormbook.org/chapters/www_intracellulartrafficking/intracellulartrafficking.html.)

or the HLA-DO (B cells), which also stabilize the class II molecule and assist in peptide selection (Figure 5-8).

Stabilization allows the binding of peptides with low and high structural stability. Low-stability peptides are released from class II molecules. The interaction between high-stability peptides and the binding groove on class II molecules creates a stable peptide–class II molecule complex. Large and small peptides may bind to the open-ended class II binding cleft. Proteolytic enzymes trim the larger peptide to 10 to 30 amino acids.

DENDRITIC CELLS AND CANCER VACCINES

Tumor cells are usually not immunogenic because HLA molecules are downregulated and tumor-specific antigens cannot be presented to T cells. Vaccinologists use dendritic cell cross-priming to increase the immunogenicity of tumor cells for use in vaccines. In cross-priming, dendritic and tumor cells are obtained from the patient and purified. In the laboratory, DCs and tumor cells are mixed together and incubated for several days. DCs ingest intact tumor cells and process the appropriate antigens for presentation in the context of class I molecules. Administration of antigen-pulsed dendritic cells to the patient evokes a vigorous CD8 cytotoxic cell response to tumor cells. This concept is being used to develop autologous pulsed dendritic cell vaccines against tumors. From a theoretical perspective, dendritic cell vaccines could be used to treat all cancers. However, clinical experience shows that at the present time, the efficacy of dendritic cell vaccination is limited to melanoma and renal cancer treatments.

DENDRITIC CELLS AND DISEASE

Dendritic cells may play a critical role in psoriasis. Interactions between dendritic cells and T cells play a critical role in the formation of plaques in chronic psoriasis. Plaques contain high numbers of pDCs, myeloid DCs, and inflammatory dendritic skin cells. Interactions between DCs and CD4 cells lead to the clonal expansion of CD8 cells in skin lesions. CD8 cells produce proinflammatory cytokines that are implicated in psoriasis.

Dendritic cells also play a role in the pathogenesis of human immunodeficiency virus (HIV) infections. FDCs can concentrate infectious viruses for extended periods. Moreover, FDCs promote the migration of T cells into the germinal center and the transfer of virus to T cells. At the same time, IDCs are infected and support viral replication for 45 to 60 days.

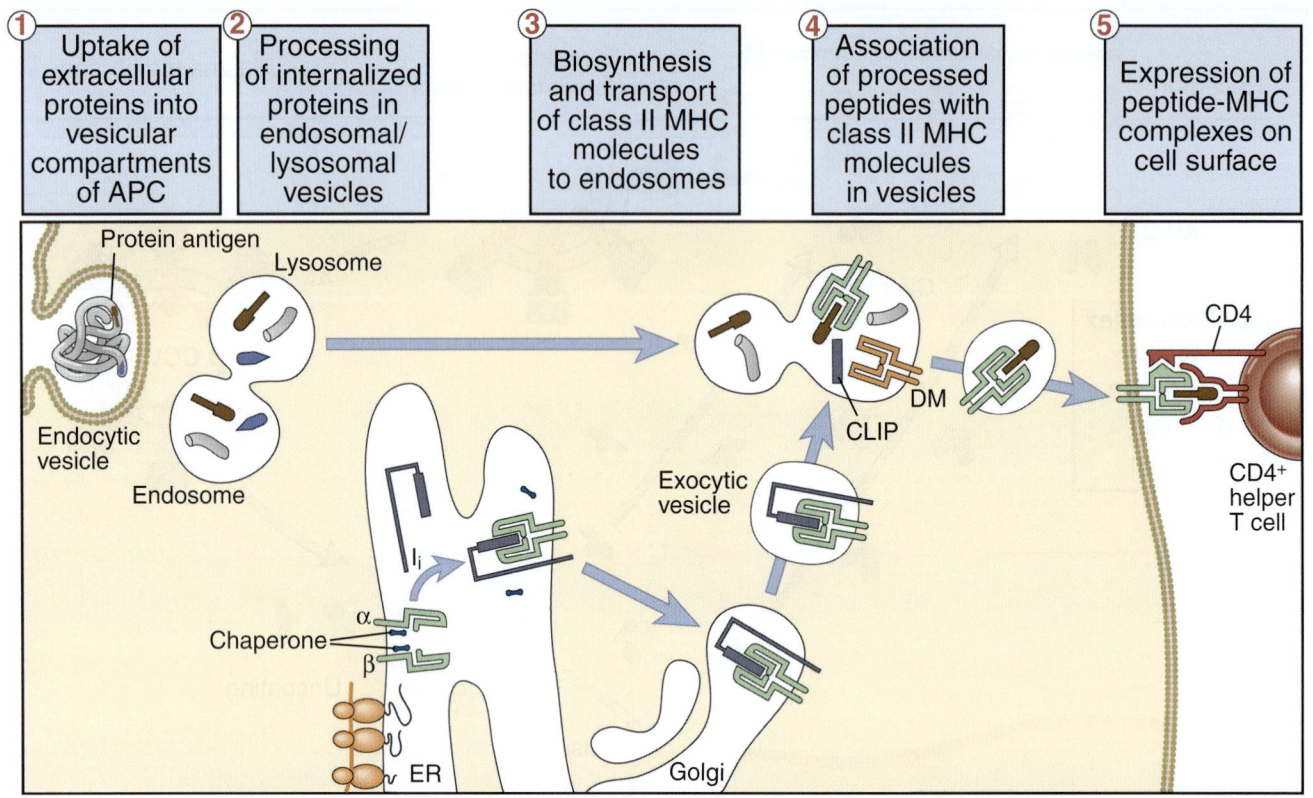

Figure 5-7

The class II major histocompatibility complex (MHC) pathway of antigen presentation. The numbered stages in processing of extracellular antigens correspond to the stages described in the text. (*APC*, antigen-presenting cell.) (From Abbas AK, Lichtman AH, Pillai S: Cellular and molecular immunology, ed 6 [updated edition], Philadelphia, 2010, Saunders.)

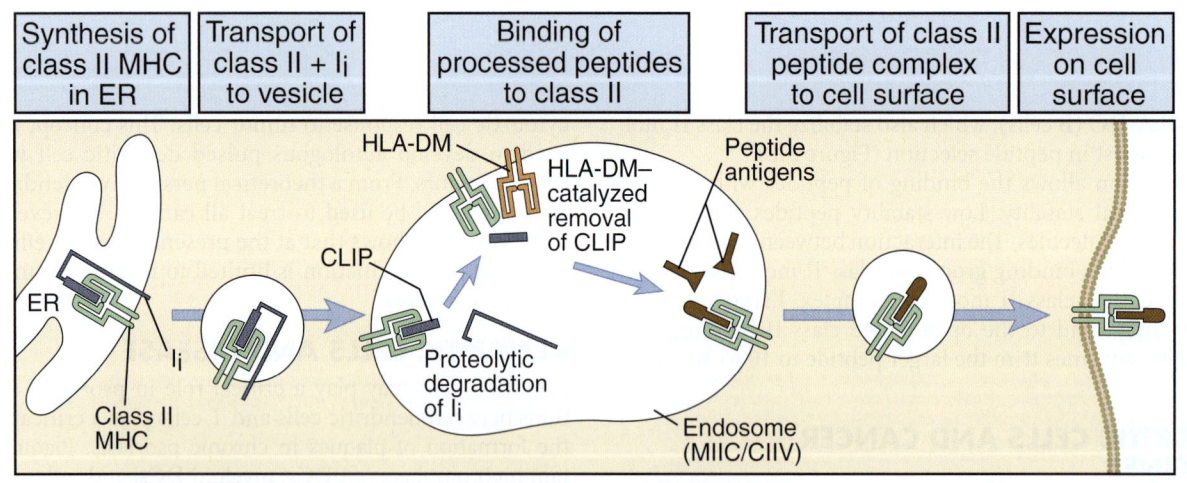

Figure 5-8

The functions of class II major histocompatibility complex (MHC)–associated invariant chains and human leukocyte antigen (HLA)–DM. Class II molecules with bound invariant chain, or class II-associated invariant chain peptide (CLIP), is transported into vesicles, where the CLIP is removed by the action of HLA-DM. Antigenic peptides generated in the vesicles are then able to bind to the class II molecules. Another class II–like protein, called HLA-DO, may regulate the DM-catalyzed removal of CLIP. (*CIIV*, class II vesicle.) (From Abbas AK, Lichtman AH, Pillai S: Cellular and molecular immunology, ed 6 [updated edition], Philadelphia, 2010, Saunders.)

SUMMARY

- Antigen-presenting cells break down large-molecular-weight antigens into 10 to 30 amino acid fragments for loading onto HLA class I and II molecules.
- Antigen-presenting cells can be either "professional" or "amateur" cells.
- Dendritic cell subsets are uniquely suited for antigen presentation.
- Antigen-presenting cells are involved in both the innate and adaptive immune responses.
- Macrophages and B cells ingest antigens by different mechanisms, but both cells process antigen using the endocytic pathway.
- The endocytic pathway is complex and involves proteolytic enzymes and HLA class II stabilizing proteins.

REFERENCES

Bénaroch P, Yilla M, Raposo G, et al: How MHC class II molecules reach the endocytic pathway, EMBO J 14(1):37, 1995.

Bieber T: The Langerhans cell: Outpost of the immune system in the epidermis, Hautarzt 37:424, 1986.

Gray D, Kosco M, Stockinger B: Novel pathways of antigen presentation for the maintenance of memory, Int Immunol 3:141, 1991.

Hart DN, McKenzie JL: Interstitial dendritic cells, Int Rev Immunol 6(2–3):127, 1990.

He XZ, Wang L, Zhang YY, et al: An effective vaccine against colon cancer in mice: Use of recombinant adenovirus interleukin-12 transduced dendritic cells, World J Gastroenterol 14(4):532, 2008.

Hsiao L, Takahashi K, Takeya M, et al: Differentiation and maturation of macrophages into interdigitating cells and their multicellular complex formation in the fetal and postnatal rat thymus, Thymus 17:219, 1991.

Morisaki T, Matsumoto K, Onishi H, et al: Dendritic cell-based combined immunotherapy with autologous tumor-pulsed dendritic cell vaccine and activated T cells for cancer patients: rationale, current progress, and perspectives, Hum Cell 16(4):175, 2003.

Nestle FO, Turka LA, Nicoloff BJ: Characterization of dermal dendritic cells in psoriasis. Autostimulation of T lymphocytes and induction of Th1 type cytokines, J Clin Invest 94(1):202, 1994.

Nonn M, Schinz M, Zumback K, et al: Dendritic cell-based tumor vaccine for cervical cancer I: in vitro stimulation with recombinant protein-pulsed dendritic cells induces specific T cells to HPV16 E7 or HPV18 E7, J Cancer Res Clin Oncol 129(9):511, 2003.

Parmentier HK, van der Linden JA, Krijnen J, et al: Human follicular dendritic cells: Isolation and characteristics in situ and in suspension, Scand J Immunol 33:441, 1991.

Szakal AK, Kosco MH, Tew JG: A novel in vivo follicular dendritic cell-dependent iccosome-mediated mechanism for delivery of antigen to antigen-processing cells, J Immunol 140:341, 1988.

Tew JG, Wu J, Qin D, et al: Follicular dendritic cells and presentation of antigen and co-stimulatory signals to B cells, Immunol Rev 156:39, 1997.

Villadangos JA, Young L: Antigen-presentation properties of plasmacytoid dendritic cells, Immunity 29(3):352, 2008.

ASSESSMENT QUESTIONS

1. Which of the following are considered tissue macrophages?
   - I. Follicular dendritic cells
   - II. Interdigitating cells
   - III. Langerhans cells
   A. I
   B. III
   C. I and II
   D. II and III
   E. I, II, and III

2. Which of the following cells is considered a "professional" antigen-presenting cell?
   A. Monocyte
   B. Endothelial cell
   C. Keratinocyte
   D. Fibroblast

3. Follicular dendritic and interdigitating dendritic cells arise from a _____ precursor cell.
   A. Lymphoid
   B. Myeloid
   C. Platelet
   D. Red blood cell

4. Which of the following are able to hold native or processed antigens on the cell surface using iccosomes?
   A. Follicular dendritic cells
   B. Interdigitating dendritic cells
   C. Plasmacytoid dendritic cells
   D. Monocytic dendritic cells

5. Which of the following is a role of the invariant chain (Ii) in antigen processing?
   - I. Directing the class II molecule to the phagosome or endosome
   - II. Preventing peptide loading of the class II molecule until it reaches the phagosome or the endosome
   - III. Preventing class I molecules from competing for low-stability peptides
   A. I
   B. III
   C. I and II
   D. II and III
   E. I, II, and III

6. What are the specialized macrophage populations found in the brain called?
   A. Glial cells
   B. Kupffer cells
   C. Osteocytes
   D. Histiocyte

CHAPTER 6

Surface Interactions Between T Cells and Antigen-Presenting Cells

LEARNING OBJECTIVES

- Discuss the clonal selection hypothesis and its relationship to the T cell receptor (TCR)
- Know the structure and functions of the α/β TCRs and γ/δ TCRs
- Define complementarity determining region
- Compare and contrast the roles of CDR1, CDR2, and CDR3 in the association of TCR with class II molecules
- Identify T cell subsets that interact with antigens presented on MHC class II molecules
- Understand the concept of somatic recombination in relationship to the TCR
- Explain the roles of *RAG-1* and *RAG-2* in the generation of TCR diversity
- Compare and contrast the junctional diversity and N- and P-nucleotide additions
- Recognize the components of the CD3 complex
- Differentiate between the signaling and nonsignaling components of the CD3 complex
- Identify TCR:MHC stabilizing molecules and their ligands
- Recognize the four critical co-stimulatory molecules and their roles in cell activation
- Compare the roles of B7-1 and B7-2 in the activation of T cell subsets
- Compare and contrast the roles of CD28 and CTLA-4 in T cell activation
- Understand how abatacept prevents T cell activation
- Understand how alefacept prevents T cell activation
- Recognize monoclonal antibodies that block TCR–HLA molecule interactions
- Explain the mechanism by which superantigens stimulate T cells
- Compare and contrast the pathophysiology of staphylococcal and streptococcal toxic shock syndrome
- Discuss the relationship between V_β isoforms and toxic shock syndrome
- Recognize the immunologic defect in hyper-IgM syndrome
- Identify the immunologic defect in Omenn syndrome

KEY TERMS

Abatacept
Alefacept
α/β T cell receptor (TCR)
B7 molecules
Complementarity determining regions (CDRs)
CD2
CD3 complex
CD4
CD8
CD11a
CD28
CD40L
Enterotoxin
γ/δ T cell receptor
Hyper-IgM syndrome
Immuno-receptor tyrosine-based activation motifs (ITAMs)
Junctional diversity
Monoclonal antibodies
Omenn syndrome
Somatic cell recombination
Superantigen
P-nucleotide additions

INTRODUCTION

In this chapter, the discussion centers on the roles of receptor interaction in the activation or deactivation of T cells. Much like starting an automobile, several signals must be given in a defined sequence to override interlocking safety systems. For example, T cell activation requires three different steps: (1) The initial step entails interaction between the lymphocyte T cell receptor (TCR) and the antigen-loaded class II molecule. (2) In the second step, a CD4 molecule binds to class II molecules and stabilizes the TCR–class II complex. (3) In the final step of the activation sequence, the CD28 of the T cell interacts with a B7 molecule on the APC (antigen-presenting cell) (Figure 6-1).

If these three interactions do not occur, the T cell becomes nonfunctional for an extended period. In some cases, nonresponsive T cells become apoptotic and die.

T cell activation is central to the elicitation of an immune response. T cells act as effector cells or direct the immune response by influencing the activity of macrophages in the inflammatory response and of B cells in the synthesis of antibodies.

CLONAL SELECTION HYPOTHESIS

In the late 1950s, MacFarland Burnet proposed the clonal selection theory, which states that antigens, rather than lymphocytes, direct the immune response. The five basic tenets of

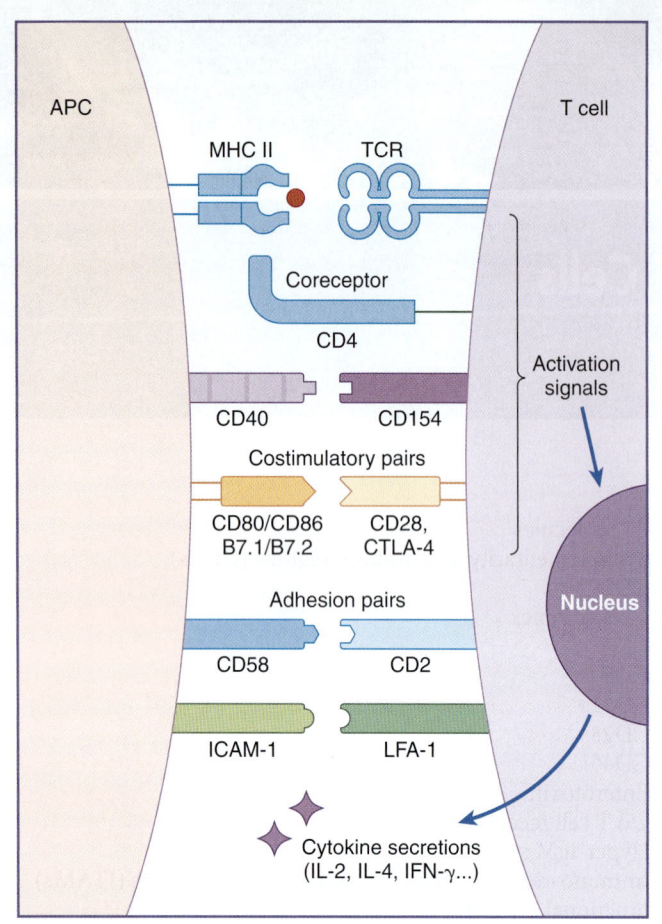

Figure 6-1

Accessory molecules involved in antigen presentation. The binding between the major histocompatibility complex (MHC)–antigen peptide complex and the T cell receptor (TCR) acts as the first signal toward induction of T cell activation. Accessory molecules increase avidity between T cells and antigen-presenting cells (APCs) by performing additional adhesive and signaling functions. Adhesion molecules, such as LFA-1 (CD11a/CD18; leukocyte function—associated antigen-1) and ICAM-1 (CD54; intracellular adhesion molecule-1), promote firm adhesion between T cells and APCs and can provide co-stimulatory signals for T cell activation. This interaction also facilitates T cell sampling of antigen in the context of MHC molecules on the surface of APCs. Additionally, T cells require further co-stimulation through binding of CD28 with either of its ligands, CD80 or CD86 (B7.1 or B7.2). If all these events transpire, full activation of the T cell occurs, leading to production of T cell cytokines and a proliferative response. (From Actor JK: Elsevier's integrated immunology and microbiology, Philadelphia, 2007, Mosby.)

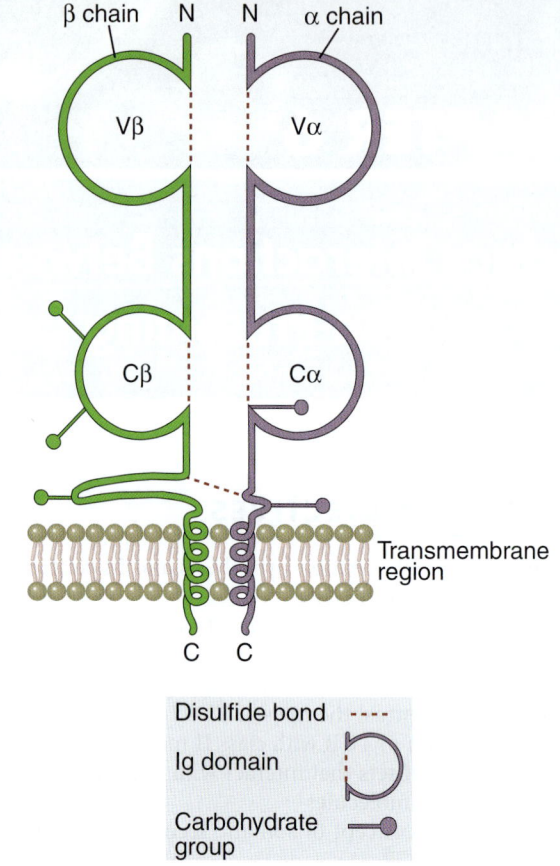

Figure 6-2

Structure of the T cell receptor. The schematic diagram of the α/β T cell receptor (TCR) shows the domains of a typical TCR-specific for a peptide–major histocompatibility complex (MHC) complex. The antigen-binding portion of the TCR is formed by Vα and Vβ domains. (From Abbas AK, Lichtman AH, Pillai S: Cellular and molecular immunology, ed 6 [updated edition], Philadelphia, 2010, Saunders. Adapted from Bjorkman PJ: MHC restriction in three dimensions: a view of T cell receptor/ligand interactions, Cell 89:167, 1997. Copyright Cell Press.)

the theory are (1) each lymphocyte has a unique receptor that binds to only one antigen; (2) the receptor must react with the antigen for cellular activation; (3) only selected clones of lymphocytes activated by antigen will divide (clonal expansion); (4) all of the daughter cells will express antigen receptors identical to the parent cell and (5) some of the daughter cells act as effector cells, and others become memory cells.

T CELL RECEPTORS

The unique antigen binding receptor on T cells is called the *T cell receptor (TCR)*. It is expressed on all T cells and exists in either α/β or γ/δ forms. The α/β TCR is expressed on peripheral blood T cells. γ/δ expressing T cells are rare in peripheral blood but are found in abundance in mucosal tissue. Each T cell has a homogeneous TCR population that recognizes a single antigen or epitope.

α/β T Cell Receptors

The TCR is a dual chain α/β heterodimer that consists of variable (V) and constant (C) regions. The structure of an α/β TCR is shown in Figure 6-2.

The V regions of the α/β-chains determine antigenic specificity by creating a three-dimensional pocket that recognizes immunogenic epitopes. The dual-chain V region pocket is created through the association of several different genes. The V_α pocket is the result of V_α genes joining with a junctional (J_α) gene. In the β-chain, a functional V_β is created by linking V_β, diversity (D_β), and J_β-domains.

Complementarity determining regions (CDRs), which are hypervariable regions in the $V_{\alpha/\beta}$-chains have actual contact with antigens. Class II molecules have six CDRs (three on each chain). The role of CDRs in binding to major histocompatibility complex (MHC) class II molecules is shown in Figure 6-3.

In the α-chains, CDR1 interacts with the N-terminal portion of the epitope. β-chain CDR1 reacts with the C-terminal portion of the peptide. CDR2s interact with the class II molecules but are not involved in antigen recognition. CDR3s are responsible for binding to the epitope presented by class II molecules. Most of the sequence variability responsible for TCR diversity is found in CDR3.

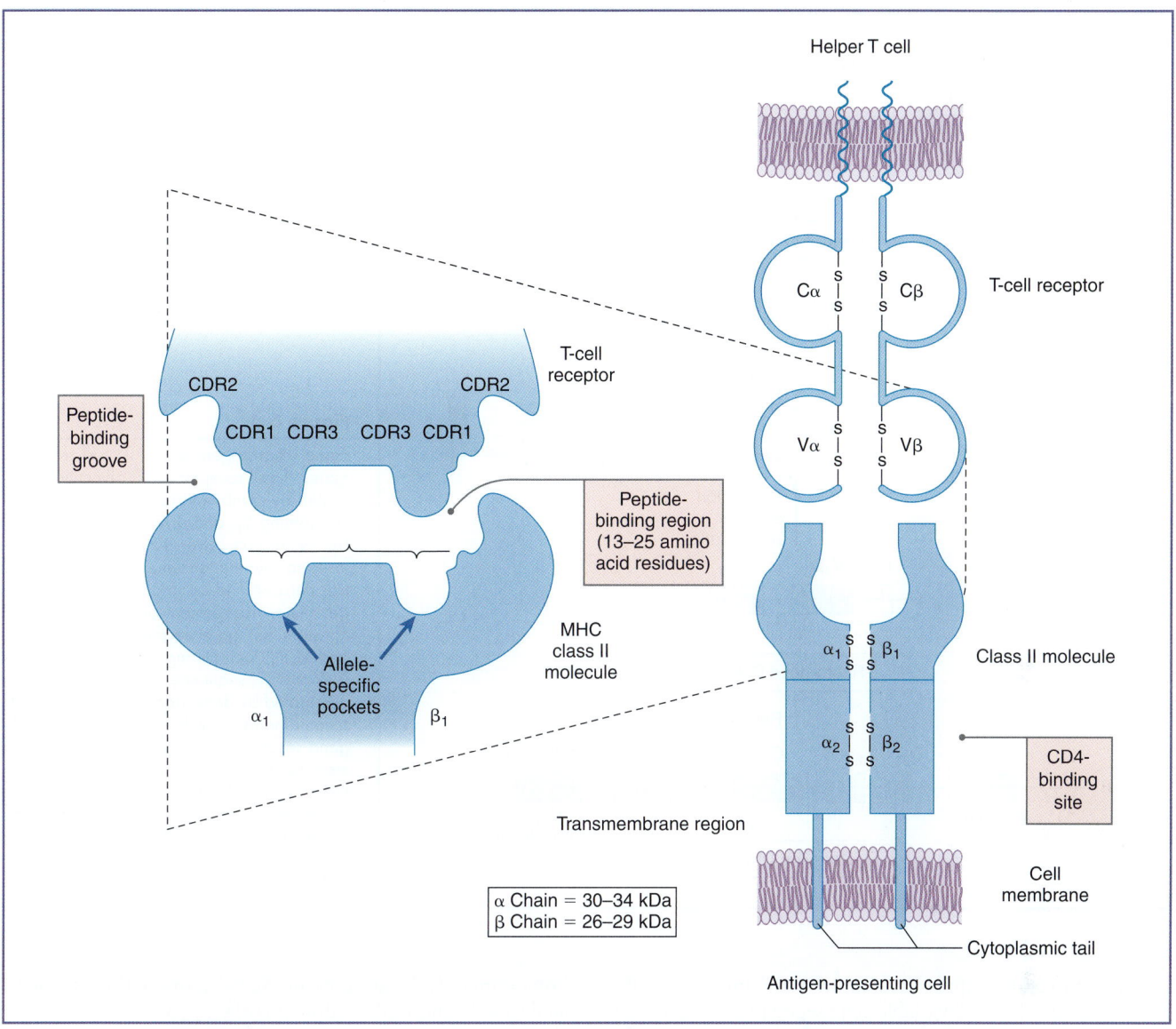

Figure 6-3

Major histocompatibility complex (MHC) class II. Processed antigenic fragments (10–30 amino acids in length) interact with the α₁- and β₁-domains on the class II molecule within the peptide-binding groove, allowing presentation to CD4+ Th cells. Interactions with the T cell receptor (TCR) are stabilized by CD4 recognition of the conserved regions on the class II molecule. (From Actor JK: Elsevier's integrated immunology and microbiology, Philadelphia, 2007, Mosby.)

In addition to V regions, each TCR has an invariant constant (C) region. The C region consists of 140 to 180 hydrophilic amino acids and continues to a short hinge region with cysteine residues that link the α-chain and the β-chain A transmembrane anchor unit, which consists of highly charged hydrophobic amino acids, is connected to a short cytoplasmic region.

γ/δ T Cell Receptors

The Tγ/δ TCR structure is similar to the α/β TCRs. These T cells are only found in the mucosa and function as a bridge between innate and adaptive immunity. CD4γ/δ T cells recognize microbial phosphorylated molecules such as isopentylpyrophosphate (IDP) and dimethylallylpyrophosphate (DMAP). Direct interaction between these molecules and the γ/δ TCR activates the T cell. Antigen processing by APCs or presentation by MHC molecules is not required for activation. A vigorous γ/δ T cell response localizes the microbe in the mucosa until an adaptive response is mounted.

ORIGIN OF T CELL RECEPTOR DIVERSITY

In the generation of TCR diversity, two factors must be considered. First, each lymphocyte has a TCR that recognizes a single epitope. Second, 10^{13} different epitopes must be recognized. If a single lymphocyte TCR recognizes only one epitope, it follows that 10^{13} lymphocyte clones are present in each of the CD4 (Th1 and Th2) and CD8 (Tc1 and Tc2) populations.

To create a repertoire of antigen-specific TCRs, alternative forms of genes present in somatic cells are rearranged in a process, called *somatic cell recombination*, by using *RAG-1 and RAG-2* recombinase activating enzymes (Figure 6-4).

In the α-chain, 70 to 80 different V_α gene products can be linked to 61 different J-chains. Simple recombination in the

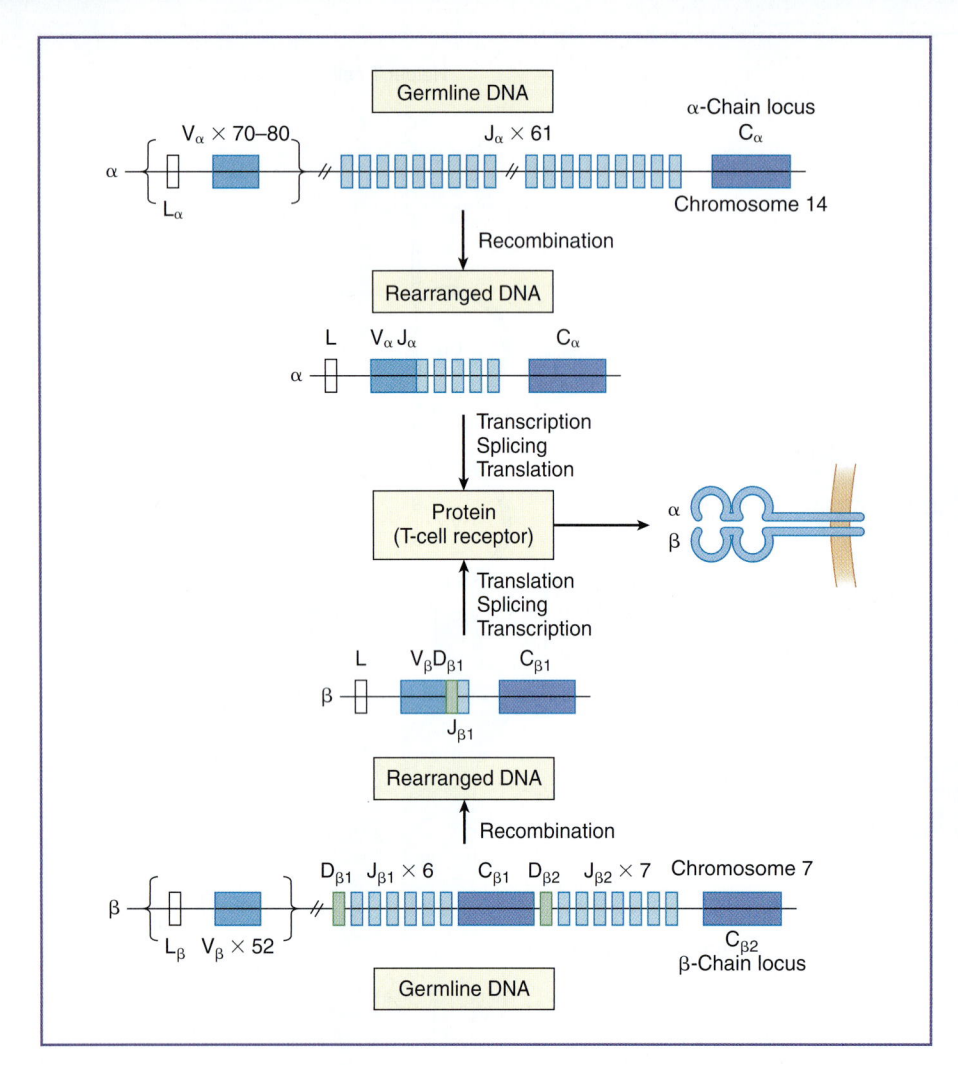

Figure 6-4

Gene rearrangement of T cell receptor genes. T cell receptor (TCR) diversity is generated by combinatorial joining of variable (V), joining (J), and diversity (D) genes and by N region diversification (nucleotides inserted by the enzyme deoxynucleotidyl transferase). The top and bottom rows show germ-line arrangement of the V, D, J, and constant (C) gene segments at the TCR-α and TCR-β loci. During T cell development, a V-region sequence for each chain is assembled by deoxyribonucleic acid (DNA) recombination. For the α-chain (top), a Vα gene segment rearranges to a Jα gene segment to create a functional gene encoding the V domain. For the β-chain (bottom), rearrangement of a Dβ, a Jβ, and a Vβ gene segment creates the functional V domain exon. (From Actor JK: Elsevier's integrated immunology and microbiology, Philadelphia, 2007, Mosby.)

α-chain can result in approximately 4.9×10^3 antigen-specific TCRs. β-chains have 52 variable gene segments, two diversity gene segments, and 13 J region genes. Recombination in the β-chain results in 1.3×10^3 unique TCRs.

Additional TCR diversity is created by alternate joining of D$_\beta$-chains, junctional flexibility, and N- and P-nucleotide additions. Alternate joining of D domains creates 5×10^3 diverse TCRs. Adding six or more amino acids to the J domains (junctional diversity) creates more TCR diversity. Random insertion of palindromic sequences at single strand breaks (P-nucleotides) or nontemplated amino acids (N-nucleotides) into the TCR coding regions also occurs. Junctional diversity and P- and N-nucleotides generate an additional 10^{11} possible TCRs. The sum of the gene re-arrangements ($4.9 \times 10^3 + 1.3 \times 10^3 + 5.3 \times 10^3 + 1.0 \times 10^{11}$) allows the immune system to respond to all known antigens.

CD3–T CELL RECEPTORS PROTEIN COMPLEX

The TCR lacks intracellular signaling capability because of short cytoplasmic tails. To transduce activation signals to the nucleus, the TCR associates with a number of signaling proteins to create the CD3 complex. The pan T cell maker CD3 is composed of five subunits (α, β, ζ, ε, and γ) proteins. In the assembly of the CD3 complex, two copies of of ζ-chains which form disulfide-linked homodimers (ζ–ζ) are present. Signal transduction is associated with the intracellular domains of ε-, γ-, and ζ-chains. These chains contain 44 to 81 amino acid sequences called *immunoreceptor tyrosine–based activation motifs* (ITAMs), which are essential to the signaling process. TCR ζ-chains have a short, nine-amino-acid transmembrane sequence and a long (113 amino acids) cytoplasmic tail with three ITAMs (Figure 6-5).

STABILIZING MOLECULES

The TCR binds to the class II molecules with low affinity. The dissociation constant (Kd) is approximately 10^{-5} to 10^{-7}M. Because of the low affinity, additional molecules are necessary to stabilize the complex (see Figure 6-1).

CD4 molecules stabilize the interaction between the TCR and the APCs expressing HLA molecules. CD4 molecules are expressed on CD4Th1 and CD4Th2 cells, macrophages, and dendritic cells. The CD4 molecule has a small transmembrane region and a cytoplasmic tail and is capable of transducing signals to the nucleus. Phosphorylation of serine residues in the cytoplasmic tail activates the *lck* or p56 kinases. These kinases play a critical role in the activation of HLA class II restricted T helper cells.

CD8 is a dual-chain heterodimer that stabilizes the interaction between CD8 cells and antigen-loaded HLA class I molecules. Extracellular CD8 domains bind to the α_3 regions on

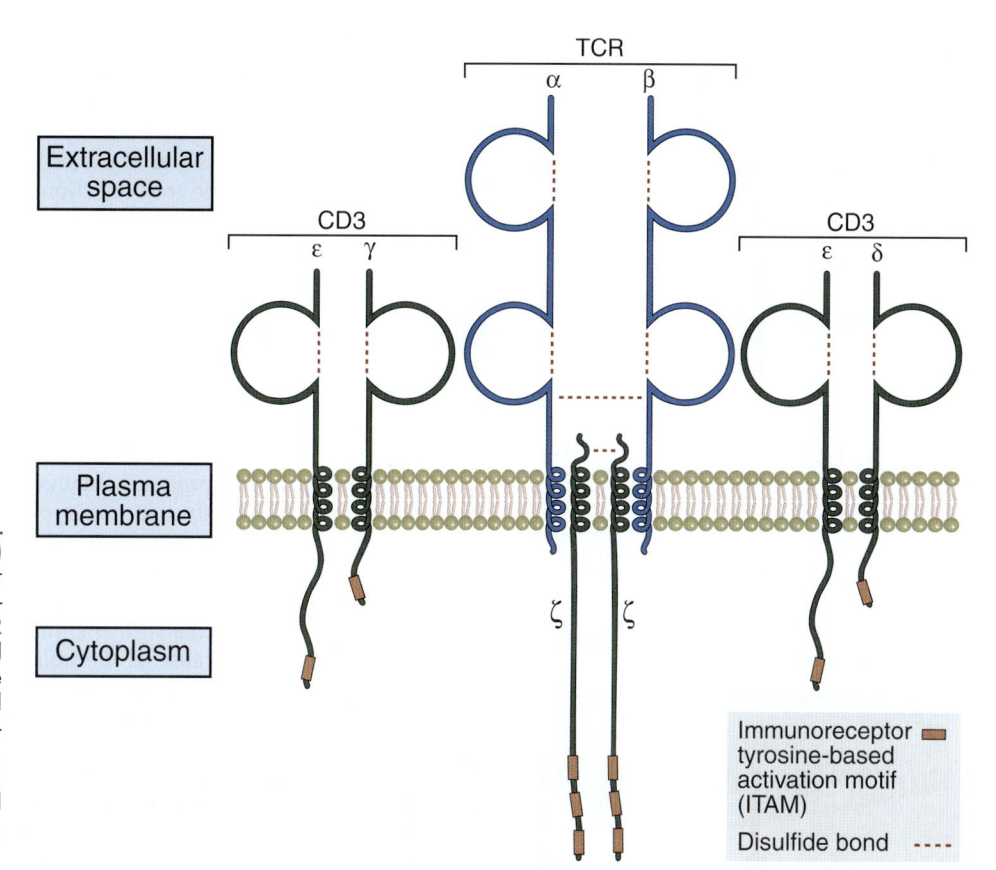

Figure 6-5
Components of the T cell receptor (TCR) complex. The TCR complex of major histocompatibility complex (MHC)–restricted T cells consists of the αβ TCR noncovalently linked to the CD3 and ζ-proteins. The association of these proteins with one another is mediated by charged residues in their transmembrane regions, which are not shown. (From Abbas AK, Lichtman AH, Pillai S: Cellular and molecular immunology, ed 6 [updated edition], Philadelphia, 2010, Saunders.)

class I molecules. The role of CD8 and endogenous antigens will be discussed in Chapter 18.

CO-STIMULATORY MOLECULES

CD28/B7 Interaction

T cells can be activated or downregulated following interaction with B7 molecules on APCs. B7-1 and B7-2 molecules are expressed on monocytes, macrophages, interstitial dendritic cells, and epithelial dendritic cells. After antigen processing, one of the two B7 isoforms is expressed, which determines the nature of the immune response. For example, expression of B7-1 activates CD4Th2 (helper cells in antibody production) and B7-2 expression activates CD4Th1 (inflammatory response).

T cells have two ligands for B7. Interactions between CD28 and B7 activate T cells. The second ligand, which binds to B7 with a high affinity, is called *cytotoxic T lymphocyte protein 4 (CTLA-4)*. Interaction between CTLA-4 and B7 downregulates T cell signaling and prevents T cell activation (Figure 6-6).

CD40 Ligand/CD40

CD40 ligand (CD40L) is a 261-amino-acid membrane glycoprotein expressed on activated CD4 lymphocytes. Expression occurs shortly after T cell activation. The natural ligand for CD40L is CD40, which is a transmembrane protein present on B cells, follicular dendritic cells, and macrophages. CD40–CD40L interactions play an important role in the amplification of the immune response and the production of antibodies. Ligation stimulates the secretion of interleukin 12 (IL-12) from the APCs. In turn, IL-12 activates CD4Th1, CD8, and natural killer (NK) cells and amplifies the immune response.

In the production of antibodies, T and B cells are brought into close proximity. CD40/CD40L ligation between T and B cells induces B cell activation, differentiation, isotypic switching, and the generation of memory cells.

CD2/CD58

CD2 is a glycoprotein present on 90% to 95% of mature T cells and NK cells. Lymphocyte function-associated antigen (LFA-3 or CD58) on APCs is the principal ligand for CD2. Both molecules are adhesion factors that strengthen the interactions between T cells and APCs. Ligation results in the production of proteins that regulate the cellular response to IL-2.

CD11a/CD18/CD54

Integrins are a family of molecules that facilitate the adhesion of T cells to molecules on APCs. CD11a is an α_1 integrin subunit that associates with an β_2-integrin subunit (CD18) to form LFA-1. LFA-1 is a glycoprotein expressed on all leukocytes. The LFA-1 ligand is intercellular adhesion molecule 1 (ICAM-1) on APCs. Interaction between these adhesion factors plays a critical role in T cell activation, T cell mobility, and control of autoimmune diseases.

AGENTS THAT BLOCK T CELL RECEPTOR–ANTIGEN PRESENTING CELL INTERACTIONS

Biotechnology-derived immunotherapeutic agents disrupt or prevent interactions between the TCR or co-stimulatory molecules and the receptors on APCs. Monoclonal antibodies and fusion proteins that prevent T cell activation are shown in Table 6-1.

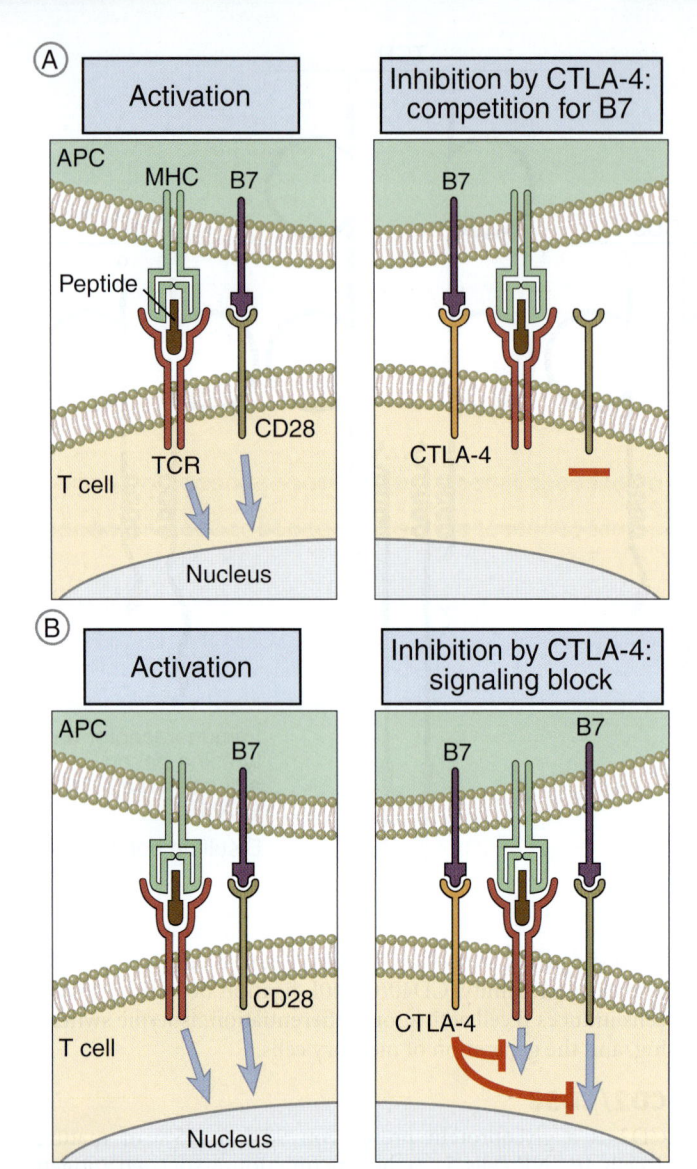

50 CHAPTER 6 SURFACE INTERACTIONS BETWEEN T CELLS AND ANTIGEN-PRESENTING CELLS

Figure 6-6
Mechanisms of action of the inhibitory receptor cytotoxic T lymphocyte protein 4 (CTLA-4). CTLA-4 may inhibit T cell responses by competitively preventing CD28 binding to B7 costimulators **(A)**, or by generating inhibitory signals (e.g., by associated phosphatases) that attenuate activation via the T cell receptor (TCR) and CD28 **(B)**. (From Abbas AK, Lichtman AH, Pillai S: Cellular and molecular immunology, ed 6 [updated edition], Philadelphia, 2010, Saunders.)

Blockade of T Cell Receptor Interactions

Laboratory-derived monoclonal antibodies (muromomab, teplizumab, and visilizumab) bind to CD3 on activated T cells. Blocking antibodies prevent the interaction between CD3 and the class I or II molecules and are thus useful in preventing recipient graft rejection and, in rare cases, the graft rejecting the host.

Blockade of Co-Stimulatory Molecule Interactions

The interaction between co-stimulatory factors on T cells and APCs can be blocked by biotechnology-derived fusion proteins or monoclonal antibodies. To create a fusion protein, two genes are fused in the laboratory and inserted into an expression vector such as a bacterium or yeast. When translated, the fusion protein contains the active portions of both proteins. Currently, two fusion proteins are used to block the interaction between co-stimulator molecules on T cells and APCs.

Abatacept is a co-stimulator inhibitor in a new class of drugs called *disease modifying antirheumatic drugs (DMARDs)*. In patients with rheumatoid arthritis, T cell activation is the major cause of the inflammatory response in the synovium. Abatacept consists of an Fc region from the immunoglobulin G (IgG) antibody and the extracellular domain of CTLA-4. The CTLA-4 fusion protein physically blocks the interaction between CD28 and the B7 on APCs. Failure to engage CD28 drives activated T cells into apoptosis.

Alefacept is another fusion protein indicated for psoriasis vulgaris, an autoimmune skin disease. Activated CD4, CD8, and memory cells are found in the skin lesions. Alefacept prevents T cell activation and reduces the severity of the lesions. The fusion protein consists of LFA-3 (CD58) linked to the distal end of an antibody molecule. Interactions between the soluble alefacept and the T cell CD2 molecule block the binding of CD2 to the CD58 on APCs.

Monoclonal antibodies, which inhibit co-stimulatory molecules, are also indicated for the treatment of psoriasis. For example, efalizumab blocks interactions between the CD11a component of LFA-1 and the adhesion factors on APCs. Again, downregulation of T cells reduces the severity of skin lesions.

ABERRANT INTERACTIONS BETWEEN TCR AND CLASS II MOLECULES

Superantigens

Superantigens are molecules that indiscriminately stimulate up to 20% of all T lymphocytes (normal response to antigen stimulates only 0.01% of T cells), which release massive amounts of proinflammatory cytokines such as tumor factor–α (TNF-α). When released into blood, high levels of TNF-α cause life threatening hypovolemic shock and organ failure.

Table 6-1 Biologic Reagents That Block Interactions between T Cells and Antigen-Presenting Cells

Name	Origin	Reagent Type	Target	Application
Muromonab	Mouse	Monoclonal antibody	CD3	Transplant rejection
Teplizumab	Humanized	Monoclonal antibody	CD3	Autoimmune diseases
Visilizumab	Humanized	Monoclonal antibody	CD3	Graft-versus-host reaction
Alefacept		Fusion protein	CD2	Psoriasis
Abatacept		Fusion protein	CD28	Rheumatoid arthritis
Efalizumab	Humanized	Monoclonal antibody	CD11a	Plaque psoriasis

Superantigens stimulate CD4 cells by a unique mechanism. T cells and APCs are brought into direct contact by the bridging of the constant region of class II molecules and the variable segments of the TCR β-chain (V_β). Superantigen binding is unique, however, in that it occurs outside the normal binding cleft (Figure 6-7).

Staphylococcal and streptococcal superantigens have been implicated in food poisoning, exfoliative dermatitis in infants (scalded skin syndrome), cellulitis, scarlet fever, and toxic shock syndrome. *Staphylococcus aureus* secretes five enterotoxins (SEA, SEB, SEC2, SEE, and TSST-1). Enterotoxins are similar to exotoxins but usually only cause moderate to severe diarrhea. All staphylococcal enterotoxins can cause the symptoms of food poisoning, but only SEA and SEB are involved in exfoliative dermatitis. Toxic shock syndrome is associated with the TSST-1, SEB, or SEC2 superantigens.

In the last 20 years, an increase has been seen in the incidence of streptococcal toxic shock syndrome associated with necrotizing fasciitis or myositis. The etiologic agents are invasive Group A streptococcal strains such as *Streptococcus pyogenes*. These strains produce three different superantigens (SPE-A, SPE-B, and SPE-C) and numerous pyogenic toxins. SPE-A is specifically associated with streptococcal toxic shock syndrome (sTSS). Streptococcal and staphylococcal superantigens act in a similar manner.

TOXIC SHOCK SYNDROME AND TAMPON USE

An association between superabsorbent tampons and toxic shock syndrome has been reported in the literature. In 1979, a tampon manufacturer changed the normal tampon cotton matrix to a highly absorbent polyacrylate. The new matrix concentrated water, magnesium, iron, and oxygen and enhanced the growth of *Staphylococcus* or *Streptococcus*, which are part of the normal vaginal flora. Increased magnesium concentrations triggered the production of TSST-1 or SPE-A. The toxin enters the blood by two mechanisms. (1) First, vaginal epithelial cells have TSST-1 receptors that translocate the toxin across the vaginal wall and into the bloodstream. (2) Second, high-absorbency tampons decrease moisture in the vaginal

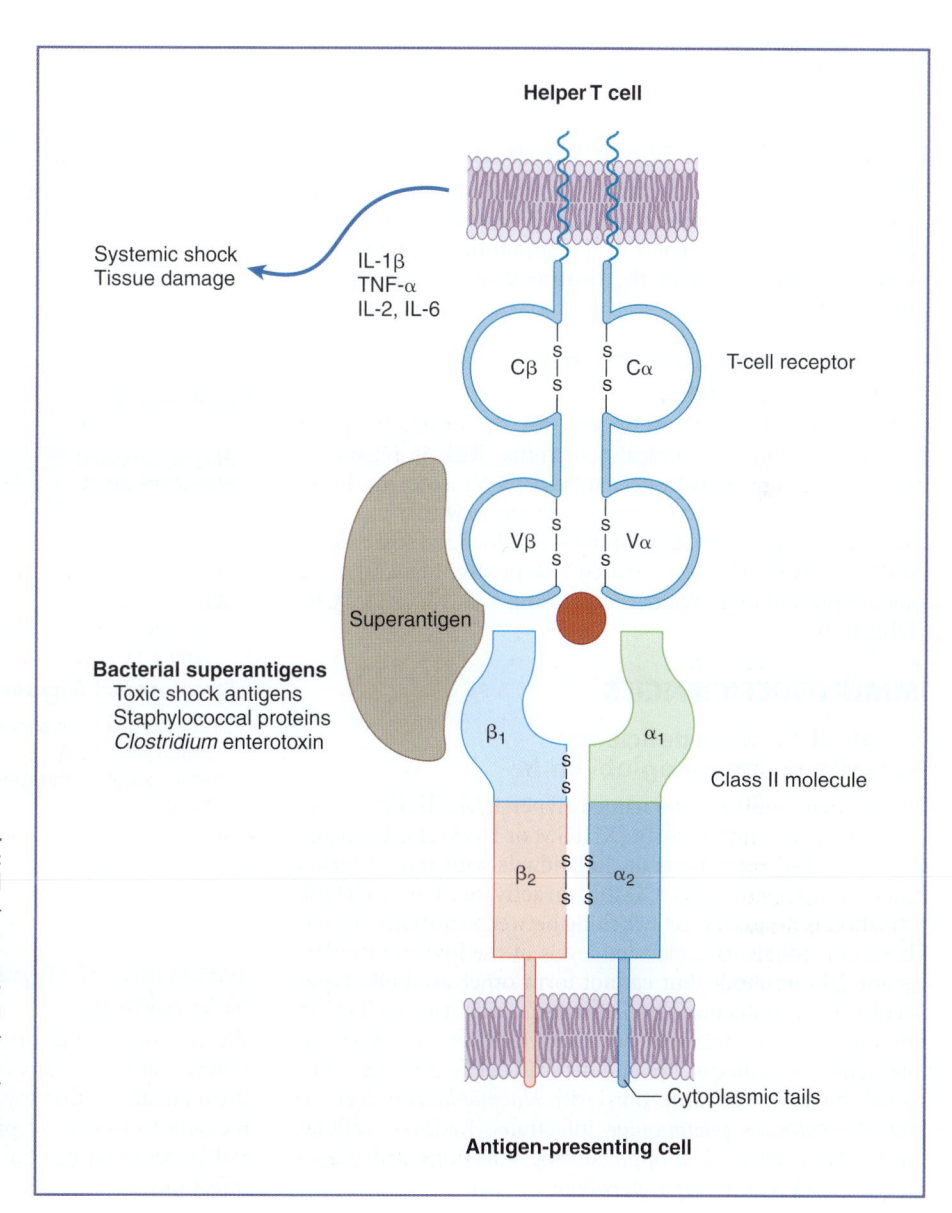

Figure 6-7
Superantigens. T cells of various antigenic specificities are activated when bacterial superantigens cross-link major histocompatibility complex (MHC) class II molecules with common T cell receptor (TCR) Vβ regions. All T cells that express that particular Vβ region are subject to activation, causing massive release of cytokines and subsequent symptoms of shock and host injury. This occurs regardless of antigen specificity and the peptide that fills the MHC class II groove. (From Actor JK: Elsevier's integrated immunology and microbiology, Philadelphia, 2007, Mosby.)

walls. During tampon removal, the vaginal wall is often torn allowing TSST-1 and SPE-A direct access to the bloodstream. In the 12 months following the release of the product into the market, 1200 cases of toxic shock syndrome and significant mortality occurred. Subsequently, the polyacrylate tampon was removed from the market in 1983, and thereafter the incidence of toxic shock syndrome has decreased significantly.

TOXIC SHOCK SYNDROME

Staphylococcal toxic shock syndrome is characterized by rapid onset (within 8–12 hours) of fever, vomiting, diarrhea, hypovolemic shock, and multi-organ failure. Death usually occurs within 24 to 36 hours. Superantigen-activated T cells produce high levels of cytokines such as TNF-α and IL-1. These cytokines plus TSST-1 promote vascular permeability and fluid leakage into tissue and severe diarrhea. As a result of electrolyte and fluid loss, less blood is available for the heart to pump. The significant reduction in cardiac output results in hypovolemic shock. Reduced tissue perfusion eventually damages the kidneys, heart, and lungs. Cardiac failure results in death.

Streptococcal superantigens and pyogenic toxins evoke different toxic shock symptomology. sTSS is characterized by adult respiratory distress syndrome, shock, and renal failure. Between 30% and 70% of patients die in spite of aggressive medical treatment.

Treatment of Toxic Shock Syndrome

The goal of pharmacotherapy is to eradicate the infective agent. Careful consideration must be given to the identification of the etiologic agent and the antibiotic resistance patterns. Antibiotics used in the treatment of toxic shock are shown in Table 6-2.

V$_\beta$ Isoforms and Superantigen-Induced Clinical Symptoms

Only select individuals are at risk for the development of superantigen-induced clinical symptoms. Risk is related to the presence of genetically determined TCR V$_\beta$ isoforms. Fifty-two possible V$_\beta$ genes exist. Only individuals with a V$_\beta$2 TCR have are at high risk for developing staphylococcal toxic shock syndrome. Similarly, an increased risk of streptococcal toxic shock is present in individuals expressing V$_\beta$8, 12, or 14 TCRs (Table 6-3).

IMMUNODEFICIENCIES

X-Linked Immunodeficiency with Hyper-Immunoglobulin M

The original syndrome was named Hyper-IgM (HIGM). However, the most common form (XHIGM or HGM1) is inherited as an X-linked recessive trait. Individuals with HIGM lack a functioning CD40 ligand (CD40L) on activated T cells. CD40L activation is necessary for switching between antibody classes. These individuals have elevated levels of the high-molecular-weight IgM antibody, but cannot form other antibody types necessary for protection against bacteria and viruses. CD4Th1 immunity also is impaired because CD40L is necessary for interaction with monocytes and dendritic cells. Affected individuals have repeated infections with *Haemophilus influenzae* and *Streptococcus pneumoniae* infections. Reduced cellular immunity is reflected in opportunistic infections with *Pneumocystis carinii* and *Cryptosporidium*.

Table 6-2 Antibiotics Indicated for Treatment of Toxic Shock Syndrome

Antibiotic	Indication	Mechanism of Action
Linezolid	Treatment of both staphylococcal and streptococcal infections Bacteriostatic for *Staphylococcus* and bactericidal for *Streptococcus*	Blocks formation of 70S ribosome
Clindamycin	Treatment of group A invasive streptococcal infections	Blocks formation of 50S ribosomal subunit
Daptomycin	Treatment of staphylococci and group A streptococci	Binds to bacterial membranes and causes rapid membrane potential depolarization
Aqueous penicillin G	Treatment of staphylococcal and streptococcal infections	Cell wall inhibitor
Nafcillin	Treatment of penicillin-resistant staphylococcal infections	Cell wall inhibitor
Vancomycin	Treatment of methicillin-resistant staphylococcal infections	Cell wall inhibitor

Table 6-3 Staphylococcal and Streptococcal Superantigens

Staphylococcal Superantigens	TCR V$_\beta$
SEA	V$_\beta$3,11
SEB	V$_\beta$3,12,14,15,17,20
SEC2	V$_\beta$12,13,14,15,17,20
SEE	V$_\beta$5.1,6.1,6.3, 8.18
Staphylococcal toxic shock syndrome (TSST-1)	V$_\beta$2
Streptococcal Superantigens	**TCR V$_\beta$**
Streptococcal toxic shock syndrome SPE-A	V$_\beta$8,12,14
Streptococcal erythrogenic toxin SPE-B	V$_\beta$8
SPE-C	V$_\beta$1,2,5.1,10

Treatment of Hyper-Immunoglobulin M Syndrome

The goal of pharmacotherapy is to prevent infections. Intravenous or subcutaneous immunoglobulin replacement remains the mainstay of therapy. Treatment significantly decreases the incidence of lower respiratory tract infections such as bacterial pneumonia but has no effect on upper respiratory tract infections.

OMENN SYNDROME

Omenn syndrome is an autosomal recessive form of severe combined immunodeficiency (SCID). Neonates with Omenn syndrome have a missense mutation in *RAG-1* and *RAG-2* genes that assemble TCR VDJ and VJ genes. This defect blocks the generation of mature T cells and some B cells. Infants lack CD3 and α/β TCR expressing cells. However, large numbers of γ/δ T cells are found in skin. Desquamation of skin is often evident. Affected children usually do not survive without bone marrow transplantation.

SUMMARY

- T cell receptors are present on all T cells and interact with antigen-loaded class I and class II molecules.
- A TCR recognizes only a single epitope or antigen, and each lymphocyte has a homogeneous population of TCRs.
- Molecules expressed on APCs skew the response to an antibody-mediated or cell-mediated immune response.
- Interactions between co-stimulatory molecules and the appropriate ligands are required for T cell activation.
- Toxic shock syndrome is caused by a superantigen interacting with a TCR and a class II molecule.

REFERENCES

Altmann A, Mustelin T, Coggeshall KM, et al: T lymphocyte activation: A biological model of signal transduction, Crit Rev Immunol 10:348, 1990.

Anderson ME, Siahaan TJ: Targeting ICAM-1/LFA-1 interaction for controlling autoimmune diseases: Designing peptide and small molecule inhibitors, Peptides 24(3):487, 2003.

Brady RL, Barclay AN: The structure of CD4, Curr Top Microbiol 205:1, 1996.

Brenner MB, McLean J, Dialynas DP, et al: Identification of a putative second T cell receptor, Nature 322(6075):145, 1986.

Chien YH, Jores R, Crowley MP, et al: Recognition by γ/δ T cells, Annu Rev Immunol 14:511, 1996.

Damle NK, Linsley PS, Ledbetter JA, et al: Direct helper T cell-induced B cell differentiation involves interaction between T cell antigen CD28 and B cell activation antigen B7, Eur J Immunol 21(5):1277, 1991.

Davis MM, Bjorkman PJ: T cell antigen receptor genes and T cell recognition, Nature 334(6181):395, 1988.

DeLibero G: Sentinel function of broadly reactive human γ/δ T cells, Immunol Today 22:22, 1997.

Engel I, Letourneur F, Houston JT, Ottenhoff TH, Klausner RD: T cell receptor structure and function: Analysis by expression of portions of isolated subunits, Adv Exper Med Biol 323:1, 1992.

Garcia KC, Degano M, Stanfield RL, et al: An α/β T cell receptor structure at 2.5 A and its orientation in the TCR-MHC complex, Science 274(5285):209, 1996.

Garcia KC, Teyton L, Wilson IA, et al: Structural basis of T cell recognition, Annu Rev Immunol 17:369, 1999.

Gollob JA, Li J, Kawasaki H, et al: Molecular interaction between CD58 and CD2 counter-receptors mediates the ability of monocytes to augment T cell activation by IL-12, J Immunol 157(5):1996, 1886.

Gollob JA, Ritz J: CD2-CD58 interaction and the control of T cell interleukin-12 responsiveness. Adhesion molecules link innate and acquired immunity, Ann NY Acad Sci 795:71, 1996.

Haas W, Pereira P, Tonegawa S, et al: γ/δ cells, Annu Rev Immunol 11:637, 1993.

Harrison SC, Wang J, Yan Y, et al: Structure and interactions of CD4, Cold Spring Harb Symp Quant Biol 57:541, 1992.

June CH, Bluestone JA, Nadler LM, et al: The B7 and CD28 receptor families, Immunol Today 15:321, 1994.

Kehry MR: CD40-mediated signaling in B cells, J Immunol 156:2345, 1996.

Leahy DJ: A structural view of CD4 and CD8, FASEB J 9:17, 1995.

Panina-Bordignon P, Fu XT, Lanzavecchia A, et al: Identification of HLA-DR α-chain residues critical for binding of the toxic shock syndrome toxin superantigen, J Exp Med 176(6):1779, 1992.

Raulet DH: T-cell immunity. How γ/δ T cells make a living, Curr Biol 4(3):246, 1994.

San José E, Sahuquillo AG, Bragado R, et al: Assembly of the TCR/CD3 complex: CD3 ε/δ and CD3 ε/γ dimers associate indistinctly with both TCR α and TCR β-chains. Evidence for a double TCR heterodimer model, Eur J Immunol 28(1):12, 1998.

Stuber E, Strober W, Neurath M, et al: Blocking the CD40L-CD40 interaction in vivo specifically prevents the priming of T helper 1 cells through the inhibition of interleukin 12 secretion, J Exp Med 183(2):693, 1996.

van der Merwe PA, Barclay AN, Mason DW, et al: Human cell-adhesion molecule CD2 binds CD58 (LFA-3) with a very low affinity and an extremely fast dissociation rate but does not bind CD48 or CD59, Biochemistry 33(33):10149, 1994.

Zimmerman T, Blanco FJ: Inhibitors targeting the LFA-1/ICAM-1 cell-adhesion interaction: Design and mechanism of action, Curr Pharm Des 14(22):2128, 2008.

Zumla A: Superantigens, T cells, and microbes, Clin Infect Dis 15:313, 1992.

ASSESSMENT QUESTIONS

1. Which of the following is a characteristic of the T cell receptor (TCR)?
   I. Is present on all T cells
   II. Has dual-chain structure
   III. Recognizes antigen bound to class I and class II molecules
   A. I
   B. III
   C. I and II
   D. II and III
   E. I, II, and III

2. To which of the following can some genetic diversity in the TCR be attributed?
   I. Differences in the ζ-chain
   II. Recombination in α/β-chains
   III. Alternate joining of J-chains
   A. I
   B. III
   C. I and II
   D. II and III
   E. I, II, and III

3. Which of the following occurs after the interaction between CD40 and CD40L?
   I. Secretion of interleukin 12 (IL-12)
   II. Activation of CD4 and CD8
   III. B cell differentiation
   A. I
   B. III
   C. I and II
   D. II and III
   E. I, II, and III

4. Superantigens are molecules that:
   I. Interact with class I molecules
   II. Interact with class II molecules and TCR outside the binding groove
   III. Indiscriminately activate T cells
   A. I
   B. III
   C. I and II
   D. II and III
   E. I, II, and III

5. Which of the following components of the CD3 complex lacks signaling capacity?
   A. TCR
   B. ε-chain
   C. γ-chain
   D. ζ-chain

6. Which of the following is activated by the interaction between CD28 and B7-1?
   A. CD4Th2 cells
   B. CD4Th1 cells
   C. CD8 cells
   D. Natural killer (NK) cells

CHAPTER 7

Intracellular Signaling and T Cell Activation

LEARNING OBJECTIVES

- Define autocrine signaling
- Define paracrine signaling
- Draw the immunologic synapse showing primary and secondary components
- Explain the function of adaptor proteins
- Discuss the advantages of T cell receptor (TCR) clustering
- Identify the three transcription factors necessary for interleukin 2 (IL-2) synthesis
- Recognize the signaling pathways activated by T cell receptor–human leukocyte antigen (TCR–HLA) engagement
- Identify the signaling pathway activated by CD28–B7 interactions
- Explain the relationship between the Ras–MAP kinase and Rac–JNK pathways and the transcription factors for IL-2
- Explain the relationship between the PLCγ1 calcium-dependent pathway and PLCγ1–DAG/PKC pathway and the transcription factors for IL-2
- Identify the signaling pathways activated by CD28–B7 engagement
- Compare the mechanisms by which cyclosporine and tacrolimus inhibit T cell signaling
- Recognize the mechanism by which sirolimus inhibits T cell signaling
- Compare and contrast the structure of high-affinity and low-affinity IL-2 receptors
- Explain the role of autocrine signaling in the restriction of an immune response to a specific antigen
- Recognize the two monoclonal antibodies that block the engagement of soluble IL-2 with the high-affinity receptor
- Identify the immunologic defect in X-linked severe combined immunodeficiency (SCID)

KEY TERMS

AP-1 complex
Autocrine signaling
Cyclosporine A
Fos
Immunologic synapse
Jun
NFAT
Nuclear paracrine factor-κB (NF-κB)
Phospholipase C
Phosphokinase C
Ras
Sirolimus
Tacrolimus

INTRODUCTION

An immune response requires the activation and proliferation of antigen-stimulated T cell clones. Surface interactions initiate intracellular signaling that results in the synthesis of numerous proinflammatory cytokines, survival factors, and growth factors. One of the most important growth factors is interleukin 2 (IL-2), a 15,500-kDal protein produced by activated T cells. IL-2 has both autocrine and paracrine functions. In autocrine signaling, activated T cells produce IL-2, which binds to receptors on the same cell to initiate T cell growth and proliferation. Soluble IL-2 can react with nearby activated T cells expressing IL-2 receptors (paracrine signaling) as well. IL-2 is also required for the survival and function of regulatory T cells that damper the response to self-antigens.

SIGNALING PATHWAYS FOR INTERLEUKIN 2 SYNTHESIS

Engagement of the TCR–HLA molecules and CD28–B7 molecules activates several signaling pathways, which culminate in the translocation of three nuclear transcription factors (NFAT, NF-κB, and an AP-1 complex consisting of Fos and Jun proteins). In the nucleus, transcription factors bind to the promoter regions of IL-2 genes, which begin the transcription of messenger ribonucleic acid (RNA) and the translation of IL-2 protein. The pathways involved in the synthesis of IL-2 are shown below.

Pathways Activated by TCR–HLA Interactions

- Ras–MAP kinase (MAPK) pathway
- Rac–JNK pathway
- PLCγ1 calcium-dependent pathway
- PLCγ1–DAG/PKC pathway

Pathways Activated by CD28–B7 Interactions

- PI-3 kinase pathway

IMMUNOLOGIC SYNAPSE

T cell receptor (TCR)–mediated signaling is initiated by a structure known as the *immunologic synapse* or the *supramolecular activation cluster (SMAC)*. The synapse is a "bull's eye–like" structure with the engaged TCR–HLA class I or II molecules and CD28–B7 molecules clustered in the center (Figure 7-1).

Molecular clustering serves three purposes: (1) TCRs engage antigen-loaded HLA molecules with an intermediate affinity. Although these complexes only survive for short periods, they can transduce an activation signal to the nucleus. However, successful activation of T cells requires serial and sustained engagement of TCR–HLA complexes. (2) In the clustered arrangement, multiple TCRs interact with small numbers of antigen-loaded HLA molecules on antigen-presenting cells (APCs). (3) Clustering also congregates multiple cytoplasmic immuno receptor tyrosine-based activation motifs (ITAMs) near adaptor proteins, which are necessary for downstream signaling. Following the engagement of CD4 or CD8 with invariant HLA molecule domains, leukocyte-specific protein tyrosine (lck kinase) is activated and phosphorylates ITAMs. Activated ITAMs serve as "docking stations" for adaptor proteins.

ADAPTOR PROTEINS

Adaptor proteins form short-lived complexes with other proteins to transduce membrane activation signals to the major cytoplasmic signaling pathways. The most studied adaptor protein is zeta (ζ)-chain associated protein of 70 kDal (Zap-70). Phosphorylation of two ITAMs on TCR ζ-molecules creates a "docking site" for ZAP-70. CD4-activated or CD8-activated lck phosphorylates ZAP-70, which becomes an active kinase. ZAP-70 phosphorylates phospholipase Cγ1 and another adaptor protein called *linker for activation of T cells (LAT)*.

Phosphorylated LAT serves two functions: (1) It provides a "docking site" for growth factor receptor-bound protein 2 (Grb-2) and its associated protein son of sevenless (SOS). (2) The GrB-2–SOS complex activates Ras, the initiating signal in the MAPK pathway. LAT also activates phosphokinase Cγ1 (PKC), the initiating signal for the NF–κB pathway.

THE RAS–MAPK PATHWAY

One component of the AP-1 transcription factor complex necessary for the synthesis of IL-2 is a product of the Ras–MAPK pathway. Rat **s**arcoma protein (Ras) is a small G protein, which is regulated by guanosine diphosphate (GDP) and guanosine triphosphate (GTP) in the cytoplasm. GTP activates the Ras protein. Hydrolysis of GTP and removal of a phosphate inactivates Ras (Figure 7-2). In T cell activation, Ras transduces signals from the surface receptor to the MAPK pathway. Hydrolysis of GTP is controlled by the presence or absence of Grb–SOS.

When activated, Ras attaches to the membrane and undergoes a conformational change that allows the activation of MAP kinases. The principal kinase in the pathway is an extracellular signal-regulated kinase called *ERK*. ERK phosphorylates a small protein called *ELK*, which initiates the transcription of the Fos protein—one component of the AP-1 complex (Figure 7-3).

THE RAC–JNK PATHWAY

The second component (Jun protein) of the AP-1 complex is activated in the Rac–JNK pathway. Protein kinase B, also known as *Rac protein kinase*, is activated by a GDP–GTP exchange protein called *Vav*. Activated Rac (GATP) phosphorylates the c-Jun N terminal kinase (JNK) which subsequently adds a phosphate to c-Jun. The association of Fos and Jun creates a functional AP-1 complex, which acts as an early transcriptional activator.

AP-1 regulates the production of gene products necessary for T cell division (see Figure 7-2) and the synthesis of IL-2. The creation of the AP-1 provides the first of the three separate nuclear transcription signals necessary for IL-2 synthesis.

CALCIUM AND PLC SIGNALING PATHWAY

The second nuclear transcription factor (NFAT) necessary for synthesis of IL-2 is a product of the calcium–PLC signaling pathway. In the pathway, phospholipaseγ1 activated by LAT catalyzes the cleavage of membrane phosphatidylinositol-4, 5-bisphosphate (PIP$_2$) to yield two second messengers: inositol-1, 4, 5-trisphosphate (IP$_3$) and diacylglycerol (DAG). In turn, these molecules activate two distinct pathways.

In the calcium-dependent pathway, IP$_3$ translocates to the endoplasmic reticulum and releases stored intracellular calcium. To maintain cellular homeostasis and replenish intracellular calcium stores, the cell activates a membrane ion channel called *calcium release activated channel (CRAC)*, which allows an influx of calcium from the external milieu. Some calcium binds to a regulatory protein called *calmodulin*. The calcium–calmodulin complex activates a phosphatase called *calcineurin*. This enzyme activates the nuclear factor of activated T cells (NFAT) protein, which translocates to the nucleus. NFAT provides the second transcription signal for IL-2 synthesis (Figure 7-4).

PLCγ1–DAG/PKC PATHWAY

Nucleotide factor–κB (NF-κB), the third nuclear transcription factor, is a product of the calcium-independent PLCγ1–DAG/PKC pathway. Membrane-attached DAG activates phosphokinase C (PKC). The activated PKC kinase adds phosphates to a number of different target molecules, which form a trimolecular complex that removes an inhibitor from NF-κB. NF-κB is a peliotropic transcription factor that promotes cell growth, cell survival, and the synthesis of IL-2 (Figures 7-4 and 7-5).

CD28–B7 SIGNALING PATHWAY

NF-κB is also the downstream target of CD28–B7 signaling. In the activation pathway, ITAMs on the cytoplasmic tails of CD28 are phosphorylated and recruit PI-3 kinase. The PI-3 kinase activates a number of different pathways, including the Ras–MAP and Jak–STAT (Janus tyrosine kinase–signal transducer activator of transcription) signaling pathways. In the Jak–STAT pathway, PI-3 kinase phosphorylates Jak1 and recruits STATs to the cytoplasmic tail of CD28. In turn, Jak1 phosphorylates STATs, which are released into the cytoplasm. Dimerization of phosphorylated STATs allows translocation to the nucleus and activation of multiple genes. The Jak–STAT pathway is much simpler and shorter than other pathways, and the cellular response is extremely rapid. The PI-3 phosphorylates at position 3 on the inositol ring creating PI-3, 4, 5-triphosphate (PI-3, 4, 5), which accelerates the removal of the inhibitor of NF-κB.

AGENTS THAT INHIBIT T CELL RECEPTOR SIGNALING

Several therapeutic agents inhibit T cell signaling and downregulate immune responses. Cyclosporine A (CsA) is used as prophylaxis to prevent organ rejection or severe, active

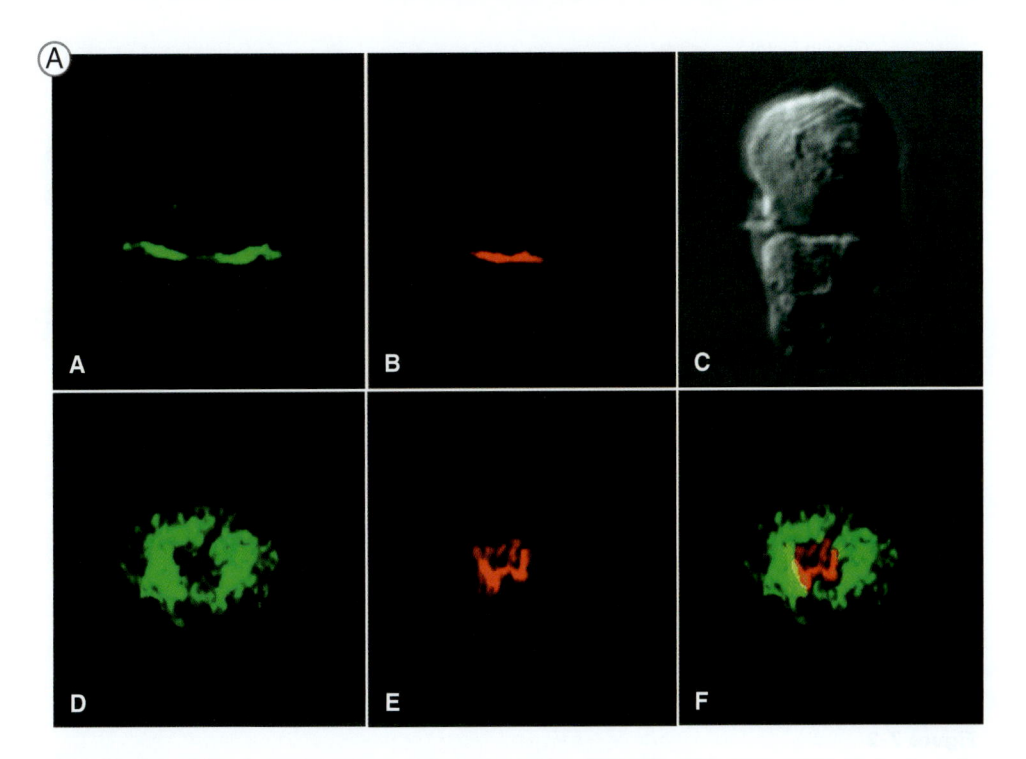

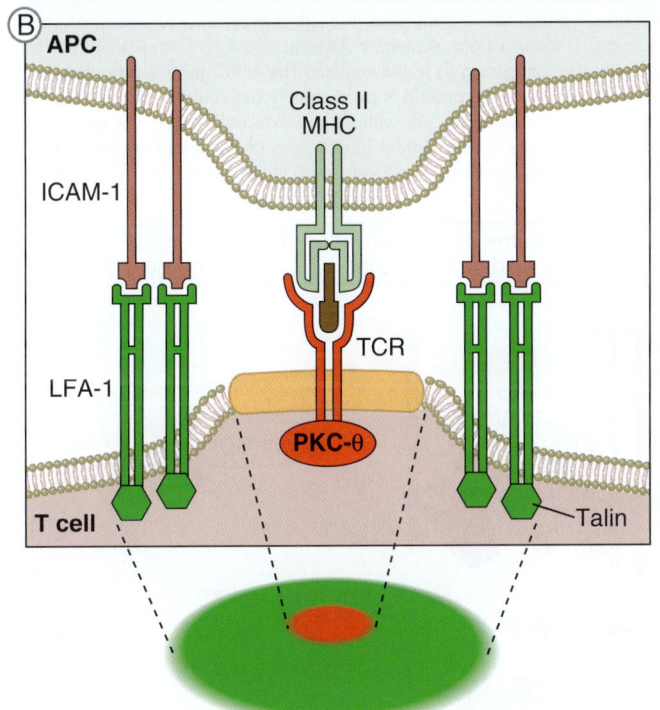

CHAPTER 7 INTRACELLULAR SIGNALING AND T CELL ACTIVATION   57

Figure 7-1

The immunologic synapse. **A,** Two views of the immunologic synapse in a T cell–APC (antigen-presenting cell) conjugate (*shown as a Nomarski image in panel C*). Talin, a protein that associates with the cytoplasmic tail of the LFA-1 integrin was revealed by an antibody labeled with a green fluorescent dye, and PKC-θ, which associates with the TCR complex, was visualized by antibodies conjugated to a red fluorescent dye. **Panels A and B,** A two-dimensional optical section of the cell contact site along the x-y axis, revealing the central location of PKC-θ, and the peripheral location of talin, both in the T cell. **Panels D–F,** A three-dimensional view of the entire region of cell-cell contact along the x-z axis. Note, again, the central location of PKC-θ and the peripheral accumulation of talin. **B,** A schematic view of the synapse, showing talin and LFA-1 in the p-SMAC (green) and PKC-θ and the TCR in the c-SMAC (red). (In Abbas AK, Lichtman AH, Pillai S: Cellular and molecular immunology, ed 6 [updated edition], Philadelphia, 2010, Saunders. Reprinted with permission from Macmillan Publishers Ltd.; Monks CRF, Freiburg BA, Kupfer H, et al: Three dimensional segregation of supramolecular activation clusters in T cells, *Nature*, 395:82–86, 1998.)

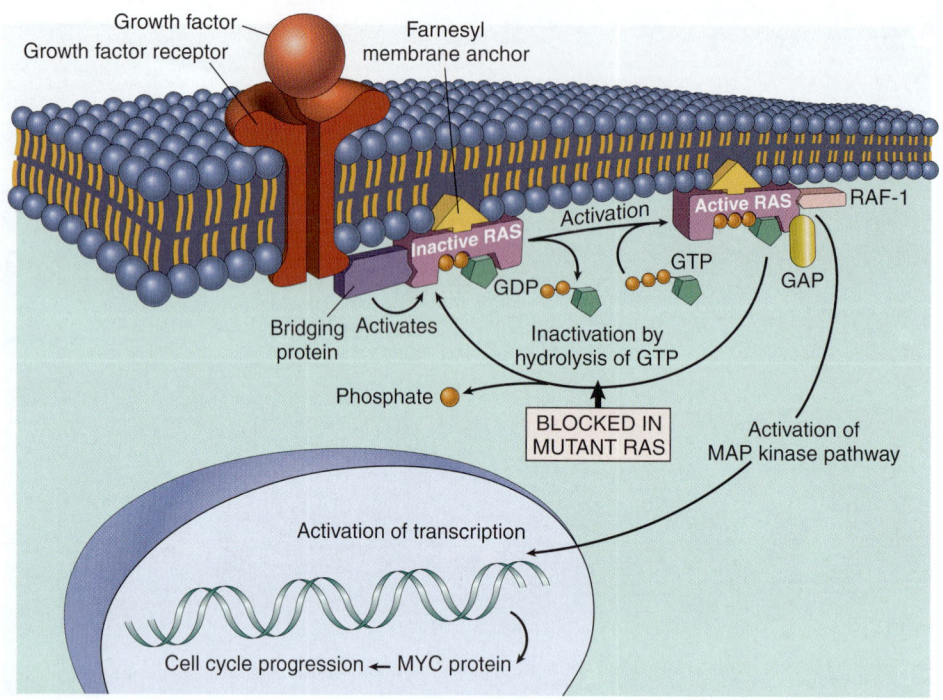

CHAPTER 7 INTRACELLULAR SIGNALING AND T CELL ACTIVATION

Figure 7-2

Model for action of *RAS* genes. When a normal cell is stimulated through a growth factor receptor, inactive (GDP-bound) RAS is activated to a GTP-bound state. Activated RAS recruits RAF-1 and stimulates the MAP-kinase pathway to transmit growth-promoting signals to the nucleus. The *MYC* gene is one of several targets of the activated RAS pathway. The mutant RAS protein is permanently activated because of inability to hydrolyze GTP, leading to continuous stimulation of cells without any external trigger. The anchoring of RAS to the cell membrane by the farnesyl moiety is essential for its action, and drugs that inhibit farnesylation can inhibit RAS action. (From Vinay K: Robbins basic pathology, ed 8, Philadelphia, 2003, Saunders.)

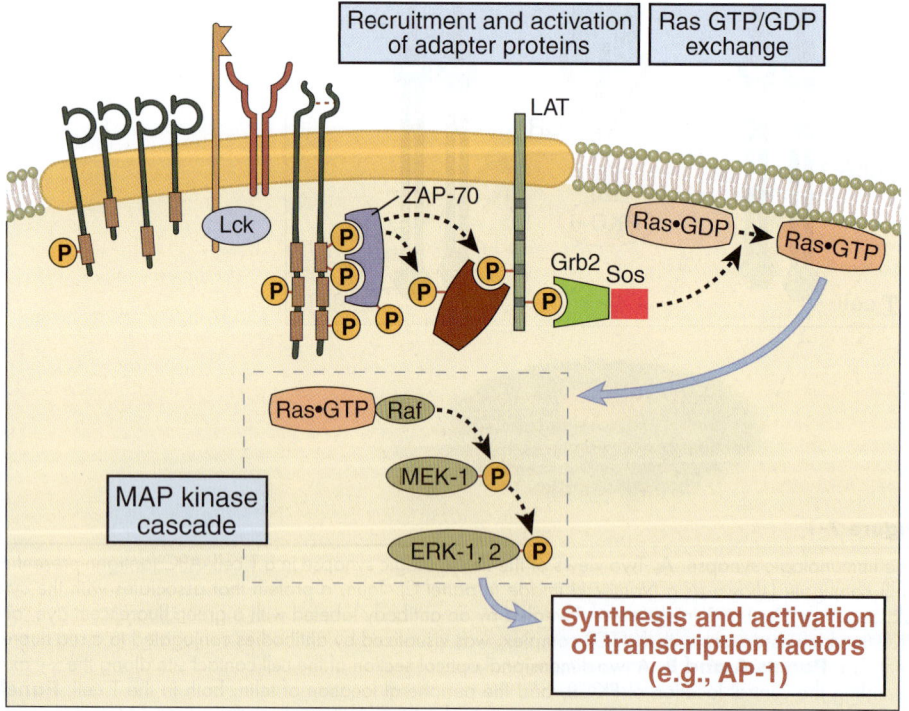

Figure 7-3

The Ras–MAP kinase pathway in T cell activation. ZAP-70 that is activated by antigen recognition phosphorylates membrane-associated adapter proteins (such as LAT), which then bind another adapter, Grb-2, which provides a docking site for the GTP–GDP exchange factor SOS. SOS converts Ras GDP to Ras GTP. Ras GTP activates a cascade of enzymes, which culminates in the activation of the MAP kinase ERK. A parallel Rac-dependent pathway generates another active MAP kinase, JNK (*not shown*). (From Abbas AK, Lichtman AH, Pillai S: Cellular and molecular immunology, ed 6 [updated edition], Philadelphia, 2010, Saunders.)

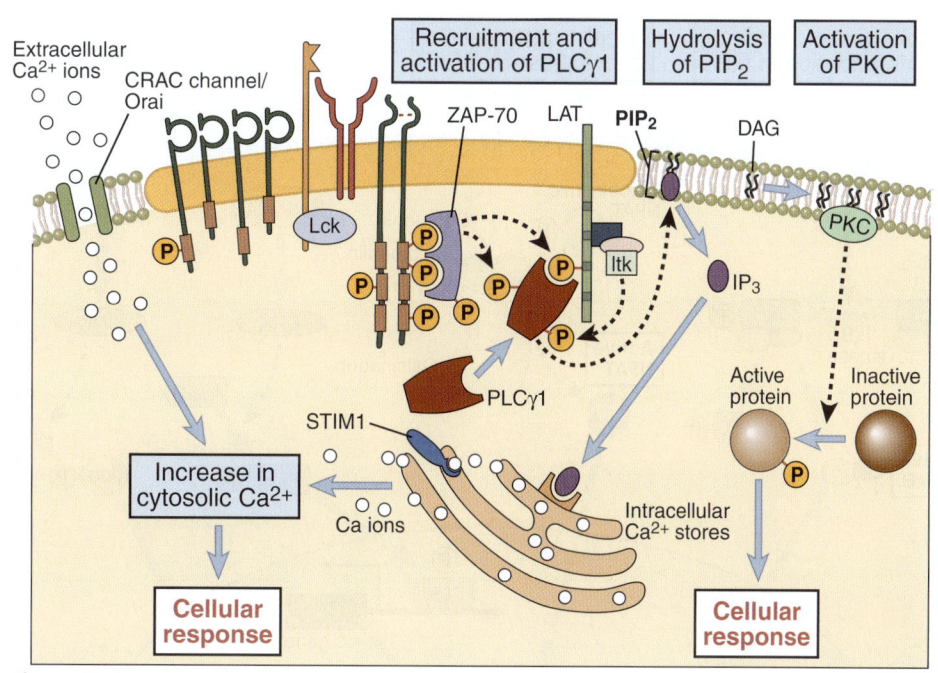

Figure 7-4

T cell signaling downstream of PLC-γ1. The LAT (linker for activation of T cells) adapter protein that is phosphorylated on T cell activation binds the cytosolic enzyme PLC-γ1, which is phosphorylated by ZAP-70 and other kinases, such as Itk, and activated. The active PLC-γ1 hydrolyzes membrane PIP_2 to generate IP_3, which stimulates an increase in cytosolic calcium and DAG, which activates the enzyme PKC. Depletion of endoplasmic reticulum (ER) calcium is sensed by stromal interaction molecule 1(STIM1), which induces the opening of the calcium release activated channel (CRAC) that facilitates the entry of extracellular calcium into the cytosol. Orai is a component of the CRAC channel. Increased cytosolic calcium and phosphokinase C (PKC) then activate various transcription factors, leading to cellular responses. (From Abbas AK, Lichtman AH, Pillai S: Cellular and molecular immunology, ed 6 [updated edition], Philadelphia, 2010, Saunders.)

---

rheumatoid arthritis. Although the exact mechanism has not been clearly defined, it is believed that CsA binds to a protein called *cyclophilin* in the cytoplasm. The complex blocks T cell activation by inhibiting calcineurin phosphatase. As a result, NFAT is not translocated to the nucleus, and IL-2 is not synthesized.

Cyclosporine has serious and life-threatening side effects, including neural, hepatic, and renal toxicity. Neurotoxicity is usually mild and manifests as tremors, but seizures have been described. Cyclosporine A–induced cholestasis and hepatocyte destruction are characteristic of hepatotoxicity. In the kidney, CsA produces a dose-dependent vasoconstriction of renal arteries, which results in mild-to-moderate renal dysfunction. Manifestations of renal dysfunction include a reduced glomerular filtration rate, increased sodium resorption, and hypertension.

Tacrolimus (FK506) has replaced CsA as an anti-rejection agent. It is 10- to 100-fold more active than CsA and has less toxicity. Tacrolimus binds to a cytoplasmic protein called *FK506-binding protein 12 (FKBP-12)* and blocks the activity of calcineurin (Table 7-1) in the calcium–PKC signaling pathway.

INTERLEUKIN 2 RECEPTORS

Autocrine IL-2 stimulation of high-affinity IL-2 receptors is necessary for T cell growth and proliferation. High-affinity IL-2 receptors are only expressed on activated T cells and consist of three chains (α, β, and γ). α-chains and β-chains bind IL-2 and are involved in intracellular signaling. The γ-chain serves as a support structure and is common to a number of cytokine receptors (IL-2, IL-4, IL-7, IL-9, and IL-15).

AGENTS THAT BLOCK AUTOCRINE INTERLEUKIN 2 SIGNALING

Sirolimus has a biochemical structure similar to CsA and tacrolimus, but it blocks T cell activation by preventing autocrine IL-2 signaling from the high-affinity receptor to the nucleus. In the signaling pathway, sirolimus binds to cytoplasmic FKBP-12 but does not block the activity of calcineurin. Rather, a bi-molecular complex binds to a third protein called *rapamycin-associated protein (RAP)*. The three-component complex inactivates the protein target of rapamycin (TOR), which is important in accelerating cell division.

Monoclonal antibodies are also used to block the interaction between the high-affinity receptor and the soluble IL-2. Antibody blockade of the IL-2 receptor prevents T cell growth, and proliferation and induces T cell apoptosis (Table 7-2).

Basiliximab is a monoclonal antibody directed at the IL-2 receptor α-chain (also known as *IL-2R-α-chain*, CD25, or TAC). Another humanized monoclonal antibody, called *daclizumab*, also is directed at the IL-2R-α-chain. Both antibodies have proven useful in the treatment of acute rejection of transplanted kidneys.

60 CHAPTER 7 INTRACELLULAR SIGNALING AND T CELL ACTIVATION

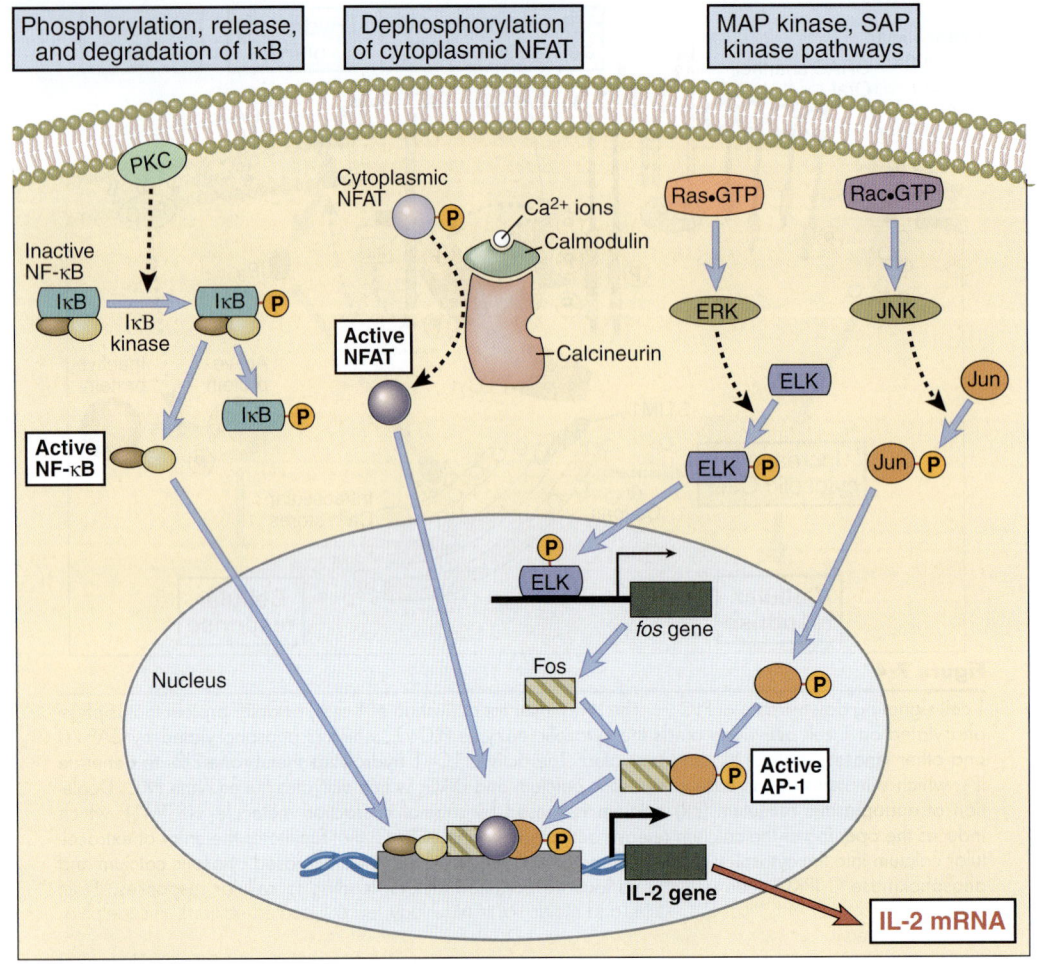

Figure 7-5

Activation of transcription factors in T cells. Multiple signaling pathways converge in antigen-stimulated T cells to generate transcription factors that stimulate expression of various genes (in this case, the interleukin 2 [IL-2] gene). The calcium–calmodulin pathway activates NFAT (nuclear factor of activated T cells), and the Ras and Rac pathways generate the two components of AP-1. Less is known about the link between T cell receptor (TCR) signals and NF-κB activation. (NF-κB is shown as a complex of two subunits, which, in T cells, are typically the p50 and p65 proteins, named for their molecular sizes in kiloDaltons [kDa].). PKC is important in T cell activation, and the PKC-θ isoform is particularly important in activating NF-κB. These transcription factors function coordinately to regulate gene expression. Note also that the various signaling pathways are shown as activating unique transcription factors, but considerable overlap may be present, and each pathway may play a role in the activation of multiple transcription factors. (From Abbas AK, Lichtman AH, Pillai S: Cellular and molecular immunology, ed 6 [updated edition], Philadelphia, 2010, Saunders.)

Table 7-1 Fungal Immunosuppressive Agents That Inhibit T Cell Activation and Signaling

Immunosuppressive Agent	Source	Mechanism
Cyclosporine A	Cyclic peptide produced by *Tolypocladium inflatum*	Inhibits calcineurin
Tacrolimus (FK506)	Macrolide produced by *Streptomyces tsukubaensis*	Inhibits calcineurin
Sirolimus	Produced by *Streptomyces hygroscopicus*	Inhibits IL-2 receptor signal transduction

Modifed from Actor JA: Immunology and immunobiology, Philadelphia, 2007, Elsevier.

DEFECTIVE T CELL SIGNALING AND IMMUNODEFICIENCIES

X-Linked Severe Combined Immunodeficiency

X-linked severe combined immunodeficiency (SCID) is a life-threatening primary immunodeficiency, which is characterized by a lack of T and B lymphocytes or by dysfunctional lymphocytes. Most infants with the disease die within 1 year as a result of recurrent infections by opportunistic pathogens. Several defects in cellular signaling have been described. In X-linked SCID, the major defect is an inability to synthesize a receptor γ-chain, which is part of the IL-2 high-affinity receptor and a number of different IL receptors (IL-2, IL-4, IL-7, IL-9, and IL-15). Engagement of these receptors is critical to lymphocyte activation, synthesis of different types of antibodies, TCR re-arrangements,

Table 7-2 Monoclonal Antibodies That Inhibit Soluble Interleukin 2 Binding to Receptors

Name	Origin	Reagent Type	Target	Application
Basiliximab	Chimeric	Monoclonal antibody	IL-2R α-chain (CD25 or TAC)	Prevention of acute organ rejection
Daclizumab	Humanized	Monoclonal antibody	ILR-2 α-chain	Prevention of acute kidney rejection

and natural killer (NK) cell development. X-linked SCID is the most common form of immunodeficiency, affecting 1 in 50,000 to 100,000 births.

ZAP-70 Immunodeficiency

The ZAP-70 protein kinase is expressed on T cells and is associated with the CD3 ζ-chain of the TCR complex. Dysfunctional ZAP proteins cannot phosphorylate ITAMs, which are critical to the initiation of the signaling process and for T cell differentiation. Mutations in Zap-70 are responsible for a rare autosomal recessive form of SCID in humans. This syndrome is characterized by CD8 cells and CD4 cells that are refractory to T cell stimulation.

Treatment of Severe Combined Immunodeficiency

Unfortunately, treatment options for SCID are limited to isolating the patient to protect against microbial infections. Aggressive broad-spectrum antimicrobial treatment must be initiated at the first sign of infection. Affected individuals may also receive intravenous immunoglobulin replacement therapy. The only cure for the disease is bone marrow transplantation or, in select cases, gene therapy.

SUMMARY

- Interleukin 2 (IL-2) synthesis is essential for T cell stimulation.
- IL-2 synthesis requires the activation of three different transcription factors produced in five different signaling pathways.
- Cyclosporine and tacrolimus block the activation of the transcription factors for IL-2.
- Autocrine IL-2 stimulation is required for the growth and proliferation of T cells.
- Sirolimus blocks the signaling from the high-affinity IL-2 receptor.

REFERENCES

Bonnevier JL, Mueller DL: Cutting edge: B7/CD28 interactions regulate cell cycle progression independent of the strength of TCR signaling, J Immunol 169(12):6659, 2002.

Brini AT, Harel-Bellan A, et al: Cyclosporin A inhibits induction of IL-2 receptor alpha chain expression by affecting activation of NF-κB-like factor(s) in cultured human T lymphocytes, Eur Cytokine Netw 1(3):131, 1990.

Buss WC, Stepanek J, et al: Proposed mechanism of cyclosporine toxicity: inhibition of protein synthesis, Transplant Proc 20(Suppl 3):863, 1988.

Davis DM, Dustin ML: What is the importance of the immunological synapse? Trends Immunol 25(6):323, 2004.

Gallo EM, Cante-Barrett K, Crabree GR, et al: Lymphocyte calcium signaling from membrane to nucleus, Nat Immunol 7(1):25, 2006.

Hogan PG, Chen L, Nardone J, Rao A: Transcriptional regulation by calcium, calcineurin, and NFAT, Genes Dev 17(18):2205, 2003.

Kuhns MS, Davis MM, Garcia KC, et al: Deconstructing the form and function of the TCR/CD3 complex, Immunity 24(2):133, 2006.

Li Y, Sedwick CE, Hu J, Altman A, et al: Role for protein kinase Ctheta (PKCtheta) in TCR/CD28-mediated signaling through the canonical but not the non-canonical pathway for NF-κB activation, J Biol Chem 280(2):1217, 2005.

Nelson BH, Willerford DM: Biology of the interleukin-2 receptor, Adv Immunol 70:1, 1998.

Oum JH, Han J, Myung H, Hleb M, Sharma S, Park J: Molecular mechanism of NFAT family proteins for differential regulation of the IL-2 and TNF-alpha promoters, Mol Cells 13(1):77, 2002.

Paliogianni F, Raptis A, Ahuja SS, et al: Negative transcriptional regulation of human interleukin 2 (IL-2) gene by glucocorticoids through interference with nuclear transcription factors AP-1 and NF-AT, J Clin Invest 91(4):1481, 1993.

Palmer BF, Toto RD: Severe neurologic toxicity induced by cyclosporine A in three renal transplant patients, Am J Kidney Dis 18(1):116, 1991.

Rudolph MG, Stanfield RL, Wilson IA: How TCRs bind MHCs, peptides, and coreceptors, Annu Rev Immunol 24:419, 2006.

Samelson LE: Signal transduction mediated by the T cell antigen receptor: The role of adapter proteins, Annu Rev Immunol 20:371, 2002.

Sugamura K, Asao H, Kondo M, et al: The interleukin-2 receptor gamma chain: Its role in the multiple cytokine receptor complexes and T cell development in XSCID, Annu Rev Immunol 14:179, 1996.

Thomson AW, Whiting PH, Simpson JG: Cyclosporine: Immunology, toxicity and pharmacology in experimental animals, Agents Actions 15(3–4):306, 1984.

Weil R, Israel A: Deciphering the pathway from the TCR to NF-κB, Cell Death Differ 13(5):826, 2006.

ASSESSMENT QUESTIONS

1. Self-stimulation of IL-2 receptors is called:
   A. Paracrine stimulation
   B. Autocrine stimulation
   C. Hormonal stimulation
   D. Neuronal stimulation

2. Which of the following is *not* a transcription factor for IL-2?
   A. AP-1
   B. NFAT
   C. NF-κB
   D. Zap-70

3. In the phospholipase Cγ1 pathway, which of the following is responsible for the release of calcium from intracellular stores?
   A. Inositol 1,4,5, triphosphate
   B. Diacetylglycerol
   C. Phosphokinase C
   D. NFAT

4. Which of the following therapeutic agents block the activation of calcineurin?
   A. Cyclosporine
   B. Sirolimus
   C. Basiliximab
   D. Corticosteroids

5. The major defect in X-linked severe combined immunodeficiency is an:
   A. Inability to synthesize receptor α-chains
   B. Inability to synthesize receptor γ-chains
   C. Inability to synthesize receptor β-chains
   D. Inability to synthesize the Tac protein

6. Which of the following pathways' downstream target is NF-κB?
   I. Ras–MAP kinase (MAPK) pathway
   II. Calcium-independent DAG–PKC signaling pathway
   III. PI-3 kinase pathway
   A. I
   B. III
   C. I and II
   D. II and III
   E. I, II, and III

CHAPTER 8

B Cell Activation and Signaling

LEARNING OBJECTIVES

- Describe the structure of the B cell receptor (BCR) complex
- Differentiate between the signaling and nonsignaling components of the BCR
- Define the role of CD2 in intracellular signaling
- Explain the usefulness of BCR cross-linking in the intracellular signaling process
- Identify the intracellular signaling pathways activated by cross-linked BCRs
- Recognize the definition of thymus-dependent (TD) antigen
- Identify the definition of a thymus-independent (TI) antigen
- Compare and contrast the molecular structure of TD and TI antigens
- Explain the interactions between TI types I and II antigens and cellular ligands
- Compare and contrast the antibody responses elicited by TI types I and II antigens
- Explain the role(s) of the B lymphocyte stimulator (BLyS) in B cell differentiation to plasma cells
- Identify the role of CD22 in B cell regulation
- Examine the role of atacicept in blocking B cell differentiation
- Explain how belimumab and epratuzumab inhibit B cell differentiation
- Recognize the key immunologic defect in early-onset X-linked agammaglobulinemia (XLA) and its role in intracellular signaling
- Describe treatment modalities commonly used to treat XLA

KEY TERMS

B cell receptor (BCR)
B lymphocyte stimulator (BLyS)
Brutons tyrosine kinase (BTK)
Plasma cell
Thymus-dependent (TD) antigens
Thymus-independent (TI) antigens
Type I thymus-independent antigens
Type II thymus-independent antigens
X-linked agammaglobulinemia

INTRODUCTION

B cells are the major effector cells in an antibody-mediated immune response. The production of antibodies to protein antigens often requires interactions among T cells, B cells, and monocytes. The response is termed *thymus-dependent (TD) antibody production*. B cells are activated by the engagement of two receptors on the cell surface. However, some antigens can initiate antibody production without antigen processing or the help of T cells. These antigens are termed *thymus-independent (TI) antigens*. The activation of B cells may require the engagement of one or more receptors. As a consequence of intracellular signaling, B cells differentiate into antibody-producing plasma cells.

B CELL RECEPTOR COMPLEX

In the initial stage of B cell activation, antigens react with the membrane B cell receptor (BCR), which is a monomeric form of an antibody called immunoglobulin M (IgM; see Chapter 9). Monomeric IgM consists of two mu (μ)–heavy chains and two kappa (κ)– or lambda (λ)–light chains. M–heavy chains have four constant regions (C_H1–C_H4) and one variable domain (V_H). Light chains are connected to the µ-chains and have one constant C_L domain and one V_L domain. Within the variable regions of both heavy and light chains are hypervariable regions. The combination of hypervariable regions in the heavy and light chains creates a three-dimensional pocket that determines antigen specificity (Figure 8-1). Each B cell expresses a homogeneous population of BCRs that recognize only one antigen. Therefore, 1×10^{13} B cell clones are needed to respond to all known antigens.

The BCR has a short intracytoplasmic tail and cannot transduce signals to the nucleus. To transduce signals, the BCR forms complexes with invariant immunoglobulin-alpha (Ig-α) and immunoglobulin-beta (Ig-β) molecules, which contain multiple immunoreceptor tyrosine-based activation motifs (ITAMs).

B CELL RECEPTOR SIGNALING

Activating signals are initiated by the cross-linkage of two BCRs by multi-valent antigens. Cross-linkage of two BCRs brings activated a sarcoma (v-src) kinase into the proper position for the activation of cellular signaling. The v-src enzyme phosphorylates the tyrosine residues on the Ig-α and Ig-β ITAMs (Figure 8-2). Phosphorylated ITAMs also act as "docking sites" for syk, an enzyme analogous to ZAP-70 in T cells. Syk activates two downstream signaling pathways whose products promote the synthesis of antibodies.

In one pathway, phosphorylation of phospholipase Cγ2 (the B cell isoform of phospholipase 1) activates the PLC calcium-dependent and DAG pathways. Activation results in the translocation of nuclear factor of activated T cells (NFAT) and

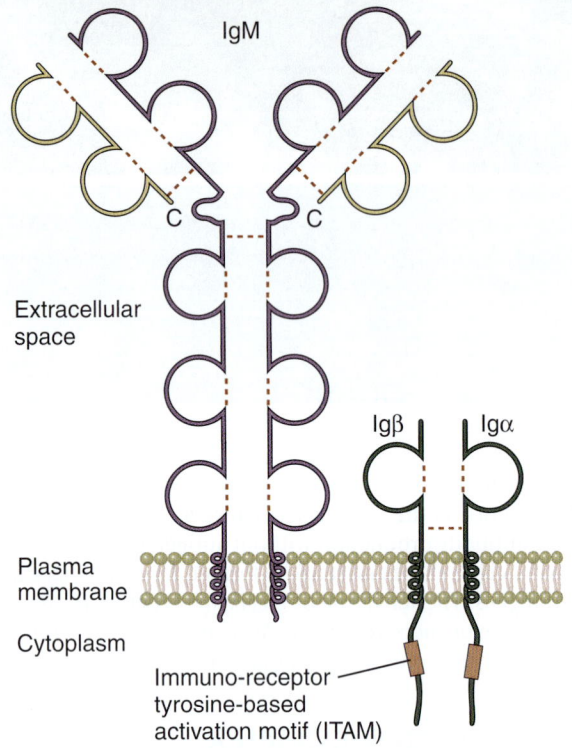

Figure 8-1

B cell antigen receptor complex. Membrane immunoglobulin M (IgM) on the surface of mature B cells is associated with the invariant Ig-α and Ig-β molecules, which contain immuno-receptor tyrosine-based activation motifs (ITAMs) in their cytoplasmic tails that mediate signaling functions. Note the similarity to the T cell receptor (TCR) complex. (From Abbas AK, Lichtman AH, Pillai S: Cellular and molecular immunology, ed 6 [updated edition], Philadelphia, 2010, Saunders.)

nuclear factor–kappaB (NF-κB) to the nucleus. In a second pathway, phosphorlyation of an adaptor protein called SLP-65 (SH-2 binding leukocyte protein) allows interaction with Btk and Grb kinases. The Grb–SLP-65 complex recruits SOS (son of sevenless), which acts as a guanosine triphosphate–guanosine diphosphate (GTP–GDP) exchange protein that activates Ras and Rac. In turn, the MAP (mitogen-activated protein) kinase and the JNK (c-Jun N terminal kinase) pathways are activated with translocation of AP-1 to the nucleus. In B cells, AP-1 accelerates for cell division, which creates B memory cells and B cell differentiation into plasma cells.

AMPLIFICATION OF THE B CELL SIGNAL

Like T cells, B cells require a second signal for activation. The second signal is provided by a B cell co-receptor complex that consists of CR2, CD19, and CD81 (TAPA-1). The CR2 molecule recognizes a decay product of complement called C3d that is bound to large-molecular-weight antigens or bacteria. Complement is a series of serum proteins that can be activated by polysaccharides (innate immunity) or antigen–antibody complexes (acquired immunity). Complement is discussed in detail in Chapter 11.

Amplification occurs when the multi-valent antigen binds to CD2 and cross-links multiple BCRs. Engagement of the BCR and CR2 activates a lyn kinase that phosphorylates the Ig-α and Ig-β ITAMs. Binding also reorients CD19 and CD81 to bring them into proximity with Ig-α and Ig-β ITAMs (Figure 8-3).

Phosphorylation of CD19 activates a PI-3 kinase, which initiates the Ras–MAP and Jak–STAT signaling pathways that stimulate B cell differentiation, survival, and growth.

THYMUS-DEPENDENT ANTIGENS

Some antigens require the help of T cells for the stimulation of B cells to produce antibodies. In the parafollicular cortex (T cell zone) of the lymph node, dendritic cells process and present antigens in the context of class II molecules. Antigens are presented to CD4Th2 cells. At this point, the T cell is activated but does not know which B cell needs help to produce antibodies.

B cell activation occurs in the lymph node B cell zone. The unprocessed antigens that activated the T cell bind to antigen-specific BCRs. After interaction between the BCR and antigens, B cells internalize, process, and present epitopes in the context of class II molecules (Figure 8-4).

Under the influence of chemokines, B cells translocate to T cell–rich zones. T cells and B cells come together, and B cells present antigens in the context of class II molecules to the T cell receptors (TCRs) on the activated T cell. As a consequence, activated T cells begin to help B cells to produce antibodies. Secondary signals from CD28–B7-1 and CD40–CD40L interactions are necessary to amplify the help from T cells. Small-molecular-weight cytokines produced by CD4Th2 cells cause the proliferation and differentiation of B cells in defined foci. Within 4 to 7 days, cytokine-stimulated B cells migrate back to lymph node follicles, where they form germinal centers containing proliferating B cells, memory B cells, and plasma cells. A summary of T helper cell–mediated B cell activation is shown in Figure 8-5.

THYMUS-INDEPENDENT ANTIGENS

Antigens that do not require the help of T cells to initiate antibody production are termed *thymus-independent (TI)* antigens. B cells that respond to TI antigens are found in the spleen, bone marrow, peritoneal cells, and mucosa. In the spleen, specialized subsets of marginal-zone B cells interact with the native, unprocessed TI antigens bound to the surface of marginal-zone macrophages. In the peritoneum and mucosa, another specialized B cell population, called *B-1 cells*, recognizes TI antigens. B-1 cells are derived from the fetal liver and may represent a separate B cell lineage. Both marginal-zone B cells and B-1 cells produce natural antibodies that are important in the defense against encapsulated bacteria.

In general, TI antigens are linear carbohydrate molecules and have repeating epitopes that engage and cross-link multiple BCRs. On the basis of the necessity for ancillary or secondary receptor interactions, TI antigens can be classified into type I or type II antigens. Bacterial endotoxins, glycolipids, and nucleic acids are type I antigens and require interaction with a BCR and a second signal to activate B cells. Type II antigens directly cross-link multiple BCRs to activate B cells. Natural and synthetic polysaccharides are considered type II antigens. Both type I and type II antigens elicit antibody production, but they are poor inducers of memory cells.

Type I Thymus-Independent Antigens

Lipopolysaccharide (LPS) endotoxins are normal constituents of a gram-negative bacterial cell wall and are released when the bacterium dies or is killed by antibiotics. Endotoxins consist of three domains: (1) the O-polysaccharide region, (2) a core

Figure 8-2

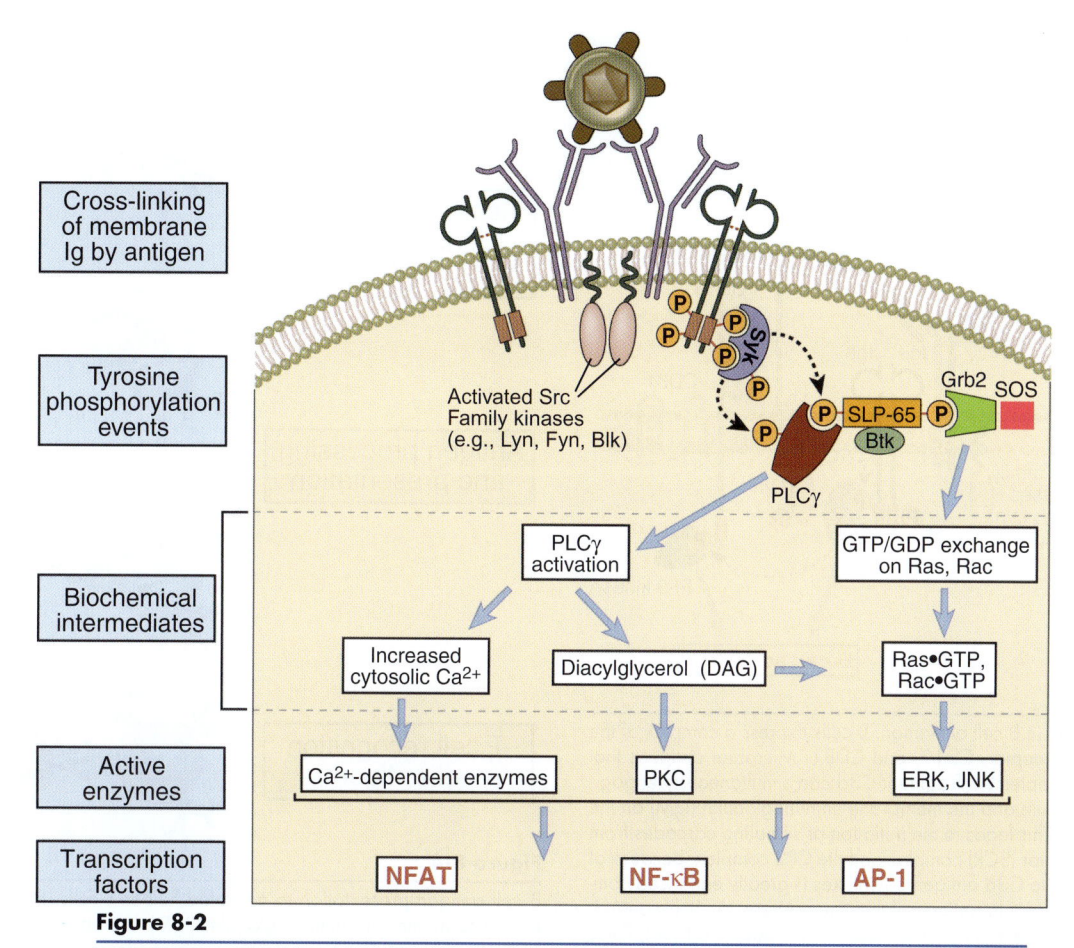

Signal transduction by the B cell receptor (BCR) complex. Antigen-induced cross-linking of membrane immunoglobulin (IgM) on B cells leads to clustering and activation of Src-family tyrosine kinases and tyrosine phosphorylation of the immuno-receptor tyrosine-based activation motifs (ITAMs) in the cytoplasmic tails of the Ig-α and Ig-β molecules. This leads to docking of Syk and subsequent tyrosine phosphorylation events as depicted. Several signaling cascades follow these events, as shown, leading to the activation of several transcription factors. These signal transduction pathways are similar to those described in T cells. (From Abbas AK, Lichtman AH, Pillai S: Cellular and molecular immunology, ed 6 [updated edition], Philadelphia, 2010, Saunders.)

region, and (3) lipid A. The outer O-polysaccharide contains repeating immunogenic epitopes of three to five units that evoke an antibody response. The core polysaccharide region is intermediate between the O-region and lipid A. It contains d-manno-oct-2-ulosonic acid and glycerol-d-manno-heptose. The membrane-anchoring domain, or lipid A, consists of a highly conserved, phosphorylated dimer of N-acetylglucosamine with five to seven attached fatty acids. Both the O-region and lipid A bind to receptors on mammalian cells.

Endotoxin-induced B cell stimulation requires interaction with two receptors. The O-region polysaccharide reacts with antigen-specific BCRs. Lipid A binds to a Toll-like receptor (TLR-4) that has associated ITAMs. In some instances, endotoxins binding is nonspecific and multiple B cell clones are stimulated (polyclonal B cell activation) to produce an antibody called IgM.

Type II Thymus-Independent Antigens

Type II antigens are polysaccharide antigens with repeating epitopes that cross-link multiple BCRs to stimulate B cell activation. For example, capsular polysaccharides from the highly virulent *Pneumococcus*, *Haemophilus*, and *Meningococcus* species are classic type II antigens. Antibodies resulting from type II antigen stimulation are usually low-affinity antibodies, called *natural antibodies*, which are produced without overt exposure to antigens.

PLASMA CELL DIFFERENTIATION

The driving forces for B cell differentiation into plasma cells are two cytokines produced by T cells, monocytes, dendritic cells, and macrophages. (1) One cytokine, called the *B lymphocyte stimulator (BLyS)*, interacts with the TACI (membrane-activated calcium–modulator cyclophilin ligand-interactor) and the BLyS-receptor 3 (BLySR3). Engagement of BLyS with its ligands promotes B cell survival and differentiation into plasma cells. (2) The second cytokine is a proliferation-inducing ligand (APRIL), which binds to the B cell maturation antigen (BCMA). APRIL acts a co-stimulator of B cell proliferation and supports antibody switching from one class to another (Figure 8-6).

PLASMA CELL LONGEVITY

Depending on the nature of the antigen, plasma cells are either short lived or long lived. Short-lived plasma cells are generated during TI responses and allow rapid production of protective

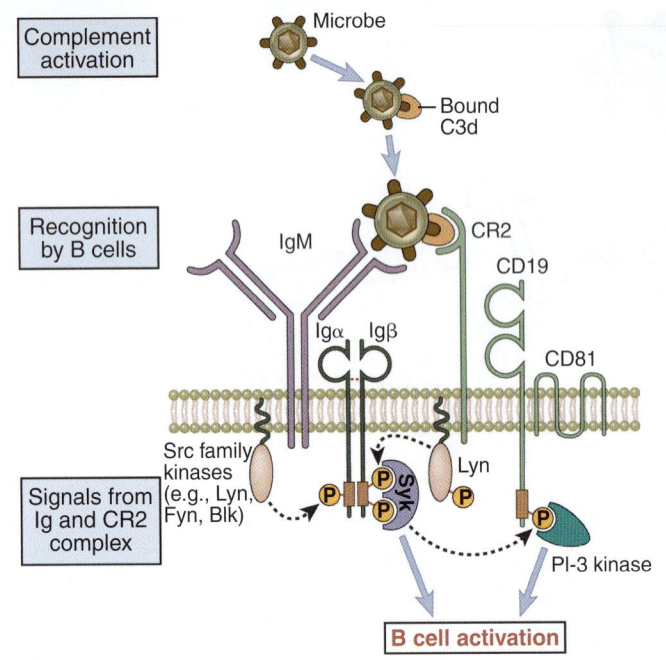

Figure 8-3
Role of complement in B cell activation. B cells express a complex of the CR2 complement receptor, CD19, and CD81. Microbial antigens that have bound the complement fragment C3d can simultaneously engage both the CR2 molecule and the membrane immunoglobulin (IgM) on the surface of a B cell. This leads to the initiation of signaling cascades from both the B cell receptor (BCR) complex and the CR2 complex, because of which the response to C3d antigen complexes is greatly enhanced compared with the response to antigen alone. (From Abbas AK, Lichtman AH, Pillai S: Cellular and molecular immunology, ed 6 [updated edition], Philadelphia, 2010, Saunders.)

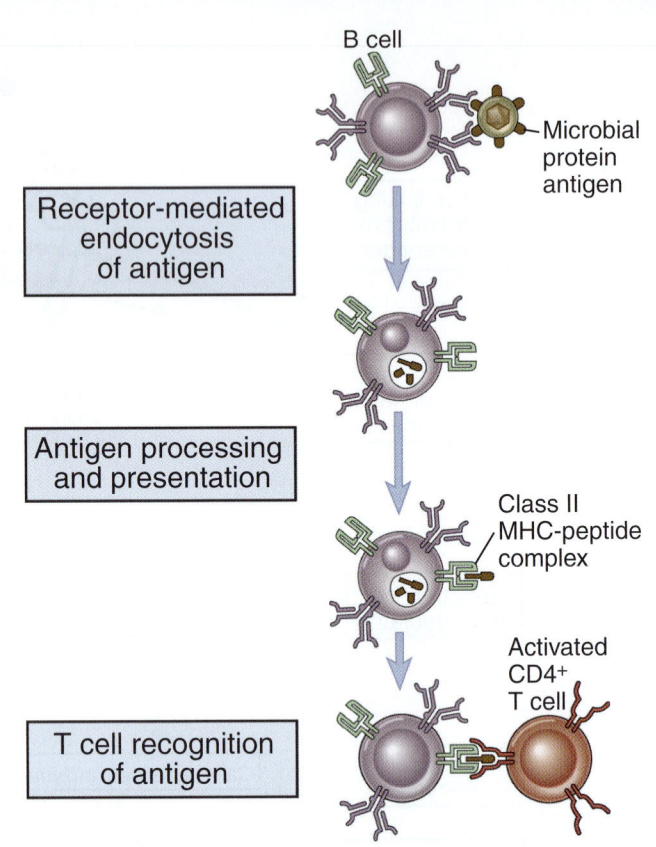

Figure 8-4
B cell antigen presentation to activated helper T cells. Protein antigens bound to membrane immunoglobulin (IgM) are endocytosed and processed, and peptide fragments are presented in association with class II HLA molecules. Activated helper T cells recognize the MHC-peptide complexes and then stimulate B cell responses. Activated B cells also express co-stimulators (e.g., B7 and CD28 molecules) that enhance helper T cell responses. (From Abbas AK, Lichtman AH, Pillai S: Cellular and molecular immunology, ed 6 [updated edition], Philadelphia, 2010, Saunders.)

antibodies to *Pneumococcus*, *Haemophilus*, and *Meningococcus*. These plasma cells are localized in secondary lymphoid tissue such the splenic periarteriolar lymphoid sheath (PALS) and lymph node germinal centers. Long-lived plasma cells are generated after stimulation by TD antigens. Approximately 7 weeks after immunization with a TD antigen, plasma cells in the germinal center migrate to bone marrow and become long-lived plasma cells. These cells continue to produce antibodies for months or years and provide protection against previously encountered antigens. Approximately 80% of antibodies directed at TD antigens found in serum are produced by long-lived plasma cells in bone marrow.

AGENTS THAT BLOCK B CELL DIFFERENTIATION INTO PLASMA CELLS

Blockade of B cell differentiation into plasma cells is an important goal of therapy. Inhibition of B cell differentiation can involve the use of fusion proteins or monoclonal antibodies. For example, atacicept is a soluble recombinant fusion protein that contains the binding portion of the B cell TACI receptor that binds both BLyS and APRIL and the distal portion of an antibody molecule. The fusion protein binds and neutralizes soluble BLyS and APRIL cytokines before they can react with stimulatory ligands on the B cell surface. Atacicept has been used successfully in the treatment of systemic lupus erythematosus (SLE) and rheumatoid arthritis.

Two monoclonal antibodies directly prevent B cell differentiation. Belimumab is a humanized monoclonal antibody directed at soluble BLyS. It is currently in clinical trials for the treatment of SLE. Epratuzumab, another humanized monoclonal antibody, is directed at CD22 expressed on the surface on B cells. Antibody engagement of CD22 activates the protein tyrosine phosphatase called SHP1, a negative regulator of BCR signaling. Epratuzumab is useful in the treatment of non-Hodgkin's lymphoma and SLE (Table 8-1).

IMMUNODEFICIENCIES

Bruton Agammaglobulinema (X-Linked Agammaglobulinemia)

In 1952, Colonel Ogden Bruton, an Army pediatrician, reported the first known immunodeficiency. The patient was a 9-year-old boy, who had no measurable antibody levels. The immune defect was originally named *Bruton agammaglobulinemia*. Additional studies showed that 90% of the patients were male, and the name was changed to *X-linked agammaglobulinemia (XLA)*, or *early-onset agammaglobulinemia*. Patients with this immunodeficiency have recurrent episodes of otitis media, pneumonia, and sinusitis caused by *Streptococcus pneumoniae* or *Haemophilus influenzae*. Diarrhea caused by *Giardia* and *Campylobacter* is also common.

CHAPTER 8 B CELL ACTIVATION AND SIGNALING 67

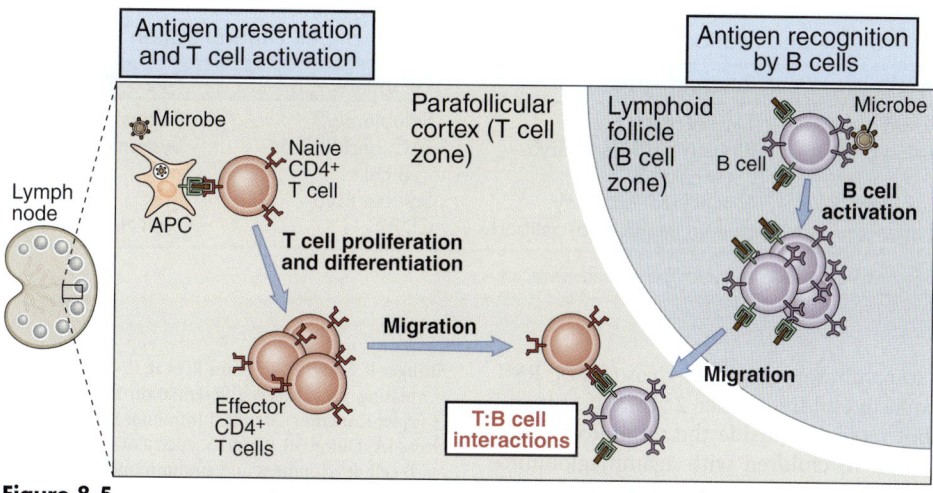

Figure 8-5

The interactions of helper T cells and B cells in lymphoid tissues. CD4+ helper T cells recognize processed protein antigens displayed by professional antigen-presenting cells (APCs) and are activated to proliferate and differentiate into effector cells. These effector T cells begin to migrate toward lymphoid follicles. Naive B lymphocytes, which reside in the follicles, recognize the antigens in this site and are activated to migrate out of the follicles. The two cell populations come together at the edges of the follicles and interact. (From Abbas AK, Lichtman AH: Basic immunology: functions and disorders of the immune system, ed 2 [updated edition], Philadelphia, 2006, Saunders.)

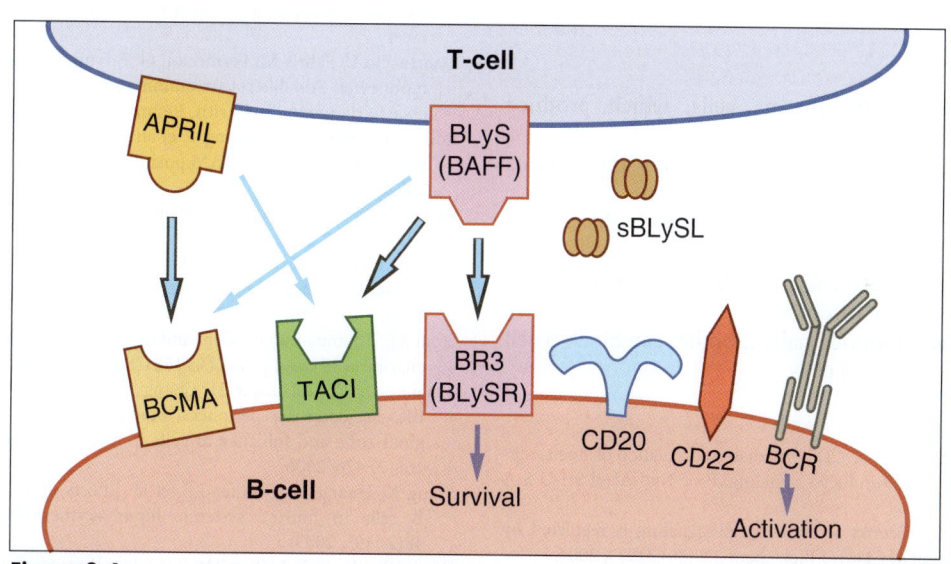

Figure 8-6

The interaction between a T cell–derived cytokine called the *B lymphocyte stimulator (BLyS)* and a proliferation-inducing ligand (APRIL) and their receptors on B cells. BLyS interacts with TACI (membrane-activated calcium-modulator cyclophilin ligand-interactor) and the BLyS-receptor 3 (BLySR3). Engagement of BLyS with its ligands promotes B cell survival and differentiation into plasma cells. APRIL binds to the B cell maturation antigen (BCMA).

The incidence of XLA is unclear; an estimated frequency of 1 per 250,000 live births is considered to be an underestimation.

The immunologic defect has been mapped to the Bruton's kinase gene (*BTK*) which is important in B cell maturation and intracellular signaling pathways. In the maturation process, the pro–B cell is the first committed cell in the B cell lineage that is sensitive to interleukin 7 (IL-7). When stimulated with IL-7, the pro–B cell re-arranges BCR heavy chains to increase the antigen-binding repertoire. *BTK* controls the rearrangement of the μ-chain. A dysfunctional *BTK* gene restricts the μ-chain re-arrangements, which limits the antigen specificity of the BCR. As a consequence, patients with early-onset agammaglobulinemia fail to respond to most antigens.

Treatment of Early-Onset Agammaglobulinemia

To restore normal antibody levels, patients are treated with pooled immunoglobulin administered by the intravenous or the subcutaneous route. Most preparations contain antibodies to bacterial agents and reduce the incidence of pneumonia, meningitis, and intestinal infections. Some intravenous immunoglobulin preparations (RSV-IVIG) contain high

Table 8-1. Fusion Proteins and Monoclonal Antibodies That Inhibit B Cell Differentiation

Name	Origin	Reagent Type	Target	Application
Atacicept	Fusion protein	TACI receptor	Soluble BLyS	Relapsing multiple sclerosis (RMS)
BR3-Fc	Fusion protein	Binding portions of BLyS-receptor 3	TACI and BR3 on B cells	Systemic lupus erythematosis (SLE)
Belimumab	Humanized	Monoclonal antibody	Soluble BLyS	SLE
Epratuzumab	Humanized	Human monoclonal antibody	CD22	Non-Hodgkin's lymphoma and SLE

TACI, membrane-activated calcium–modulator cyclophilin ligand-interactor.

levels of antibodies to respiratory syncytial virus (RSV). RSV infections are common in children under 2 years of age, and usually, RSV does not replicate outside the respiratory tract. However, RSV infection in children with agammaglobulinemia can cause a fatal pneumonia. A more directed therapy for RSV infection is palivizumab, a humanized monoclonal anti-RSV antibody. It is licensed for use in high-risk infants with chronic lung disease and congenital heart diseases.

In patients with chronic sinus infections and respiratory infections, long-term broad-spectrum antibiotic therapy is indicated. Oral antibiotics such as amoxicillin, amoxicillin/clavulanate, and cefuroxime axetil can be used. Intravenous ceftriaxone may be required to treat chronic pulmonary infection or pneumonia.

SUMMARY

- B cells differentiate into plasma cells, which produce antibodies.
- B cell response to protein antigens requires interactions among T cells, B cells, and macrophages.
- B cells can trap, process, and present antigens in the context of class II molecules.
- Endotoxins and polysaccharides can directly activate B cells by cross-linking surface receptors.
- Fusion proteins and monoclonal antibodies can block B cell differentiation into plasma cells.

REFERENCES

Aruffo A, Kanner SB, Sgroi D, et al: CD22-mediated stimulation of T cells regulates T-cell receptor/CD3-induced signaling, Proc Natl Acad Sci U S A 89(21):10242, 1992.

Cherukuri A, Carter RH, Brooks S, et al: B cell signaling is regulated by induced palmitoylation of CD81, J Biol Chem 279(30):31973, 2004.

Cherukuri A, Cheng PC, Sohn HW, et al: The CD19/CD21 complex functions to prolong B cell antigen receptor signaling from lipid rafts, Immunity 14(2):169, 2001.

Dall'Era M, Chakravarty E, Wallace D, et al: Reduced B lymphocyte and immunoglobulin levels after atacicept treatment in patients with systemic lupus erythematosus: Results of a multicenter, phase Ib, double-blind, placebo-controlled, dose-escalating trial, Arthritis Rheum 56(12):4142, 2007.

Ettinger R, Sims GP, Robbins R, et al: IL-21 and BAFF/BLyS synergize in stimulating plasma cell differentiation from a unique population of human splenic memory B cells, J Immunol 178(5):2872, 2007.

Gross JA, Dillon SR, Mudri S, et al: TACI-Ig neutralizes molecules critical for B cell development and autoimmune disease. Impaired B cell maturation in mice lacking BLyS, Immunity 15(2):289, 2001.

Hartung HP: Atacicept: A new B lymphocyte-targeted therapy for multiple sclerosis, Nervenarzt 80(12):1462, 2009.

Kawasaki A, Tsuchiya N, Fukazawa T, et al: Analysis on the association of human BLYS (BAFF, TNFSF13B) polymorphisms with systemic lupus erythematosus and rheumatoid arthritis, Genes Immun 3(7):424, 2002.

Otipoby KL, Andersson KB, Draves KE, et al: CD22 regulates thymus-independent responses and the lifespan of B cells, Nature 384(6610):634, 1996.

Pleiman CM, D'Ambrosio D, Cambier JC, et al: The B-cell antigen receptor complex: Structure and signal transduction, Immunol Today 15(9):393, 1994.

Quartuccio L, Fabris M, Ferraccioli G: B lymphocyte stimulator (BLyS) and monocytes: Possible role in autoimmune diseases with a particular reference to rheumatoid arthritis, Reumatismo 56(3):143, 2004.

Rolli V, Gallwitz M, Wossning T, et al: Amplification of B cell antigen receptor signaling by a Syk/ITAM positive feedback loop, Mol Cell 10(5):1057, 2002.

Smith KG, Fearon DT: Receptor modulators of B-cell receptor signalling—CD19/CD22, Curr Top Microbiol Immunol 245(1):195, 2000.

Snapper CM, Mond JJ: A model for induction of T cell-independent humoral immunity in response to polysaccharide antigens, J Immunol 157(6):2229, 1996.

Stein KE: Thymus-independent and thymus-dependent responses to polysaccharide antigens, J Infect Dis 1651(Suppl):S49, 1992.

Vugmeyster Y, Seshasayee D, Chang W, et al: A soluble BAFF antagonist, BR3-Fc, decreases peripheral blood B cells and lymphoid tissue marginal zone and follicular B cells in cynomolgus monkeys, Am J Pathol 168(2):476, 2006.

Wang X, Huang W, Schiffer LE, et al: Effects of anti-CD154 treatment on B cells in murine systemic lupus erythematosus, Arthritis Rheum 48(2):495, 2003.

Weng WK, Jarvis L, LeBien TW: Signaling through CD19 activates Vav/mitogen-activated protein kinase pathway and induces formation of a CD19/Vav/phosphatidylinositol 3-kinase complex in human B cell precursors, J Biol Chem 269(51):32514, 1994.

Zanetti M, Glotz D: Considerations on thymus-dependent and -independent antigens in acquired and natural immunity, Ann Inst Pasteur Immunol 139(2):192, 1988.

ASSESSMENT QUESTIONS

1. Which of the following are characteristics of a thymus-independent type II antigen?
    I. Lipopolysaccharide endotoxins
    II. Cross-links B cell receptors (BCRs)
    III. Stimulates B cells to produce low affinity antibodies
   A. I
   B. III
   C. I and II
   D. II and III
   E. I, II, and III

2. B cell differentiation to plasma cells is driven by a cytokine called:
   A. BLyS
   B. PALS
   C. TACI
   D. BCMA

3. Which of the following is a biotechnology-derived fusion protein that blocks B cell differentiation into plasma cells?
   A. Abatacept
   B. Alefacept
   C. Atacicept
   D. Efalizumab

4. Which of the following is a characteristic of the B cell receptor?
    I. Resembles an immunoglobulin M (IgM) antibody
    II. Binds to only one type of antigen
    III. Signals to activation pathways
   A. I
   B. III
   C. I and II
   D. II and III
   E. I, II, and III

5. Which of the following interactions are required to produce antibodies to a thymus-dependent antigen?
    I. Antigen and a BCR
    II. CD2 and antigen-bound C3d
    III. B cell class II molecules and the T cell receptor (TCR) on activated T cells
   A. I
   B. III
   C. I and II
   D. II and III
   E. I, II, and III

6. Thymus-independent type I antigens stimulate B cells to produce antibodies by:
   A. Cross-linking BCRs
   B. Binding to BCRs and Toll receptors
   C. Binding to BCRs and CR2
   D. Binding to class II antigens

CHAPTER 9

Antibodies

LEARNING OBJECTIVES

- Describe the basic structure of antibodies
- Discuss the function of the variable and hypervariable portion of antibodies
- Identify the functions of the C_H1–C_H3 regions
- Recognize the definition of the complementarity-determining regions (CDRs)
- Compare and contrast antibody affinity and avidity
- Compare and contrast the structure and antigen-binding capability of Fab and F(ab')$_2$
- Describe the usefulness of Fab fragments in treating drug overdoses
- Compare and contrast the structure and function of immunoglobulin M (IgM) and IgG
- Identify the structure and biologic functions of IgG subclasses
- Identify the clinical implications of IgG subclasses
- Compare and contrast the structure and function of IgA and secretory IgA (sIgA)
- Understand the mechanism used to transport IgA to the exterior
- Understand the role of mucosal-associated lymphoid tissue (MALT) and sIgA in vaccination
- Relate the structure and function of IgD
- Restate the biologic function of IgE
- Locate the IgE C_H4 domain
- Identify the definition of an anamnestic response
- Understand the mechanisms involved in the generation of an anamnestic response
- Understand the role of cytokines in isotypic switching
- Discuss the immunologic defects in transient hypogammaglobulinemia of infancy (THI)
- Discuss the immunologic defects associated with common variable immunodeficiency (CVID)
- Identify symptoms and immunologic defects associated with hyperimmunoglobulinemia E (Job syndrome)
- Describe the drugs used to treat Job syndrome
- Understand the pathophysiology of multiple myeloma
- Define monoclonal antibody
- Describe Bence Jones proteins
- Identify the drugs used to treat multiple myeloma
- Understand the pathophysiology of Waldenström's macroglobulinemia

KEY TERMS

Affinity
Avidity
Anamnestic response
Bence Jones proteins
Complementarity-determining regions (CDRs)
Fab
F(ab')$_2$
Fc
IgM
IgG
IgA
IgD
IgE
Isotypes
Multiple myeloma
Waldenström's macroglobulinemia

INTRODUCTION

Antibodies are soluble proteins produced by plasma cells. They are normally found in peripheral blood and external body fluids such as saliva, tears, and colostrums. Antibodies neutralize viruses or mark antigens or microbes for destruction by phagocytosis or complement lysis. A number of different synonyms for antibodies exist. When serum is placed in an electrical field, blood proteins migrate at different rates, depending on size and charge. Small-molecular-weight albumins migrate rapidly, whereas globulin fractions migrate more slowly. Antibodies are localized in the slow-migrating gamma (γ) fractions and are termed *gammaglobulins*. Ultra-centrifugation also can be used to separate immunoglobulins on the basis of size. On the basis of the sedimentation rate (Svedberg units) in a centrifugal field, antibodies are divided into three different molecular weights: (1) the 7S antibody fraction with a molecular weight of 150,000, (2) the 11S fraction with a molecular weight of 300,000, and (3) the 19S fraction with a molecular weight of 900,000.

ANTIBODY STRUCTURE

Antibodies have a basic structure which consists of pairs of heavy (H) and light (L) chains. Each heavy chain has a molecular weight of 50,000 Daltons. The weight of light chains is approximately 25,000 Daltons. Disulfide bonds link heavy

CHAPTER 9 ANTIBODIES

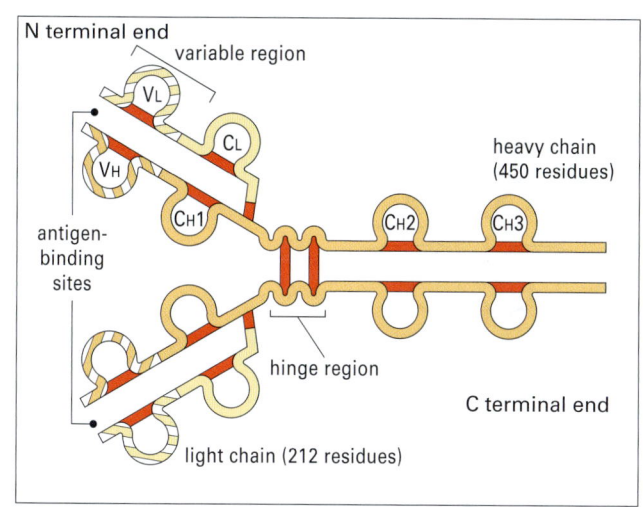

Figure 9-1

The N terminal end of immunoglobulin G (IgG) is characterized by sequence variability (V) in both the heavy and light chains, referred to as the V_H and V_L regions, respectively. The rest of the molecule has a relatively constant (C) structure. The constant portion of the light chain is termed the C_L region. The constant portion of the heavy chain is further divided into three structurally discrete regions: C_H1, C_H2, and C_H3. These globular regions, which are stabilized by intrachain disulfide bonds, are referred to as *domains*. The sites at which the antibody binds antigen are located in the variable domains. The hinge region is a segment of heavy chain between the C_H1 and C_H2 domains. Flexibility in this area permits the two antigen-binding sites to operate independently. There is close pairing of the domains except in the C_H2 region. Carbohydrate moieties are attached to the C_H2 domains. (From Roitt I, Brostoff J, Male D, et al: Immunology, ed 7, Philadelphia, 2006, Mosby.)

chains and attach light chains to heavy chains. Heavy and light chains consist of several different globular domains that have constant or variable amino acid sequences (Figure 9-1).

Heavy-chain constant domains are called *constant regions* (C_H1, C_H2, and C_H3). Heavy-chain C_H1 segments are linked to the variable (V_H) domain, which is part of the antigen-combining site. The C_H2 region is the hinge region that ensures antibody flexibility—the larger the hinge region, the more flexible is the antibody (Figure 9-2). Flexibility is essential because epitopes are often widely spaced on protein molecules or microbes. Attachment to cellular receptors is facilitated by the antibody C_H3 region. However, some antibody subpopulations express an additional heavy-chain region (C_H4) that restricts binding to select cells.

Light chains attached to the heavy chains also have constant (C_L) and variable region (V_L) domains. The V_L domain contributes to antigen binding. These 24-kiloDalton (kDal) light chains are covalently linked to heavy chains via disulfide bonds.

Antibody specificity is determined by the association of V regions from both heavy and light chains. In essence, V segments form a three-dimensional pocket that is the mirror image of the antigen that elicited its production (Figure 9-3).

Within the antigen-binding pocket, small 10-amino-acid hypervariable regions determine specificity at the molecular level. Amino acid sequences that form the three-dimensional antigen pocket are termed *complementarity-determining regions (CDRs)*. Each heavy- and light-chain variable region contains three CDRs.

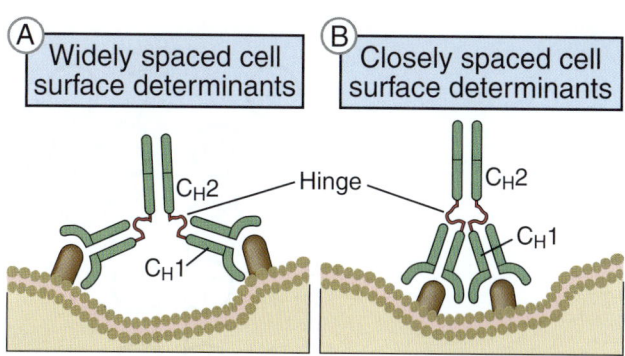

Figure 9-2

Flexibility of antibody molecules. The two antigen-binding sites of an immunoglobulin (Ig) monomer can simultaneously bind to two determinants separated by varying distances. **A**, An immunoglobulin molecule is depicted binding to two widely spaced determinants on a cell surface. **B**, The same antibody is binding to two determinants that are close together. This flexibility is mainly caused by the hinge regions located between the C_H1 and C_H2 domains, which permit independent movement of antigen-binding sites relative to the rest of the molecule. (From Abbas AK, Lichtman AH, Pillai S: Cellular and molecular immunology, ed 6 [updated edition], Philadelphia, 2010, Saunders.)

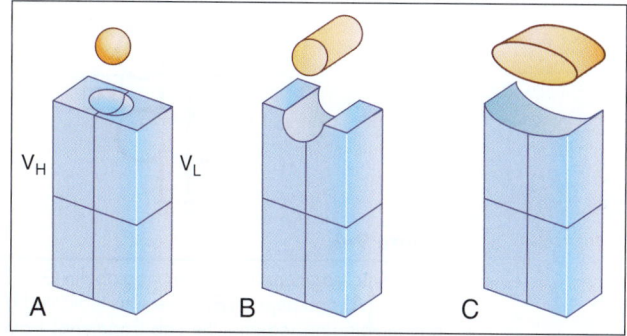

Figure 9-3

Antigens can bind in pockets or grooves or on extended surfaces in the binding sites of antibodies. Schematic representations of the different types of binding sites in a Fab fragment of an antibody are shown: *left*, pocket; *center*, groove; *right*, extended surface.

AFFINITY AND AVIDITY

Antibody binding is described in terms of affinity and avidity. The binding strength or affinity is the result of the interaction between an antibody and a single antigenic determinant. From a practical perspective, antibody affinity is important in determining the rate at which an infection is terminated. Antibodies with high affinity will tightly bind lower concentrations of microbes and quickly terminate an infection. Low-affinity antibodies are most efficient when large antigen concentrations are present, which means that it takes longer to terminate the infections. Antibody avidity is dependent on the number of antibody-combining sites and the number of epitopes in a single antigen. It is the combined strength of multiple interactions between antibodies and epitopes. Avidity will always be geometrically higher than the affinity.

ANTIBODY FRAGMENTS

Porter delineated antibody structure by digesting antibodies with proteolytic papain and pepsin. Papain cleaves the heavy-chain C_H2 domains above the disulfide bonds that connect

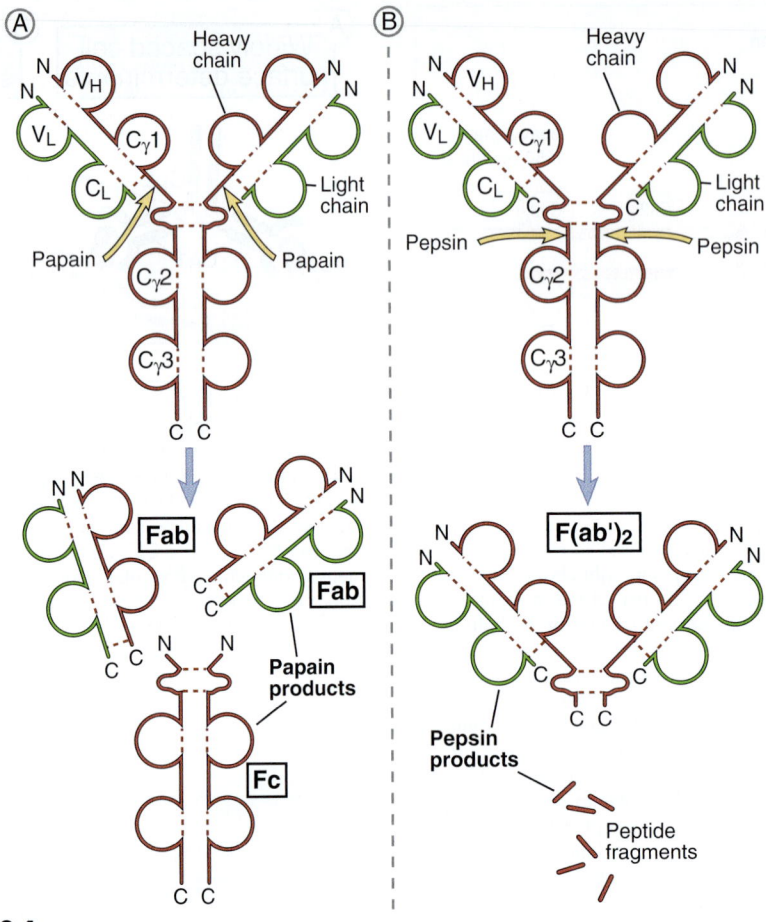

Figure 9-4

Proteolytic fragments of an immunoglobulin G (IgG) molecule. IgG molecules are cleaved by the enzymes papain (**A**) and pepsin (**B**) at the sites indicated by arrows. Papain digestion allows the separation of two antigen-binding regions (the Fab fragments) from the portion of the IgG molecule that binds to complement and Fc receptors (the Fc fragment). Pepsin generates a single bivalent antigen-binding fragment, F(ab')$_2$. (From Abbas AK, Lichtman AH, Pillai S: Cellular and molecular immunology, ed 6 [updated edition], Philadelphia, 2010, Saunders.)

heavy chains and yields three different fragments. The resultant pieces are identical in structure and consist of constant and variable regions of heavy (V$_H$ and C$_H$1) and light (V$_L$ and C$_L$) chains linked by disulfide bonds. These two fragments, each having a molecular weight of 60,000, are called *Fab* (fragment antigen binding). Each Fab binds a single antigen. The remaining fragment, which consists of C$_H$2 and C$_H$3 heavy-chain units, is easily crystallized and is called *Fc* (fraction crystallized). Later studies showed that the Fc portion of antibodies binds to receptors (FcR) on immunocompetent cells (Figure 9-4).

Pepsin cleaves IgG heavy chains at a point below the disulfide bond that links two heavy chains. The resulting fragment consists of two Fab linked together by heavy-chain disulfide bonds. The large-molecular-weight fragments are called F(ab')$_2$. Each F(ab')$_2$ can bind two antigens. The remainder of the antibody is reduced to small peptide fragments that have no biologic function.

CLINICAL USEFULNESS OF FAB FRAGMENTS

Fab fragments are used in the clinic to treat select drug overdoses and envenomations. For example, Fab fragments are commonly used to treat digoxin overdoses or North American *Crotalidae* (rattlesnake) envenomations. Fab fragments neutralize the drug or the venom in blood, and the resulting equilibrium shifts away from target cell binding. Since the molecular weight of the antigen–Fab complexes are usually less than 65,000 molecular weight (MW), they pass through the kidneys and are eliminated in urine. Patients usually begin to recover within 30 minutes of receiving a bolus of Fab fragments.

ANTIBODY ISOTYPES

The five antibody isotypes (IgM, IgG, IgA, IgD, and IgE) are differentiated by the chemical structure of the heavy chain. Antibody isotypes have different molecular structures, have different affinity constants, appear at different times in an immune response, and have different functions (Figure 9-5).

Immunoglobulin M Isotype

Immunoglobulin M (IgM, or 19S) is the antibody formed during the initial response to an antigen or microbe. Following antigen stimulation, IgM-producing plasma cells migrate from the lymph node to bone marrow, where they become long-lived plasma cells. A 5- to 10-day lag time occurs before IgM antibodies appear in blood, and peak IgM levels occur at 21 days. During the response, memory B cells are also produced,

CHAPTER 9 ANTIBODIES   73

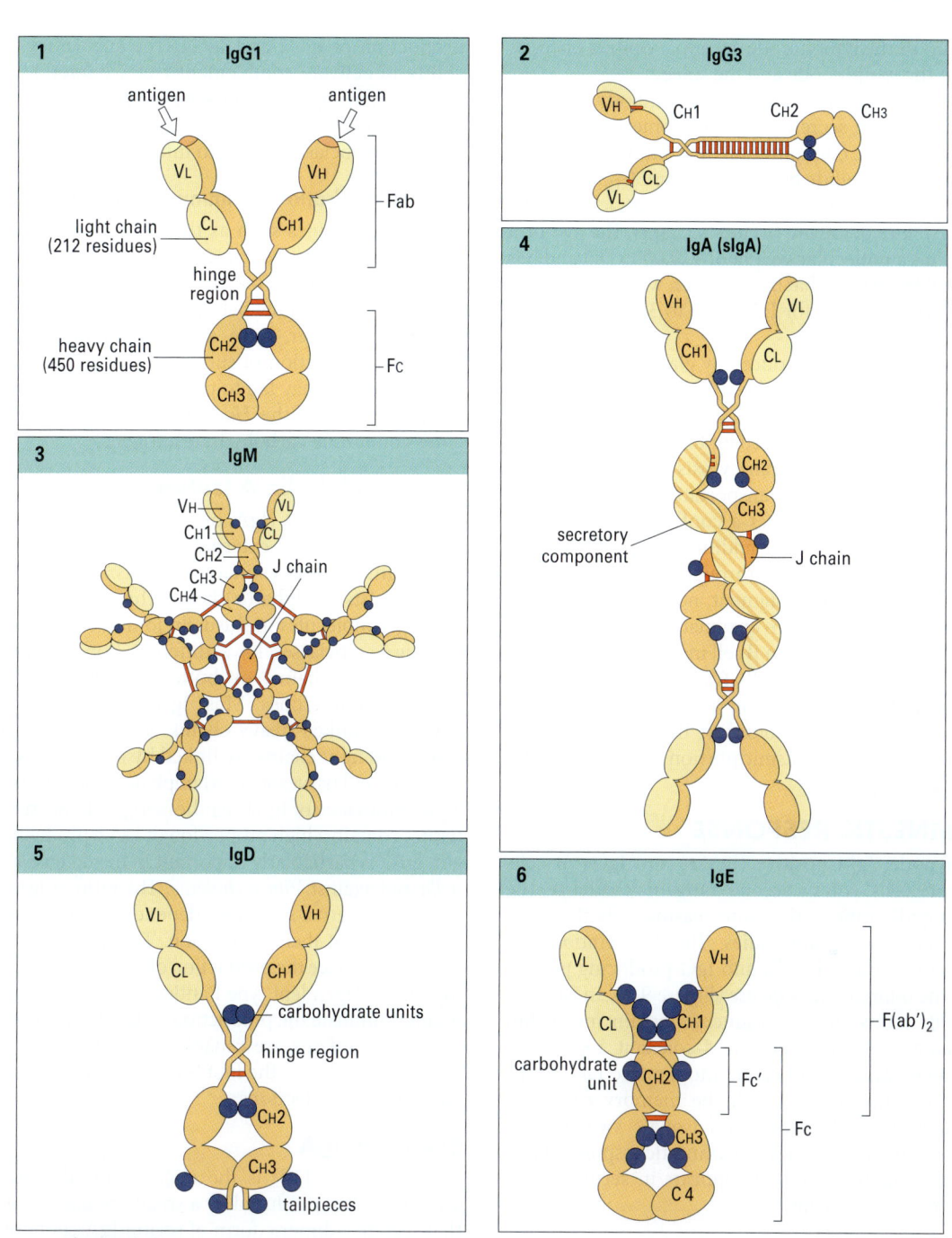

Figure 9-5

Carbohydrate side chains are shown in blue. Inter–heavy (H)–chain disulfide bonds are shown in red, but interchain bonds between H and light (L) chains are omitted. **1,** A model of IgG1 indicating the globular domains of H and L chains. Note the apposition of the C_H3 domains and the separation of the C_H2 domains. The carbohydrate units lie between the C_H2 domains. **2,** Polypeptide chain structure of human IgG3. Note the elongated hinge region. **3,** IgM H- chains have five domains with disulfide bonds cross-linking adjacent C_H3 and C_H4 domains. The possible location of the J chain is shown. IgM does not have extended hinge regions, but flexion can occur about the C_H2 domains. **4,** The secretory component of sIgA is probably wound around the dimer and attached by two disulfide bonds to the C_H2 domain of one IgA monomer. The J chain is required to join the two subunits. **5,** This diagram of IgD shows the domain structure and a characteristically large number of oligosaccharide units. Note also the presence of a hinge region and short octapeptide tailpieces. **6,** IgE can be cleaved by enzymes to give the fragments F(ab')$_2$, Fc, and Fc'. Note the absence of a hinge region. (From Roitt I, Brostoff J, Male D, et al: Immunology, ed 7, Philadelphia, 2006, Mosby.)

and they remain in the lymph node germinal centers or recirculate between the lymph node and the spleen.

IgM has the basic heavy- or light-chain antibody structure but exists in pentameric, secretory, and monomeric configurations. In the pentameric configuration, five antibody units are covalently linked by disulfide bonds at adjacent C_H3 domains. An additional molecule, called a *J-chain*, also is attached to the penultimate cysteines of the mu (μ) heavy chains. The five-unit IgM molecule has a molecular weight of 970,000 kDal and has 10 antigen-combining sites that bind antigen with high avidity. In serum, the normal range for IgM is 85 to 350 mg/100 mL, and the half-life is 5 to 6 days.

Secretory IgM (sIgM) is produced by glandular-associated B cells. During synthesis, a specialized J-chain is added to the molecule. The J chain serves two functions. Along with the Fc portion of the antibody, it is required for binding to the poly-Ig receptors (pIgRs) that mediate transcytosis through epithelial cells. In addition to its role in transportation to the exterior, the addition of the J chain causes a conformational change in the molecule, which allows the addition of an 83,000-MW fragment of the pIgR as it traverses through epithelial cells into extracellular fluids. The pIgR fragment, now called the *secretory piece*, protects the sIgM from enzymatic degradation.

Monomeric IgM is localized in B cell membranes and functions as a B cell antigen receptor (BCR). The membrane form has an additional 41 amino acids in a C_H4 domain, and 25 hydrophobic amino acids are found in the transmembrane portion. The remaining cytoplasmic portion contains 16 polar amino acids (see Chapter 8).

THE ANAMNESTIC RESPONSE

In the lymph node, IgM-positive (IgM+) and IgG+ B cells serve as memory cells. After a second antigenic challenge, the IgG+ B cells rapidly differentiate into plasma cells that produce antigen-specific IgG antibodies. The proliferation and differentiation of memory B cells into IgG-producing plasma cells is called the *anamnestic response* (Figure 9-6). In isotypic switching, light chains and V_H segments remain intact, but γ-chain–constant regions replace IgM-constant regions in the final antibody structure to create monomeric IgG. IgM+ memory cells function to replenish the memory cell pool. They undergo rapid proliferation and isotype switching to become IgG+ memory cells. In the anamnestic response, large concentrations of high-affinity IgG appears in serum 1 to 3 days after exposure to antigens.

Immunoglobulin G Isotype

Immunoglobulin G (IgG, or 7S) antibodies consist of two H chains and two L chains. Unlike IgM, the smaller IgG is able to penetrate extracellular and intracellular spaces. IgG binds antigens with both high affinity and low avidity. Normal adult serum levels range from 640 to 1350 mg/100 mL. In peripheral blood, the IgG antibody population has an average half-life of 23 days and is the only isotype that crosses the placenta.

Immunoglobulin G Subclasses

Subclasses IgG1, IgG2, IgG3, and IgG4 are differentiated on the basis of the size of the hinge region, position of interchain disulfide bonds, and molecular weight. IgG3 has a molecular weight of 170 kDal, whereas the other subtypes have a molecular weight of 146 kDal. IgG1 and IgG3 are usually produced in response to proteins. Carbohydrate antigens elicit the production of IgG2 and IgG4. The subclasses differ in their ability to activate complement (see Chapter 11) or bind and react to Fc receptors on phagocytic cells. Complement activation by IgG1 and IgG3 is 40 times higher than that by IgG2. The IgG4 subclass appears to inhibit complement activation.

Clinical Implications of Immunoglobulin G Subtype

Common vaccines such as those for *Haemophilus*, *Pneumococcus*, and *Neisseria meningitides* require a vigorous IgG2 response for host protection. In most infants, synthesis of IgG2 and IgG4 begins between 2 and 4 months of age. Some children, however, have a developmental block that prevents the production of subclasses until 2 and 6 years of age. These children may fail to produce protective antibodies after administration of the *Haemophilus* and meningococcal vaccines containing carbohydrate antigens.

Immunoglobulin A Isotype

Immunoglobulin A (IgA, or 11S) is a dimeric antibody found in both serum and external secretions such as tears, saliva colostrums, and intestinal secretions. The basic dimeric IgA unit consists of alpha (α) heavy chains and two light chains. Two IgA molecules are usually joined together by a J-chain. Two IgA subclasses have different bonding between heavy chains, light chains, or both and resistance to proteases secreted by microbes. Most IgA1 is found as a dimer with covalently linked heavy chains. In the IgA2 form, both the heavy and light chains are linked by ionic bonds.

Lymphoid tissues such as lymph nodes and the spleen contain a predominance of IgA1-synthesizing cells. Secretory lymphoid tissues contain a high proportion of IgA2-producing cells. In the gut, IgA2 is particularly important in the defense against *Salmonella* and against *Vibrio cholerae*. The ratio of IgA subclasses in serum or external secretions depends on the nature of the antigens that elicit their production. Thymus–dependent antigens (proteins) induce the production of IgA1 antibodies. Conversely, thymus-independent type I antigens (lipopolysaccharide endotoxins) stimulate the production of IgA2 antibodies.

Human infants are capable of synthesizing IgA at 2 to 3 weeks of age. IgA is the first line of defense against respiratory and intestinal infections.

Secretory IgA

Secretory IgA (11S) is the major antibody found in bodily secretions. It is produced by a small population of plasma cells that secrete a dimeric form of serum IgA containing a J chain. The transport of IgA from blood to external fluids is identical to that described for secretory IgM. IgA binds to a polymeric Ig Fc receptor (pIgR) on the internal surface of epithelial cells. Endocytosis creates intracellular vesicles containing IgA–pIgR complexes. The secretory piece, which is a cleavage fragment of pIgR, is added to the IgA in the intracellular vesicles. The secretory piece coils around IgA and prevents its digestion in the acidic external fluids. During exocytosis, a fragment of the secretory piece is removed, and free sIgA is secreted into external fluids. In external fluids, sIgA is dimeric with a J chain and the secretory piece. The transport process for IgA is shown in Figure 9-7.

Clinical Importance of Secretory IgA

Lymphocytes producing sIgA are localized in the mucosal associated lymphoid tissue (MALT). Because the MALT is interconnected, stimulation of one mucosal surface ultimately

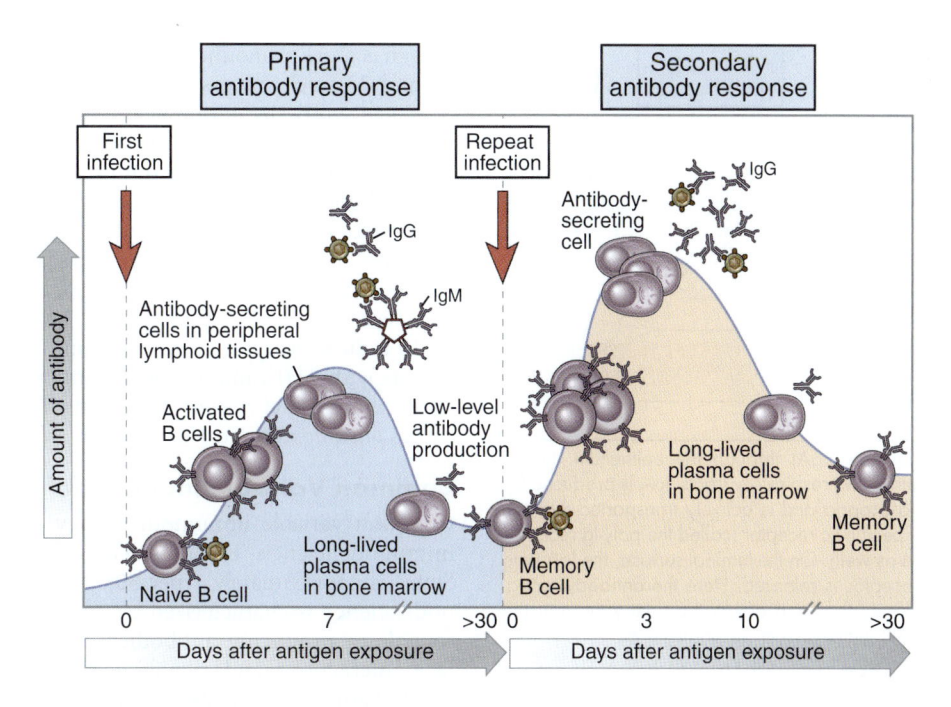

Feature	Primary response	Secondary response
Time lag after immunization	Usually 5–10 days	Usually 1–3 days
Peak response	Smaller	Larger
Antibody isotype	Usually IgM > IgG	Relative increase in IgG and, under certain situations, in IgA or IgE
Antibody affinity	Lower average affinity, more variable	Higher average affinity (affinity maturation)
Induced by	All immunogens	Only protein antigens
Required immunization	Relatively high doses of antigens, optimally with adjuvants (for protein antigens)	Low doses of antigens; adjuvants may not be necessary

Figure 9-6

In a primary immune response, naïve B cells are stimulated by the antigen, become activated, and differentiate into antibody-secreting cells that produce antibodies specific for the eliciting antigen. Some of the antibody-secreting plasma cells survive in bone marrow and continue to produce antibodies for long periods. Long-lived memory B cells are also generated during the primary response. A secondary immune response is elicited when the same antigen stimulates these memory B cells, leading to more rapid proliferation and differentiation and production of greater quantities of specific antibody than are produced in the primary response. The principal characteristics of primary and secondary antibody responses are summarized in the table. These features are typical of T cell–dependent antibody responses to protein antigens. (From Abbas AK, Lichtman AH, Pillai S: Cellular and molecular immunology, ed 6 [updated edition], Philadelphia, 2010, Saunders.)

provides protection to all mucosal surfaces. The mechanism for providing protection to all mucosal surfaces is simple. Antigen-stimulated MALT lymphocytes enter the lymph and migrate to a regional lymph node. Antigen-specific IgA-producing B cells from the lymph node enter the bloodstream and localize in all mucosal lymphoid tissues, thereby providing widely distributed protection. Vaccine makers make use of this interconnection for their purposes. For example, intranasal administration of attenuated influenza vaccine stimulates the MALT and provides protection to all respiratory mucosal surfaces.

Immunoglobulin D (IgD)

Immunoglobulin D (IgD) is composed of two delta (δ) heavy chains and two light chains. IgD is bound to B cells via the Fc receptor or is free in serum. Because it has a half-life of 2 to 3 days, the plasma concentration is less than 1% of the total immunoglobulin in serum.

Emerging evidence suggests that IgD-producing B cells are auto-reactive lymphocytes that have escaped clonal deletion. IgD-expressing B cells may actually represent a separate lineage of B cells called *B-1 lymphocytes*. Autoantibodies produced by these lymphocytes react with epithelial tissue, red

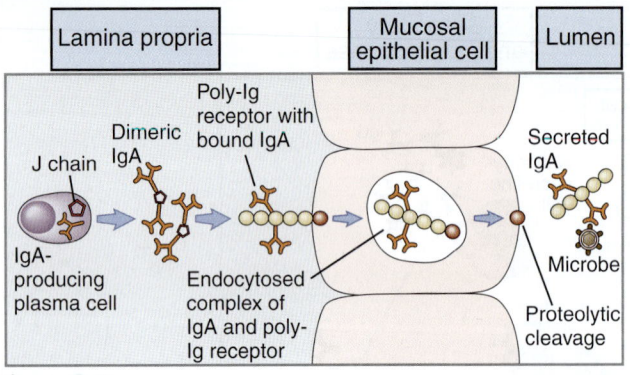

Figure 9-7

Transport of immunoglobulin A (IgA) through the epithelium. In the mucosa of the gastrointestinal and respiratory tracts, IgA is produced by plasma cells in the lamina propria and is actively transported through epithelial cells by an IgA-specific Fc receptor (called the poly-Ig receptor because it recognizes IgM as well). On the luminal surface, the IgA with a portion of the bound receptor is released. Here the antibody recognizes ingested or inhaled microbes and blocks their entry through the epithelium. (From Abbas AK, Lichtman AH: Basic immunology: functions and disorders of the immune system, ed 2 [updated edition], Philadelphia, 2006, Saunders.)

blood cell membranes, cellular receptors and, single-stranded or double-stranded deoxyribonucleic acid (DNA) and cause autoimmune disease. Autoantibodies produced by B-1 lymphocytes mediate disorders such as systemic lupus erythematosus (SLE), myasthenia gravis, autoimmune hemolytic anemia, and idiopathic cytopenia purpura.

Immunoglobulin E

Immunoglobulin E (IgE) is the major mediator of asthma, urticaria, and rhinitis, which are classified as immediate allergic reactions. IgE is similar to IgG in structure, but IgE has two unique features: (1) The epsilon (ε) heavy chain has a high (12%) carbohydrate content and has an additional constant region (C_H4). The unique C_H4 region restricts IgE binding to high-affinity receptors (Fcε-RI) on basophiles and mast cells, which contain preformed granules of heparin and histamine.

Antigen-induced cross-linkage of receptor-bound IgE initiates a process that culminates in the release of histamine and heparin, which increase vascular permeability and promote contraction of smooth muscle. In addition to a role in allergic reactions, IgE plays a critical role in the immune response to parasites such as *Schistosoma mansoni* and *Trichinella spirillum*. Histamine induces muscular contractions in the intestine, which aid in the expulsion of parasites.

PRIMARY IMMUNODEFICIENCIES

Transient Hypogammaglobulinemia of Infancy

In most infants, transient hypogammaglobulinemia of infancy (THI) is short lived and related to the catabolism rate of passively acquired maternal antibodies that provide protective immunity in the infant. Rapid catabolism of maternal antibodies may occur before the infant can synthesize his or her own antibodies. The lack of antibodies creates a "physiologic antibody trough" that puts the infant at risk for infection. The trough is more pronounced in premature babies born between 26 and 32 weeks of gestation. At 3 to 6 months, the infant begins to synthesize antibodies.

Some infants also have a developmental block that prevents both IgG and IgA synthesis until reaching the age of 6 years. The pathophysiology of the developmental block is not fully delineated, but it may be caused by the aberrant synthesis of cytokines. Infants with THI have increased synthesis of tumor necrosis factor alpha (TNF-α), TNF-β, and interleukin 10 (IL-10). Increased TNF suppresses the IgG and IgA responses. IL-10 induces isotypic switching from the IgG family to IgD. Infants with THI cannot produce antibodies to carbohydrate antigens and are at risk for developing infections with *Streptococcus pneumoniae* and *Haemophilus influenzae* type B.

Common Variable Immunodeficiency

Common variable immunodeficiency (CVID) is a primary immunodeficiency. The prevalence of CVID in the United States is approximately 1 per 50,000 live births. This immunodeficiency is characterized by a paucity of B cells that are capable of producing antibodies. Molecular defects in surface interactions and signaling pathways are common in CVID pathways. Patients have reduced numbers of cell surface CD40, which is critical to B cell proliferation. Defective protein kinase C activation and tyrosine phosphorylation also are found in the BCR signaling pathway. Individuals with CVID have recurrent infections with *Haemophilus influenzae*, *Streptococcus pneumoniae*, *Moraxella catarrhalis*, and *Staphylococcus aureus*. Some patients also may have infections by uncommon pathogens such as *Pneumocystis carinii*, *Giardia lamblia*, and *Mycoplasma pneumoniae*.

Treatment of IgG Immunodeficiencies

For most primary immunoglobulin immunodeficiencies, the cycle of recurrent infections can be interrupted by immunoglobulin replacement therapy. However, patients with IgG subclass immunodeficiency are usually not treated with immunoglobulin replacement therapy unless they fail to respond to both protein and polysaccharide antigens. Aggressive antibiotic therapy is indicated for preventing *S. pneumoniae* and *H. influenzae* infections. Patients with immunoglobulin deficiencies also have a high frequency of *G. lamblia* infections, which require a course of metronidazole to reduce diarrhea.

Selective IgA Deficiency

IgA deficiency is a common immunodeficiency with an estimated frequency between 1 per 200 and 1 per 1000 live births. In children, recurrent infections are not normally associated with IgA deficiency, which can be attributed to a compensatory mechanism involving secretory IgM. Many adults with IgA deficiency, however, have recurrent otitis media, sinusitis, bronchitis, and gastrointestinal (GI) infections. Between 10% and 40% of adults also have anti-IgA antibodies and have severe allergic or immune complex reactions following administration of immunoglobulins during replacement therapy.

Defects in IgA production may be the result of an intrinsic B cell defect; inadequate or defective CD4+ helper T cells; excessive IgA suppressor cells; and the suppressive effects of maternal IgA. The presence of anti-IgA antibodies in patients also suggests that a break occurs in peripheral tolerance.

Treatment of IgA Deficiency

No treatment for IgA deficiency is currently available. Antibiotic treatment of sinopulmonary and GI infections are indicated. To boost immunity, patients can be immunized with the pneumococcal polysaccharide vaccine. However, not all patients are capable of mounting an immune response to carbohydrate antigens.

Hyperimmunoglobulinemia E (Job Syndrome)

Job syndrome consists of a constellation of eczematous dermatitis, recurrent skin boils, skin abscesses, and cystic lung disease caused by *S. aureus*. Patients also have coarse facial features as well as abnormalities in the skeleton, connective tissue, and dentition.

Several immunologic defects are associated with Job syndrome. A reversal of the Th1:Th2 ratio in peripheral blood is seen. Th2 cells and IL-4 are elevated, which results in isotypic switching to IgE production. The low number of Th1 with defective production of cytokines and adhesion factors impairs inflammatory responses.

Treatment of Job Syndrome

Each clinical problem is usually treated separately. Topical steroids and tacrolimus are used to control skin eruptions. Drug coverage for staphylococcal infections is dependent on whether the *Staphylococccus* is resistant or sensitive to common cell wall inhibitors.

PLASMA CELL DYSCRASIAS

Multiple Myeloma

Multiple myeloma is a neoplasm within the marrow of the axial skeletal system. It is characterized by the uncontrolled proliferation of a single plasma cell clone. In bone marrow, proliferation of plasma cells causes soft tissue masses (plasmacytomas). Because the plasmacytoma is derived from a single plasma cell clone, antibodies have the same isotype, antigen specificity, and affinity constant. These antibodies are called *monoclonal antibodies* because they are produced by a single B cell clone and have striking homogeneity. Some free antibody light chains are found in serum from patients with multiple myeloma. Light chains excreted into urine are termed *Bence Jones proteins,* thus named after the British physician who first described the proteins.

Bone destruction is also associated with multiple myeloma. High levels of IL-6 produced by a plasmacytoma cause the release of osteoclast-stimulating factor (OSF). Activated osteoclasts destroy the mineralized bone matrix and release calcium into blood.

Bone marrow destruction often results in compression fractures of the spine and weight-bearing bones. Increased calcium levels in the blood also damage the kidneys. Kidney failure is the leading cause of death in patients with multiple myeloma.

Treatment of Multiple Myeloma

Treatment of multiple myeloma is complicated. Several combinations of chemotherapeutics have been used to reduce the tumor mass. The most commonly used regimen is melphalan and prednisone. However, quicker therapeutic results have been reported with a combination of vincristine, Adriamycin, and dexamethasone (VAD) therapy. Bisphosphonates are also administered to increase bone healing and prevent hypocalcemia.

Waldenström's Macroglobulinemia

Waldenström's macroglobulinemia is a rare non-Hodgkin's lymphoma, which causes an overproduction of monoclonal IgM. IgM levels above 40 g/L increase the viscosity of serum. Hyperviscosity causes headaches, confusion, dizziness, and deafness.

Treatment of Waldenström's Macroglobulinemia

Plasmapheresis is used to reduce the levels of serum IgM and restore normal viscosity. Maintenance plasmapheresis may be required to keep the patient asymptomatic. Chemotherapy must also be used to control the proliferation of IgM-secreting cells.

SUMMARY

- Antibodies are the first line of defense against exogenous antigens.
- Antibodies mark the targets for destruction by phagocytosis or complement lysis.
- The five different antibody isotypes differ in structure and function.
- On second exposure to an antigen, an anamnestic response occurs, with isotypic switching from IgM to IgG.
- Secretory IgA and IgM are found in external secretions and are the first line of defense against respiratory pathogens.
- IgE is the antibody that is involved in immediate allergic reactions such as asthma, urticaria, and rhinitis.
- Transient or variable immunoglobulin deficiencies increase the risk of infections with *Streptococcus pneumoniae*, *Haemophilus influenzae* type B, and *Staphylococcus aureus*.
- Multiple myeloma is a B cell malignancy that is characterized by destruction of skeletal bone and the production of monoclonal antibodies.

REFERENCES

Almogren AB, Senior W, Loomes LM, et al: Structural and functional consequences of cleavage of human secretory and human serum immunoglobulin A1 by proteinases from *Proteus mirabilis* and *Neisseria meningitidis*, Infect Immun 71(6):3349, 2003.

Bjornson AB, Detmers PA: The pentameric structure of IgM is necessary to enhance opsonization of *Bacteroides thetaiotaomicron* and *Bacteroides fragilis* via the alternative complement pathway, Microb Pathog 19(2):117, 1995.

Brewer JW, Corley RB: Late events in assembly determine the polymeric structure and biological activity of secretory IgM, Mol Immunol 34(4):323, 1997.

Burton DR, Woof JM: Human antibody effector function, Adv Immunol 51:1, 1992.

Fallgreen-Gebauer E, Gebauer W, Bastian A, et al: The covalent linkage of secretory component to IgA. Structure of sIgA, Biol Chem Hoppe Seyler 374(11):1023, 1993.

Fonseca R, Bergsagel PL, Drach J, et al: International Myeloma Working Group molecular classification of multiple myeloma: Spotlight review, Leukemia 23(12):2210, 2009.

Gotz H, Kirschbaum R: Immunoglobulins gamma D (IgD) and gamma E (IgE). Structure, function and clinical importance [translation], Med Klin 66(51):1749, 1971.

Gould HJ, Sutton BJ, Beavil AJ, et al: The biology of IGE and the basis of allergic disease, Annu Rev Immunol 21:579, 2003.

Harris LJ, Larson SB, MacPherson A: Comparison of intact antibody structures and the implications for effector function, Adv Immunol 72:191, 1999.

Krivan G, Gacs G, et al: Hyperimmunoglobulinemia E (Job) syndrome [translation], Orv Hetil 132(7):369, 1991.

Porter RR: Separation and isolation of fractions of rabbit gamma-globulin containing the antibody and antigenic combining sites, Nature 182(4636):670, 1958.

Schur PH: IgG subclasses—a review, Ann Allergy 58(2):89–96, 99, 1987.

Shakib F, Stanworth DR: Human IgG subclasses in health and disease. (A review). Part II, Ric Clin Lab 10(4):561, 1980.

ASSESSMENT QUESTIONS

1. Which of the following antibodies is the first antibody produced during an immune response?
   A. IgM
   B. IgE
   C. IgA
   D. IgD

2. IgE antibodies bind to:
   I. Basophiles
   II. Mast cells
   III. Monocytes
   A. I
   B. III
   C. I and II
   D. II and III
   E. I, II, and III

3. Which of the following antibodies is found in external secretions?
   A. IgD
   B. IgG
   C. sIgA
   D. IgE

4. Bone destruction in multiple myeloma patients is caused by:
   A. Activation of osteoclasts
   B. Activation of osteoblasts
   C. Production of IL-4
   D. Production of IL-2

5. Which of the following antibody fragments can bind two antigens?
   A. Fc
   B. Fab
   C. F(ab')$_2$
   D. Fd

6. Antibody isotypes are differentiated on the basis of:
   I. Heavy chain structure
   II. Light chain structure
   III. Variable region of light chains
   A I
   B. III
   C I and II
   E. II and III
   F. I, II, and III

CHAPTER 10

Antibody Diversity

LEARNING OBJECTIVES

- Recognize the three theories that explain antibody diversity
- Compare and contrast genes that code for light chains and heavy chains
- Recognize the key features of combinatorial diversity
- Explain the biologic function of complementarity regions 1, 2, and 3
- Discuss the role of the recognition signal sequence (RSS) in recombination
- Relate the biologic significance of the 12/23 rule in the recombination of V(D)J genes
- Understand the role of *RAG-1* and *RAG-2* in recombination
- Identify the role of the Artemis enzyme in recombination
- Understand how messenger ribonucleic acid (mRNA) slicing attaches C regions to VJ or VDJ
- Define junctional diversity
- Relate junctional diversity to the antigen-combining pocket
- Compare and contrast recombination events conferring diversity in the T cell receptor (TCR), B cell receptor (BCR), and antibodies
- Compare and contrast the functions of P-nucleotides and N-nucleotides in generating junctional diversity
- Identify the definition of allelic exclusion
- Explain the role of affinity maturation in immune response

KEY TERMS

Affinity maturation
Allelic exclusion
Artemis
Combinatorial diversity
Deoxynucleotidyl transferase
Junctional diversity
Ligase
Messenger ribonucleic acid (mRNA) splicing
Nonhomologous end joining
One turn–two turn rule
P-nucleotides and N-nucleotides
RAG enzymes
Recognition signal sequences
Somatic mutation
Signal joints

INTRODUCTION

Three theories have been put forth to explain antibody diversity, which allows B cells to generate an antibody repertoire capable of reacting with a wide range of antigens: (1) The *germ-line theory* postulates that separate genes exist for each antibody molecule and that the antibody repertoire is largely inherited. (2) The *deoxyribonucleic acid (DNA) rearrangement theory* proposes that a limited number of genes undergo genetic rearrangements to create antibody populations. (3) Finally, the *somatic mutation theory* proposes that a limited number of inherited genes undergo mutations to general antibody repertoires. In vivo and in vitro studies have demonstrated that both the DNA rearrangement theory and the somatic mutation theory provide the most plausible explanations for antibody diversity.

Antibodies are encoded by different germ-line genetic loci. Variable (V) region, joining (J) region, and constant (C) region gene products are assembled into a functional antibody. Variable portion genes (V) code for amino acids that constitute the framework regions of the variable region, and three hypervariable complementarity-determining regions (CDR1, CDR2, and CDR3). The hypervariable regions form the three-dimensional antigen-binding pocket. Antibody specificity is determined by the specific amino acid sequences in CDR3. The joining (J) segment is, in reality, part of the V region and provides some of the framework for the antigen-binding pocket. Only heavy chains have an additional diversity (D) gene.

Antibody diversity is generated from the large number of V, J, D, and C genes available for recombination. Light-chain loci have 30 to 35 genes encoding for the variable (V_L) regions (Table 10-1). Five to seven genes code for J_L segments in kappa (κ) or lambda (λ) light chains, respectively. Lambda and kappa light chains have one highly conserved constant region.

Heavy chains are larger than the light chains. A hundred genes code for heavy-chain variable (V_H) regions. Diversity (D) genes (N=23) are inserted between V and J genes. J genes (N=5) are linked to the constant region (N=5). The constant region may be from one of the five antibody isotypes (mu [μ], gamma [γ], alpha [α], epsilon [ε], or delta [δ]). An assembled heavy chain consists of VJDC gene products (Figure 10-1).

COMBINATORIAL DIVERSITY

The rearrangement of genes takes advantage of recognition signal sequences (RSS) flanking the V, J, and D sequences. The RSSs consist of a heptamer (5'CACAGTG-3') followed by either 12 bases (RSS 12) or 23 bases (RSS 23) and an AT-rich nonamer (5'-ACAAAAACC-3'). Genes can only recombine when they are located on the same side of the chromosome. RSSs align genes on the same side of the DNA because the spacer placement also corresponds to one (12 AA) or two turns (23 AA) of DNA. This recombination restriction is called the *12/23 rule* or the *one turn–two turn* rule. Only RSS 12 and RSS 23 segments can combine.

Table 10-1 Number of Genes Coding for V, D, J, and C Regions in Light and Heavy Chains

	Kappa Light Chains	Lambda Chains	Heavy Chains
Variable segments	30	35	100
Diversity segment	0	0	23
Joining segment	5	7	5
Constant region	1	1	5*
Potential different antibodies	150	245	115,000

*Constant region for immunoglobulin G (IgG), IgM, IgA, IgD, and IgE. Total possible antibodies based on recombination of lambda, kappa, and heavy chains: $150 \times 245 \times 115{,}500 = 4{,}226{,}255{,}000 = 4.2 \times 10^9$.

LIGHT CHAIN VJ RECOMBINATION

The two types of antibody light chains are called *lambda* and *kappa* light chains. A single antibody can have either two kappa light chains or two lambda light chains, but not both. Recombination of light chain V and J provides the simplest example of recombination. V_L RSSs have a 23-base spacer on the 3' end. Joining genes have a 12-base RSS on the 5' end.

Light chain V and J coding genes or exons are separated by a single intron, and the assembly of the light chain requires only one recombination event. *RAG-1* and *RAG-2* enzymes, which are part of a recombinase family, facilitate the recombination of genes. Tetrameric complexes of *RAG-1* and *RAG-2* bind to 23-base RSSs on a V_L gene and a 12-base spacer on the J_L gene and bring the genes close. As the genes move closer, a large loop, called a *signal joint*, is created. The loop contains introns located between the two coding genes. As the signal joint is deleted from the chromosome, *RAG-1* nicks one strand of the double-stranded DNA between the coding gene and the RSS heptamer. The 3'OH group from the nicked strand reacts with 5'OH on the same strand to form a hairpin. *RAG-1* then attacks the second strand and forms another strand-specific hairpin curve (Figure 10-2).

The hairpins must be removed from the coding ends before V and J genes can be ligated. The opening of the hairpins is facilitated by a nuclease called *Artemis* and DNA-dependent kinase (DNA-PK). Using ligase IV, the double strands are tied together by using a specialized process called *nonhomologous end joining (NHEJ)*. The process is nonhomologous because strand breaks are ligated without requiring a template.

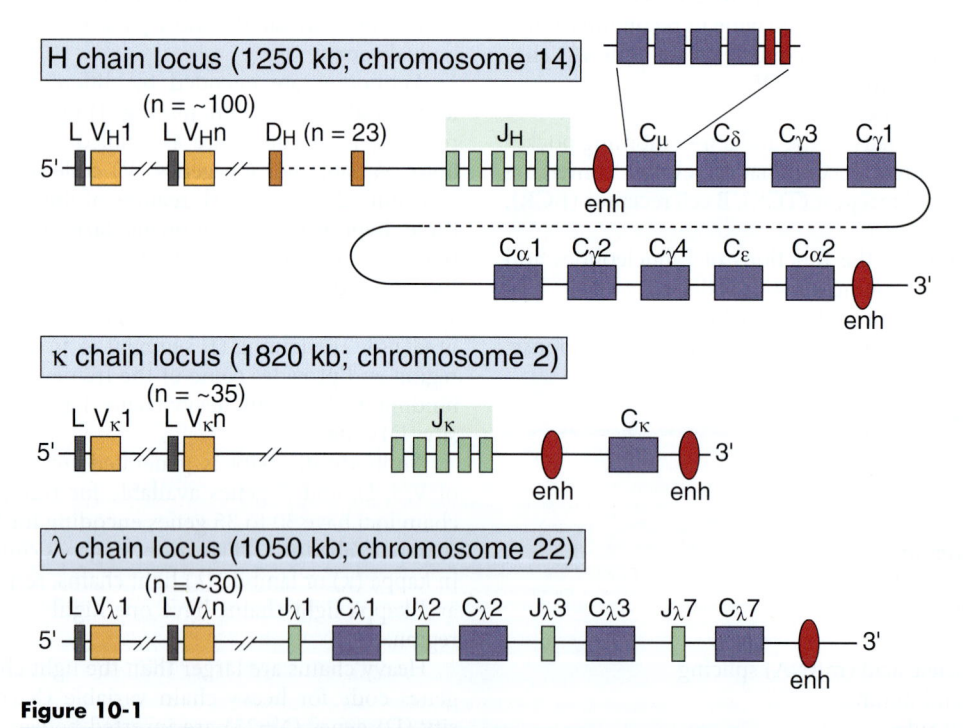

Figure 10-1

Germ-line organization of human immunoglobulin (Ig) loci. The human heavy chain, κ-light chain, and λ-light chain loci are shown. Only functional genes are shown; pseudogenes have been omitted for simplicity. Exons and introns are not drawn to scale. Each C_H gene is shown as a single box but is composed of several exons, as illustrated for C_H. Gene segments are indicated as follows: *L*, leader (often called signal sequence); *V*, variable; *D*, diversity; *J*, joining; *C*, constant; *enh*, enhancer. (From Abbas AK, Lichtman AH, Pillai S: Cellular and molecular immunology, ed 6 [updated edition], Philadelphia, 2010, Saunders.)

CHAPTER 10 ANTIBODY DIVERSITY 81

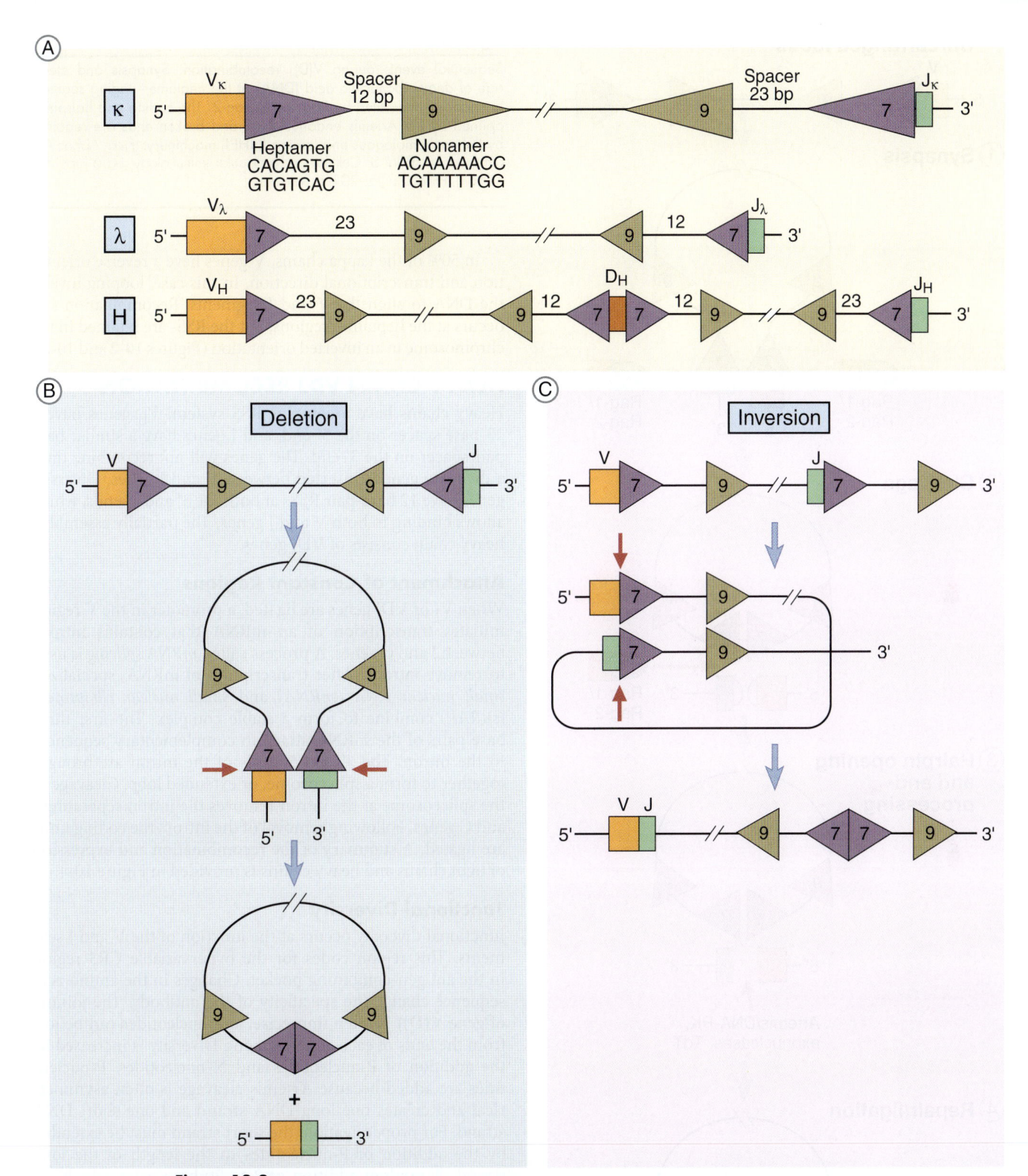

Figure 10-2

V(D)J recombination. The deoxyribonucleic acid (DNA) sequences and mechanisms involved in recombination in the Ig gene loci are depicted. The same sequences and mechanisms apply to recombinations in the T cell receptor (TCR) loci. **A,** Conserved heptamer (7-bp) and nonamer (9-bp) sequences, separated by 12-bp or 23-bp spacers, are located adjacent to V and J exons (for κ- and λ-loci) or to V, D, and J exons (in the H-chain locus). The V(D)J recombinase recognizes these recombination signal sequences and brings the exons together. **B,** Recombination of V and J exons may occur by deletion of intervening DNA and ligation of the V and J segments. **C,** Or, it may occur if the V gene is in the opposite orientation, by inversion of the DNA followed by ligation of adjacent gene segments. Red arrows indicate the sites where germ-line sequences are cleaved prior to their ligation to other Ig or TCR gene segments. (From Abbas AK, Lichtman AH, Pillai S: Cellular and molecular immunology, ed 6 [updated edition], Philadelphia, 2010, Saunders.)

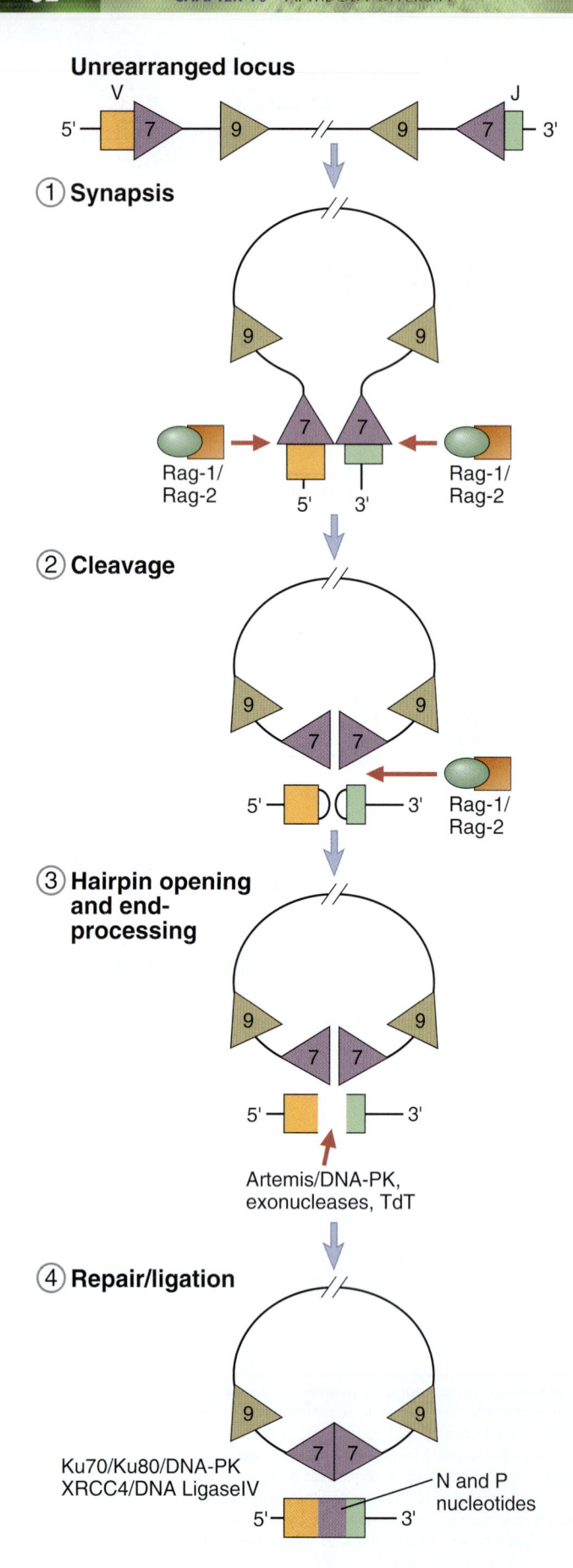

Figure 10-3

Sequential events during V(D)J recombination. Synapsis and cleavage of deoxyribonucleic acid (DNA) at the heptamer–coding segment boundary is mediated by Rag-1 and Rag-2. The coding end hairpin is opened by the Artemis endonuclease, and broken ends are repaired by the nonhomologous end joining (NHEJ) machinery. (From Abbas AK, Lichtman AH, Pillai S: Cellular and molecular immunology, ed 6 [updated edition], Philadelphia, 2010, Saunders.)

In 50% of the kappa chains, V genes have a reverse orientation and transcriptional direction. In this case, looping inverts the DNA to align the V and J segments. Recombination still occurs at the heptamer regions, but the RSSs are retained in the chromosome in an inverted orientation (Figures 10-2 and 10-3).

HEAVY CHAIN VDJ RECOMBINATION

Heavy chains have a complex RSS system. V_H genes have a 23-base spacer on the 5′ end, and J genes have a similar base pair spacer on the 3′ end. The genes will not recombine until a diversity gene is inserted between V and J genes. Diversity genes have 12 base-pair RSSs at both the 3′ and 5′ ends, which allows binding to both V and J genes. The partially assembled heavy chain consists of VDJ genes.

Attachment of Constant Regions

When VJ or VDJ genes are ligated, a promoter in the V region initiates transcription of an mRNA that contains introns between J and C genes. A process called *mRNA splicing* is used to remove introns. After transcription of mRNA, specialized *small nuclear RNA (snRNA)* and *small nuclear riboprotein (snRAP)* combine to form a stable complex. The first three base pairs of the snRNA attach to complementary sequences in the intron. The 3′ and 5′ ends of the intron are brought together to form a spliceosome, or extended loop. Cleavage of the spliceosome at the intron removes the intron separating J and C genes. Following removal of the intron, the coding units are ligated. A summary of the recombination and expression of light chains and heavy chains is provided in Figure 10-4.

Junctional Diversity

Junctional diversity occurs at the junction of the V and J segments. This region codes for the hypervariable CR3 region in the antigen-combining pocket. Changes in the amino acid sequence change the specificity of the antibody. The joining of gene V(D)J is often imprecise, and nucleotides can be lost from the ends of each gene segment. Diversity is increased by the addition of P-nucleotides and N-nucleotides. P-nucleotides are added because Artemis cleavage is often asymmetrical and creates one long DNA strand and one short DNA strand. For proper ligation, the short strand must be extended by the addition of P-nucleotides to the length of the long strand. A random addition of 2 to 20 base pairs, which are called *N-nucleotides*, also occurs. The addition of N-nucleotides changes the amino acid sequence in the hypervariable CR3 region. Addition of P-nucleotides and N-nucleotides is mediated by a unique enzyme called *terminal deoxynucleotidyl transferase* (Figure 10-5).

Nucleotides also can be removed from J genes during recombination. Following the cleavage of hairpin turns, endonucleases may inadvertently remove sequences from the exon.

CHAPTER 10 ANTIBODY DIVERSITY

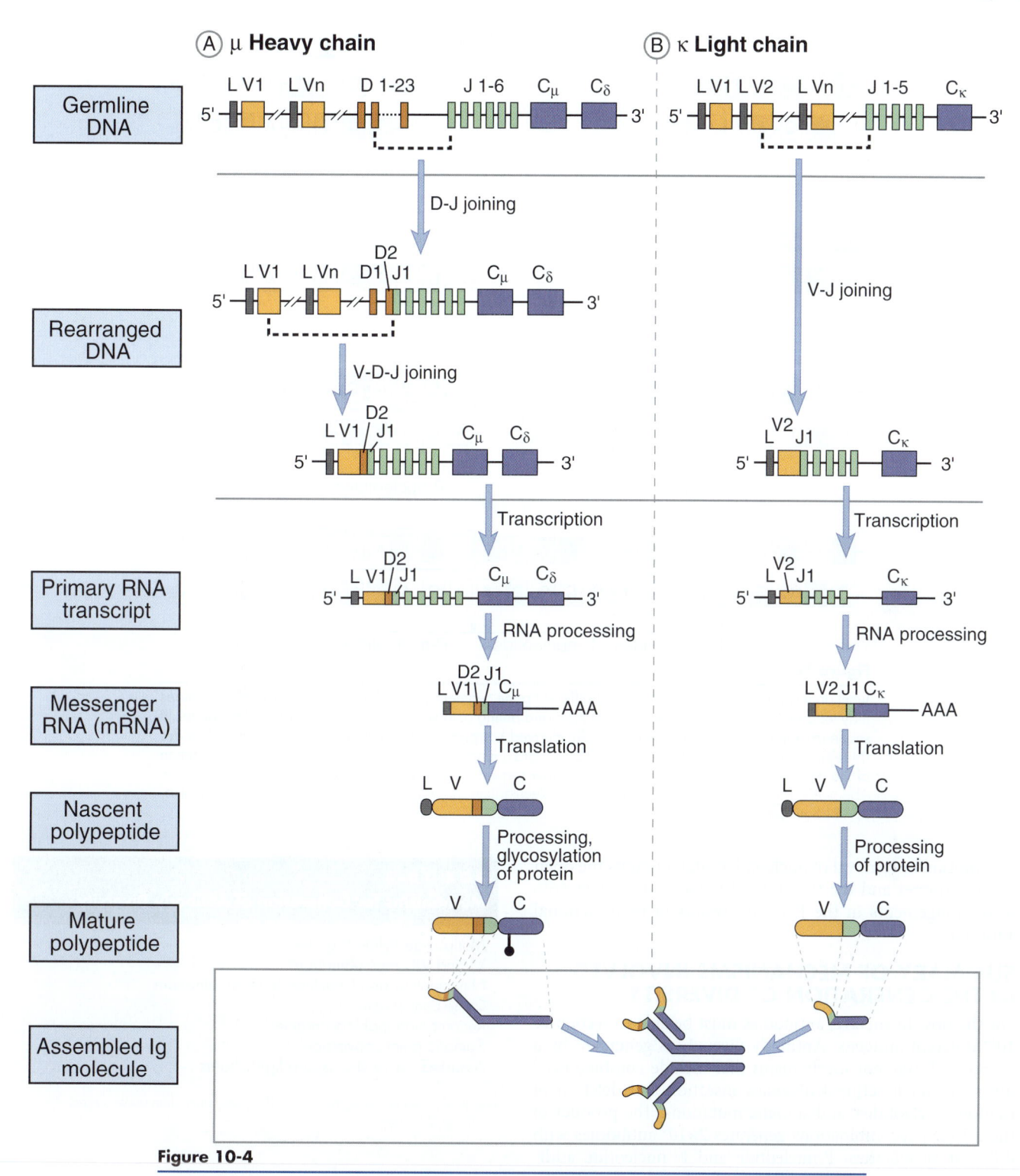

Figure 10-4

Immunoglobulin (Ig) heavy-chain and light-chain gene recombination and expression. The sequence of deoxyribonucleic acid (DNA) recombination and gene expression events is shown for the Igμ heavy chain (**A**) and the Igκ light chain (**B**). In the example shown in A, the V region of the μ heavy chain is encoded by the exons V1, D2, and J1. In the example shown in B, the V region of the κ-chain is encoded by the exons V1 and J1. (From Abbas AK, Lichtman AH, Pillai S: Cellular and molecular immunology, ed 6 [updated edition], Philadelphia, 2010, Saunders.)

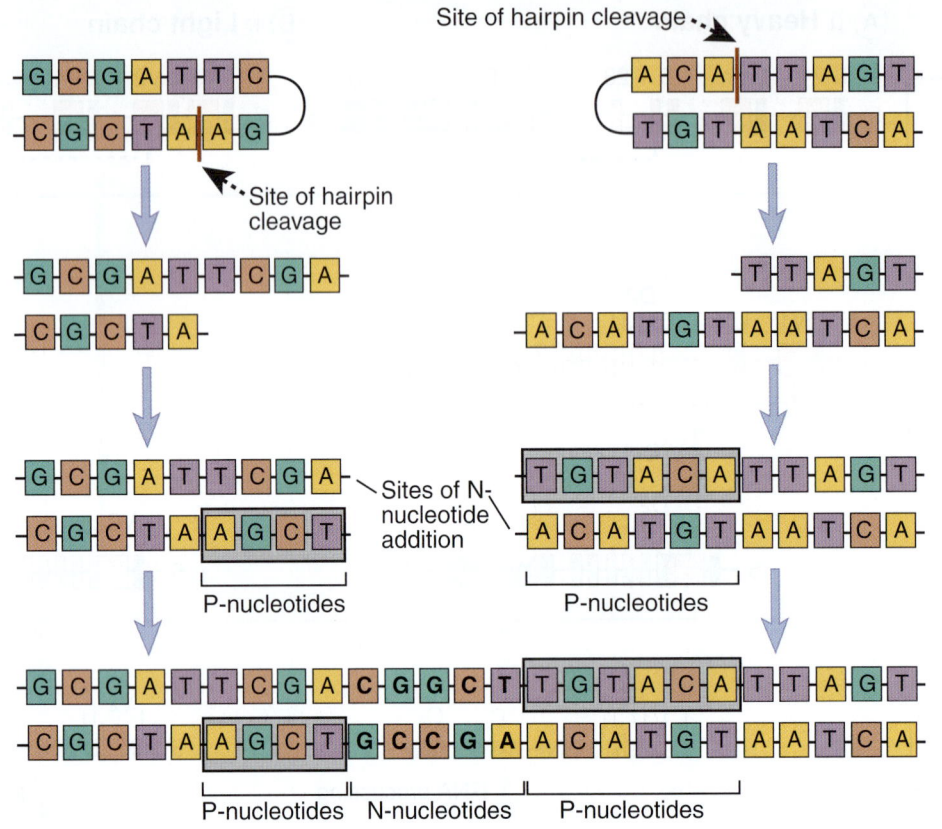

Figure 10-5

Junctional diversity. During the joining of different gene segments, the addition or removal of nucleotides may lead to the generation of novel nucleotide and amino acid sequences at the junction. Nucleotides (P sequences) may be added to asymmetrically cleaved hairpins in a templated manner. Other nucleotides (N regions) may be added to the sites of VD, VJ, or DJ junctions in a nontemplated manner by the action of the enzyme TdT. These additions generate new sequences that are not present in the germ-line. (From Abbas AK, Lichtman AH, Pillai S: Cellular and molecular immunology, ed 6 [updated edition], Philadelphia, 2010, Saunders.)

Addition or removal of nucleotides often disrupts the open reading frames and the structure of the antibody. Over 66% of rearrangements in the J regions results in nonfunctional antibodies.

SUMMARY OF MECHANISMS INVOLVED IN THE GENERATION OF DIVERSITY

For the host to survive, antibodies must be able to recognize 10^{13} different antigens. Antibody diversity is generated by a number of different mechanisms that include combinatorial diversity and junctional diversity, insertion and deletion of random nucleotides, and somatic mutations. The product of these V(D)J recombinations generates 2×10^9 antibodies with different specificities. P-nucleotide and N-nucleotide additions and somatic mutations account for 1×10^4 different antibodies (Box 10-1).

ALLELEIC EXCLUSION

Since both maternal and paternal V(D)J and C genes are inherited, an antibody-producing B cell is diploid. Genes from only one parent (heavy) are rearranged to produce antibodies. H-chain genes from the other parent are excluded or not productively rearranged. *Allelic exclusion* is the term used to describe antibody production from a single rearranged set of parental genes.

BOX 10-1
Mechanisms for Generation of Antibody Diversity

Mutiple–germ-line V genes
VJ and VJD recombinations
N-nucleotide and P-nucleotide recombinations
Gene conversion
Recombinational inaccuracies
Somatic point conversion
Assorted heavy chains and light chains

Modified from Male D, Brostoff J, Roth DB, et al: Immunology, ed 7, 2006, Mosby.

AFFINITY MATURATION

Somatic hypermutation of V genes occurs in B cells in germinal centers. In V genes, "hotspots" in the hypervariable region are present and are easily mutated. Mutations in the V region CDRs create IgM B cell receptors (BCRs) with increased affinity for antigen.

During antigen-driven B cell expansion, these cells are preferentially stimulated to produce high-affinity antibodies. This process is termed *affinity maturation*.

SUMMARY

- Antibodies must be diverse to interact with 10^{13} different antigens.
- Diversity is localized in the variable (V) and joining (J) regions of the antigen-binding site.
- Combinatorial diversity and junctional diversity, combined with additional somatic mutations, generate antibodies with a wide range of antigen specificities.
- During an immune response, the antibody affinity will increase as a consequence of mutations in the B cell genome.

REFERENCES

Burton DR, Woof JM: Human antibody effector function, Adv Immunol 51:1, 1992.

Early P, Hood L: Allelic exclusion and nonproductive immunoglobulin gene rearrangements, Cell 24(1):1, 1981.

Gould HJ, Sutton BJ, Beavil AJ, et al: The biology of IGE and the basis of allergic disease, Annu Rev Immunol 21:579, 2003.

Jeske DJ, Jarvis J, Milstein C, et al: Junctional diversity is essential to antibody activity, J Immunol 133(3):1090, 1984.

Jung D, Alt FW: Unraveling V(D)J recombination: Insights into gene regulation, Cell 116(2):299, 2004.

Kalmanovich G, Mehr R: Models for antigen receptor gene rearrangement. III. Heavy and light chain allelic exclusion, J Immunol 170(1):182, 2003.

Komori T, Sugiyama H: N sequences, P nucleotides and short sequence homologies at junctional sites in VH to VHDJH and VHDJH to JH joining, Mol Immunol 30(16):1393, 1993.

Lewis SM: P nucleotides, hairpin DNA and V(D)J joining: Making the connection, Semin Immunol 6(3):131, 1994.

Meier JT, Lewis SM: P nucleotides in V(D)J recombination: A fine-structure analysis, Mol Cell Biol 13(2):1078, 1993.

Milstein C: Affinity maturation of antibodies, Immunol Today 12(2):93, 1991.

Schmale J, Costea N, Dray S, et al: Allelic exclusion of light chain allotypes in rabbit IgM cold agglutinins, Proc Soc Exp Biol Med 130(1):48–50, 1969.

ASSESSMENT QUESTIONS

1. V(D)J gene recombination would be included in the definition of:
   A. Combinatorial diversity
   B. Junctional diversity
   C. Somatic mutation
   D. P-nucleotide additions

2. Which of the following are characteristics of diversity (D) genes?
   I. Have 12 base-pair sequences at each end
   II. Join V and J genes in antibody heavy chains
   III. Join V and J genes in antibody heavy and light chains
   A. I
   B. III
   C. I and II
   D. II and III
   E. I, II, and III

3. In the recombination of light chain V and J regions, which of the following removes the hairpin curves in DNA?
   A. Ligase IV
   B. Artemis
   C. RAG-1 and RAG-2
   D. Recognition signal sequences

4. Which of the following is used to join the V(D)J and constant (C) region genes?
   A. Signal joint
   B. RAG-1
   C. P-nucleotide addition
   D. mRNA splicing

5. The rearrangement of antibody genes from one parent and nonproductive rearrangement of genes from the other parent is called:
   A. Junctional diversity
   B. Affinity maturation
   C. Allelic exclusion
   D. Hypervariable exclusion

6. Which of the following theories provides the most plausible explanations for antibody diversity?
   I. Germ-line theory
   II. DNA rearrangement theory
   III. Somatic mutation theory
   A. I
   B. III
   C. I and II
   D. II and III
   E. I, II, and III

CHAPTER 11

Complement

LEARNING OBJECTIVES

- Recognize the biologic functions of the complement cascade
- Identify the components of the classic complement pathway
- Discuss the roles of anaphylatoxin in an immune response
- Recognize the biologic function of C2b
- Name the complement components in classic pathway C3 convertase
- Relate complement activation to microbial insolubility, osponization, and phagocytosis
- Recognize the three different anaphylatoxins generated in complement pathways
- Identify the components and function of the membrane attack complex (MAC)
- Differentiate between the classic complement pathway and the alternative complement pathway
- Describe the unique structure and function of C9
- Identify the molecules involved in the control of the classic recognition complex
- Describe the function of proteins that inhibit the activation of the classic antigen recognition, activation, and MAC steps
- Analyze the role of C3 in the activation of the alternative complement pathway
- Name the components of the C3 convertase in the alternative complement pathway
- Recognize the proteins that control the activation of the alternative C3 convertase
- List the seven molecules expressed on mammalian cell membranes that inhibit complement activation
- Identify the role of complement in B cell activation
- Identify the role of complement in the generation of memory cells
- Describe the immunologic defect in hereditary angioneurotic edema (HANE)
- Design a successful treatment regimen for HANE
- Describe the immunologic defects in paroxysmal nocturnal hemoglobulinuria (PNH)
- Design a treatment regimen for PNH

KEY TERMS

Activation complex
Anaphylatoxin
Antigen recognition complex
Alternative complement pathway
C1 esterase inhibitor (C1INH)
C3 convertase
C4 binding protein (C4BP)
C5 convertase
CD59
Classic complement pathway
Complement receptor I
Decay accelerating factor (DAF)
Factor H
Factor I
Hereditary angioneurotic edema
Homologous restriction factor (HRF)
Membrane activation complex
Membrane cofactor protein (MCP)
Metastable C3
Paroxysmal nocturnal hemoglobulinuria
Properdin
S protein (vitronectin)

INTRODUCTION

Complement is a family of more than 20 plasma proteins that includes enzymes, proenzymes, enzyme inhibitors, and glycoproteins. Components interact in cascades and assist in the resolution of a microbial infection. For example, fragments indirectly render the microbe insoluble and draw phagocytic cells to the area of infection. Other fragments coat the microbe and act as opsonins, which promote phagocytosis. In a third function, complement components create lesions in the microbial cell wall that result in osmotic lysis. Complement fragments also provide the second signal necessary for B cell activation.

Three different complement cascades have been described—classical, alternative, and the mannose-binding lectin (MBL) pathways (see Chapter 2). Only the classic pathway requires an antibody for complement activation. In the MBL and alternative pathways, complement components are directly activated by highly conserved microbial antigens.

CLASSIC COMPLEMENT PATHWAY

The classic pathway was the first described using sheep red blood cells (SRBCs) coated with anti-SRBC immunoglobulin M (IgM). Over a number of years, nine complement proteins were found to be involved in the cascade. These proteins interact in the following sequence: Ab:C142356789. On the basis of function, the classic cascade is subdivided into recognition, activation, and membrane attack complexes.

Recognition Complex

The recognition complex consists of antibody (Ab) and C1. The C1 component is a complex of three proteins (C1q, r, and s). C1q is composed of polypeptide chains with a triple helix "collagen-like" amino terminus and a globular structure at the carboxyl terminus (Figure 11-1). C1r and C1s are inactive serine esterases.

When the antibody binds to the antigen, a conformational change occurs in the hinge region, which exposes complement receptors. Although both IgG and IgM can activate the complement cascade, IgM is more efficient because of the proximity of multiple hinge regions. In the initial step of complement activation, C1q bridges two hinge regions. In the next step, C1r and C1s associate to form a tetrameric complex (two molecules of each protein), which binds to C1q. In the presence of calcium, C1r activates the serine esterase activity of C1s.

Activation Complex

Activated C1s cleaves multiple C4 and C2 molecules. C4 is a large 210-kDal trimeric polypeptide, which contains an unusual thioester group. C4 is cleaved into C42a and C4b. C4a is a soluble protein that attracts phagocytic cells into the area where complement is being fixed. The C4b fragment is coupled to the microbial cell. Cleavage of C2 results in the production of C2a and C2b. The larger C2a (75-kDal) fragment remains in contact with C4b to create an AbC4b2a complex on the cell surface. Plasmin cleavage of the smaller, soluble C2b fragment creates a kinin, which causes leakage of fluid from vessels and tissue edema.

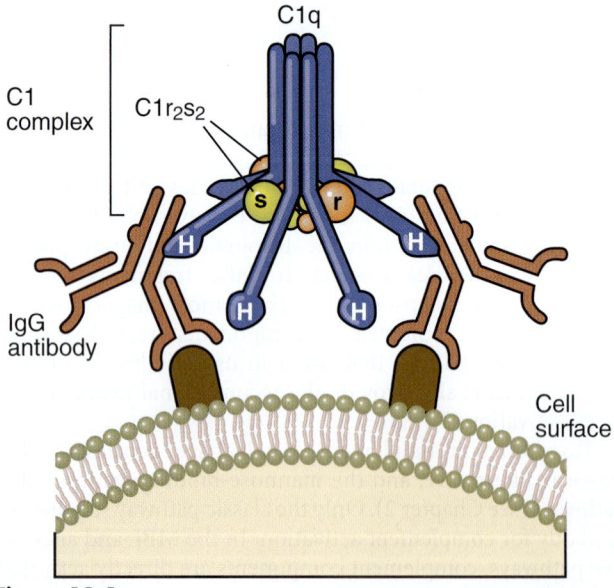

Figure 11-1
Structure of C1. C1q consists of six identical subunits arranged to form a central core and symmetrically projecting radial arms. The globular heads at the end of each arm, designated H, are the contact regions for immunoglobulin. C1r and C1s form a tetramer composed of two C1r and two C1s molecules. The ends of C1r and C1s contain the catalytic domains of these proteins. One C1r$_2$s$_2$ tetramer wraps around the radial arms of the C1q complex in a manner that juxtaposes the catalytic domains of C1r and C1s. (From Abbas AK, Lichtman AH, Pillai S: Cellular and molecular immunology, ed 6 [updated edition], Philadelphia, 2010, Saunders.)

C3 Convertase

The C4b2a complex, or C3 convertase, catalyzes the cleavage of C3 into C3a and C3b. This is the most important step in the complement cascade and occurs in the classic, alternative, and MBL pathways. C3b is a highly unstable molecule that has a unique thioester that allows covalent binding to a microbial cell. Some C3b fragments bind to the target cell, where they act as opsonins. In the classic pathway, most C3b is found in an AbC4bC2aC3b complex on the cell surface, which is called the *C5 convertase*.

The soluble C3a fragment acts as an anaphylatoxin. By definition, an anaphylatoxin is a molecule that induces the movement of eosinophils and phagocytic cells (chemotaxis) toward increasing concentrations of C3a (Figure 11-2). Anaphylatoxins also release histamine and heparin from basophils and mast cells. Histamine and heparin cause vasoconstriction and increased vascular permeability, which reduce the solubility of microbes or antigen–antibody complexes.

Membrane Attack Complex

The C5 convertase cleaves C5 into C5a and C5b fragments. The C5b binds to the cell surface and serves as a platform for the membrane attack complex (MAC), which consists of C5bC6789 (Figure 11-3). C5a is the most potent anaphylatoxin (100–1000 times more potent than C3a) in the complement cascade.

Binding of the C6C7 component creates a trimolecular, lipophilic complex, which is inserted into cell membranes. C8 also is inserted into the microbial cell wall or membrane, further increasing the stability of the C5b678 complex (Figure 11-3). Polymerized C9 is inserted into the cell membrane and creates pores in the cell membrane that cause osmotic lysis (Figure 11-4).

Control of the Classic Complement Cascade

Inadvertent or aberrant complement activation is controlled by soluble proteins that inhibit the antigen recognition, activation, and membrane attack complexes.

Control of the Recognition Complex

C1 esterase inhibitor (C1INH) is a soluble protein that inhibits C1 activation by disassociating C1r and C1s and preventing the activation of C4 (Figure 11-5).

Control of the Activation Complex

The C4 binding protein (C4BP) is a plasma protein that inhibits the classic and MBL complement pathways by blocking the interaction between C4b and C2a (Table 11-1).

Control of the Membrane Attack Complex

S Protein (vitronectin) is a plasma protein that associates C5bC6C7 with C8.

ALTERNATIVE PATHWAY OF COMPLEMENT ACTIVATION

Because it is inherently unstable, serum C3 spontaneously fragments into C3a and C3b. Metastable C3b covalently binds to highly conserved microbial polysaccharides (e.g., inulin, zymosan) and lipopolysaccharides (Figure 11-6).

Activation Complex

Binding of C3b causes a conformational change that exposes a binding site for factor B. On the cell surface, factor B complexes with C3b. Factor D, a serine protease, cleaves factor B into a soluble Ba and a Bb fragment. The C3bBb fragment becomes a C3 convertase, which is stabilized by another molecule called *properdin*.

Some C3b is liberated by the novel convertase and binds to the complex itself, creating a C3bBbC3b. The new complex acts as a C5 convertase that hydrolyzes the alpha chain, liberating C5a and C5b (Figure 11-7). C5b catalyzes the formation of the MAC.

Control Mechanisms for the Alternative Pathway

Soluble factor H downregulates the alternative pathway by inactivating soluble or bound C3b and amplifying the decay of the C3bBb complex. Factor I is a serine protease that cleaves C3b and C4b and prevents further activation of complement.

MAMMALIAN CELL INACTIVATION OF COMPLEMENT

Activated C3b from either the classic pathway or the alternative pathway can bind to mammalian cell membranes and activate the complement MAC. To prevent lysis, mammalian cells express molecules that inactivate individual complement components or accelerate the destruction of C3 convertases formed by the classic and alternative pathways. The following are known membrane-bound complement inhibitors:

- Factor H binds to sialic residues on cell membrane and inactivates C3b inadvertently bound to cells.
- Membrane cofactor protein (MCP; CD46), in combination with other proteins, inactivates C4b.
- Decay accelerating factor (DAF; CD55) is a glycoprotein that is anchored in the membrane by a covalent linkage to glycosylphosphatidylinositol (GPI). It functions to disassociate the C3 convertases by releasing C2a from the AbC4bC2a complex in the classic pathway and C3b and Bb in the alternative pathway (Figure 11-8).
- Complement receptor 1 (CR1) is found on erythrocytes and inhibits the formation of the classic and alternative pathway C3 convertase. It often acts in concert with DAF.
- Membrane cofactor protein (MCP or CD56) is a single-chain glycoprotein that interacts with membrane-bound factor I to cleave C3b and C4b.
- CD59 is a GPI-linked protein that binds to C8 and C9 and inhibits complement-mediated lysis of red blood cells, platelets, and leukocytes (Figure 11-9).
- Homologous restriction factor (HRF) is a 20,000–molecular weight (MW) protein that inhibits the interaction of the C8 and C9 terminal complement components.

COMPLEMENT, B CELL ACTIVATION, AND IMMUNOLOGIC MEMORY

Assuming a multi-valent antigenic molecule, two signals are necessary to activate B cells. The second signal is provided by a B cell co-receptor complex that consists of CR2, CD19, and CD81 (TAPA-1). The complement C3d decay fragment binds to the B cell CD2 molecule. At the same time, other epitopes bind to the B cell receptor (BCR). Complement binding activates kinases, which phosphorylate the CD19 cytoplasmic tail and activation of PI-3 signaling pathway.

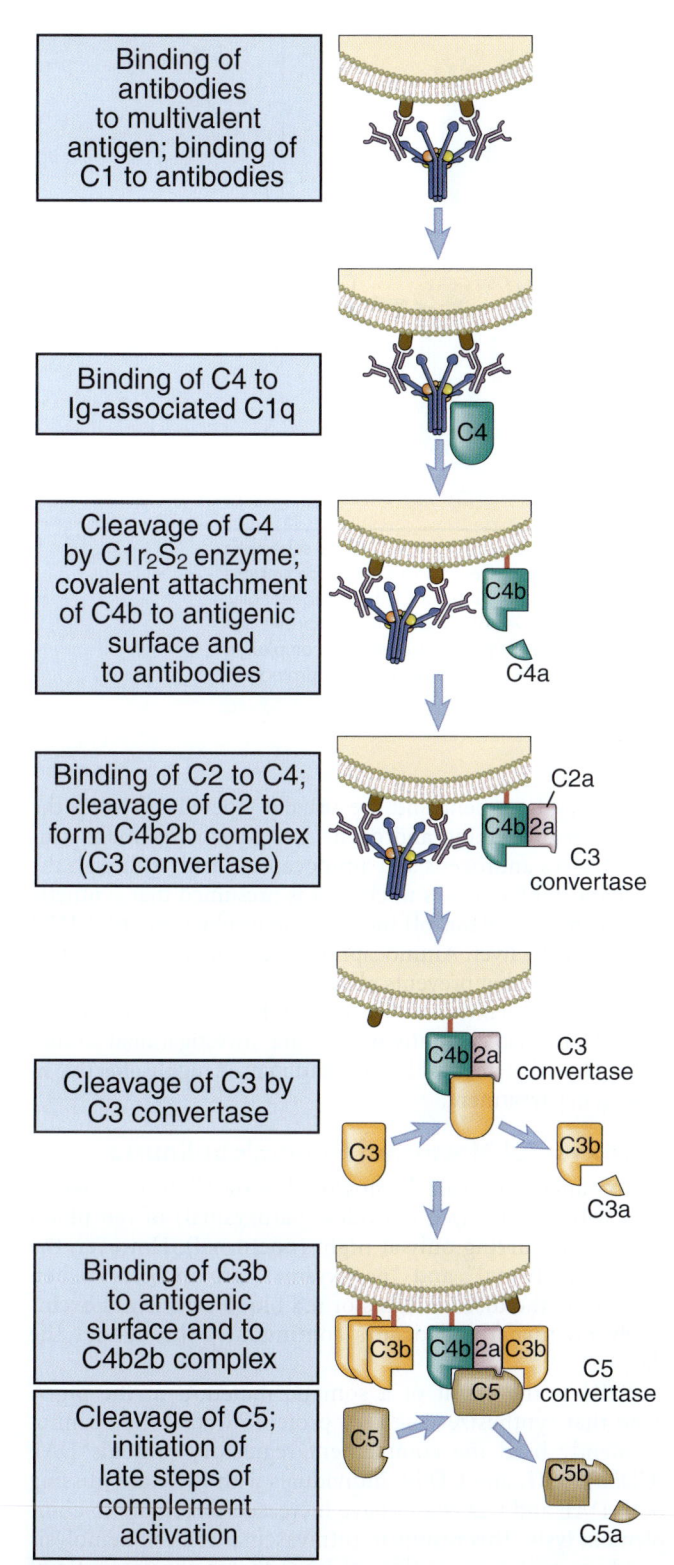

Figure 11-2

The classic pathway of complement activation. Antigen–antibody complexes that activate the classic pathway may be soluble, fixed on the surface of cells (*as shown*), or deposited on extracellular matrices. The classic pathway is initiated by the binding of C1 to antigen-complexed antibody molecules, which leads to the production of C3 and C5 convertases attached to the surfaces where the antibody was deposited. The C5 convertase cleaves C5 to begin the late steps of complement activation. (From Abbas AK, Lichtman AH, Pillai S: Cellular and molecular immunology, ed 6 [updated edition], Philadelphia, 2010, Saunders.)

Steps shown in figure:
- Binding of antibodies to multivalent antigen; binding of C1 to antibodies
- Binding of C4 to Ig-associated C1q
- Cleavage of C4 by C1r₂S₂ enzyme; covalent attachment of C4b to antigenic surface and to antibodies
- Binding of C2 to C4; cleavage of C2 to form C4b2b complex (C3 convertase)
- Cleavage of C3 by C3 convertase
- Binding of C3b to antigenic surface and to C4b2b complex
- Cleavage of C5; initiation of late steps of complement activation

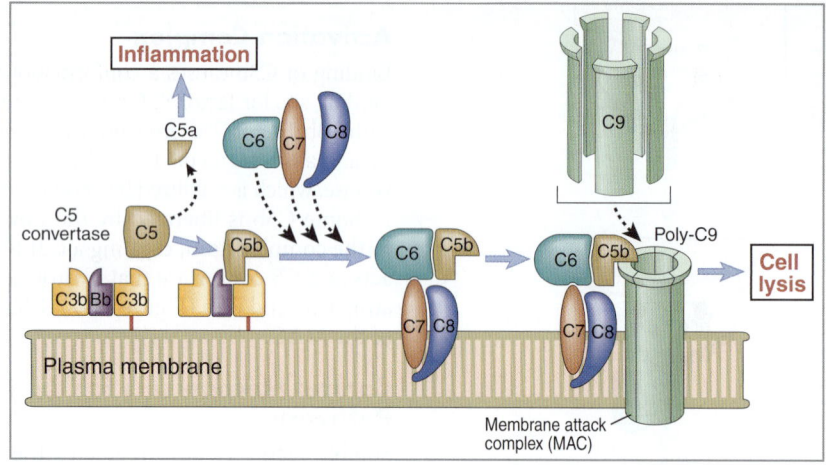

Figure 11-3

Late steps of complement activation and formation of the membrane attack complex (MAC). A schematic view of the cell surface events leading to formation of the MAC is shown. Cell-associated C5 convertase cleaves C5 and generates C5b, which becomes bound to the convertase. C6 and C7 bind sequentially, and the C5b,6,7 complex becomes directly inserted into the lipid bilayer of the plasma membrane, followed by stable insertion of C8. Up to 15 C9 molecules may then polymerize around the complex to form the MAC, which creates pores in the membrane and induces cell lysis. C5a released on proteolysis of C5 stimulates inflammation. (From Abbas AK, Lichtman AH, Pillai S: Cellular and molecular immunology, ed 6 [updated edition], Philadelphia, 2010, Saunders.)

Immunologic memory is also potentiated by the complement decay products iC3b and C3dg. Antigens coated with these fragments bind to iccosomes on follicular dendritic cells. Iccosome-bound antigens continually stimulate B cells which differentiate into plasma and memory cells.

COMPLEMENT DEFICIENCIES

Hereditary Angioneurotic Edema

In addition to its role in complement activation, C1 INH inhibits the activation of the clotting, kinin, and plasmin pathways (Figure 11-10). In the absence of C1 INH, precursors are converted to plasmin, bradykinin, and coagulation pathways. Activated C2 kinins allow fluid to escape into tissue, causing edema.

Hereditary angioneurotic edema (HANE) is caused by C1 INH deficiency. During a clinical episode, well-circumscribed edema is localized to the face, tongue, and larynx (Figure 11-11). Edema in the larynx is often severe and restricts normal breathing.

Over 66% of patients with HANE require emergency medical intervention during a clinical episode of laryngeal edema. Without adequate medical treatment, 33% of these patients die during a clinical episode.

Inherited and acquired forms of HANE exist. The inherited form is an autosomal dominant trait and appears during the first decade of life. It is characterized by normal levels of nonfunctional C1 INH. Acquired HANE is often associated with lymphoproliferative disorders or the presence of specific autoantibodies directed toward the C1 INH molecule. Most patients with acquired HANE have increased catabolism of C1 INH, which is reflected in the low serum levels of C1 INH.

Treatment of Hereditary Angioneurotic Edema

Oral androgens, anabolic steroids, and antifibrinolytic agents are commonly used to treat HANE. In cases of acquired C1 INH deficiency, glucocorticosteroids are effective as an emergency treatment and are usually tapered off when the patient begins taking androgens. Long-term treatment usually involves androgens and aminocaproic acid. Although the mechanism of action is unclear, it is presumed that synthetic androgens (e.g., danazol) increase the production of C1 INH and C4 by the liver. Aminocaproic acids function as an antifibrolytic agent that prevents plasmin activation.

Pooled human C1 INH concentrate and recombinant C1 INH are also currently undergoing investigational studies in the United States and Europe and may be highly effective in emergency treatment.

Paroxysmal Nocturnal Hemoglobulinuria

Paroxysmal nocturnal hemoglobulinuria (PNH) is associated with short, rapid episodes (paroxysmal) of red blood cell lysis occurring only at night (nocturnal). However, the terms "nocturnal" and "paroxysmal" are incorrect when describing the disease. Lysis of red blood cells is not exclusively nocturnal and occurs continuously throughout the day.

PNH is the result of a somatic mutation in the pig-A gene that synthesizes the GPI protein. Mutant GPI cannot covalently bind the complement regulatory proteins DAF (CD55), HRF, and CD59. Individuals with PNH are missing both DAF and CD59 and have increased sensitivity to complement lysis. This results in intravascular red cell hemolysis and hematoglobinuria (loss of iron) that is characteristic of the disease.

The absence of CD59 on platelets also contributes to recurrent thrombosis that is often fatal in individuals with PNH. MAC localization on platelets creates membrane pores that allow exovesiculation of platelet vesicles. These vesicles, which localize on the platelet surface, contain a membrane receptor for coagulation factor VI. Activation of the clotting sequence creates thrombi, which localize in the mesenteric, hepatic, and cerebral veins.

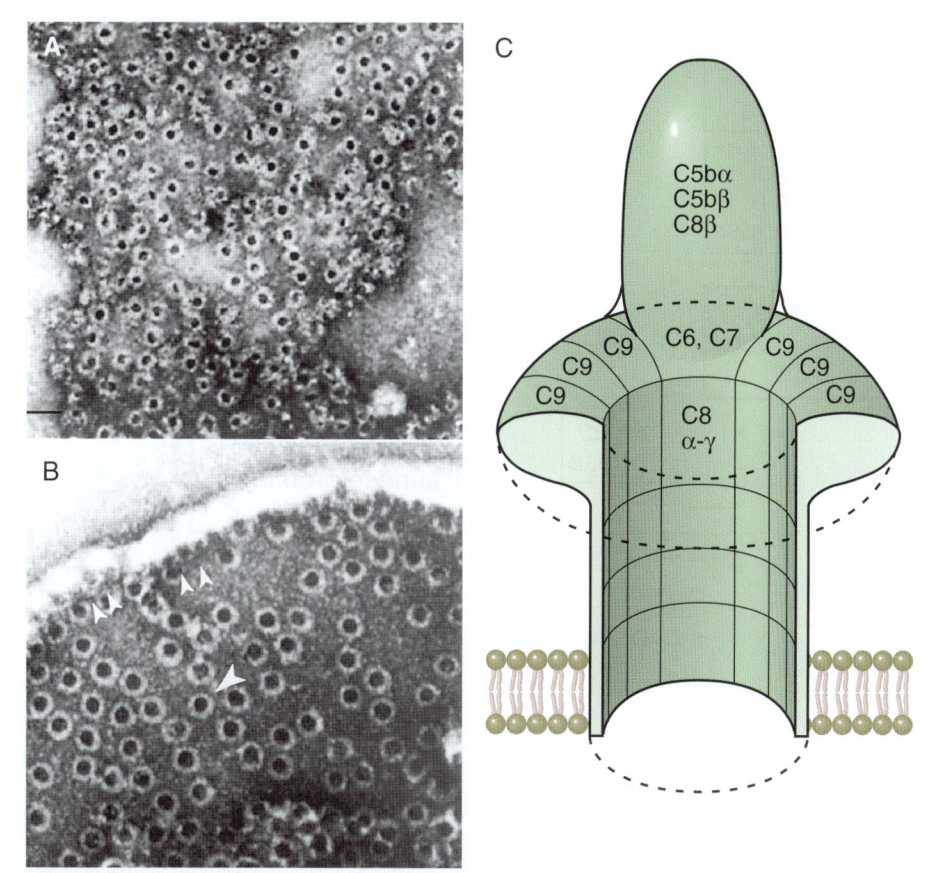

CHAPTER 11 COMPLEMENT 91

Figure 11-4
Structure of the membrane attack complex (MAC) in cell membranes. **A,** Complement lesions in erythrocyte membranes are shown in this electron micrograph. The lesions consist of holes approximately 100Å in diameter that are formed by poly-C9 tubular complexes. **B,** For comparison, membrane lesions induced on a target cell by a cloned cytotoxic T lymphocyte (CTL) line are shown in this electron micrograph. The lesions appear morphologically similar to complement-mediated lesions, except for a larger internal diameter (160Å). CTL-induced and natural killer (NK) cell–induced membrane lesions are formed by tubular complexes of a polymerized protein (perforin), which is homologous to C9. **C,** A model of the subunit arrangement of the MAC is shown. The transmembrane region consists of 12 to 15 C9 molecules arranged as a tubule, in addition to single molecules of C6, C7, and C8 α- and γ-chains. The C5bα, C5bß, and C8ß chains form an appendage that projects above the transmembrane pore. (From Abbas AK, Lichtman AH, Pillai S: Cellular and molecular immunology, ed 6 [updated edition], Philadelphia, 2010, Saunders. From Podack ER: Molecular mechanisms of cytolysis by complement and cytolytic lymphocytes, J Cell Biochem 30:133, 1986. Copyright 1986 Wiley-Liss. Reprinted by permission of Wiley-Liss, Inc., a subsidiary of John Wiley & Sons, Inc.)

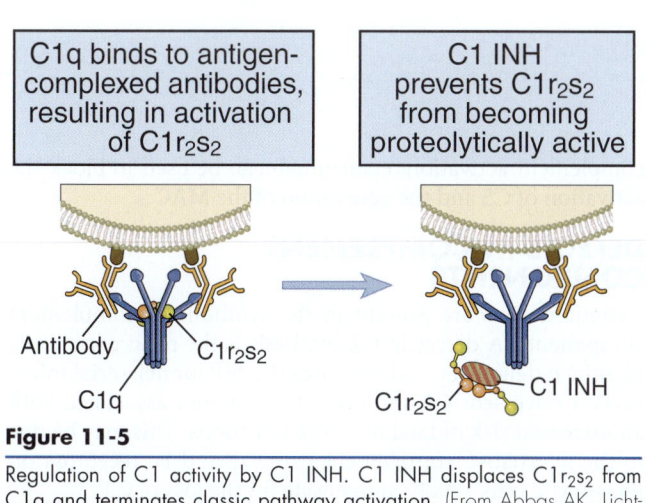

Figure 11-5
Regulation of C1 activity by C1 INH. C1 INH displaces $C1r_2s_2$ from C1q and terminates classic pathway activation. (From Abbas AK, Lichtman AH, Pillai S: Cellular and molecular immunology, ed 6 [updated edition], Philadelphia, 2010, Saunders.)

Table 11-1 Molecules and Receptors That Inhibit Complement Activation

Receptor	Interacts with	Function
C1 esterase inhibitor	C1r, C1s	Binds to C1r and C1s and disassociates them from C1q
C4 binding protein	C4b	Binds C4b and displaces C2
Membrane cofactor protein (MCP, CD46)	C3b, C4b	Cofactor for factor I mediated cleavage of C4b
Decay accelerating factor (DAF)	C4b, C2a	Displaces C2a from C4b
Factor I	C4b, C3b	Cleaves C3b and C4b
Factor H	C3b	Binds C3b
Complement receptor type 1 (CR1, CD35)	C3b, C4b, iC3B	Promotes dissociation of C3 convertase

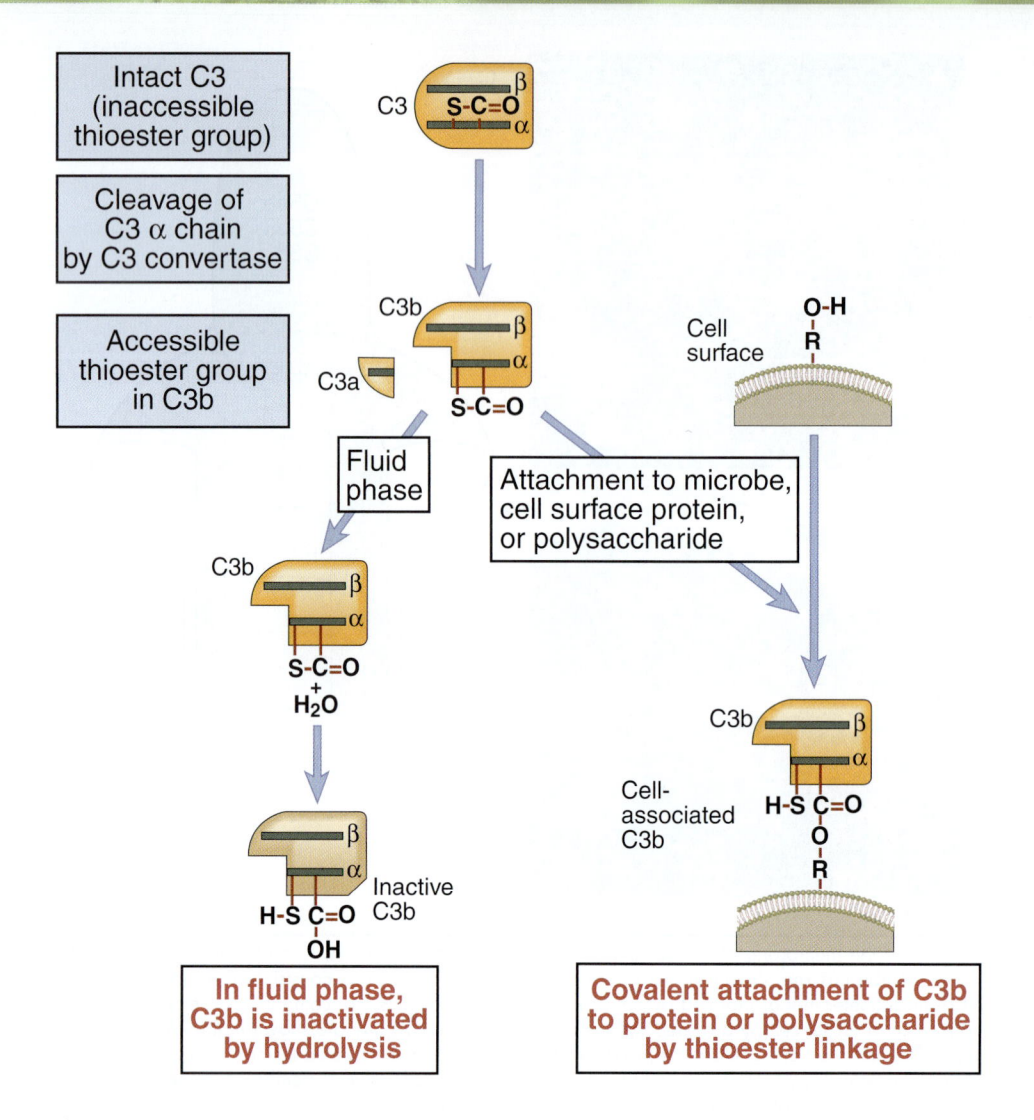

Figure 11-6

Internal thioester bonds of C3 molecules. A schematic view of the internal thioester groups in C3 and their role in forming covalent bonds with other molecules is shown. Proteolytic cleavage of the α-chain of C3 converts it into a metastable form in which the internal thioester bonds are exposed and are susceptible to nucleophilic attack by oxygen (*as shown*) or nitrogen atoms. The result is the formation of covalent bonds with proteins or carbohydrates on the cell surfaces. C4 is structurally homologous to C3 and has an identical thioester group. (From Abbas AK, Lichtman AH, Pillai S: Cellular and molecular immunology, ed 6 [updated edition], Philadelphia, 2010, Saunders.)

Treatment of Paroxysmal Nocturnal Hemoglobulinuria

In the treatment of PNH, clinicians must deal with five separate problems: (1) the lack of red blood cells, (2) deficient erythropoiesis, (3) increased thrombosis, (4) loss of iron (hematoglobinuria), and (5) persistent complement activation. Transfusion of packed red blood cells can replace lost cells. Androgens and recombinant erythropoietin are commonly used to accelerate erythropoiesis. Thrombotic complications are reduced by standard therapy, which includes heparin and maintenance doses of common anticoagulants. Iron loss is corrected by the administration of supplemental iron. To reduce complement activation, eculizumab can be used to block the activation of C5 and the generation of the MAC.

DEFECTS IN COMPLEMENT COMPONENTS

Genetic defects are present in the synthesis of complement components. A defect in C2 synthesis is the most commonly identified deficiency and increases the risk for neisserial infections. Conversely, C2 and C4 defects are not associated with an increased risk of fatal bacterial infections. This may be due to the alternative complement pathway and Fc receptors on phagocytic cells which compensate for the loss of C2.

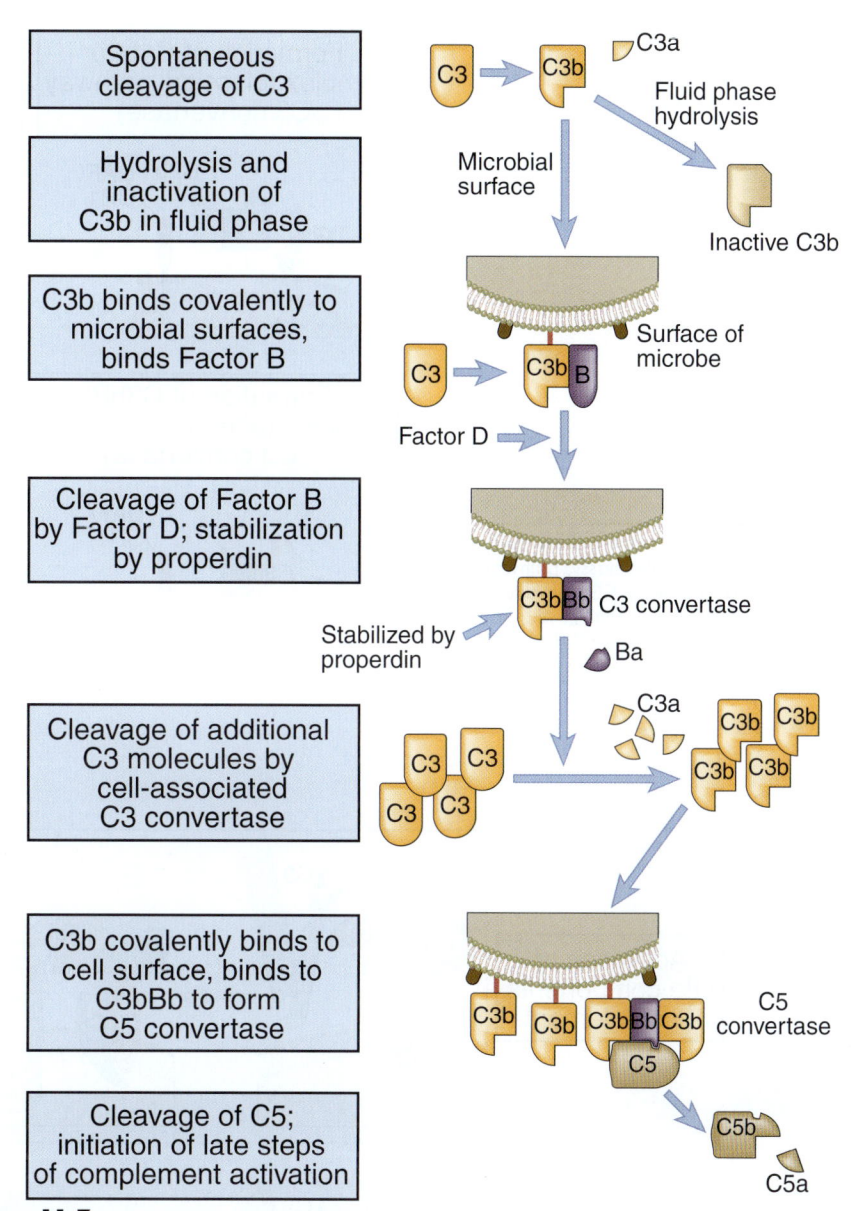

Figure 11-7

The alternative pathway of complement activation. Soluble C3 in plasma undergoes slow, spontaneous hydrolysis of its internal thioester bond, which leads to the formation of a fluid-phase C3 convertase (not shown) and the generation of C3b. If the C3b is deposited on the surfaces of microbes, it binds factor B and forms the alternative pathway C3 convertase. This convertase cleaves C3 to produce more C3b, which binds to the microbial surface and participates in the formation of a C5 convertase. The C5 convertase cleaves C5 to generate C5b, the initiating event in the late steps of complement activation. (From Abbas AK, Lichtman AH, Pillai S: Cellular and molecular immunology, ed 6 [updated edition], Philadelphia, 2010, Saunders.)

Deficiencies in complement components that form or stabilize the classic or alternative C3 convertase increase the risk of pyogenic (pus-forming) infections with streptococcal and staphylococcal species. Individuals with a C3 deficiency usually have recurrent infections of the respiratory tract, gut, and skin.

Life-threatening meningitis is associated with defects in properdin, factor H, factor I, and the complement MAC. Properdin deficiencies are usually X linked, and meningococcal infections are usually fatal.

Treatment of Complement Deficiencies

Individuals with C2, properdin, factor H, factor I, or complement MAC deficiency have a significant risk of developing meningococcal infections. Vaccination is indicated to create high levels of protective antibodies. In the choice of vaccines, the age of the individual and the meningococcal serotype should be considered.

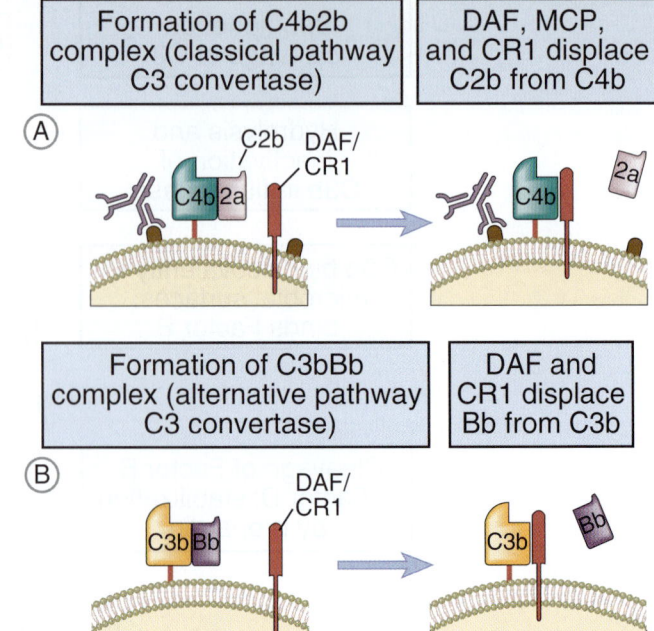

Figure 11-8
Inhibition of the formation of C3 convertases. Several membrane proteins present on normal cells displace either C2a from the classic pathway C3 convertase (**A**) or Bb from the alternative pathway C3 convertase (**B**) and stop complement activation. (From Abbas AK, Lichtman AH, Pillai S: Cellular and molecular immunology, ed 6 [updated edition], Philadelphia, 2010, Saunders.)

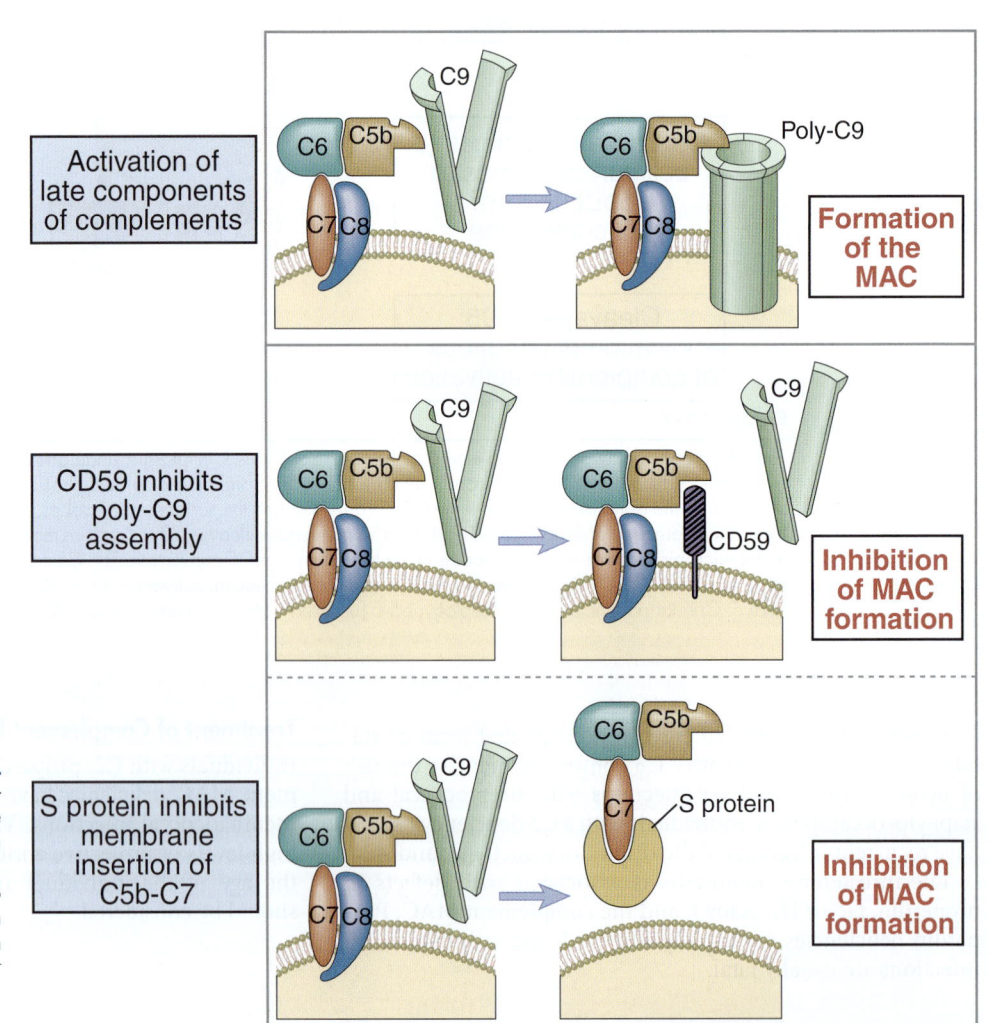

Figure 11-9
Regulation of formation of the membrane attack complex (MAC). The MAC is formed on cell surfaces as an end result of complement activation. The membrane protein CD59 and S protein in the plasma inhibit formation of the MAC. (From Abbas AK, Lichtman AH, Pillai S: Cellular and molecular immunology, ed 6 [updated edition], Philadelphia, 2010, Saunders.)

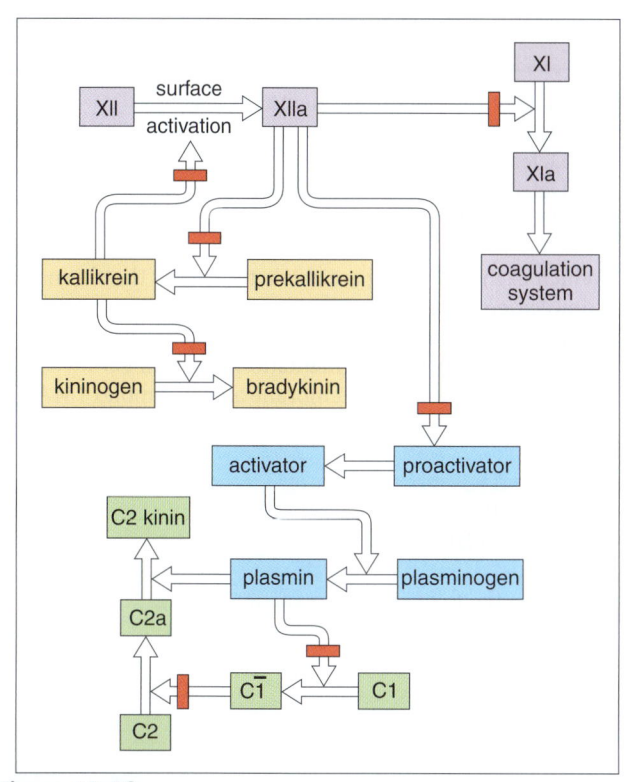

Figure 11-10

C1 inhibitor (C1INH) is involved in the inactivation of elements of the kinin, plasmin, complement, and clotting systems, all of which may be activated following the surface-dependent activation of factor XII. The points at which C1INH acts are shown in red. Uncontrolled activation of these pathways results in the formation of bradykinin and C2 kinin, which induce edema. (From Roitt I, Brostoff J, Male D, et al: Immunology, ed 7, Philadelphia, 2006, Mosby.)

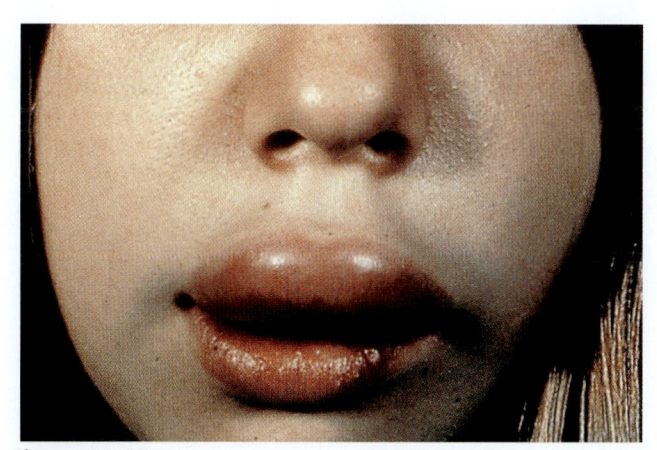

Figure 11-11

The clinical appearance of hereditary angioedema, showing the local transient swelling that affects mucous membranes. (From Roitt I, Brostoff J, Male D, et al: Immunology, ed 7, Philadelphia, 2006, Mosby.)

SUMMARY

- The complement system consists of 9 proteins that interact in cascades to resolve microbial infections.
- Three different cascades have been described. Only the classic cascade requires antibodies for activation.
- Complement components play critical roles in the immobilization of microbes, opsonization, chemotaxis, and B cell activation.
- Hereditary angioneurotic edema is caused by failure to regulate complement activation.
- Paroxysmal nocturnal hemoglobulinuria (PNH) is caused by lack of membrane-bound complement inhibitors.
- Complement deficiencies in C2, alternative pathway components, or the membrane attack complex (MAC) increase the risk of life-threatening neisserial infections.

REFERENCES

Carroll MC: The complement system in regulation of adaptive immunity, Nat Immunol 5(10):981, 2004.

Carroll MC: The role of complement and complement receptors in induction and regulation of immunity, Annu Rev Immunol 16:545, 1998.

Chaplin H Jr: Review: The burgeoning history of the complement system 1888-2005, Immunohematology 21(3):85, 2005.

Colten HR, Rosen FS: Complement deficiencies, Annu Rev Immunol 10:809, 1992.

Davitz MA: Decay-accelerating factor (DAF): A review of its function and structure, Acta Med Scand Suppl 715:111, 1987.

Gotze O, Muller-Eberhard HJ: The C3-activator system: An alternate pathway of complement activation, J Exp Med 134(3 Pt 2):90s, 1971.

Jasin HE: Human heat labile opsonins: Evidence for their mediation via the alternate pathway of complement activation, J Immunol 109(1):26, 1972.

Liszewski MK, Farries TC, Lublin DM, et al: Control of the complement system, Adv Immunol 61:201, 1996.

Loos M: Bacteria and complement—a historical review, Curr Top Microbiol Immunol 121:1, 1985.

Pickering MC, Cook HT: Translational mini-review series on complement factor H: Renal diseases associated with complement factor H: Novel insights from humans and animals, Clin Exp Immunol 151(2):210, 2008.

Roozendaal R, Carroll MC: Emerging patterns in complement-mediated pathogen recognition, Cell 125(1):29, 2006.

Thurman JM, Holers VM: The central role of the alternative complement pathway in human disease, J Immunol 176(3):1305, 2006.

Sahu A, Sunyer JO, Moore WT, et al: Structure, functions, and evolution of the third complement component and viral molecular mimicry, Immunol Res 17(1–2):109, 1998.

Sunyer JO, Zarkadis IK, Lambris JD: Complement diversity: A mechanism for generating immune diversity? Immunol Today 19(11):519, 1998.

Walport MJ: Complement. First of two parts, N Engl J Med 344(14):1058, 2001.

Walport MJ: Complement. Second of two parts, N Engl J Med 344(15):1140, 2001.

ASSESSMENT QUESTIONS

1. Which of the following are functions of complement?
   I. Opsonization
   II. Cell lysis
   III. B cell activation
   A. I
   B. III
   C. I and II
   D. II and III
   E. I, II, and III

2. The classical pathway C3 convertase consists of:
   A. AbC1
   B. AbC1C4bC2a
   C. C3bBb
   D. AbC1C4aC2bC3b

3. Which of the following are membrane-expressed molecules that inhibit complement deposition on mammalian cells?
   I. Decay accelerating factor (CD55)
   II. C4 binding protein
   III. C1 esterase inhibitor
   A. I
   B. III
   C. I and II
   D. II and III
   E. I, II, and III

4. Hereditary angioneurotic edema is caused by:
   A. Defective C1 esterase
   B. Defective CD59
   C. Defective C1 esterase inhibitor
   D. Defective homologous restriction factor

5. Which of the following are characteristics of the alternative complement pathway?
   I. C4 activation
   II. Spontaneous fragmentation of serum C3
   III. Formation of a membrane attack complex (MAC)
   A. I
   B. III
   C. I and II
   D. II and III
   E. I, II, and III

6. Which of the following is an anaphylatoxin?
   A. C3a
   B. C4b
   C. C2a
   D. C5b

CHAPTER 12

Phagocytosis and Intracellular Killing

LEARNING OBJECTIVES

- Restate the role of precipitin reaction in phagocytosis
- Define the zone of equivalence
- Identify the three different antibody Fc receptors in phagocytic cell membranes
- Compare and contrast pinocytosis and phagocytosis
- Explain the respiratory burst
- Identify the role of superoxide dismutase in the generation of hydrogen peroxide (H_2O_2)
- Define the reactive oxygen species
- Compare and contrast intracellular killing of microbes by superoxide (O_2^-), H_2O_2, and hydroxyl ($OH-$) radicals
- Identify the role of myeloperoxidase in intracellular killing
- Differentiate between oxygen-dependent intracellular killing and oxygen-independent intracellular killing
- Recognize the constituents of primary, secondary, and tertiary granules
- Explain the relationship between chronic inflammation and cancer
- Understand the alternative mechanism for generating mutagenic nitrosoamines or N-nitrosoamides
- Explain why catalase-producing and peroxidase-producing bacteria can survive oxygen-dependent intracellular killing
- Recognize the immunologic defect in Gaucher's disease
- Design a therapeutic regimen to treat Gaucher's disease
- Recognize the immunologic defect in chronic granulomatous disease (CGD)
- Analyze the importance of cytochrome b588 in respiratory burst
- Design acceptable treatment modalities for CGD
- Identify the fungal species that commonly infect patients with myeloperoxidase (MPO) deficiency
- Explain the relationship between CR3 and leukocyte adhesion deficiency type I

KEY TERMS

Catalase
Chronic granulomatous disease
Gaucher's disease
Myeloperoxidase
Oxygen-dependent intracellular killing
Oxygen-independent intracellular killing
Peroxidase
Phagocytosis
Pinocytosis
Reactive oxygen species
Respiratory burst
Singlet oxygen
Superoxide dismutase

INTRODUCTION

Phagocytosis and intracellular killing comprise the final step in the resolution of extracellular microbial infections. Phagocytic cells express receptors for the Fc domain of bound antibody and opsonizing complement fragments. After binding to the receptors, antigens or intact microbes are ingested and destroyed by oxygen-dependent and oxygen-independent killing mechanisms. As a prelude to phagocytosis, microbes are rendered insoluble by the chemical properties of the antigen–antibody complexes and the action of anaphylatoxins.

PRECIPITATION OF ANTIGEN–ANTIBODY COMPLEXES

Phagocytosis is more efficient when antigen–antibody complexes are insoluble. The molar concentration of antigens and antibodies in plasma determines immune complex solubility. In the early phase of the immune response to the foreign protein, few antibodies are directed at antigens, and the very small immune complexes can pass through the kidney. As the concentration of antibodies increases, the ratio of antibodies to antigens decreases, and very large immune complexes are formed. When equimolar concentrations of antigens and antibodies are present (the equivalence zone), large complexes are deposited in small capillaries and in the renal glomeruli. Deposition of immune complexes is augmented by anaphylatoxins released during complement activation.

CELLULAR RECEPTORS FOR COMPLEMENT

CR1 Complement Receptor

The CR1 complement receptor (CD35) is expressed on a number of blood cells, including polymorphonuclear leukocytes, monocytes or macrophages, and follicular dendritic cells. These receptors are single-chain membrane proteins with multiple short consensus receptors (SCRs). Binding of complement fragments occurs some distance from the cell. The CR1 complement receptor recognizes C3b, iC3b, and C4b.

CR2 Complement Receptor (CD21)

The CR2 membrane glycoprotein receptor (CD21) binds the complement decay fragments iC3b and C3dg. CR2 is expressed by follicular dendritic cells in the germinal centers and serves to trap antigen–antibody complexes on iccosomes.

CR3 Complement Receptor (Mac-1, CD11b/CD18)

Complement receptor type 3 (CR3, Mac-1, and CD11b/CD18) is found on monocytes, neutrophils, natural killer (NK) cells, and dendritic cells. CR3 is composed of α and β chains. The CD11b receptor interacts with cell-bound iC3b to initiate phagocytosis. CD18 forms the β_2-chain of CD11a, CD11b, and CD11c (leukocyte adhesion molecule). CD18 is the major component of lymphocyte function–associated antigen 1 (LFA-1), macrophage antigen 1 (Mac-1), and CD4 integrins, which bind leukocytes to the capillary endothelium.

Fc Receptors for Immunoglobulin G

Three different immunoglobulin G (IgG) receptors (CD64, CD16, and CD32) are expressed on phagocytic cells. Fc-gamma receptor I (FcγRI or CD64) is a high-affinity, isotype-restricted receptor that is present on most phagocytic cells, eosinophils, and dendritic cells. CD16 (Fc receptors FcγRIIIa and FcγRIIIb) is a low-affinity Fc receptor expressed on neutrophils, NK cells, eosinophils, and macrophages. The CD32 receptor is expressed on B lymphocytes and cells of macrophage or monocyte lineage. It is also known as a low-affinity Fc-gamma receptor II (FcγRII), which binds immune complexes.

INGESTION OF ANTIGENS OR MICROBES

Endocytosis is a general term describing a process by which cells absorb external material by engulfing it with the cell membrane. Endocytosis is usually subdivided into pinocytosis and phagocytosis. If the antigen is a small-molecular-weight protein or a polysaccharide, the cell membrane invaginates in a process called *pinocytosis*, and the protein or carbohydrate is placed in a fluid-filled sack called a *vesicle*. Large-molecular-weight antigens or intact microbes are internalized by a different form of endocytosis, which is called *phagocytosis*. During phagocytosis, the membrane envelopes the particle to form an internal vacuole termed *phagosome*.

INTRACELLULAR KILLING OF BACTERIA

In the phagosome, bacteria are killed by two different mechanisms. One mechanism is dependent on the presence of oxygen, a respiratory burst, and the generation of reactive oxygen species. The second mechanism (which is independent of oxygen) uses preformed granules containing proteolytic enzymes to kill microbes.

Oxygen-Dependent Respiratory Burst

Following the ingestion of microbes, an oxygen-dependent respiratory burst occurs, with rapid production of singlet oxygen (O_2^-) and hydrogen peroxide (H_2O_2) and energy in the form of adenosine triphosphate (ATP). In the oxidative phosphorylation pathway, nicotinamide adenine dinucleotide phosphate (NADPH) oxidase generates singlet oxygen as it transfers electrons to the cytochrome system.

$$2O_2 + NADPH \rightarrow 2O_2^- + NADP^+ + H^+$$

Electrons are transported through the cytochrome system by a series of oxidation reduction reactions to generate both singlet oxygen (O_2^-) and ATP. A cytochrome known as *cytochrome b588* is the major producer of singlet oxygen.

Some singlet oxygen is released into the phagosome as free radical oxygen. Most singlet oxygen, however, interacts with an enzyme called *superoxide dismutase*, which converts singlet oxygen to oxygen (O_2) and H_2O_2.

$$2O_2^- + 2H^+ \rightarrow O_2 + H_2O_2$$

Additional dismutations occur between O_2^- and H_2O_2 to form hydroxyl (OH^-) radicals. Singlet oxygen can also participate in other reactions. O_2^- can react with nitric oxide (NO^-) to form peroxynitrite anion ($ONOO^-$) or the conjugate acid ($ONOOH$). The reactive peroxynitrite molecule also can react with phenolic compounds, proteins, lipids, and deoxyribonucleic acid (DNA). A slow decomposition of protonated peroxynitrite ($ONOOH^+$) produces hydroxyl radicals, protons, and peroxynitrous acid.

The major reactive oxygen species (singlet oxygen, hydrogen peroxide, and hydroxyl radicals) are toxic to microbes. Singlet oxygen disrupts bacterial cell walls. Hydrogen peroxide and hydroxyl radicals attack cell membranes and also cause damage to bacterial DNA.

Myeloperoxidase (MPO) catalyzes an additional microbial killing mechanism. MPO is stored in the azurophilic granules of neutrophils and the lysosomes of monocytes. Fusion of the granules and phagosome membranes deposits MPO into the phagosome. In the presence of a halide, which is usually Cl^-, MPO interacts with hydrogen peroxide to form hypochlorous acid. The acid pH kills the microbe and dissolves the cell walls.

The reaction is shown below:

$$Cl^- + H_2O_2 + MPO \rightarrow H_2O + OCl^-$$

A summary of the oxygen-dependent killing process is shown in Figure 12-1.

Oxygen-Independent Intracellular Killing

Oxygen-independent intracellular killing uses preformed cytoplasmic granules containing antimicrobial agents. Primary, secondary, and tertiary granules fuse with the phagosome membrane and empty their contents into the phagosome. Each type of granule has a different array of cytotoxic molecules that have different microbial targets.

Primary granules fuse with the phagosome membrane and secrete a number of antimicrobial agents, including proteinases, and lysozyme. Lysozyme attacks the bacterial cell wall at the beta 1, 4 glucosidic linkages between N-acetyl muramic acid and N-acetylglucosamine residues and destroys the integrity of the cell wall.

Secondary granules are usually smaller than primary granules and deposit lactoferrin and a unique family of proteins called *defensins* into the phagosome. Lactoferrin chelates iron and prevents bacterial synthesis of heme-containing cytochromes. Defensins are a family of small cationic proteins that induce osmotic lysis by forming pores in bacterial cell walls.

Tertiary granules also are abundant in phagocytic cells. These granules contain gelatinase, acetyltransferase, and lysozyme.

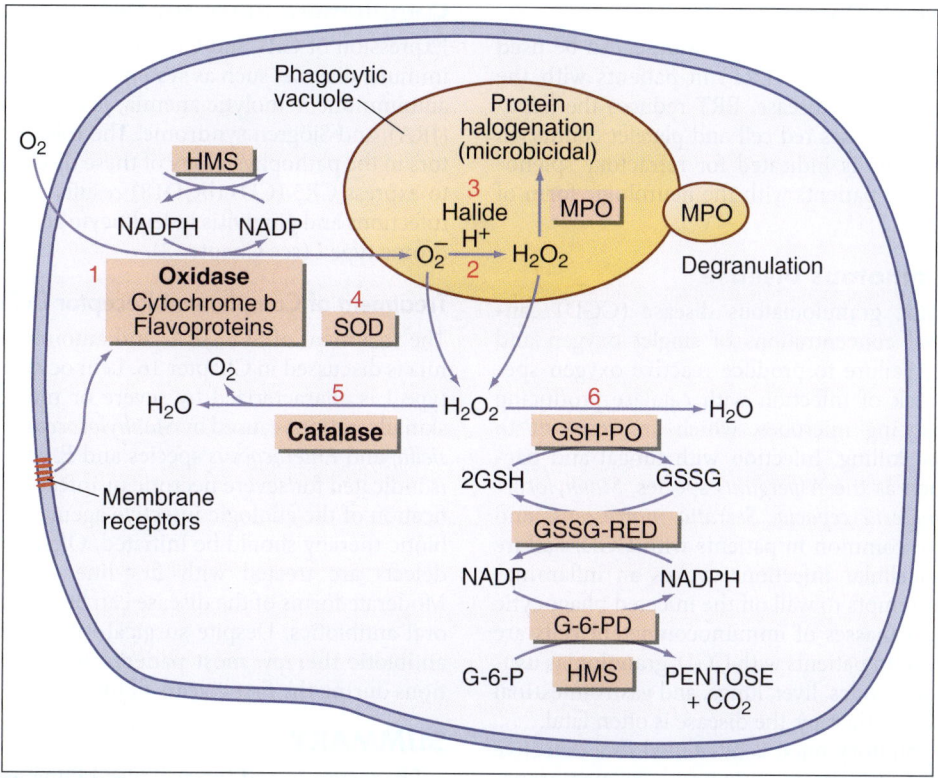

Figure 12-1

Oxygen-dependent killing by phagocytic cells. **1,** Liberation of singlet oxygen by NAD and cytochrome system, and conversion of singlet oxygen. **2,** Conversion of singlet oxygen to hydrogen peroxide. **3,** Myeloperoxidase formation of hypochlorous acid and bacterial protein halogenation. **4,** Superoxide dismutase. **5,** Catalase. **6,** Breakdown of hydrogen peroxide by glutathione peroxidase (GSH-PO) and reduced glutathione (GSSG-RED).

INFLAMMATION, TISSUE DAMAGE, AND CANCER

As a consequence of continual or chronic inflammation, reactive oxygen species and hypochlorous acid leak from the phagocytic cell and injure host tissue. Chemical reactions in the injured tissue transform reactive oxygen species into mutagens, which cause changes in host cell DNA. In one chemical reaction, highly mutagenic chloramines also are created when primary amines react with hypochlorous acid. In another reaction, activation of nitric oxide synthase converts L-arginine to citrulline with the liberation of NO^-. Reactions between NO^- and O_2 generate dinitrogen trioxide (N_2O_3). In turn, this compound reacts with water to form mutagenic nitrates. Other reaction products interact with secondary amines or amides in protein to form mutagenic N-nitrosamines or N-nitrosoamides.

Cancers may arise as a result of rapid cell division, which is usually part of the tissue repair process. In the repair process, normal cells and cells with mutated DNA undergo cell division at the same rate. Expansion of the mutated cell population and subsequent changes in the genome of mutated cells cause the uncontrolled division and development of cancerous cells.

Microbial Evasion of Intracellular Killing

Bacteria have developed mechanisms to prevent intracellular killing. Some aerobic bacteria produce catalase and peroxidase, which break down H_2O_2 into water and oxygen. These bacteria can live and replicate within the phagosome.

The catalase reaction is as follows:
$$2H_2O_2 \rightarrow 2H_2O + O_2$$
The peroxidase reaction is as follows:
$$H_2O_2 + 2H^+ \rightarrow H_2O$$

IMMUNODEFICIENCIES ASSOCIATED WITH PHAGOCYTOSIS

Gaucher's Disease

In Gaucher's disease, patients have a deficiency in β-glucosidase or glucosylceramidase, which is necessary for the intracellular degradation of senescent red blood cells—a normal function of macrophages and monocytes. As a consequence, glucocerebroside (a membrane lipid component) accumulates in phagocytic cells in the liver, spleen, bone marrow, lymph nodes, and alveolar capillaries. The high lipid concentration inhibits protein kinase C that is necessary for macrophage activation and phagocytosis.

Non-neurologic and neurologic forms of the disease exist. Non-neurologic disease is common in adult Ashkenazi Jews and is characterized by hepatosplenomegaly, pancytopenia, and skeletal disease. Neurologic forms of the disease occur in infants and are characterized by seizures, epilepsy, learning disabilities, and dementia.

Treatment of Gaucher's Disease

Imiglucerase, a recombinant glucocerebrosidase, can be used in enzyme replacement therapy (ERT) in patients with the non-neurologic form of the disease. ERT reduces the hepatosplenomegaly and increases red cell and platelet counts. In some cases, splenectomy is indicated for refractory splenomegaly. ERT efficacy in patients with the neurologic form of the disease is variable.

Chronic Granulomatous Disease

Patients with chronic granulomatous disease (CGD) cannot generate normal concentrations of singlet oxygen and hydrogen peroxide. Failure to produce reactive oxygen species increases the risk of infection with catalase-producing or peroxidase-producing microbes, which are resistant to oxygen-independent killing. Infection with fungal and bacterial pathogens such as the *Aspergillus* species, *Staphylococcus aureus*, *Burkholderia cepacia*, *Serratia marcescens*, and *Nocardia* species are common in patients with CGD. Failure to resolve the intracellular infections evokes an inflammatory response that attempts to wall off the infected phagocytic cells. These spherical masses of immunocompetent cells are known as *granulomas*. In patients with CGD, granulomas usually form in the lymph nodes, liver, lungs, and gastrointestinal tract. Despite aggressive therapy, the disease is often fatal.

The defective respiratory burst is attributed to a defective cytochrome b588. This cytochrome is composed of membrane-bound (gp91phox and gp22phox) and cytosolic (p47phox, p67phox, and p40phox) components. In patients with CGD, gp91phox or p47phox proteins are defective, and the cytochrome is inactive.

Treatment of Chronic Granulomatous Disease

Administration of antibiotics is necessary to control infections. Acceptable medical treatment includes first-line antibiotics such as trimethoprim-sulfamethoxazole (antibacterial), and itraconazole (antimycotic). Patients with active disease and granuloma often benefit from parenteral antibiotics and intravenous corticosteroids. Interferon-gamma (IFN-γ) treatment is recommended for patients who have some residual O_2^- production. Human stem cell transplantation is the only available curative therapy. At this juncture, 24 patients have undergone transplantations with moderate success.

Myeloperoxidase Deficiency

MPO deficiency is relatively common (1 per 2000 to 1 per 4000 live births). In most individuals with MPO deficiency, *Staphylococcus* and *Escherichia coli* can be killed by using oxygen-independent mechanisms. Fungi, however, pose a more serious problem. *Candida* species such as *C. albicans*, *C. krusei*, *C. stellatoidea*, and *C. tropicalis* survive in MPO-deficient phagocytic cells.

Treatment of Myeloperoxidase Deficiency

Because bacterial or fungal infections are rare in patients with MPO deficiency, prophylactic antibiotic treatment is not recommended. However, individuals with both diabetes mellitus and MPO deficiency have a high risk of invasive *Candida* infections. After identification of the infectious fungi, prompt and aggressive antibiotic therapy should be initiated.

Complement Receptor Deficiency

Expression of CR1 and CR2 receptor is associated with autoimmune diseases such as systemic lupus erythematosus (SLE), autoimmune hemolytic anemia, juvenile rheumatoid arthritis (JRA), and Sjögren syndrome. The role of complement receptors in the pathophysiology of these diseases is unclear. Failure to express CR3 (CD11bCD18) results in recurrent cutaneous infections and gingivitis in leukocyte adhesion deficiency syndrome type I (see Chapter 2).

Treatment of Complement Receptor Deficiency

The treatment of SLE, JRA, and autoimmune hemolytic anemia is discussed in Chapter 16. Leukocyte adhesion deficiency type I is characterized by severe or moderate gingivitis and skin ulcerations caused by *Staphylococcus*, *Pseudomonas*, *Klebsiella*, and *Enterococcus* species and *E. coli*. Surgical treatment is indicated for severe necrotic or infected tissue. After identification of the etiologic infective agent, microbe-specific antibiotic therapy should be initiated. Often, patients with severe defects are treated with first-line intravenous antibiotics. Moderate forms of the disease can be treated with appropriate oral antibiotics. Despite surgical intervention and aggressive antibiotic therapy, most patients succumb to virulent infections during the first 2 years of life.

SUMMARY

- Phagocytosis and intracellular killing are the final steps in the resolution of extracellular microbial infections.
- Intracellular killing involves oxygen-dependent and oxygen-independent intracellular killing mechanisms.
- Chronic inflammation and leakage of reactive oxygen species and hypochlorous acid from phagocytic cells increases the risk of deoxyribonucleic acid (DNA) mutations and cancer.
- Failure to generate reactive oxygen species allows catalase-producing or peroxidase-producing bacteria to survive and replicate in phagosomes.

REFERENCES

Campo López C, Calabuig Alborch JR, Aguilar Jiménez J, et al: Skeletal manifestations of Gauchers disease: A report of two cases, An Med Interna 21(4):179, 2004.

Cech P, Papathanassiou A, Boreux G, et al: Hereditary myeloperoxidase deficiency, Blood 53(3):403, 1979.

Cech P, Stalder H, Widmann JJ, et al: Leukocyte myeloperoxidase deficiency and diabetes mellitus associated with Candida albicans liver abscess, Am J Med 66(1):149, 1979.

Gresham HD, McGarr JA, Shackelford PG, et al: Studies on the molecular mechanisms of human Fc receptor-mediated phagocytosis. Amplification of ingestion is dependent on the generation of reactive oxygen metabolites and is deficient in polymorphonuclear leukocytes from patients with chronic granulomatous disease, J Clin Invest 82(4):1192, 1988.

Karnovsky ML, Badwey JA: Respiratory burst during phagocytosis: An overview, Methods Enzymol 132:353, 1986.

Koppenol WH, Butler J: Mechanism of reactions involving singlet oxygen and the superoxide anion, FEBS Lett 83(1):1, 1977.

Wolf JE, Ebel LK: Chronic granulomatous disease: Report of case and review of the literature, J Am Dent Assoc 96(2):292, 1978.

ASSESSMENT QUESTIONS

1. Which of the following is *not* generated during an oxygen-dependent respiratory burst?
   A. H_2O_2
   B. ONOO-
   C. ONOOH
   D. H_2SO_4

2. Oxygen-independent killing is associated with:
   I. Fusion of preformed granules with phagosome membrane
   II. Activation of the cytochrome system
   III. Conversion of L-arginine to citrulline
   A. I
   B. III
   C. I and II
   D. II and III
   E. I, II, and III

3. Which of the following are characteristics of phagocytosis?
   I. Ingestion of large-molecular-weight antigens or intact microbes
   II. Membrane envelopment of the antigen or intact microbe
   III. Ingestion of low-molecular-weight antigens
   A. I
   B. III
   C. I and II
   D. II and III
   E. I, II, and III

4. Gaucher's disease is associated with:
   A. Defective respiratory burst
   B. Defective phosphatidylinositol synthesis
   C. Defective cytochrome b588
   D. Defective phagocytosis

5. Chronic granulomatous disease is caused by:
   I. Defective singlet oxygen production
   II. Defective cytochrome b588
   III. Defective H_2O_2 production
   A. I
   B. III
   C. I and II
   D. II and III
   E. I, II, and III

6. Myeloperoxidase (MPO) catalyzes the production of:
   A. Singlet oxygen
   B. H_2O_2
   C. Hypochlorous acid
   D. L-arginine

CHAPTER 13

Antibodies and In Vivo Therapy

LEARNING OBJECTIVES

- Discuss the problems associated with the use of animal antisera
- Explain the immunologic mechanisms involved in the evolution of serum sickness
- Recognize the constituents of fractionated immunoglobulin (Ig)
- Identify the conditions and diseases treated with intravenous immunoglobulin (IVIG)
- Identify the signs and symptoms of idiopathic thrombocytopenic purpura (ITP)
- Recognize the immunologic mechanism involved in ITP
- Explain the role of IVIG in inhibiting the progression of ITP
- Discuss the pathophysiology of Kawasaki disease
- Explain the relationship between IVIG and complement in Kawasaki disease
- Recall the role of pooled Ig in treatment of Rh blood group incompatibility
- Identify the role of IVIG in the downregulation of T cell–mediated autoimmune diseases
- Compare and contrast the advantages and limitations of pooled human Ig, and monoclonal antibodies
- Compare and contrast DNA de novo synthesis and the nucleic acid salvage pathways
- Explain the biologic basis for HAT (hypoxanthine-aminopterin-thymidine) selection
- Compare and contrast murine, chimeric, humanized, and human monoclonal antibodies
- Recall the guidelines used in the generic names for monoclonal antibodies used in immunotherapy
- Using the naming guidelines, describe how murine, humanized, and human monoclonal antibodies are designated
- Define bi-specific antibodies
- Recognize the characteristics of bi-functional and flex antibodies
- Define single-chain variable fragments (scFv)
- Restate the three critical issues in the development of radiolabeled antibodies
- Identify two antibodies used for the treatment of non-Hodgkin's lymphoma

KEY TERMS

Active immunity
Chimeric antibodies
Classic nucleic acid pathway
Erythroblastosis fetalis
HAT selection
Hybridoma
Humanized monoclonal antibodies
Idiopathic thrombocytopenic purpura
Kawasaki disease
Monoclonal antibody
Nucleic acid salvage pathway
Passive immunity
Serum sickness
Single-chain variable fragment (scFv) protein

INTRODUCTION

Immunity can be generated by active or passive means. *Active immunity* results from exposure to microbes such as *Streptococcus* and *Pneumococcus* or vaccination with dead or weakened microbes. In contrast, the administration of antibodies to correct an immunodeficiency or provide short-term immunity against microbial infections is called *passive immunity*. Transfer of antibodies in colostrum from mother to child or administration of pooled immunoglobulins are examples of natural and artificial passive immunity.

HETEROLOGOUS ANTISERA TO PROVIDE PASSIVE IMMUNITY

The administration of antibodies to provide passive immunity is not a new concept. In the 1890s, Emil von Behring introduced the concept of passive immunity for the treatment of diseases. He demonstrated that equine polyvalent antiserum was efficacious in the treatment of diphtheria infections in children. In the early 1900s, equine antiserum therapy was used to treat streptococcal pneumonia, bacterial meningitis, and *Haemophilus* infections. By 1950, antibody therapy had been supplanted by antibiotics, which were cheaper to produce. However, equine antisera are still used for the neutralization of anthrax, tetanus, gas gangrene and diphtheria exotoxins; snake venoms; and the rabies virus. Immunogenicity is a major problem associated with heterologous antisera. Anaphylaxis and serum sickness have been frequently encountered in their use.

Serum Sickness

Serum sickness is caused by the administration of large amounts of any foreign protein. Within 7 to 10 days after administration, an immunoglobulin M (IgM) antibody response to the foreign protein develops. When equal molar concentrations of antigens and antibodies are generated, large complexes settle out in the internal elastic lamina of arteries and perivascular regions. Activation of the complement cascade and the release of cytotoxic factors from endothelial cells cause the necrosis of the capillary vessels in the skin and kidneys.

Patients develop clinical manifestations of fever, arthralgia, lymphadenopathy, and skin eruptions. Serious side effects also have been reported as a consequence of antibody therapy. High concentrations of infused antibody (0.5 to 2.0 mg/kg) can cause renal failure, aseptic meningitis, and thrombosis.

POOLED HUMAN IMMUNOGLOBULIN

To reduce the morbidity associated with heterologous antisera, fractionated human immunoglobulin is now used as a therapeutic agent. Pooled human immunoglobulin is prepared from a panel of 3000 to 10,000 donors and contains 95% intact, unmodified IgG with trace amounts of IgA and IgM. Preparations also contain the macrophage–granulocyte stimulating factor, interleukin 1 (IL-1), and complement regulators.

Initially, pooled human immunoglobulin was administered by the intramuscular (IM) route. Although effective in reducing the frequency of infections, it was difficult to maintain optimal antibody levels in blood. In 1981, intravenous preparations of human immunoglobulin (IVIG) became available. IVIG allows the infusion of large volumes of antibodies while reducing the cost and the pain associated with intramuscular administration.

IVIG has been used to treat immunodeficiencies, human immunodeficiency virus (HIV) infection in infants, lymphoproliferative malignancies, and infections in low-birth-weight infants. It is also used to treat a wide range of autoimmune diseases such as myasthenia gravis, systemic lupus erythematosus, and autoimmune neuropathies (Box 13-1).

IVIG is particularly useful in the treatment of diseases such as idiopathic thrombocytopenic purpura (ITP) and Kawasaki disease and for the prevention of erythroblastosis fetalis.

Idiopathic Thrombocytopenic Purpura

ITP is a pediatric disease that is associated with low platelet counts. Children often present with bruises all over the body, bleeding gums, and, occasionally, a bleeding nose. Patients with persistently low platelet counts are also at high risk of intracranial hemorrhage.

ITP is an autoimmune disease characterized by antibody-coated platelets. In most cases, coated platelets bind to Fc receptors on macrophages in the spleen and liver. Following phagocytosis, platelets are destroyed by the oxidative killing mechanism. In a small proportion of patients, the liver fails to remove the platelets, and circulating antibody–platelet immune complexes are created. Complexes localize in arterioles and capillaries, occluding vessels and causing tissue ischemia. Vessels in the heart, kidney, brain, pancreas, and spleen are common targets for immune complex deposition.

Treatment of Idiopathic Thrombocytopenic Purpura

Administration of IVIG reduces autoantibody levels and disease symptoms. The mechanism is both simple and elegant. Pooled IVIG saturates specialized neonatal Fc receptors (FcRn) on endothelial cells. When the receptor is engaged, IgG is internalized by pinocytosis and recycled to the cell surface, thus preventing lysosomal degradation (Figure 13-1).

In contrast, serum autoantibodies binding to other Fc receptors on the same cells are internalized and destroyed, thereby arresting the disease process but not curing the disease.

Kawasaki Disease

Kawasaki disease is a self-limiting, febrile disease that is characterized by vasculitis of peripheral and coronary vessels. Patients present with a persistent rash, conjunctivitis, and lymphadenopathy. Individuals with Kawasaki disease have a high risk of heart failure, pericarditis, mitral or aortic valve insufficiency, and rupture of the coronary artery. In the last 5 years, Kawasaki disease has emerged as the leading cause of heart disease in the United States. Although the etiology of the disease is unclear, an immune response to a viral (parvovirus

---

BOX 13-1
Diseases Treated with Pooled Human Immunoglobulin

Immune thrombocytopenia
Guillain-Barré syndrome
Kawasaki disease
Dermatomyositis
Kidney transplants with ABO blood group incompatibility
Sjögren syndrome
Common variable immunodeficiency
Chronic lymphocytic leukemia
Pediatric human immunodeficiency virus (HIV) infection
Alzheimer's disease
Systemic lupus erythematosus (SLE)

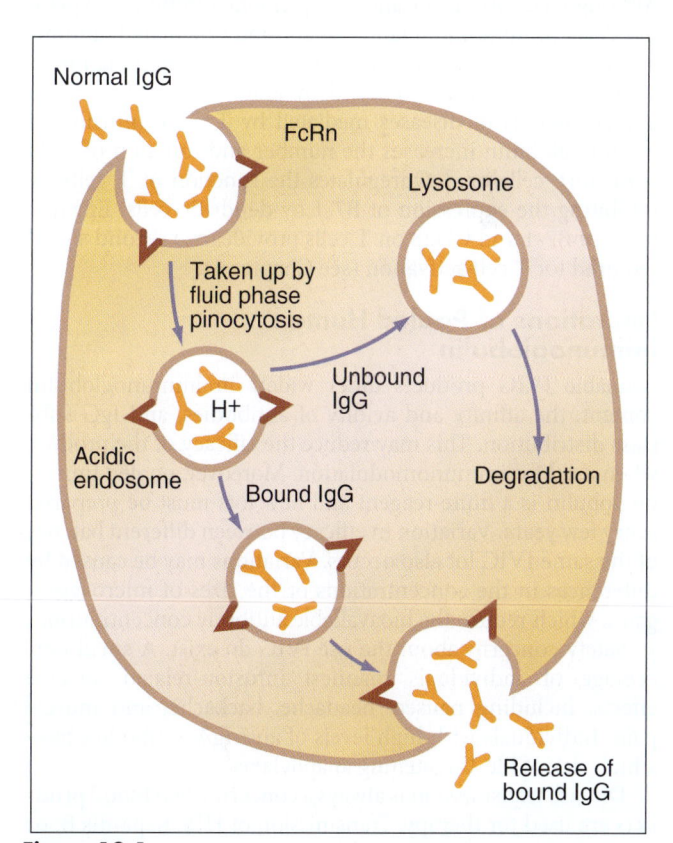

Figure 13-1

The role of FcRn in recycling normal IgG after administration of pooled immunoglobulin preparations.

B19 or cytomegalovirus) or bacterial (*Yersinia*) infection is believed to activate an autoimmune response to vascular endothelial cells and cardiac myosin.

Treatment of Kawasaki Disease

Infusion of IVIG reduces the symptoms by inhibiting the formation of a C3 convertase. Microaggregates within the IVIG displace C3b from tissue-bound immune complexes to the fluid phase, which downregulates the inflammatory response. IVIG also downregulates an inflammatory response by scavenging the anaphylatoxins (C3a and C5b) via low-affinity F(ab')$_2$ receptors in microaggregated immunoglobulin. In children with early disease, one regimen of IVIG may reduce the symptoms and progression of the disease for several years.

Erythroblastosis Fetalis

Pooled immunoglobulin is also used to prevent erythroblastosis fetalis in neonates caused by Rh factor incompatibility between mother and child (see Chapter 3). Generally, the mother is Rh negative (Rh−) and the fetus is Rh positive (Rh+). Spillage of fetal blood into the maternal circulation elicits an immune response that destroys the infant's blood cells. When the fetal bone marrow cannot compensate for the destruction of red blood cells, severe anemia occurs. Administration of RhoGAM (anti-Rh) is sufficient to prevent the stimulation of the maternal immune response to Rh+ red blood cells from the fetus.

INTRAVENOUS IMMUNOGLOBULIN AND T CELL–MEDIATED AUTOIMMUNE DISEASES

Although Fc saturation and complement inhibition explain the IVIG immunomodulation of antibody-mediated autoimmune diseases, it does not account for the downregulation of autoimmune diseases mediated by auto-reactive T cells. In animal models of diseases mediated by T cells, infusion of immunoglobulin increases the number and function of CD4 regulatory cells or downregulates the function of T cells by inhibiting the expression of B7-1 by dendritic cells. Engagement of B7-1 and CD28 on T cells provides the second signal required for T cell activation (see Chapter 6).

Limitations of Pooled Human Immunoglobulin

Available IVIG products differ widely in immunoglobulin content, the affinity and avidity of antibodies, and IgG subclass distribution. This may reduce the efficacy of the product when used for immunomodulation. Moreover, pooled immunoglobulin is a finite reagent and new lots must be prepared every few years. Variation in efficacy between different batches of the same IVIG lot also occurs. Variations may be caused by differences in the concentrations or the sizes of microaggregates, which reduce the bioavailable antibody concentration.

Safety concerns about the use IVIG do exist. A small percentage of individuals manifest infusion-related adverse effects, including nausea, headache, backache, and muscle pain. Individuals with high levels of anti-IgA antibodies have a high risk of life-threatening anaphylaxis.

Disease transmission is always a concern when blood products are used for therapy. Transmission of HIV, hepatitis B, or Creutzfeldt-Jakob syndrome prions has not been reported. However, several cases of IVIG-transmitted hepatitis C were reported before 1994. Additional antiviral measures included in the manufacturing process have reduced the possibility of hepatitis C transmission.

MONOCLONAL ANTIBODIES PRODUCED IN TISSUE CULTURE

Monoclonal antibodies are a product of recombinant DNA technology and can be produced in the laboratory. The name is derived from the fact that antibodies are produced from a population of cells that originated from a single B cell clone (monoclonal). Monoclonal antibodies have the same isotype and affinity constants for an antigen. In essence, monoclonal antibodies are a homogeneous antibody population that can be produced in the laboratory for decades.

Köhler and Milstein created the tissue culture–based system that produces homogeneous antibodies that bind to only one antigen with a high affinity. The methodology is based on the fusion of antigen-stimulated murine splenic B cells with a tissue culture–adapted, antibody-producing murine myeloma cell line. The spleen cells carry the information for antibody specificity, while the myeloma cells act as factories for the production of a specific immunoglobulin isotype. The fusion of the two types of cells creates a hybrid cell that can produce homogeneous antibodies directed at a specific antigen.

In the experimental protocol, polyethylene glycol (PEG) is used to fuse cell membranes. At best, the fusion is non-specific and creates different products that include B cell–B cell fusions; B cell–myeloma cell fusions; and myeloma cell–myeloma cell fusions. The next step selects the B cell–myeloma cell fusions for expansion and study. Selection is necessary to prevent overgrowth by tissue culture–adapted myeloma cells and myeloma cell–myeloma cell fusion products.

HAT (Hypoxanthine–Aminopterin–Thymidine) Selection

Selection takes advantage of different nucleic acid synthesis pathways. The classic de novo pathway is a complex pathway that produces folic acid. In turn, folic acid serves as a single carbon methyl donor in the synthesis of nucleotides. The nucleic acid salvage pathway provides a second conduit for DNA synthesis. In this pathway, thymidine and hypoxanthine are recycled into new nucleotides. Recycling requires the presence of an enzyme called *hypoxanthine-guanine phosphorylribosyl transferase (HPRT+)*.

Selection of B cell–myeloma cell hybrids is facilitated by the use of medium that contains hypoxanthine–aminopterin, and thymidine (HAT). Murine B cells have both classic and salvage pathways. As a consequence of several mutational events in the myeloma cells, the *HPRT* gene is inactivated, and they can only synthesize DNA by the classic pathway. In the HAT selection process, aminopterin (a folic acid inhibitor) blocks the production of DNA by the classic de novo pathway and kills the myeloma cells.

Since B cell–myeloma cell hybrids have both classic and de novo synthesis pathways, they survive the selection process. The surviving cells are known as *hybridomas*.

Hybridomas are placed in 96-well microtiter plates and are allowed to grow for 1 to 3 weeks. Each well is tested for the presence of antibodies. Cultures producing antibodies are cloned in agar to isolate single-cell hybridomas. Each hybridoma is expanded from the single B cell clone and retested for antibody production. The original protocol for the production of monoclonal antibodies is shown in (Figure 13-2).

Production of murine monoclonal antibodies solved the problem of limited reagents, but the immunogenicity problem remained unsolved. When administered to humans, murine monoclonal antibodies are considered foreign and generate an antibody response that neutralizes the monoclonal antibodies before they can reach their target. In addition, a risk of developing serum sickness exists.

MONOCLONAL ANTIBODIES WITH REDUCED IMMUNOGENICITY

The immunogenicity of murine monoclonal antibodies has been reduced by additional genetic engineering. For example, chimeric antibodies are composed of murine V_H and V_L domains and constant domains from human IgG. These

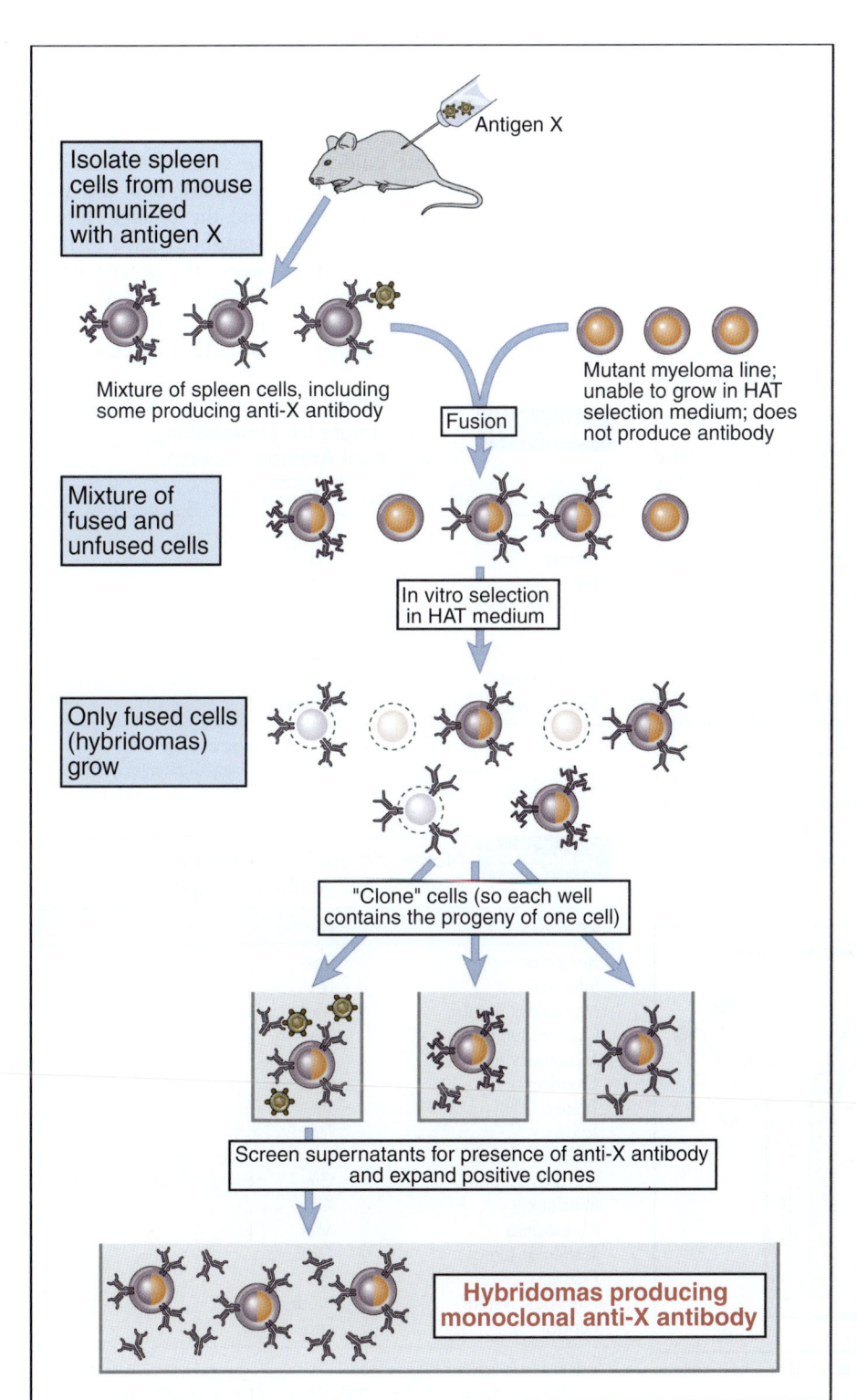

Figure 13-2

The protocol for generating murine monoclonal antibodies. (From Abbas AK, Lichtman AH, Pillai S: Cellular and molecular immunology, ed 6 [updated edition], Philadelphia, 2010, Saunders.)

monoclonal antibodies contain only 33% murine protein. Humanized monoclonal antibodies contain only 5% murine or rat protein, which is located in the hypervariable regions or the complementarity-determining regions (CDRs) of heavy and light chains (Figure 13-3).

CDRs are short amino acid sequences found in the antibody hypervariable region that actually come in contact with antigens. Despite the reduction in murine proteins, monoclonal antibodies often elicit an immune response. The immunogenicity problem was solved by the introduction of human monoclonal antibodies.

Chimeric Antibodies

To produce chimeric antibodies, murine hybridomas are produced by the classic method described above. The genes coding for the murine variable region of heavy and light chains are isolated from the hybridoma and amplified by polymerase chain reaction (PCR). Constant-region genes of human heavy and light chains also are amplified. After insertion of human and murine genes into a plasmid and transfection into bacteria, chimeric antibodies are produced as inclusion bodies. Following lysis of the cells, the chimeric antibodies are purified for in vivo use. Antibody aggregation and limited growth of antibody-producing bacteria restrict the usefulness of bacterial expression systems.

Humanized Antibodies

Humanized monoclonal antibodies are derived from murine hybridomas. However, genes coding for the six murine CDRs (three each on heavy and light chains) are amplified by PCR and inserted into a plasmid vector. Genes for human variable and constant regions also are inserted into the same vector. Transfected bacteria or transformed human B cells produce humanized monoclonal antibodies.

Human Monoclonal Antibodies

It has now become possible to produce human monoclonal antibodies in transgenic mice. In these animals, the murine immune system has been inactivated and replaced by megabase-sized yeast artificial chromosome (YAC) carrying the genes for IgG1–IgG4. Repeated stimulation of the mice produces a robust response of antibodies with high affinity for antigens. B cells isolated from the draining lymph nodes or spleen are fused with myeloma cells. Following HAT selection and hybridoma expansion in 96-well microtiter plates, supernatant fluids are tested for antibody production. These laboratory-created human monoclonal antibodies have high affinity for antigens and have elimination kinetics that are identical to natural antibodies.

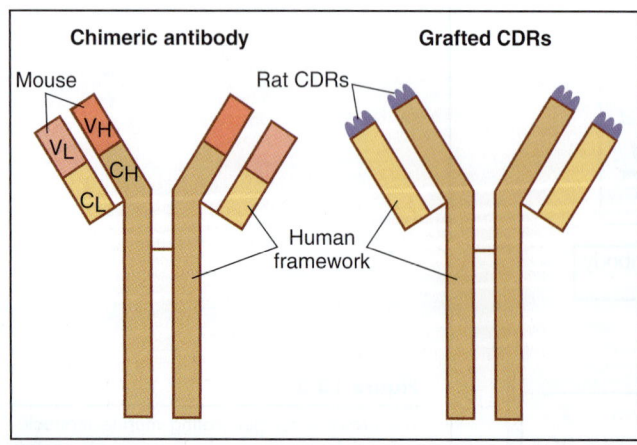

NOMENCLATURE FOR MONOCLONAL ANTIBODIES

Generic names of monoclonal antibodies provide information about the nature of the antibody, the animal source, and the antibody target. The World Health Organization Committee on Nonproprietary Names and the Adopted Name Council have published guidelines for monoclonal antibody nomenclature (Table 13-1 and Table 13-2).

According to these guidelines, the suffix designates the product as a monoclonal antibody (mab), and the prefixes show the monoclonal origin and the biologic target. For example, Humira, a monoclonal antibody used to treat autoimmune rheumatoid arthritis, carries the generic name *adalimumab*. The name explains that the agent is a monoclonal antibody (*mab*) of human origin (*u*), which targets a component of the immune system (*lim*). Another example is

Table 13-1 Nomenclature for Designating Monoclonal Antibody Source

Source	Name
Human	u
Mouse	o
Rat	a
Hamster	e
Primate	i
Chimeric	xi
Humanized	zu
Rat/mouse	axo

Modified from Smith BT: Concepts in immunology and immunotherapeutics, Bethesda, MD, 2003, American Society of Health-System Pharmacists.

Table 13-2 Nomenclature for Designating Monoclonal Antibody Target

Source	Name
Bacterial	Bac
Infection	Les
Musculoskeletal	Mol
Colonic tumor	Col
Mammary tumor	Man
Ovarian	Gov
Tumor	Tu
Toxin	Tox
Immune system	Lim
Cardiovascular	Cir
Interleukin	Kin
Melanoma	Mel
Testicular tumor	Got
Prostate	Pro
Nervous system	Neur
Fungal	Fug

Modified from Smith BT: Concepts in immunology and immunotherapeutics, Bethesda, MD, 2003, American Society of Health-System Pharmacists.

Figure 13-3 Generation of chimeric and humanized antibodies by genetic engineering.

Omnitarg, or *pertuzumab*, which is a monoclonal antibody (*mab*) that is humanized (*zu*) and targets tumor cells (*tu*). Pertuzumab is highly effective in blocking HER-2 receptors expressed on breast cancer cells, thus preventing estrogen-induced cell proliferation. The choice of the prefix has no rules, but it is usually a distinct syllable compatible with the other designations. For ease of pronunciation, the final consonant of the target designation is dropped when the source designation also begins with a consonant (e.g., *basiliximab*). A representative list of therapeutic monoclonal antibodies is provided in Table 13-3.

NOVEL ANTIBODY CONFIGURATIONS

Fab Fragments

Using molecular biology techniques, it is possible to construct monoclonal antibody fragments that consist solely of Fab or F(ab')$_2$. *Abciximab*, a chimeric Fab fragment, is commonly used to inhibit platelet clumping after angioplasty. *Afelimomab*, which is undergoing clinical trials for the treatment of sepsis or septic shock, is composed of F(ab')$_2$ antibody fragments.

Bi-Specific Antibodies

Bi-specific antibodies can be generated by genetic engineering and the fusion of two antibody-producing hybridomas to form a quadroma. Antibodies produced by the quadroma have a normal Y-shaped IgG configuration. Bi-specific antibodies combine heavy and light chains of one monoclonal antibody with one specificity with the heavy and light chains of another monoclonal antibody with a different specificity. Therefore, a single antibody can react with two different antigens because bi-specific antibodies have two different sets of CDRs.

Bi-Functional Antibodies

Antibodies or antibody fragments can be constructed in a number of different formats by using recombinant DNA technology. Tetravalent antibodies are the most common format used in cancer immunotherapy. Two antibodies react with target molecules on the cancer cell surface, while the other antibodies react with cytotoxic T cells or natural killer (NK) cells. Antibody-mediated cross-linkage of cytotoxic cell receptors activates cytotoxic T and NK cells that lyse tumor cells.

Flex antibodies are a unique subset of tetravalent antibodies that have linker segments between the antigen-combining sites. Because of their increased flexibility, they can react with antigens that are distant from one another on the same cell.

Single-Chain Fab Variable Fragments and Phage Display

Genetic information coding for antibody-variable regions can be gleaned from naïve B cells and used to construct genetic libraries. Library construction uses common molecular biology techniques such as reverse transcription of messenger ribonucleic acid (mRNA) to create complementary DNA (cDNA) and PCR, which amplify the variable regions in heavy and light chains. These antibody-variable regions (antigen-combining sites) called *single-chain variable fragments (scFv)* can be expressed in the protein coat of bacterial viruses, or bacteriophages (Figure 13-4).

Libraries from tonsillar B cells have created 10^7 to 10^{10} different antibody fragments with micromolar-binding affinities.

ScFv are generated by a multiple-step protocol. In the first step, mRNA coding for V_H and V_L are isolated from naïve B cells, hybridomas, or B cells from persons immunized against a specific pathogen. Using reverse transcription, cDNA is

Table 13-3 Selected Monoclonal Antibodies Currently Used for Immunotherapy

Generic Name	Nature of Monoclonal	Target	Indication
Abciximab	Chimeric	GPIIb/IIIa	Anti-platelet, post-angioplasty
Adalimumab	Human	Tumor necrosis factor (TNF)	Rheumatoid arthritis
Alemtuzumab	Humanized	CD52	B cell chronic lymphocytic leukemia
Basiliximab	Chimeric	CD25	Organ rejection
Bevacizumab	Humanized	Vascular endothelial growth factor (VEGF)	Metastatic colon cancer
Cetuximab	Chimeric	Epidermal growth factor (EGF) receptor	Solid tumors
Daclizumab	Humanized	CD25	Acute renal graft rejection
Eculizumab	Humanized	C5	Paroxysmal nocturnal hemoglobulinuria (PNH)
Efalizumab	Humanized	CD11a	Severe plaque psoriasis
Gemtuzumab ozogamicin	Humanized	CD33	Acute myelogenous leukemia
Ibritumomab tiuxetan	Murine	CD20	B cell lymphoma
Infliximab	Chimeric	TNF	Rheumatoid arthritis, Crohn's disease
Muromonab-CD3	Murine	CD3	Acute organ rejection
Natalizumab	Humanized	Alpha 4-integrin	Relapsing multiple sclerosis
Omalizumab	Humanized	Immunoglobulin E (IgE)	Asthma, allergies
Palivizumab	Humanized	F-glycoprotein	Respiratory syncytial virus (RSV)
Panitumumab	Human	EGF receptor	EGF-R-expressing metastatic colorectal cancer
Ranibizumab	Humanized	VEGF	Macular degeneration
Rituximab	Chimeric	CD20	B cell leukemia
Tositumomab	Murine	CD20	B cell lymphoma
Trastuzumab	Humanized	Herceptin receptor	Breast cancer, non–small cell lung cancer

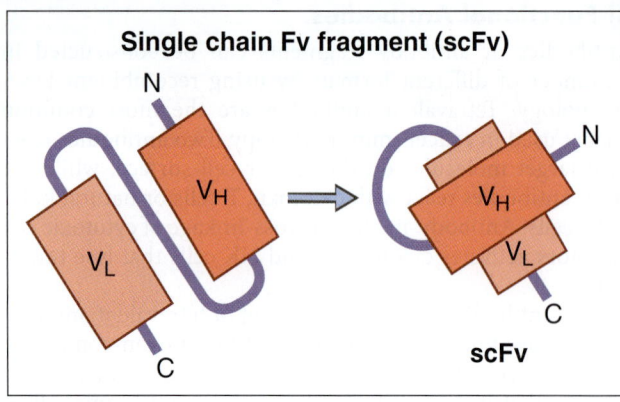

Figure 13-4
Genetically engineered single-chain variable fragment (scFv).

created for the V_H and V_L chains. To link variable heavy and light chain regions, nucleotides coding for repeating units of glycine and serine $(Gly_4Ser)_3$ are added to the DNA.

ScFv are expressed in a nonlytic M13 filamentous phage. DNA coding for the scFv are inserted into phage DNA at a site coding for the phage protein coat. *Escherichia coli*, a gram-negative bacterium, is a receptive host for phage replication. The secreted M13 phage displays scFv in the phage coat. Soluble phage is recovered and tested for antigen binding. Only a small number of expressed scFV may react with an antigen of interest because expression is a reflection of the amino acids in the variable region. Phage expressing scFv and high antigen-binding affinity for the antigen of interest is eluted and used to infect new *E. coli*. Using the M13 phage display expression system, large amounts of antigen-specific scFv (20–400 mg/L) can be produced by *E. coli* within a short period.

Many advantages as well as disadvantages to the use of scFv exist. One of the advantages is the excellent pharmacokinetics for tissue penetration. The disadvantages are that scFv are monovalent and have a high off-rate and poor target retention time. To increase retention time, multimeric scFv have been genetically engineered. Reductions in the glycine and serine $(Gly_4Ser)_3$ linker create scFv which are bivalent (diabodies), trivalent (triabodies), or tetravalent (tetrabodies).

ScFv are now being introduced into clinical trials. Pexelizumab, a humanized scFv directed at C5, has been shown to decrease tissue damage following an acute myocardial infarction and coronary artery bypass graft (CABG) surgery.

RADIOIMMUNOTHERAPY

Radioisotopes with moderately high energy can be linked to monoclonal antibodies. In reagent design, the overriding issues are affinity of the antibody for the target, isotope energy level, and half-life. Radioisotopes are coupled directly with the antibody via a tyrosine residue or bound directly to the antibody Fc by a chelator. Only five radioisotopes are used in radioimmunotherapy. These isotopes include (1) rhenium 186, (2) yttrium-90, (3) indium-111, (4) iodine-131, and (5) technetium-99. All have a half-life between 6 hours and 8 days and energy levels between 100 Kev and 375 Kev.

Two radiolabeled antibodies have been used extensively in treating patients with relapsed, refractory low-grade, and transformed non-Hodgkin's lymphoma (NHL). 131-I tositumomab and 90-Y ibritumomab are murine monoclonal antibodies directed at CD20 expressed on 95% of B cell lymphomas.

Inherent toxicities and risks are associated with the use of these radiolabeled antibodies, which include prolonged myelosuppression, myelodysplastic syndrome, and acute myelogenous leukemia. Toxicity is reduced when the anti-CD20 is combined with fludarabine or with fludarabine and cyclophosphamide.

A preloading delivery system, which reduces toxicity, also is used to deliver radioactivity to tumor cells. The protocol takes advantage of the high-binding affinities between *biotin* (vitamin H or B_7) and an egg protein called *avidin*. In the laboratory, biotin is coupled with a tumor-specific antibody. After the biotinylated antibodies are administered and bind to tumor cells, free avidin is administered in low concentrations. Avidin binds with high affinity to both bound and unbound biotinylated antibodies without saturating all of the biotin receptor sites on the antibodies. Non–tumor-cell-bound, soluble antibodies with biotin-avidin localize in the liver and are ingested by Kupper cells. After clearance of non-bound antibodies, radiolabeled avidin is added, and it binds almost irreversibly to the biotinylated tumor cell–bound antibodies. Radiolabeled antibodies are internalized, and the tumor cell is destroyed.

SUMMARY

- Antisera produced in animals are rarely used in clinical medicine because of immunogenicity and the risk of anaphylaxis or serum sickness.
- Pooled human immunoglobulin is used to treat immunodeficiencies and various disease states.
- Pooled human immunoglobulin is a finite source of antibodies, and different production lots vary in the concentration of antibodies and efficacy.
- Pooled human immunoglobulin is gradually being replaced by antibodies produced in vitro by using recombinant DNA technology.

REFERENCES

Anderson MJ, Woods VL Jr, Tani P, et al: Autoantibodies to platelet glycoprotein IIb/IIIa and to the acetylcholine receptor in a patient with chronic idiopathic thrombocytopenic purpura and myasthenia gravis, Ann Intern Med 100(6):829, 1984.

Ashrafi AH, Wang J, Stockwell CA, et al: Kawasaki disease: Four case reports of cardiopathy with an institutional and literature review, Pediatr Dev Pathol 10(6):491, 2007.

Billetta R, Lobuglio AF: Chimeric antibodies, Int Rev Immunol 10(2–3):165, 1993.

Callahan CW Jr, Musci MN Jr, Santucci TF Sr, et al: Cefaclor serum sickness-like reactions: Report of a case and review of the literature, J Am Osteopath Assoc 85(7):450, 1985.

Fengtian H, Yongzhan N, Baojun C, et al: Production of phage-displayed anti-idiotypic antibody single chain variable fragments to MG7 monoclonal antibody directed against gastric carcinoma, Chin Med Sci J 17(4):215, 2002.

Kaplan C: Diopathic thrombocytopenic purpura, autoantibodies, autoantigens. An overview, Ann Med Interne (Paris) 143(6):371, 1992.

Kohler G, Milstein C: Continuous cultures of fused cells secreting antibody of predefined specificity, Nature 256:495, 1975.

Kontermann RE, Volkel T, Korn T: Production of recombinant bispecific antibodies, Methods Mol Biol 248:227, 2004.

Lewis AP, Crowe JS: Generation of humanized monoclonal antibodies by "best fit" framework selection and recombinant polymerase chain reaction, Year Immunol 7:110, 1993.

Nolan O, O'Kennedy R: Bifunctional antibodies: Concept, production and applications, Biochim Biophys Acta 1040(1):1, 1990.

ASSESSMENT QUESTIONS

1. Which of the following are characteristics of active immunity?
   I. Transfer of antibodies from mother to child
   II. Direct antigenic stimulation of the immune system
   III. Vaccination
   A. I
   B. III
   C. I and II
   D. II and III
   E. I, II, and III

2. Idiopathic thrombocytopenic purpura is caused by:
   A. Autoantibodies to smooth muscle
   B. Autoantibodies to platelets
   C. Antibodies that cross-react with heart muscles
   D. Administration of foreign protein

3. In HAT selection, B cell–myeloma cells survive because they:
   A. Have only the nucleic acid salvage pathway
   B. Have only the classic de novo DNA synthesis pathway
   C. Have two nucleic acid synthesis pathways
   D. Have a mutated HPRT enzyme

4. Which of the following monoclonal antibodies have the least amount of murine protein?
   A. Chimeric
   B. Humanized
   C. Bifunctional
   D. Human

5. Which of the following is *not* a characteristic of monoclonal antibodies?
   A. Produced by B cells expanded from a single B cell clone
   B. Finite reagent
   C. Homogeneous isotype
   D. Homogeneous affinity constants

6. Which of the following is the leading cause of heart disease in the United States?
   A. Systemic lupus erythematosus
   B. Myasthenia gravis
   C. Kawasaki disease
   D. Lymphoproliferative diseases

CHAPTER 14

Antibodies and In Vitro Research and Diagnostic Assays

LEARNING OBJECTIVES

- Recognize the components of a flow cytometry (FCM)
- Compare and contrast forward and side scatter measurements
- Differentiate between absorbance and emission spectra
- Identify common fluorochromes used in lymphocyte enumeration
- Understand the concept of dual labeling and four-quadrant analyses
- Compare and contrast the components of a flow cytometer and a fluorescence-activated cell sorter (FACS)
- Explain the lateral flow technology used in home pregnancy tests
- Compare and contrast the direct, indirect, and sandwich enzyme-linked immunosorbent assay (ELISA) formats
- Explain Western blotting
- Recognize the function of sodium dodecyl sulfate in Western blotting
- Explain polyacrylamide gel electrophoresis
- Restate the major limitation of Western blotting

KEY TERMS

Enzyme-linked immunosorbent assay (ELISA)
Flow cytometer (FCM)
Fluorescence-activated cell sorter (FACS)
Sodium dodecyl sulfate
Western blotting

INTRODUCTION

Polyclonal and monoclonal antibodies are used in a wide range of in vitro assays in many different formats. The formats of the technology range from sophisticated flow cytometry (FCM) to simple enzyme-linked immunosorbent assay (ELISA). Data from antibody-facilitated assays are often used to support a tentative clinical diagnosis, evaluate disease progress, and provide prognostic information. In vitro assays are also used to determine the presence of bacteria, viruses, and antigens in biologic fluids. Increased hormone levels characteristic of disease states or pregnancy are determined by antibody-facilitated assays.

FLOW CYTOMETRY

A flow cytometer consists of four components: (1) a fluidics system, (2) single or dual lasers, (3) optical detectors, and (4) an on-board computer system that collects and analyzes data. As part of FCM, cells are placed in a fluidic system that contains sheath fluid or saline. Using hemodynamic focusing, cells are concentrated at a nozzle and passed in a single file through a laser (the interrogation point) at a rate of several thousand cells per second. Lasers are usually of high-power, water-cooled argon or krypton. The computer records each cell as a dot on a linear or logarithmic "x–y" graph. As the cell is passed through the interrogation point, light is scattered in all directions. One optical detector collects forward, or low-level, light scatter. *Forward scatter* is laser light that passes around the cells and is roughly proportional to cell size. An optical detector converts the light passing around the cell to voltage impulses, which are stored in the computer. In essence, small cells generate small voltages, and large cells generate large voltages. Another detector collects light scattered from the laser at a 90-degree angle, which is called *side scatter*. Side scatter is a measure of the internal complexity or granularity of a cell. Since peripheral blood cells vary in both size and granularity, a linear plot of side scatter versus forward scatter is used to separate peripheral blood cells into lymphocyte, monocyte, and granulocyte populations (Figure 14-1).

Enumeration of Lymphocyte Subpopulations

Lymphocyte phenotyping (lymphocyte subset enumeration) is a routine test used to screen for immunodeficiencies, evaluate disease progress, support a tentative diagnosis, and provide prognostic information. In patients with acquired immuno deficiency syndrome (AIDS), FCM is used to monitor CD4 cell numbers.

An inverse correlation exists between CD4 numbers and the risk for specific bacterial and fungal infections. Clinicians use CD4 data to determine when and what type of prophylactic antibiotic therapy should be implemented. FCM is also used to differentiate between acute B cell leukemia (ABCL) and myelogenous leukemia, to diagnose chronic lymphocytic leukemia (CLL), and to differentiate between hairy cell leukemia and mantle cell lymphoma.

Proper identification and classification of hematopoietic neoplasms are critical because treatment of leukemia and lymphoma are radically different. For example, CLL is usually treated with nucleoside analogues and alemtuzumab directed at CD52 expressed by leukemic cells. First-line therapy for hairy cell leukemia is chlorodeoxyadenosine (2-CdA). Conversely, mantle cell lymphoma is treated with hyperfractionated cyclophosphamide, doxorubicin, vinblastine, and dexamethasone, with or without rituximab.

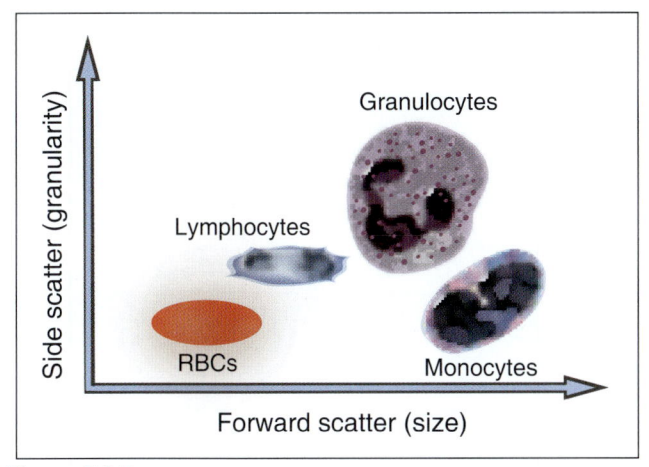

Figure 14-1

A schematic showing the flow cytometric segregation of peripheral blood cells based on size and granularity.

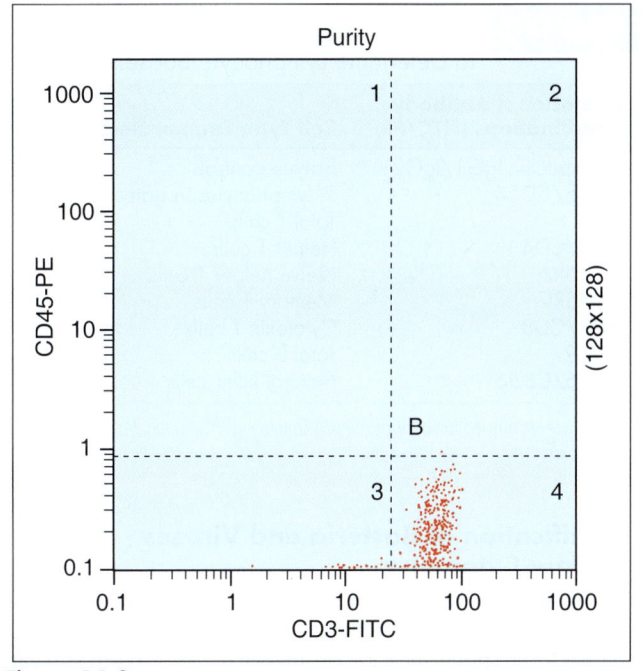

Figure 14-2

Flow cytometric analyses using dual labeling with CD3-FITC (fluorescein isothiocyanate) and CD45-PE (phycoerythrin). Cells staining with CD3-FITC are shown in the lower right quadrant. Each dot in the quadrant represents a single lymphocyte. Since there are no cells staining with CD45-PE (*upper left quadrant*), the lymphocyte population is essentially pure.

Dual staining of malignant cells has some prognostic value. For example, patients with ABCL have a poor prognosis if the malignant cells express CD10, CD34, and CD13. Conversely, the prognosis is excellent and so is response to chemotherapy when ABCL cells express CD45, CD135, and CD34.

In the enumeration of lymphocytes, size and granularity limits are used to draw an electronic "gate" around the lymphocyte population. Any subsequent data are derived solely from the "gated" area. The presence of lymphocytes in the gated area is verified by using fluorochrome-labeled monoclonal antibodies. Fluorochromes have high intensity and minimal overlapping spectra. As labeled antibodies pass the interrogation point, the fluorochrome absorbs light (excitation) at a specific wavelength. When the excited fluorochrome returns to a ground state, light is emitted at a different wavelength. Using mirrors and filters, the emitted light is delivered to photomultiplier detectors. In the detectors, fluorescence is converted to voltage intensity and stored in the computer as a dot on an x–y graph. Fluorescence yields information on the number of cells with fluorochrome, and the fluorochrome intensity is an index of the number of fluorescent markers per cell.

Although numerous fluorochromes can be used in FCM, fluorescein isothiocyanate (FITC) and phycoerythrin (PE) are commonly used in laboratory studies. FITC is a fluorescein derivative that is easily conjugated to antibodies via primary amines. In most conjugations, three to six FITC molecules are covalently linked to a single antibody. FITC is excited at 488 nanometer (nm) by an argon laser, and light is emitted at 530 nm. PE is a large-molecular-weight protein commonly found in cyanobacteria and red-green algae. Only one molecule of PE can be conjugated to an antibody. It is maximally excited at 533 nm and emits a very bright light at 570 nm.

To verify the percent of lymphocytes in the "gated" population, cells are labeled with two different antibodies—usually CD45-PE and CD3-FITC. The former is a pan-leukocyte marker, and the latter reacts only with T cells. Using a histogram of FITC versus PE immunofluorescence, cells are electronically placed into four quadrants: (1) Cells lacking both markers are placed in the lower left quadrant. (2) Cells expressing only the CD45 marker are placed in the upper left quadrant. (3) CD3-positive cells are shown in the lower right quadrant. (4) Cells expressing both markers are placed in the upper right quadrant. Generally, 95% of lymphocytes are found in the lower right quadrant (Figure 14-2).

After the lymphocyte population is verified, total T cell, CD4, and B cell populations can be enumerated using dual staining techniques, as shown in Table 14-1. Dual-color immunofluorescence enumerations of the peripheral blood CD4 subset are shown in Figure 14-3. Cells are incubated with two monoclonal antibodies conjugated to two different fluorochromes. FITC-conjugated antibodies are directed at CD3, and PE is linked to an anti-CD4 antibody. Dual-labeled CD4 helper/amplifier cells are shown in the upper right quadrant. The study is repeated using CD3–CD8 dual staining for T cytotoxic cells and CD16–CD56 staining for natural killer (NK) cells. B cells are identified by staining with anti-CD19.

FLUORESCENCE-ACTIVATED CELL SORTER

With several modifications, the flow cytometer can act as a fluorescence-activated cell sorter (FACS) capable of isolating pure populations of cells. In the FACS configuration, a vibrating mechanism breaks the cell stream into individual droplets immediately after they exit a nozzle. Droplets meeting the sorting criteria in terms of fluorescence are given a positive or negative electrical charge. For example, cells coated with FITC-labeled anti-CD3 can be isolated by giving the cells a positive charge as they pass through the laser. The charged droplet passes through deflection plates that have a positive or negative charge. Depending on the droplet's polarity, cells are deflected to the right or to the left into collection vessels. Uncharged cells are not deflected, and they enter a waste stream (Figure 14-4). Purified CD3 cells can be used in assays that assess the function of T cells.

Table 14-1 Minimum Monoclonal Panel Used to Determine Lymphocyte Subsets

Monoclonal Antibody Combinations (FITC/PE)	Cell Type Enumerated
Nonspecific IgG1/IgG2	Isotype control
CD45/CD14	% lymphocytes in gated region
CD3	Total T cells
CD3/CD4	Helper T cells
CD45RA	Naïve helper T cells
CD45RO	Memory T cells
CD3/CD8	Cytotoxic T cells
CD19	Total B cells
CD16/CD56	Natural killer cells

FITC, Fluorescein isothiocyanate; *IgG*, immunoglobulin G; *PE*, phycoerythrin.

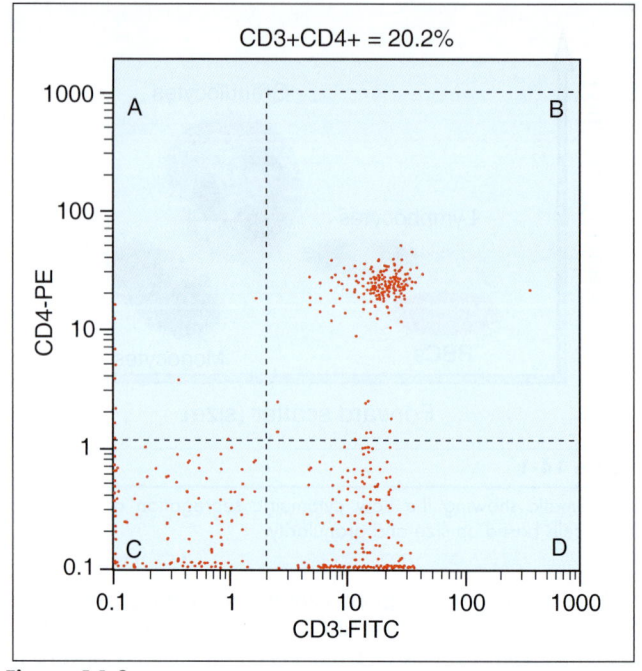

Figure 14-3
Dual staining of lymphocytes to determine the percentage of CD4 cells. Lymphocytes are dual stained with CD3-FITC (fluorescein isothiocyanate) and CD4-PE (phycoerythrin). Dual-stained cells appear in the upper right quadrant. The percentage of CD4 cells is 20.2%

Identification of Bacteria and Viruses by Flow Cytometry

FCM is often used in clinical microbiology because of its high sensitivity, specificity, and quick turnaround time. Bacteria and bacterial spores have a size range of 0.25 to 3.0 μm and can be detected in biologic fluids by using forward scatter measurements. Gated bacterial populations can be identified by labeled monoclonal antibodies directed at genus-specific antigens. FCM has been used to detect *Salmonella*, *Mycobacteria*, *Brucella*, *Mycoplasma*, *Legionella*, and *Escherichia coli* in biologic fluids. The method is extremely sensitive and can detect 10 to 100 bacteria/mL of sample. Other direct fluorochromes or substrates can be used to discriminate among viable, viable but non-culturable, and nonviable organisms. FCM also offers a rapid alternative for viral identification. Extracellular and intracellular viral antigens can be detected in biologic fluids. FCM has been useful in the rapid diagnosis of blood-borne cytomegalovirus (CMV), which is a common infection in transplant recipients and patients with AIDS. Identification of intracellular viruses is more difficult. Studies on infected cells require permeabilization to allow the entry of labeled antibodies into the cytoplasm. Since FCM requires isolated cells, it is best suited to the study of respiratory infections by using bronchoalveolar lavage fluids.

IMMUNOCHROMATOGRAPHIC TESTS

Pregnancy Testing

Most immunochromatographic test formats use lateral flow through a semi-permeable membrane. Antibodies are used as both capture and detection agents. The prototypic assay is the home pregnancy test that detects human chorionic gonadotropin (hCG) in urine. hCG is secreted by the developing placenta following conception and can be detected (5–50 mIU/mL) after 1 week of gestation.

In the test, urine is drawn through a membrane by capillary action into three distinct zones (reaction, test, and control zones). If the urine contains hCG, the color-labeled murine monoclonal antibodies react with hCG in the reaction zone, and the complex migrates to the test zone. Unlabeled polyclonal antibodies in the test zone recognize a second epitope on hCG. Labeled antibodies bound to hCG localize in the test zone, and the colored band suggests a positive test. Labeled and unlabeled antibodies continue to migrate into the control zone, which contains antimurine antibody. A colored band in the control zone confirms the proper capillary migration of urine. Positive reactions in both test and control zones confirm a positive test for elevated hCG (Figure 14-5).

ENZYME-LINKED IMMUNOSORBENT ASSAY

ELISA is a diagnostic tool that can be used to detect either antigens or antigen-specific antibodies in a biologic sample. In the simplest format, antigens are immobilized in 96-well microtiter plates. Test antibodies are then added to the mixture. To begin the detection process, an enzyme ligand is bound to the antibodies. After the removal of unbound antibodies and the unbound ligand, an enzyme substrate is added to produce a visible color change. Since the only variable in the assay is the concentration of antigens, the intensity of the color is directly proportional to the antigen concentration. Newer formats use fluorochrome or enzyme-conjugated antibodies to increase the sensitivity of the assay (Figure 14-6).

Several alternative ELISA formats include the indirect assay and the sandwich assay. In the indirect assay, antigens are immobilized, and unlabeled primary antibodies are incubated with the antigens. After the removal of the unbound antibodies, enzyme-conjugated secondary antibodies directed at the Fc region of the primary antibodies are added to the mixture. Addition of a colorimetric enzyme substrate (see Figure 14-6) yields a colorimetric endpoint.

The sandwich assay is another common ELISA format. In this configuration, antigens are captured by antibodies immobilized on a polystyrene substrate. Enzyme-conjugated antibodies directed at a second or different antigen epitope are added to the mixture. The addition of the enzyme substrate yields a visible color (Figure 14-7).

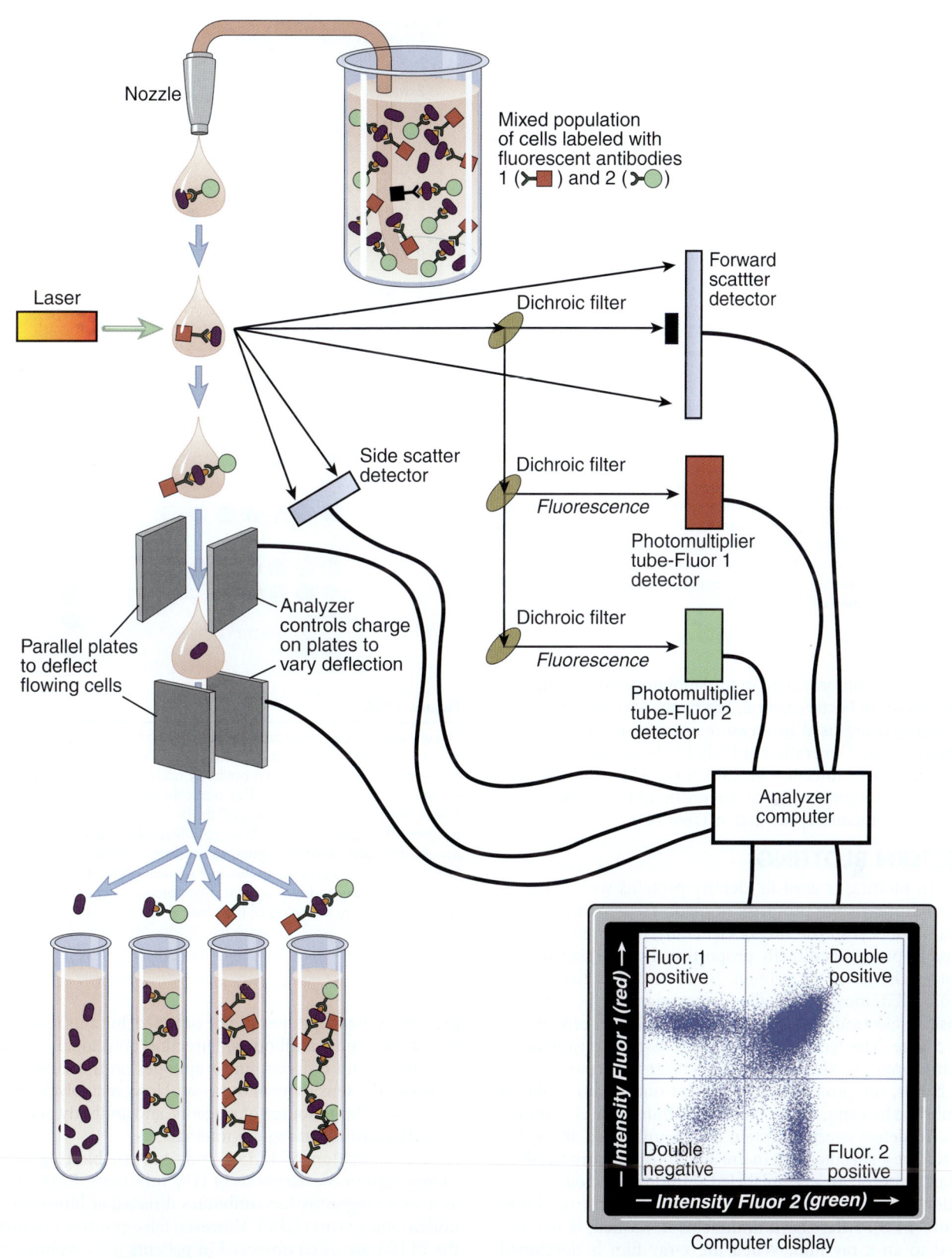

CHAPTER 14 ANTIBODIES AND IN VITRO RESEARCH AND DIAGNOSTIC ASSAYS

Figure 14-4
Principle of flow cytometry and fluorescence-activated cell sorting. The incident laser beam is of a designated wavelength, and the light that emerges from the sample is analyzed for forward scatter and side scatter as well as fluorescent light of two or more wavelengths that depend on the fluorochrome labels attached to the antibodies. The separation depicted here is based on two antigenic markers (two-color sorting). Modern instruments can routinely analyze and separate cell populations on the basis of three or more different colored probes. (From Abbas AK, Lichtman AH, Pillai S: Cellular and molecular immunology, ed 6 [updated edition], Philadelphia, 2010, Saunders.)

Figure 14-5

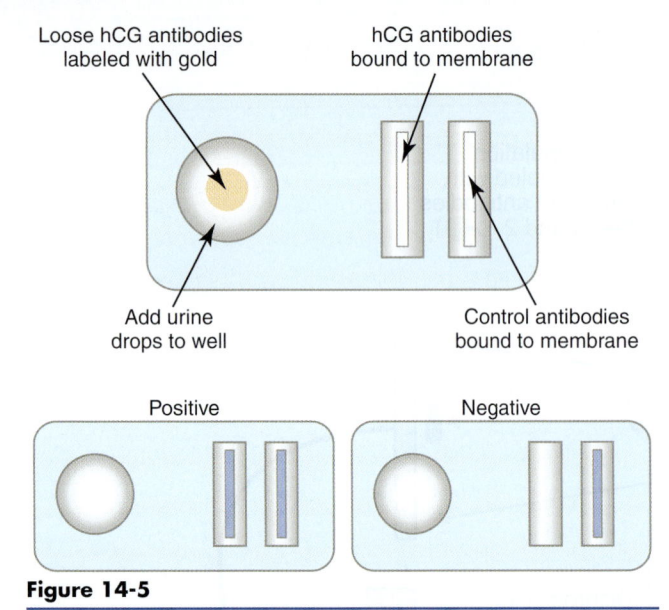

Home pregnancy test showing the reaction, test, and control zones. The reaction zone contains monoclonal antibodies directed at human chorionic gonadotropin (hCG) and linked to colloidal gold. The test zone contains membrane-fixed polyclonal antibodies directed at the second site on the hCG. The control zone contains bound polyclonal antibodies directed at the murine monoclonal antibodies. If the test is positive, both test and control zones will be colored.

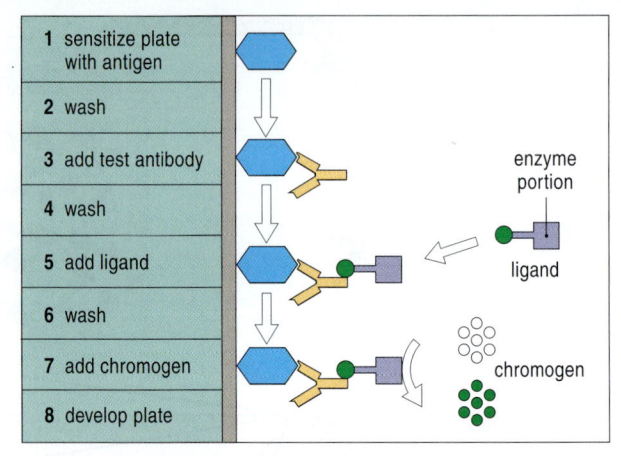

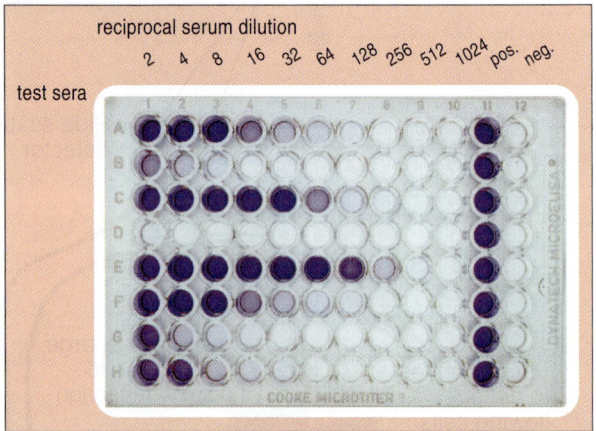

Figure 14-6

The enzyme-linked immunosorbent assay (ELISA) plate is prepared in the same way as the immunoassay up to step 4. In this system, the ligand is a molecule that can detect the antibody and is covalently coupled to an enzyme such as peroxidase. This binds the test antibody, and after the free ligand is washed away (*step 6*) the bound ligand is visualized by the addition of chromogen (*step 7*)—a colorless substrate that is acted on by the enzyme portion of the ligand to produce a colored end product. A developed plate (*step 8*) is shown in the lower panel. The amount of test antibody is measured by assessing the amount of colored end product by optical density scanning of the plate. (From Roitt I, Brostoff J, Male D, et al: Immunology, ed 7, Philadelphia, 2006, Mosby.)

ELISA is commonly used in the laboratory as an adjunct in the diagnosis of bacterial, viral, and parasitic infections. Serial ELISA assays are used to measure antigen-specific antibody levels in serum. Generally, antibody levels increase over time during an active infection and decrease when the infection abates. A representative list of diagnostic ELISA formats used in clinical medicine is provided in Table 14-2.

WESTERN BLOTTING

Western blotting is used to identify proteins within a complex mixture. In the protocol, proteins are denatured using sodium dodecyl sulfate (SDS). Generally, the amount of SDS bound to protein is directly proportional to the size and the negative charge of the protein. In an electrical field, denatured protein moves through a polyacrylamide mesh toward a positive electrode at a rate dependent on both protein size and charge. The technique is called *SDS-polyacrylamide gel electrophoresis*, or SDS-PAGE. To visualize the separated protein bands, the proteins are imprinted onto a nitrocellulose membrane by using electroblotting or transverse electrophoresis. To detect specific protein bands, unlabeled antibodies directed at a specific protein are added to the nitrocellulose. In classic protocols, a radiolabeled antibody directed at the Fc portion of the primary antibody is added to the nitrocellulose (Figure 14-8). After the immunoblot is washed, it is transferred to an x-ray film. When the x-ray film is developed, the protein bands with attached antibodies are immediately visible. Newer technology has replaced radioactivity with colorimetric dyes.

Western blotting has several limitations. Conformational epitopes are irreversibly denatured by SDS and cannot be detected. Linear epitopes can be detected, but this requires the use of polyclonal antibodies. Directing polyclonal antibodies at multiple and different linear epitopes on the same protein increases the sensitivity of the assay. However, polyclonal antibodies are a finite source of reagents, and antibody pools must be restandardized at regular intervals.

A combination of ELISA and Western blotting is commonly used in the diagnosis of HIV infections. ELISA is used as a screening assay for antibodies directed at human immunodeficiency virus (HIV). However, false-positive reactions in the ELISA are often observed in patients with syphilis, Lyme disease, hemophilia, systemic lupus erythematosus (SLE), and alcohol-related hepatitis. Western blotting, which detects HIV surface antigens, is used to confirm the ELISA results. The presence of viral antigens in biologic fluids and the presence of antibodies confirm an active HIV infection.

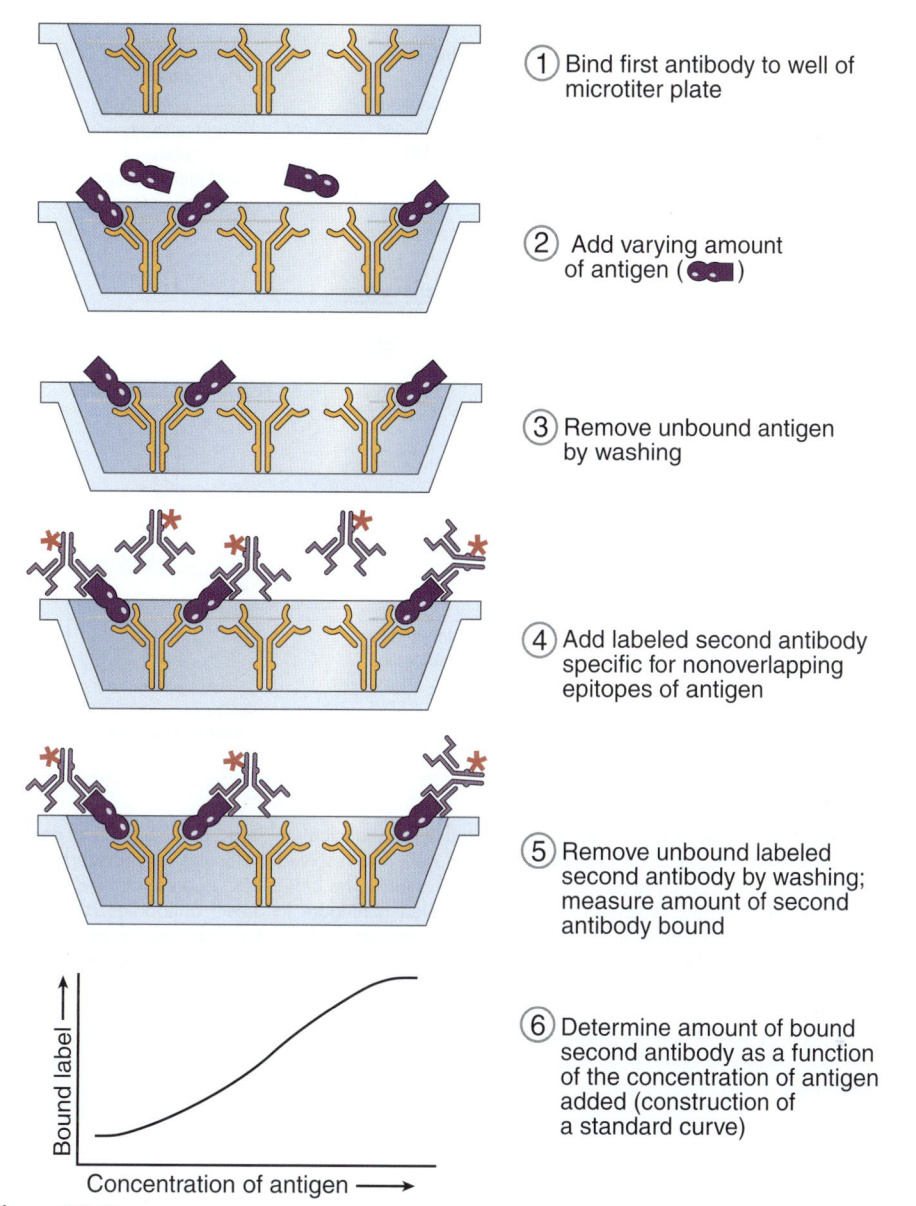

CHAPTER 14　ANTIBODIES AND IN VITRO RESEARCH AND DIAGNOSTIC ASSAYS　　115

1. Bind first antibody to well of microtiter plate
2. Add varying amount of antigen
3. Remove unbound antigen by washing
4. Add labeled second antibody specific for nonoverlapping epitopes of antigen
5. Remove unbound labeled second antibody by washing; measure amount of second antibody bound
6. Determine amount of bound second antibody as a function of the concentration of antigen added (construction of a standard curve)

Figure 14-7
Sandwich enzyme-linked immunosorbent assay (ELISA) or radioimmunoassay (RIA). A fixed amount of one immobilized antibody is used to capture an antigen. The binding of a second, labeled antibody recognizes a nonoverlapping determinant on the antigen. Addition of an appropriate substrate will allow visualization of the reaction. The amount of the secondary antibody bound is a function of the antigen concentration. (From Abbas AK, Lichtman AH, Pillai S: Cellular and molecular immunology, ed 6 [updated edition], Philadelphia, 2010, Saunders.)

Table 14-2　Diseases for Which ELISA Is Used to Support a Clinical Diagnosis

Microbe	Disease
Bordetella pertussis	Whooping cough
Borrelia burgdorferi	Lyme disease
Brucella abortus	Brucellosis
Chlamydia trachomatis	Chlamydial infections
Corynebacterium diphtheria	Diphtheria
Helicobacter pylori	Stomach ulcers
Mycoplasma pneumoniae	Atypical pneumonia
Clostridium tetani	Tetanus
Treponema pallidum	Syphilis
Legionella spp.	Legionnaires' disease
Toxoplasma gondii	Toxoplasmosis
Entamoeba histolytica	Amebiasis

ELISA, Enzyme-linked immunosorbent assay.

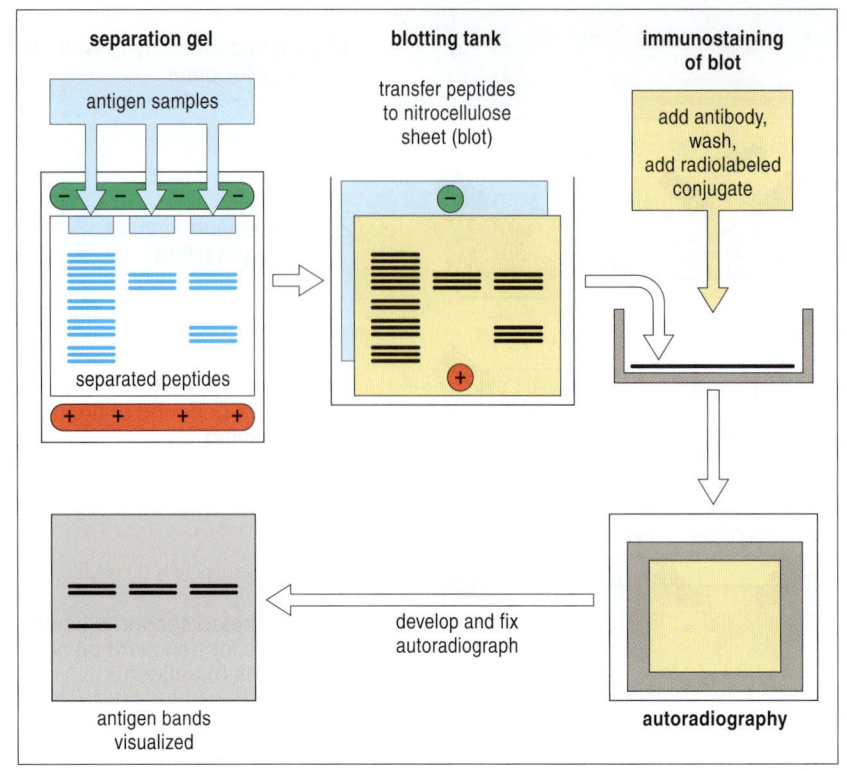

Figure 14-8

In immunoblotting, antigen samples are first separated in an analytical gel (e.g., an SDS [sodium dodecyl sulfate] polyacrylamide gel or an isoelectric focusing gel). The resolved molecules are transferred electrophoretically to a nitrocellulose membrane in a blotting tank. The blot is then treated with the antibody to the specific antigen and washed, and a radiolabeled conjugate to detect antibodies is bound to the blot. The principle is similar to that of a radioimmunoassay (RIA) or enzyme-linked immunosorbent assay (ELISA). After washing again, the blot is placed in contact with an x-ray film in a cassette. The autoradiograph is developed, and the antigen bands that have bound the antibody become visible. This immunoblotting technique can be modified for use with a chemiluminescent label or an enzyme-coupled conjugate (as in ELISA), where the bound material can be detected by treatment with a chromogen, which deposits an insoluble reagent directly onto the blot. (From Roitt I, Brostoff J, Male D, et al: Immunology, ed 7, Philadelphia, 2006, Mosby.)

SUMMARY

- Polyclonal and monoclonal antibodies are used in in vitro assays in complex (flow cytometry) or simple formats (ELISA).
- Flow cytometry is used in clinical medicine to screen for immunodeficiencies, evaluate disease progress, support a tentative diagnosis, and provide prognostic information to the clinician.
- Fluorescence-activated cell sorting is a modification of flow cytometry that allows the isolation and purification of lymphocyte subsets.
- ELISA is a solid phase immunoassay that can be used for the detection of antigens or antigen-specific antibodies.

REFERENCES

Bene MC, Kolopp Sarda MN, El Kaissauni J, et al: Automated cell count in flow cytometry: A valuable tool to assess CD4 absolute levels in peripheral blood, Am J Clin Pathol 110(3):321, 1998.

Burshtyn DN, Davidson C: Natural killer cell conjugate assay using two-color flow cytometry, Methods Mol Biol 612:89, 2010.

Duque RE, Andreeff M, Braylan RC, et al: Consensus review of the clinical utility of DNA flow cytometry in neoplastic hematopathology, Cytometry 14(5):492, 1993.

Hengel RL, Nicholson JK: An update on the use of flow cytometry in HIV infection and AIDS, Clin Lab Med 21(4):841, 2001.

Lau LG, Tan GB, Kuperan B: CD4 lymphocyte enumeration in patients with human immunodeficiency virus infection using three-colour and four-colour dual-platform flow cytometry: An inter-laboratory comparative evaluation, Ann Acad Med Singapore 31(6):765, 2002.

Subira D, Gorgolas M, Castañón S, et al: Advantages of flow cytometry immunophenotyping for the diagnosis of central nervous system non-Hodgkin's lymphoma in AIDS patients, HIV Med 6(1):21, 2005.

Weisberger J, Wu CD, Liu Z, et al: Differential diagnosis of malignant lymphomas and related disorders by specific pattern of expression of immunophenotypic markers revealed by multiparameter flow cytometry (Review), Int J Oncol 17(6):1165, 2000.

ASSESSMENT QUESTIONS

1. Which of the following antibody combinations would be used to enumerate natural killer cells?
   A. CD3 and CD4
   B. CD4 and CD8
   C. CD3 and CD8
   D. CD16 and CD56

2. In flow cytometry, forward scatter is a measurement of:
   I.   Size
   II. Granularity
   III. Expression of surface receptors
   A. I
   B. III
   C. I and II
   D. II and III
   E. I, II, and III

3. A major limitation of Western blotting is that:
   A. It cannot detect viral antigens
   B. It cannot detect hormones
   C. It cannot detect conformational epitopes
   D. It cannot denature large proteins

4. The home pregnancy test is an example of:
   A. ELISA
   B. Lateral flow immunochromatographic assay
   C. Western blotting
   D. Solid phase immunoassay

5. Which of the following are uses for flow cytometry in clinical medicine?
   A. Screening for immunodeficiencies
   B. Evaluating disease progression
   C. Supporting a tentative clinical diagnosis
   D. All of the above

CHAPTER 15

Immediate Allergic Reactions

LEARNING OBJECTIVES

- Define atopy
- Summarize the immunologic abnormalities associated with atopy
- Relate the roles of interleukin 4 (IL-4) and IL-13 in the evolution of an immediate allergic reaction
- List preformed mediators released during the early phase of an allergic response
- Compare and contrast the roles of preformed mediators in skin and lung allergic reactions
- Identify the late-phase mediators and their physiologic roles in allergic reactions
- Describe allergic rhinitis
- Identify the two common complications of allergic rhinitis
- Design a treatment regimen for allergic rhinitis
- Describe urticaria
- Design a treatment regimen for urticaria
- Explain the wheal-and-flare reaction in a skin test
- Compare and contrast urticaria and atopic dermatitis
- Identify the chemical characteristics of food allergens
- List foods that contain high histamine levels
- Explain the relationship between pollens, fruits, and oral allergy syndrome
- Define asthma
- Identify the three physiologic and immunologic components in asthma
- Identify the drugs used to control acute and chronic asthma
- List the three types of asthma that are not immunologically mediated
- Compare and contrast anaphylaxis and anaphylactoid reactions
- Identify antibiotics and therapeutic agents that cause anaphylactoid reactions
- Relate the theory behind the use of hyposensitization therapy
- Identify the major allergens in latex
- List the populations at risk for latex sensitization
- Identify the major house dust mite allergens
- Identify the roles of mite allergens in the generation of proinflammatory cytokines and immunoglobulin E (IgE) synthesis
- Identify the major cockroach-related allergens

KEY TERMS

Allergic rhinitis
Anaphylaxis
Anaphylactoid
Aspirin-induced asthma
Asthma
Atopic dermatitis
Atopy
Early-phase IgE response
Hyposensitization therapy
Infectious asthma
Late-phase IgE response
Leukotrienes
Prostaglandins
Radioallergosorbent test (RAST)
Skin test
Urticaria

INTRODUCTION

Immediate allergic reactions are mediated by the immunoglobulin E (IgE) class of antibodies, and reactions typically occur 15 to 20 minutes after exposure to an allergen. The prevalence of allergies in the United States is estimated to be between 9% and 16% of the population, or 50 million people. Over the last three decades, the incidence and severity of allergic reactions have increased substantially, and allergic diseases are now among the top three causes of illness and disability.

Allergic reactions occur in the skin (urticaria and atopic dermatitis), nose and eyes (rhinitis and conjunctivitis), lungs (asthma), and the intestine (food allergies). Clinical signs and symptoms are related to the time course, the target organ, and the nature of the pharmacologic mediators released from mast cells and basophils.

ATOPY

There is often a familial genetic tendency to develop rhinitis, urticaria, and asthma. This condition, called *atopy*, is characterized by elevated IgE levels directed at common aeroallergens or food allergens. Atopic individuals have increased numbers of CD4Th2 (T helper) cells and elevated interleukin 4 (IL-4) in peripheral blood. These abnormalities skew the immune response to IgE production. In addition, mast cells

Table 15-1 Examples of Chromosomal Locations and Genes Associated with Atopy and Asthma

Chromosomal Location	Candidate Genes	Putative Role of Gene Products in Disease
5q	Cytokine gene cluster (IL-4, IL-5, IL-13), CD14, β2-adrenergic receptor	Interleukin 4 (IL-4) and IL-13 promote immunoglobulin E (IgE) switching; IL-5 promotes eosinophil growth and activation; CD14 is a component of the lipopolysaccharide (LPS) receptor, which, via interaction with Toll receptor 4 (TLR4), may influence the balance between T_H1 and T_H2 responses to antigens; β2-adrenergic receptor regulates bronchial smooth muscle contraction
6p	Class II major histocompatibility complex (MHC)	Some alleles may regulate T cell responses to allergens
11a	FcεRI β-chain	Mediates mast cell activation
12q	Stem cell factor, interferon-gamma (IFN-γ), STAT6	Stem cell factor regulates mast cell growth and differentiation; IFN-γ opposes actions of IL-4; STAT6 mediates IL-4 signal transduction
16	IL-4 receptor α-chain	Subunit of both IL-4 and IL-13 receptors
20p	ADAM33	Metalloproteinase involved in airway remodeling
2q	DPP10	Peptidase that may regulate chemokine and cytokine activity
13q	PHF11	Transcriptional regulator involved in B cell clonal expansion and immunoglobulin expression

and basophils from atopic individuals have double the number of Fc receptors for IgE compared with nonatopic individuals. Atopic individuals also have hyperreactive airways that respond to low levels of cholinergic agonists that bind and activate acetylcholine receptors in the lung.

Although atopy is associated with genes on seven different chromosomes, single nucleotide polymorphisms in genes on chromosomes 5, 7, and 11 play a critical role in the frequency and evolution of allergic reactions (Table 15-1). These mutations increase cytokine production, expression of Fc receptors, IgE synthesis, and bronchial hyperreactivity.

Chromosome 5q genes regulate the production of cytokines (e.g., IL-4, IL-5, and IL-13). IL-4 and IL-13 drive isotypic switching to IgE production, and IL-5 promotes the growth and activation of eosinophils. IL-13 also increases bronchial mucus secretion. Tandem repeats in chromosome 11q13 are associated with polymorphisms in the FcεRI–beta chain and the number of Fc receptors expressed by mast cells and basophils. The FcεRI receptor acts as a trigger for immediate allergic reactions by stabilizing the receptor and amplifying intracellular signals. Bronchial hyperreactivity is controlled by the genes on chromosome 7.

EVOLUTION OF AN IMMEDIATE ALLERGIC REACTION

Initial Exposure to an Allergen

During initial exposure, allergens are processed by macrophages and allergenic epitopes presented to CD4Th2 cells in the context of class II molecules. In allergic or atopic individuals, T cells secrete IL-4, IL-5, and IL-13, which promote the rapid isotypic switching and IgE production by plasma cells. Secreted IgE binds specifically to Fc receptors on tissue mast cells and circulating basophils.

Second Exposure to an Allergen

Upon second exposure, the allergen cross-links two cell-bound IgEs, which initiates an energy-dependent mechanism that culminates in a biphasic immune response. The early-phase response, which occurs within 20 minutes of exposure, involves IgE–antigen interactions and is mediated by preformed pharmacologic mediators. A late-phase response, which occurs 4 to 8 hours following exposure, does not involve antibodies and is facilitated by the newly synthesized products of the arachidonic acid pathway.

Early-Phase Reactions and Preformed Mediators

In the early-phase reaction, granules containing preformed pharmacologic mediators are extruded from mast cells and basophils. The major preformed mediators include histamine, heparin, eosinophil chemotactic factor (ECF), and neutrophil chemotactic factor (NCF). Histamine is a vasoactive amine that has tissue-dependent, physiologic effects. In the skin, histamine interacts with receptors (H1 receptor) on vascular endothelial cells to create gaps between adjacent cells and increase vascular permeability (H2 receptor). Fluid from blood escapes through the gaps, causing swelling or edema in the tissue. Histamine also irritates peripheral nerve endings, causing itching and pain (pruritus). Heparin, which is also released from mast cells and basophils, potentiates the tissue edema by binding to antithrombin and preventing the activation of the normal coagulation pathway.

In the lung, histamine reacts with H1 receptors on smooth muscle in the bronchioles. Muscular contraction of the airways reduces the airway diameter, impeding the flow of air. The chemotactic factors ECF and NCF act on circulating cells and cause an influx of eosinophils and granulocytes at the site of the allergic reaction. Although the role of eosinophils in allergic reactions has not been fully delineated, enzymes released from eosinophils are known to inactivate histamine.

Late-Phase Reactions and Synthesized Mediators

Mast cells and basophils synthesize and release late-phase mediators over the course of 4 to 8 hours. These mediators include prostaglandins, leukotrienes, and platelet activating factor (PAF) (Figure 15-1).

Prostaglandins and leukotrienes are the products of the arachidonic acid pathway. Two prostaglandins (PGD_2 and PGE_2) play critical roles in late-phase reactions by increasing vascular permeability, contracting smooth muscle, and acting as an NCF. Leukotrienes are 20 carbon unsaturated fatty acids (LTA4, LTB4, LTC4, LTD4, and LTE4) that cause bronchoconstriction, increased mucus production, and sustained inflammation. PAF released from polymorphonuclear cells, endothelial cells, and monocytes causes bronchoconstriction, retraction of endothelial cells, and vasodilation. Late-phase reactions occur in some, but not all, individuals.

TYPES OF IMMUNOGLOBULIN E–MEDIATED ALLERGIC REACTIONS

Asthma

Asthma is a disease characterized by partial airway obstruction that is partially reversible either spontaneously or with treatment. The hallmark of allergic asthma is an early-phase allergic response. Approximately half of the patients with asthma also have late-phase responses. Chronic airway inflammation, airway injury, and airway repair (airway remodeling) also contribute to the pathogenesis of asthma and permanent abnormalities in lung function.

Chronic asthma has an inflammatory component. Cells involved in the inflammatory response include T cells, eosinophils, and mast cells. Cytokines released from activated macrophages mediate the inflammatory process. Tumor necrosis factor alpha (TNF-α) upregulates endothelial cell adhesion factors that bind neutrophils, monocytes, and eosinophils. The accumulation of cells forms the asthma inflammatory nidus.

If the airway inflammation is not resolved, reactive oxygen species produced by inflammatory cells injure the airways, and the tissue must be repaired and restructured. The interaction between lymphocyte CD28 and dendritic cell B7 activates dendritic cells and promotes the synthesis of pro-inflammatory cytokines. In tissue, L-arginine is converted to L-ornithine, which initiates cell proliferation, collagen synthesis, smooth muscle hypertrophy, and goblet cell hyperplasia. These changes culminate in the thickening of the sub-basement membrane, subepithelial fibrosis, and permanent damage to the bronchioles.

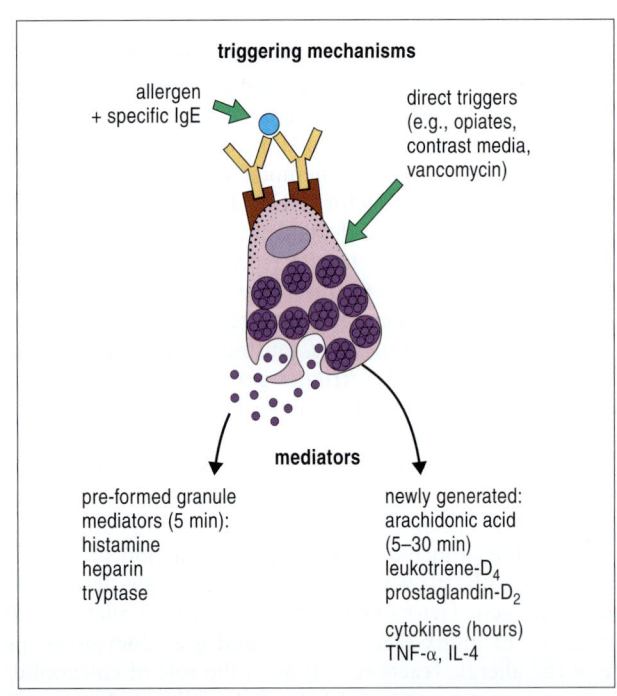

Treatment of Asthma

The clinician uses different medications to control the immediate reactions, the late-phase reaction, and chronic airway inflammation. Slow-acting β₂-agonists and oral corticosteroids are used to relieve the acute exacerbations of asthma. Therapeutics used to control long-term and chronic pulmonary symptoms are mast cells stabilizers, leukotriene antagonists, long-acting β₂-agonists, inhaled corticosteroids, and methylxanthines.

A new therapy uses a humanized monoclonal antibody, known as *omalizumab*, which is directed at IgE. It binds to soluble IgE and prevents binding to Fc receptors on mast cells and basophils. Omalizumab is usually prescribed to patients with moderate to severe asthma triggered by ubiquitous year-round allergens.

Allergic Rhinitis

Allergic rhinitis (AR) is the result of early-phase and late-phase IgE-mediated reactions and subsequent inflammation of the nasal passages, mucus membranes, nose, eyes, sinuses, and eustachian tubes. Early-phase mediators cause nasal edema, mucus secretion, itching, sneezing, and rhinorrhea. In the late phase, lymphocytes, basophils, and eosinophils accumulate in the area of an allergic reaction. Mediators released from the cellular infiltrate potentiate the inflammatory response.

AR is often complicated by sinusitis, which is infection or inflammation in any four sinus cavities in the skull. Inflammation causes the sinus lining to thicken, which impedes the flow of air or fluid. The chronic inflammation also results in the formation of nasal polyps. Usually, polyps are found in the ethmoidal sinuses located on either side of the nose between the eyes and the bridge of the nose. When the sinuses swell or the polyps impede the flow of air and fluid, bacteria begin to multiply and infect the cells lining the sinus. Acute sinusitis is usually caused by *Streptococcus pneumoniae, Haemophilus influenzae,* and *Moraxella catarrhalis.* Infections with *Staphylococcus aureus* and anaerobic bacteria are common in individuals with chronic sinusitis.

Treatment of Allergic Rhinitis

Individuals with acute or intermittent AR are treated with second-generation oral antihistamines, decongestants, nasal steroids, and leukotriene antagonists such as montelukast sodium. Intranasal antihistamines, sodium cromolyn, and anticholinergic agents are also effective in treating AR. Chronic rhinitis is treated with a short course of nasal steroids.

Figure 15-1
Mast cells release mediators after cross-linking of the immunoglobulin E (IgE) receptors on their surface. Preformed mediators are released rapidly while arachidonic acid metabolites such as leukotriene D₄ and prostaglandin D₂ are released more slowly. Mast cells can also be triggered by opiates, contrast media, vancomycin, and the complement components C3a and C5a. The mediators, which are also released by basophils, include histamine, tumor necrosis factor alpha (TNF-α), and interleulin 4 (IL-4). Histamine released by mast cells can be measured in serum following anaphylaxis or extensive urticaria, but it has a half-life of just minutes. By contrast, tryptase can be measured in serum for many hours after an anaphylactic reaction. (From Roitt I, Brostoff J, Male D, et al: Immunology, ed 7, Philadelphia, 2006, Mosby.)

Allergic Conjunctivitis

Atopic patients often develop conjunctivitis, called *allergic conjunctivitis*, which is characterized by redness, itching, and excessive tearing of the eyes. Conjunctivitis follows the same seasonal patterns of AR. *Vernal conjunctivitis* is a more serious, persistent form of conjunctivitis. It is characterized by redness and itching of the eyes, mucus production, and photophobia. In some cases, hypertrophy and edema of the upper eyelid form papillae. This form of conjunctivitis is called *giant papillary conjunctivitis*.

Treatment of Conjunctivitis

Various therapies are used to reduce the physiologic effects at different stages of AR. Artificial tear preparations are used to dilute the allergens and inflammatory mediators. Systemic or topical antihistamines reduce some symptoms.

Urticaria

Urticaria is a rash characterized by raised, flat-topped areas with associated red edematous welts (Figure 15-2).

Urticaria may be acute (6 or less weeks in duration) or chronic (6 or more weeks in duration). Acute urticaria is usually caused by food allergens such as eggs, nuts, shellfish, chocolate, tomatoes, berries, and milk. In rare instances, acute urticaria has been associated with the use of aspirin, angiotensin-converting enzyme (ACE) inhibitors, and nonsteroidal anti-inflammatory drugs (NSAIDs).

Urticaria is subdivided into types I and II on the basis of the nature of the immune response. Type I urticaria is a true IgE allergic reaction with both early and late phases. Type II urticaria is an aberrant reaction mediated by cytotoxic T cells, antibodies, complement activation, and the deposition of fibrin.

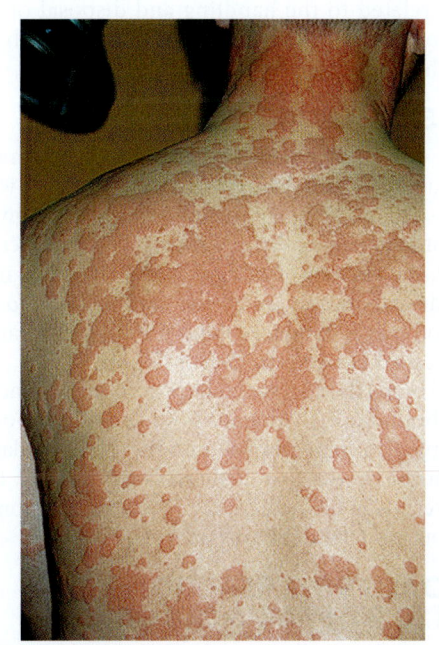

Treatment of Urticaria

Second-generation oral antihistamines, which have a minimal sedating effect, are commonly used for the treatment of IgE-mediated urticaria. Topical therapy with doxepin or capsaicin provides relief from refractory urticaria. Glucocorticosteroids are also indicated for the treatment of refractory urticaria, but their efficacy is controversial.

Atopic Dermatitis

Atopic dermatitis is a chronic, eczematous skin disease that is characterized by itching, swelling, cracking, and weeping skin lesions (Figure 15-3). Atopic dermatitis should not be confused with contact dermatitis. The former is an IgE-mediated allergic reaction, and the latter is a T cell–mediated delayed hypersensitivity reaction.

Of the two prevalent theories concerning the pathogenesis of atopic dermatitis, one postulates that allergen-stimulated Langerhans cells produce large amounts of IL-4, which causes rapid isotypic switching and the production of the IgE isotype. The second theory postulates that a topical *S. aureus* infection is the cause of atopic dermatitis. Staphylococcal superantigens stimulate Langerhans cells to produce high concentrations of IL-4 and isotypic switching.

Treatment of Atopic Dermatitis

Low- to medium-potency topical steroids are usually prescribed for the treatment of atopic dermatitis. However, calcineurin inhibitors are replacing corticosteroids because they have fewer adverse effects and can be used on all skin surfaces, including the skin on the face and neck.

ORAL ALLERGY SYNDROME

Over 25% of pollen-sensitive individuals develop burning or pruritus of the lips and tongue and edema of the buccal mucosa after ingestion of certain raw fruits and vegetables. The syndrome is an IgE-mediated early-phase reaction caused by exposure to antigens shared between pollens and fruits or

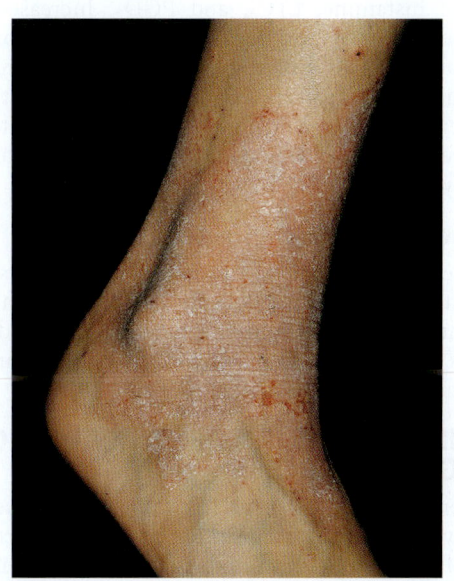

Figure 15-2
Allergic urticaria. This photo shows diffuse allergic-like skin reactions in an individual. The lesions have raised edges and develop within minutes or hours, with resolution occurring after about 12 hours. (From Roitt I, Brostoff J, Male D: Immunology, ed 6, St. Louis, 2001, Mosby.)

Figure 15-3
An atopic eczema reaction on the ankle of a child allergic to rice and eggs. (Delves PJ, et al: Roitt's essential immunology, ed 11, Oxford, 2006, Blackwell Publishing. Kindly provided by Professor J. Brostoff.)

Table 15-2	Pollens and Their Cross-Reactive Antigens
Pollen	**Cross-Reacting Antigens**
Alder	Almond, apple, celery, chery, hazelnut, peach, pear, parsley, strawberry, raspberry
Birch	Apple, carrot, cherry, pear, peach, plum, fennel, walnut, potato, wheat
Grass	Melon, tomato, watermelon, orange, wheat
Ragweed	Banana, cantaloupe, cucumber, honeydew, watermelon, zucchini, echinacea, artichoke, dandelion, hibiscus or chamomile tea
Pine	Pine nuts

Table 15-3	Allergens in Common Food Products	
Protein	**Total Percent Protein**	**Percent Allergenicity**
Egg Allergens		
Ovalbumin	54	100
Milk Allergens		
Beta lactoglobin	9	72
Casein	4	14
Soybean Allergens		
Beta conglycinin	19	74
Kunitz trypsin inhibitor	3	25
Peanuts		
Ara h1-8 proteins	17 (raw) 3 (cooked)	90
Ara h Oleoresin	Unknown	10

Modified from Metcalfe DD, Astwood JD, Townsend R, et al: Assessment of the allergenic potential of foods derived from genetically engineered crop plants, Crit Rev Food Sci Nutr, 36:S177, 1996.

vegetables. A list of pollens and their cross-reactive antigens is provided in Table 15-2.

FOOD ALLERGIES

Food allergens usually are large, water-soluble glycoproteins that are resistant to heating at 212°F and gastric proteolysis at pH 2 to pH 3. These large molecules are absorbed from the intestine and stimulate the synthesis of allergen-specific IgE. Major food allergens are peanuts, soybeans, tree nuts, milk, eggs, crustaceans, fish, and wheat (Table 15-3).

These allergens induce an early-phase response mediated by heparin and histamine, which cause vomiting, diarrhea, malabsorption, blood loss, and protein loss through the intestine. Acute urticaria, angioedema, and atopic dermatitis are also common in individuals with food allergies.

Treatment of Food Allergies

Elimination of the allergenic food from the diet is the only treatment for food allergies and other adverse food reactions.

ANAPHYLAXIS

Anaphylaxis is the most severe and often fatal allergic reaction, which involves total cardiovascular and respiratory collapse. This IgE-mediated reaction results in the massive release of histamine, LTC_4, and PGD_2. Increased vascular permeability causes a massive shift of fluids from blood into tissue within 10 minutes of exposure. The combination of vasodilation and increased vascular permeability causes hypovolemic shock and death within 15 to 60 minutes. Penicillin, bee stings, and peanuts are the most common causes of anaphylaxis.

Prevention of Anaphylaxis

Highly sensitized individuals at risk of anaphylaxis carry a self-injectable epinephrine delivery device. Epinephrine is a catecholamine that binds to α-adrenergic and β-adrenergic receptors to relax smooth muscles, decrease vascular permeability, and reduce vasodilation.

IDENTIFICATION OF AGENTS CAUSING ALLERGIC REACTIONS

If an allergic reaction is suspected, the clinician assesses the clinical symptoms and obtains skin test data to determine the source of the allergic reaction. Prick and intradermal tests are used in the diagnosis of allergies. When the prick test is used, the allergen is placed on the skin, and the skin is gently scratched or pricked. In the intradermal test, small amounts of allergen are injected subcutaneously under the skin.

If the patient is sensitive to a specific allergen, a wheal-and-flare reaction occurs at the skin test site within 15 to 20 minutes (Figure 15-4). Plasma leaking from the vessel into the skin induces edema, or swelling in the skin (wheal). Blood vessels at the periphery of the wheal then dilate, and red blood cells accumulate in the area, causing redness (flare) in the skin.

Some individuals who are at a high risk for anaphylaxis cannot have a skin test. In these cases, an in vitro radioallergosorbent test (RAST) is used to determine the presence of allergen-specific IgE. The classic RAST is actually an indirect ELISA, in which the secondary antibody is labeled with a radioisotope such as iodine-125. Because of the issues related to the handling and disposal of radioisotopes, secondary antibodies are now labeled with enzymes or fluorochromes.

HYPOSENSITIZATION THERAPY

Clinicians often implement hyposensitization therapy when allergic reactions cannot be effectively controlled with pharmacologic agents. During therapy, patients are given small amounts of allergens orally or subcutaneously. Over a period of months, the amount of allergen is increased to a maximum tolerated dose, which is called the *maintenance dose*. Hyposensitization therapy induces the synthesis of IgG antibodies, which are called *blocking antibodies* (Figure 15-5).

The IgG binds the allergen, thus preventing interaction with mast cell–bound IgE. Evidence has shown that hyposensitization therapy also increases the number of T regulatory cells that inhibit the production of allergen-specific IgE. Hyposensitization results in the reduction, but not elimination, of clinical symptoms in 60% to 90% of patients.

PSEUDOALLERGIC REACTIONS NOT MEDIATED BY IMMUNOGLOBULIN E

Symptoms similar to allergic asthma, food allergies, and anaphylaxis can be elicited by nonimmunologic reactions. Respiratory infections, exercise, and aspirin ingestion can cause asthma in some patients. High histamine levels in foods can cause symptoms consistent with a food allergy. Finally, some

CHAPTER 15 IMMEDIATE ALLERGIC REACTIONS   123

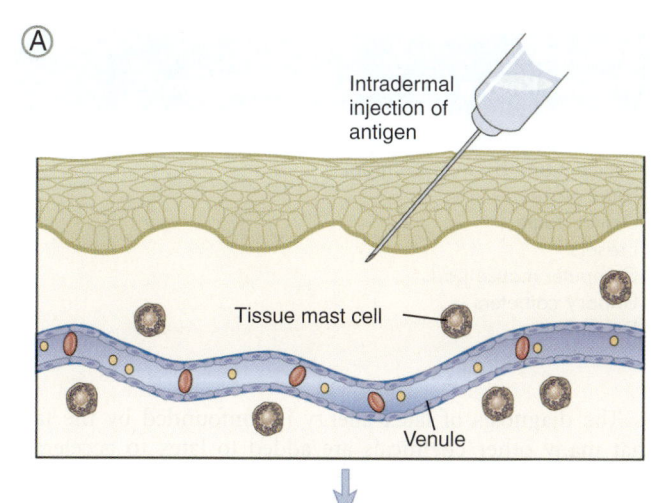

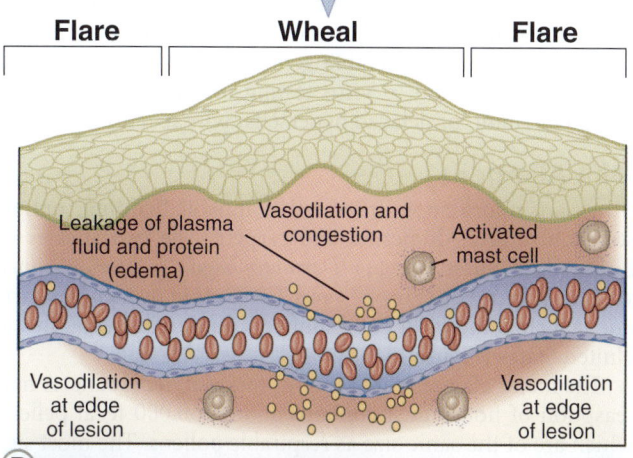

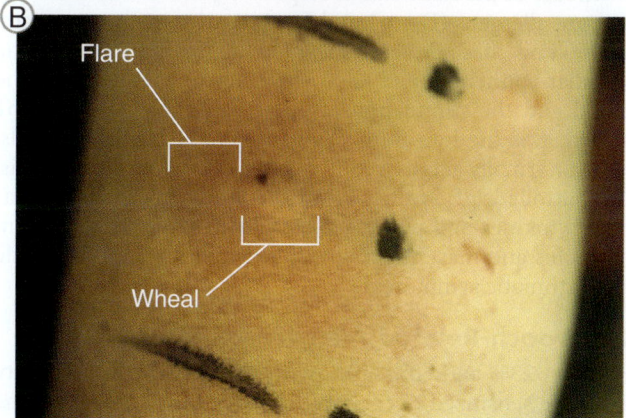

Figure 15-4
The wheal-and-flare reaction in skin. **A,** In response to antigen-stimulated release of mast cell mediators, local blood vessels first dilate and then become leaky to fluid and macromolecules, which produces redness and local swelling (a wheal). Subsequent dilation of vessels on the edge of the swelling produces the appearance of a red rim (the flare). **B,** Photograph of a typical wheal-and-flare reaction in skin in response to injection of an allergen. (In Abbas AK, Lichtman AH, Pillai S: Cellular and molecular immunology, ed 6 [updated edition], Philadelphia, 2010, Saunders. Courtesy of Dr. James D. Faix, Department of Pathology, Stanford University School of Medicine, Palo Alto, CA.)

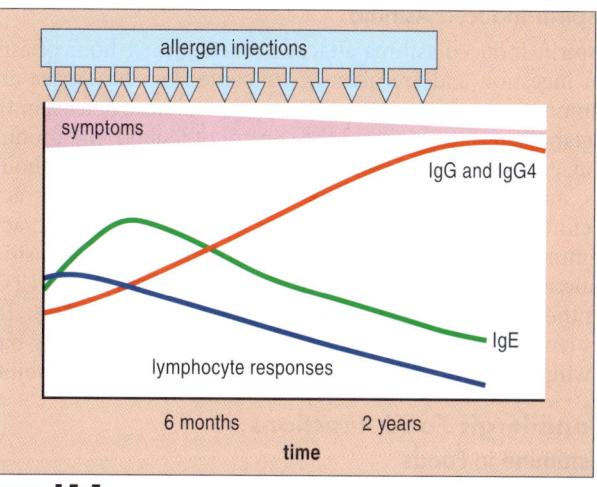

Figure 15-5
During desensitization or immunotherapy, a patient with an allergy receives regular subcutaneous injections of the relevant allergen. The immunologic changes that occur include an initial increase in immunoglobulin E (IgE) antibodies followed by a gradual decline, which in pollen-allergic patients is largely caused by a blunting of the seasonal increase. Antibodies of the IgG and specifically IgG$_4$ isotype increase progressively and may reach concentrations 10 times those present before treatment. Symptoms decline starting as early as 3 months but generally not maximally until 2 years. Changes in T cells are less well defined but include decreased in vitro response to allergens and increased production of interleukin 10 (IL-10). (From Roitt I, Brostoff J, Male D, et al: Immunology, ed 7, Philadelphia, 2006, Mosby.)

chemicals can induce anaphylactoid reactions that are similar to life-threatening anaphylaxis.

Nonallergic Asthma
Infectious Asthma
Nonallergic asthma can be caused by influenza, respiratory syncytial virus (RSV), or parainfluenza viruses. The replication of viruses often destroys the epithelial layers of the respiratory tract and exposes the sensory nerve endings. Stimulation of nerve endings by cold air or irritants causes a reflex bronchoconstriction. Asthma symptoms abate when the respiratory epithelium regenerates.

Rhinovirus and enterovirus (common cold viruses) can disrupt the control mechanisms for smooth muscle contraction by inhibiting the synthesis of the M2 muscarinic receptors. M2 receptors act in a negative feedback loop that controls the release of acetylcholine. The lack of M2 receptors allows the release of acetylcholine and increases the contraction of smooth muscle, causing symptoms that mimic asthma.

Exercise-Induced Asthma
In individuals with underlying bronchial hyperreactivity, exercise triggers an acute bronchospasm and symptoms similar to those of asthma. At rest, most individuals breathe through the nose, which serves to humidify and control the temperature in the lungs. After vigorous exercising, individuals tend to become mouth breathers. Mouth breathing evaporates water from the bronchioles, which alters airway humidity and temperature. When combined with existing airway edema, these changes induce a reflex bronchoconstriction.

Aspirin-Induced Asthma

Aspirin-induced asthma attacks occur within 1 hour of aspirin ingestion and are often accompanied by rhinorrhea and conjunctival irritation. Sensitive individual have defects in the metabolism of aspirin and the control of leukotriene production. Aspirin-sensitive individuals are poor aspirin metabolizers, and large concentrations of parental acetylsalicylic acid accumulate in the blood. In lung tissue, acetylsalicylic acid stimulates mast cells to produce leukotrienes. Aspirin-sensitive patients have a single nucleotide polymorphism in the LTC4 synthetase gene that causes the overproduction of LTC4. The C4 leukotriene is converted to LTD4 that causes airway narrowing, mucus secretion, and increased vascular permeability.

Nonallergic Food Reactions
Histamine in Foods

In sensitive individuals, severe gastrointestinal reactions occur following the ingestion of foods containing high concentrations of histamine. Eggplant, spinach, cheese, sauerkraut, vinegar, strawberry, and red wine (Chianti) contain high levels of histamine. In certain circumstances, histamine is present in tuna and mackerel. If these fish are improperly refrigerated, *Klebsiella* species decarboxylate tissue histidine to histamine, which causes a clinical syndrome called *scromboid fish poisoning*. Symptoms include diarrhea, facial flushing, dizziness, and vomiting.

Anaphylactoid Reactions

Anaphylactoid reactions are not mediated by IgE, but the symptoms mimic severe anaphylaxis. Most anaphylactoid agents activate the complement cascade or react directly with mast cells or basophils. Opiates, vancomycin, polymyxins, and ciprofloxacin are associated with anaphylactoid reactions resulting from complement activation. Activation of the complement cascade produces C3a, C4a, and C5a anaphylatoxins, which release mediators from mast cells and basophils.

Hyperosmolar radiocontrast media used in angiography reacts directly with mast cells and basophils to release pharmacologically active mediators. In addition to rashes, urticaria, angioneurotic edema, and smooth muscle spasms, some individuals develop hypotension, pulmonary edema, and cardiac arrest. Mortality from radiocontrast media–related anaphylactoid reactions is 1 to 5 per 100,000.

NEW AND NOVEL ALLERGENS
Latex Allergens

Latex is a milky fluid produced by rubber trees (*Hevea brasiliensis*) in Southeast Asia and Malaysia. The major component of latex is C1-4 polyisoprene, which is not allergenic. However, latex preparations are often contaminated with allergenic plant defense proteins called *hevein* and *hevein amine*. These allergens are carried through the manufacturing process and are present in the finished products. Latex has multiple commercial uses and is commonly found in a number of products (Box 15-1).

Persons sensitized to latex allergens develop IgE-mediated urticaria and rhinitis. Inhalation of latex allergens also causes asthma. Populations at risk for latex allergy are hospital workers and patients with spina bifida or congenital urogenital disease. An estimated 25% of the hospital workers are sensitized to latex. Because of the extensive use of urinary and intrathecal catheters, 28% to 68% of patients with spina bifida are sensitized to latex.

BOX 15-1
Products Known to Contain Latex Allergens

Condoms
Pacifiers and baby bottle nipples
Latex gloves
Dental dams
Erasers
Computer mouse pads
Urinary catheters
Diapers

The diagnosis of latex allergy is confounded by the fact that many other chemicals are added to latex to accelerate curing (thiuram, mercaptobenzothiazoles, and carbamates) and vulcanization (sulfur). These compounds elicit an irritant dermatitis caused by disruption of the skin or a delayed hypersensitivity response resembling poison ivy. Clinicians must perform in vivo and in vitro testing to differentiate among allergic, irritant, or delayed hypersensitivity reactions.

Mite Allergens

Mites are microscopic insects that inhabit bedding, upholstered furniture, draperies, and carpets. The two species of house dust mites are (1) *Dermatophagoides pteronyssinus*, which is found in Europe, and (2) *Dermatophagoides farinae*, which is the most commonly encountered species in the United States (Figure 15-6).

The major allergens are proteins found in fecal balls. A half teaspoon of house dust contains about 250,000 fecal pellets, which are of the same size as respirable pollens. The most significant allergens (Der p1 and Der p2) are cysteine proteases. In the lung, these proteases degrade the tight junctions in the vascular epithelium and allow the entry of allergens into the blood and the stimulation of an immune response. Der p1 also cleaves the low-affinity IgE receptor (CD23) on B cells, which normally acts as a control mechanism for IgE synthesis. Uncontrolled IgE synthesis and the release of proinflammatory cytokines and pharmacologically active mediators from basophils and mast cells cause contraction of smooth muscle and asthmatic symptoms.

Cockroach-Related Allergens

Between 23% and 60% of those living in crowded inner-city areas are sensitized to cockroaches. Allergens come from the saliva, fecal matter, secretions, cast skins, and dead bodies of cockroaches. The major cockroach-related allergens are Bla g1, 2, 4, and 5. However, Bla g1 is the major allergen that elicits IgE synthesis in 60% to 80% of sensitized individuals. The structure of Bla g1 is similar to that of an aspartic proteinase, but it has no enzymatic activity. The combination of sensitivity to cockroaches and repeated exposures to airborne allergens causes the increase in asthma reported in many inner-city areas.

DRUGS AND IMMEDIATE ALLERGIC REACTIONS

With the exception of penicillins (see Chapter 3) and beta lactam antibiotics, pharmaceuticals are not usually involved in IgE-mediated immediate allergic reactions. Rather, drugs may evoke delayed hypersensitivity reactions. The major lesion in addition, IL-4, IL-5, and IL-13 cause the release of cytotoxic proteins from eosinophils.

SUMMARY

- Immediate allergic reactions that occur 15 to 20 minutes after exposure to an allergen are mediated by IgE antibodies.
- Most allergic responses have an early-and late-phase reaction. Early-phase reactions are mediated by preformed histamine and heparin. Late-phase reactions are caused by the products of the arachidonic acid pathway.
- Asthma, urticaria, allergic rhinitis, and atopic dermatitis are examples of IgE-mediated allergic reactions.
- Some forms of asthma are induced by infection, exercise, and aspirin. These forms of asthma do not have an immunologic basis.
- Immediate allergic reactions can occur in the skin, lungs, or intestine.
- Food allergens differ from common aeroallergens in their chemical characteristics and response to physical stressors.
- Anaphylaxis and anaphylactoid reactions are life threatening, but only anaphylaxis is an IgE-mediated allergic reaction.
- New emerging allergens include latex, house dust mites, and cockroaches.

REFERENCES

Al-Shemari H, Bosse Y, Hudson TJ, et al: Influence of leukotriene gene polymorphisms on chronic rhinosinusitis, BMC Med Genet 9:21, 2008.

Anderson SD, Daviskas E: The mechanism of exercise-induced asthma, J Allergy Clin Immunol 106(3):453, 2000.

Blumenthal MN: The role of genetics in the development of asthma and atopy, Curr Opin Allergy Clin Immunol 5(2):141, 2005.

Coyle AJ, Wagner K, Bertrand C, et al: Central role of immunoglobulin (Ig) E in the induction of lung eosinophil infiltration and T helper 2 cell cytokine production: Inhibition by a non-anaphylactogenic anti-IgE antibody, J Exp Med 183(4):1303, 1996.

Enrique E: Immunotherapy in the treatment of food allergy. Does it have a future? Allergol Immunopathol (Madr) 37(3):143, 2009.

Gould HJ, Sutton BJ, Beavil AJ, et al: The biology of IGE and the basis of allergic disease, Annu Rev Immunol 21:579, 2003.

Kay AB: Allergy and allergic diseases. Second of two parts, N Engl J Med 344(2):109, 2001.

Litonjua AA, Lasky-Su J, Schneiter K, et al: ARG1 is a novel bronchodilator response gene: Screening and replication in four asthma cohorts, Am J Respir Crit Care Med 178(7):688, 2008.

Maddox L, Schwartz DA: The pathophysiology of asthma, Annu Rev Med 53:477, 2002.

Ono SJ: Molecular genetics of allergic diseases, Annu Rev Immunol 18:347, 2000.

Suzuki Y, Ra C: Analysis of the mechanism for the development of allergic skin inflammation and the application for its treatment: Aspirin modulation of IgE-dependent mast cell activation: role of aspirin-induced exacerbation of immediate allergy, J Pharmacol Sci 110(3):237, 2009.

Togo K, Suzuki Y, Yoshimaru T, et al: Aspirin and salicylates modulate IgE-mediated leukotriene secretion in mast cells through a dihydropyridine receptor-mediated Ca(2+) influx, Clin Immunol 131(1):145, 2009.

Wild LG, Lehrer SB: Immunotherapy for food allergy, Curr Allergy Rep 1(1):48, 2000.

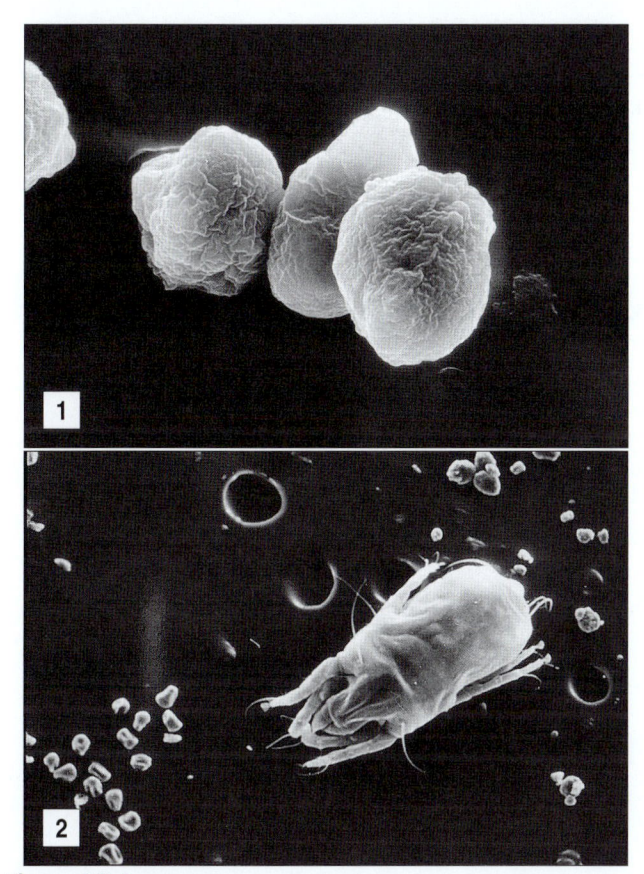

Figure 15-6

1, The dust mite is the most important source of allergen in house dust, largely as fecal particles. **2,** A mite is shown with pollen grains (*lower left*) and fecal particles (*upper right*). The mite is approximately 300 μm in length (i.e., just visible but not small enough to become airborne). Mite fecal particles are approximately 10 to 40 μm in diameter and become airborne during any disturbance of surfaces in the house. Pollen grains are similar in size to mite fecal particles (i.e., approximately 30 μm in diameter). The important allergic sources of pollen (i.e., grass, ragweed, trees) are wind pollinated, and the grains are designed to travel in the air for long distances. (From Roitt I, Brostoff J, Male D, et al: Immunology, ed 7, Philadelphia, 2006, Mosby.)

drug hypersensitivity is a morbilliform rash. By definition, a morbilliform rash consists of macules and papules of differing sizes that begin on the trunk and spread to the extremities. Rashes can occur during or after drug therapy.

IMMUNOGLOBULIN E AND PARASITIC INFECTIONS

In certain regions of the world with endemic parasitic helminthic infections, most individuals have increased CD4Th2 lymphocytes and high levels of parasite-specific IgE in serum. In the intestine, the release of preformed mediators causes violent peristaltic contractions that expel the intestinal worms. In

ASSESSMENT QUESTIONS

1. Which of the following mediators are produced during the late phase of an IgE-mediated allergic reaction?
   A. Heparin
   B. Histamine
   C. Tryptase
   D. Leukotrienes

2. Which of the following is *not* associated with atopy?
   A. Increased CD4Th2 cells
   B. Increased Fc receptors on mast cells and basophils
   C. Increased IL-4 production
   D. Increased Il-2 production

3. Allergic rhinitis is associated with:
   I. Early-phase and late-phase allergic responses
   II. Nasal polyps
   III. Bacterial infections
   A. I
   B. III
   C. I and II
   D. II and III
   E. I, II, and III

4. Which of the following is characterized by wheal-and-flare reactions in the skin?
   A. Urticaria
   B. Atopic dermatitis
   C. Allergic reactions to drugs
   D. Allergic rhinitis

5. Which of the following are attributes of food allergens?
   I. Large molecular weight glycoproteins
   II. Resistance to digestion at a low pH
   III. Resistance to heat
   A. I
   B. III
   C. I and II
   D. II and III
   E. I, II, and III

6. The major house dust mite allergen is:
   A. Der p1
   B. Bla g1
   C. Hevein
   D. C1-4 polyisoprene

CHAPTER 16

Autoimmunity

LEARNING OBJECTIVES

- Examine the relationship between thyroglobulin and iodine
- Identify the differences between T3 and T4
- Understand the hypothalamus–pituitary axis and its role in thyroid function
- Discuss the role of the thyrotropin-releasing hormone (TRH)
- Explain the function of the thyroid-stimulating hormone (TSH)
- Identify the target of the autoantibodies found in Graves' disease
- Discuss the role(s) of cytokines and fibroblasts in Graves' ophthalmopathy
- Define the term *thyroid storm*
- Design a therapy regimen to treat Graves' disease
- Compare and contrast the symptoms of Graves' disease and Hashimoto's thyroiditis
- Discuss the immunologic mechanisms that contribute to Hashimoto's thyroiditis
- Discuss the role of the intrinsic factor in vitamin B_{12} transport
- Identify the target of autoantibodies found in pernicious anemia
- Explain the role of vitamin B_{12} in red blood cell synthesis
- Design a therapy regimen to treat pernicious anemia
- Recognize the target of autoantibodies found in myasthenia gravis
- Identify the two mechanisms by which acetylcholine receptors are reduced in myasthenia gravis
- Compare and contrast ptosis and diplopia
- Design a therapy regimen to treat mild and severe myasthenia gravis
- Identify the clinical symptoms of systemic lupus erythematosus (SLE)
- List the viruses that may play a role in SLE
- Describe the two immunologic defects associated with SLE
- Design a therapy regimen to treat SLE
- Compare and contrast SLE and the "lupus-like" syndrome
- Recognize the autoantibody targets in Goodpasture syndrome
- Describe the genetic and immunologic factors that increase the risk of Goodpasture syndrome
- Design a therapy regimen to treat Goodpasture syndrome
- Define molecular mimicry
- Differentiate between the function of pancreatic alpha, beta, and delta cells
- Relate the role(s) of insulin in the body
- List the targets of autoantibodies found in type 1a diabetes
- Identify the human leukocyte antigen (HLA) alleles that increase the risk of diabetes
- List the viruses that are implicated in the onset of diabetes
- Design a drug regimen to treat diabetes
- Define ankylosing spondylitis (AS)
- List the possible microbial triggers for AS
- Explain the role of HLA-B27 in the pathophysiology of AS
- Design a treatment regimen for AS
- Compare and contrast rheumatoid arthritis and reactive arthritis
- List the microbial agents that play a role in reactive arthritis
- Define rheumatoid arthritis (RA)
- Explain the relationship between HLA alleles and RA
- Identify the six viruses that may act as triggers for RA
- Compare and contrast the roles of macrophages and fibroblasts in the pathophysiology of RA
- Define rheumatoid factor (RF)
- Understand the relationship between RF and agalactosyl antibodies
- Design a treatment regimen to treat RA
- Discuss the role of the immune system in rheumatic heart disease
- Recognize the definition of autoimmune hemolytic anemia
- Contrast the mechanisms by which α-methyldopa, penicillin, and cephalosporin cause anemia
- Identify the drugs used to treat hemolytic anemia

KEY TERMS

Acetylcholine
Acetylcholinesterase
Ankylosing spondylitis
Arthritis
Diabetes
Goiter
Goodpasture syndrome
Graves' disease
Hashimoto's thyroiditis
Intrinsic factor
Molecular mimicry
Myasthenia gravis
Pernicious anemia
RANKL (receptor activator of nuclear factor kappa-β ligand)
Reactive arthritis

Rheumatic fever
Rheumatoid factor
Systemic lupus erythematosus
Thyrotropin-releasing hormone
Thyroid-stimulating hormone

INTRODUCTION

Autoimmune diseases arise when an individual's immune system attacks his or her own tissue and organs. The immune response may be mediated by antibodies or activated lymphocytes and macrophages. These diseases are found in 5% to 7% of the population, and the disease incidence is heavily skewed toward females. In women over 65 years of age, autoimmune diseases are one of the 10 leading causes of death.

The etiology of autoimmune disease in women is multifactorial. The factors include genetic, environmental, and hormonal triggers. Individuals expressing certain human leukocyte antigen (HLA) alleles are at high risk of developing autoimmune disease. For example, individuals expressing HLA B8 and DR3 have an increased risk of developing Graves' disease. Because the onset of autoimmune diseases occurs shortly after puberty and just before the onset of menopause, estrogen particularly is thought to be one of the triggers for autoimmune disease. A wide range of different autoimmune diseases may affect a single organ (e.g., thyroid) or multiple organs (e.g., in systemic lupus erythematosus).

AUTOIMMUNE DISEASES OF THE THYROID

The function of the thyroid is to produce the hormones T3 and T4, which control physiologic functions in the cardiac, pulmonary, hematopoietic, gastrointestinal, skeletal, and endocrine systems. To produce the hormones, thyroglobulin (Tg) is synthesized by thyroid cells (thyrocytes) and stored in the follicular lumen. Iodine covalently binds to thyroglobulin tyrosine residues by using thyroperoxidase. Intracellular proteases digest thyroglobulin to produce functional triiodothyronine (T3) and thyroxin (T4), which differ only in the number of bound iodine molecules.

Synthesis of T3 and T4 is controlled by the hypothalamus–pituitary–thyroid axis. When the T3 and T4 levels fall below acceptable levels, the hypothalamus produces *thyrotropin-releasing hormone (TRH)* which travels through blood to the anterior pituitary gland. The anterior pituitary gland releases another hormone called *thyroid-stimulating hormone (TSH)*. This hormone interacts with thyrotropin receptors and stimulates iodine uptake and the production of T3 and T4 (Figure 16-1).

Thymic hormone levels are controlled by negative feedback loops. High levels of TSH act on the hypothalamus to downregulate the production of TRH. T3 and T4 also act on both the pituitary and the hypothalamus to downregulate hormone production. Autoantibodies directed at the thyroid results in either hypothyroidism or hyperthyroidism.

Graves' Disease

Graves' disease was first reported by Dr. Robert Graves in the 1830s and is the most common cause of hyperthyroidism in children and young women. The disease is caused by IgG_1 antibodies reacting with thyrotropin or TSH receptors. What causes the immune system to recognize thyroid antigens is unclear. It is conceivable that a viral infection may expose a hidden epitope in thyroid receptors.

Constant stimulation of TSH receptors causes glandular hyperplasia (goiter) and accelerated synthesis of T3 and T4. Patients often exhibit a rapid heart rate, exophthalmos, tremors, sweating, and attention deficit disorders. TSH receptors are also found in orbital cells and muscles. Reaction between the autoantibody and the TSH orbital receptor causes an inflammatory reaction called *Graves' ophthalmopathy* (Figure 16-2).

Graves' Ophthalmopathy

In the pathogenesis of Graves' ophthalmopathy, lymphocytes infiltrate the orbit of the eye and release cytokines such as tumor necrosis factor (TNF) and interleukin 1 (IL-1). These cytokines stimulate fibroblasts to secrete a glycosaminoglycan (GAG) mucopolysaccharide. GAG increases osmotic pressure in the eye, causing edema in the extraocular and retro-orbital muscles and in adipose tissue. These changes force the eyeball forward, creating bulging of the eye, or *exophthalmos*.

Thyroid Storm

In patients with undiagnosed Graves' disease, thyroid hormones often increase dramatically, which precipitates a life-threatening clinical crisis. A *thyroid storm* is precipitated by excessive stress, surgery, or sepsis. High levels of thymic hormones cause extreme tachycardia and atrial fibrillation. The mortality rate is 20%, and death occurs within 48 hours.

Treatment for Graves' Disease

Thiourea was the drug initially used to treat Graves' disease; however, it had considerable toxicity. Second-generation drugs and derivatives such as propylthiouracil and methylthiouracil, methimazole, and carbimazole have less toxicity. With the exception of methimazole, which prevents the storage of thyroid hormones, these drugs inhibit thyroperoxidase, thereby reducing the synthesis of T4 and T3.

Oral administration of radiolabeled iodine-131 is now the most common therapy for Graves' disease. The high-intensity radiation destroys thyroid cells and brings the levels of thyroid hormones into the normal range. Subtotal thyroidectomy was the treatment of choice before the advent of radioactive iodine. Methimazole therapy is indicated for those patients in whom radioactivity is contraindicated.

Hashimoto's Thyroiditis

Hashimoto's thyroiditis is the most common form of hypothyroidism, with a prevalence rate of 2% of the population of the United States. Individuals mount both an antibody response and a cellular response to thyroid tissue. The disease is caused by a break in peripheral tolerance to thyroid tissue, and the failure of regulatory cells to control auto-reactive T and B cells. About 85% to 90% of patients with Hashimoto's thyroiditis develop anti-thyroid peroxidase and anti-thyroglobulin antibodies. The inactivation of thyroperoxidase prevents the incorporation of free iodine into thyroglobulin. Elevated intracellular iodine also stimulates the maturation of dendritic cells and macrophages, which present antigens to auto-reactive CD4 and CD8 cells that have infiltrated the thyroid (Figure 16-3).

CD4Th1 cells produce IL-12, tumor necrosis factor alpha (TNF-α) and interferon gamma (INF-γ), which induce apoptosis of thyrocytes. Individuals with Hashimoto's thyroiditis also express a molecule called *Fas* on thyroid cells. The expression of the Fas molecules marks the cell for destruction by T lymphocytes.

Figure 16-1

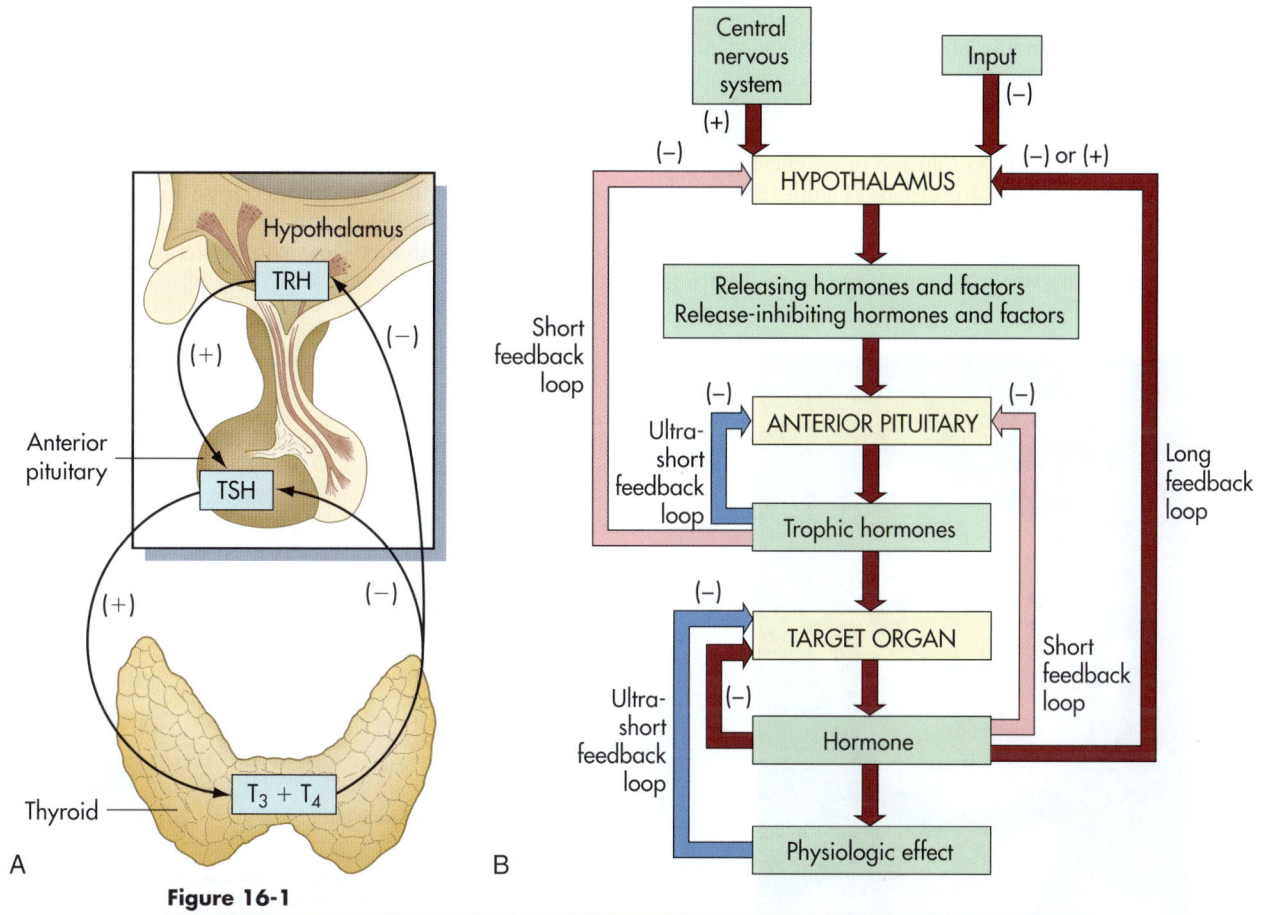

Feedback loops. **A,** Endocrine feedback loops involving the hypothalamus–pituitary gland and end organs, in this example, the thyroid gland (endocrine regulation). **B,** General model for control and negative feedback to hypothalamic–pituitary target organ systems. Negative-feedback regulation is possible at three levels: target organ (ultrashort feedback), anterior pituitary (short feedback), and hypothalamus (long feedback). (*TRH*, thyrotropin-releasing hormone; *TSH*, thyroid-stimulating hormone; T_3, triiodothyronine; T_4, tetraiodothyronine.) (From McCance KL, Huether SE: Pathophysiology: The biological basis for disease in adults and children, ed 5, St Louis, 2006, Mosby.)

Patients with Hashimoto's thyroiditis present with nonspecific symptoms such as fatigue, dry skin, and weight gain. Other symptoms include decreased sweating, deafness, peripheral neuropathy, depression, and memory loss.

Treatment for Hashimoto's Thyroiditis

Oral sodium levothyroxine, which is a synthetic thyroid hormone (T4), usually has to be taken for life by patients with Hashimoto's thyroiditis. However, the dose must be carefully titrated on the basis of the patient's needs. Some patients cannot tolerate the synthetic hormone. Natural porcine gland preparations of T3 and T4 can be used in these patients.

PERNICIOUS ANEMIA

In *pernicious anemia (PA)*, antibodies are directed at a glycoprotein known as *intrinsic factor*. These autoantibodies also neutralize any soluble intrinsic factor in the intestinal lumen.

Neutralization of the soluble intrinsic factor prevents the transport of vitamin B_{12} across the intestinal mucosa to portal blood (Figure 16-4). Without this essential vitamin, red blood cell precursors cannot divide. This results in a megaloblastic anemia characterized by the presence of immature, dysfunctional red blood cells (megaloblasts) in the blood. If untreated, PA is usually fatal after 1 to 3 years (Figure 16-5).

Treatment for Pernicious Anemia

Vitamin replacement therapy combined with folate and iron supplements is used to treat PA. Cobalamin and hydroxocobalamin are natural forms of vitamin B_{12} produced by bacterial fermentation. Both can be administered parenterally. However, hydroxocobalamin is the drug of choice because it is bioavailable for longer periods. Folate and iron supplements are included in the treatment because restoration of normal B_{12} levels triggers a rapid increase in the synthesis of red blood cells, which depletes stores of folate and iron.

MYASTHENIA GRAVIS

Myasthenia gravis (MG) is a rare disorder in which the patient exhibits progressive weakness of skeletal muscles. Individuals with the disease produce antibodies directed at postsynaptic acetylcholine receptors at the neuromuscular junctions of skeletal muscle.

Surface receptors are destroyed as a result of complement activation or are internalized and destroyed by proteolytic enzymes (Figure 16-6).

Both mechanisms decrease the number of receptors available for acetylcholine binding and the propagation of nerve impulses. Failure to propagate the nerve impulses causes fatigue and muscle weakness. Initially, muscle weakness is observed in the extraocular muscle group. Ptosis (abnormal drooping of one or both eyelids), diplopia (blurred or double vision), or both are characteristic signs of the disease (Figure 16-7).

Over a period of months, the weakness progresses from the ocular muscles to facial, jaw, tongue, and throat muscles. Without treatment, the weakness may progress to the trunk and limb muscles. MG is fatal when impairment of respiratory muscles occurs.

Treatment for Myasthenia Gravis

Depending on the severity of the disease, several different treatment strategies are used to treat MG. In mild cases, corticosteroids and acetylcholinesterase inhibitors are used. Corticosteroids downregulate the immune response, and acetylcholine inhibitors slow cholinesterase inactivation of

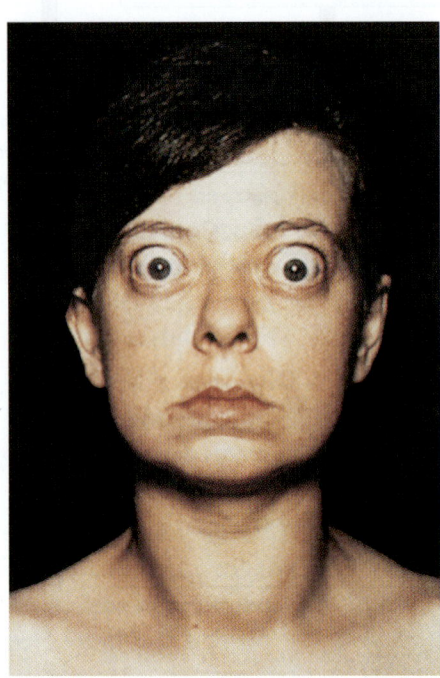

Figure 16-2

Thyrotoxicosis (Graves' disease). Note large and protruding eyeballs in association with a large goiter. (From McCance KL, Huether SE: Pathophysiology: The biological basis for disease in adults and children, ed 5, St Louis, 2006, Mosby; Seidel et al: Mosby's guide to physical examination, ed 4, St Louis, 1999.)

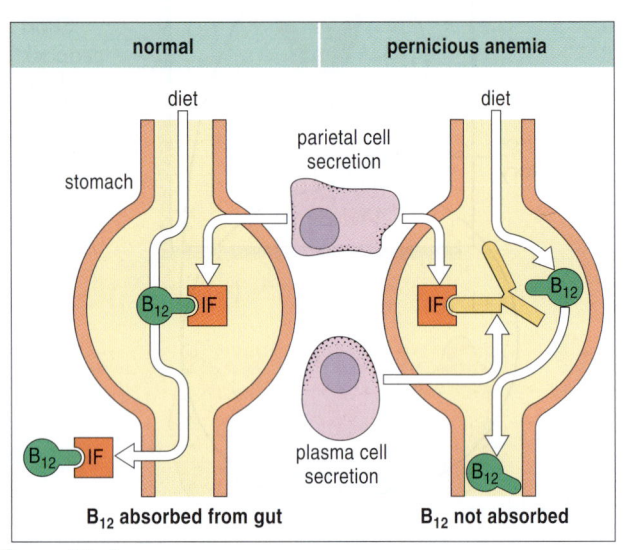

Figure 16-4

Normally, dietary vitamin B_{12} is absorbed by the small intestine as a complex with intrinsic factor (IF), which is synthesized by parietal cells in gastric mucosa. In pernicious anemia (PA), locally synthesized autoantibodies, specific for intrinsic factor, combine with intrinsic factor to inhibit its role as a carrier for vitamin B_{12}. (From Roitt I, Brostoff J, Male D, et al: Immunology, ed 7, Philadelphia, 2006, Mosby.)

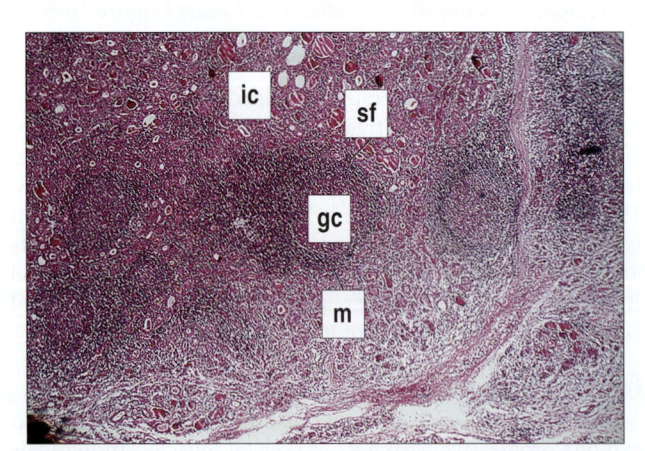

Figure 16-3

In the Hashimoto gland, the normal architecture is virtually destroyed and replaced by invading cells (ic), which consist essentially of lymphocytes, macrophages, and plasma cells. A secondary lymphoid follicle (sf), with a germinal center (gc) and a mantle of small lymphocytes (m), is present. (H&E stain, ×80. Reproduced from Woolf N. Pathology: basic and systemic, London, WB Saunders, 1998.)

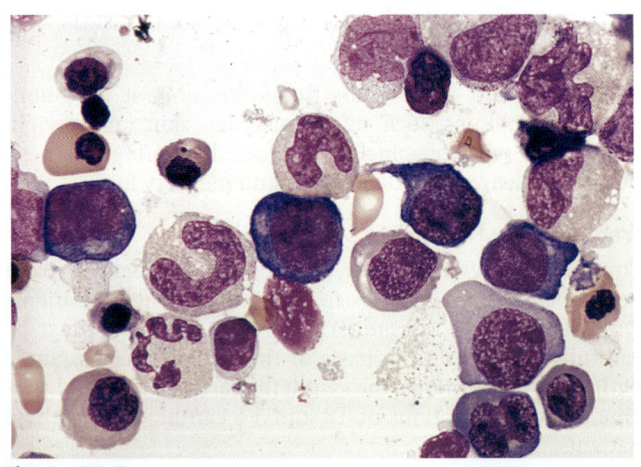

Figure 16-5

Bone marrow aspirate smear from an individual with pernicious anemia, showing megaloblastic red blood cell precursors and giant metamyelocytes. The chromatin in the red blood cell nuclei is more dispersed than in normal red blood cell precursors at comparable stage of maturation; the giant metamyelocytes have dispersed nuclear chromatin in contrast to a normal metamyelocyte, which has condensed chromatin. (Wright-Giemsa stain.) (From McCance KL, Huether SE: Pathophysiology: The biological basis for disease in adults and children, ed 5, St Louis, 2006, Mosby; Damjanov I, Linder J, editors: Anderson's pathology, ed 10, St Louis, 1996, Mosby.)

CHAPTER 16 AUTOIMMUNITY

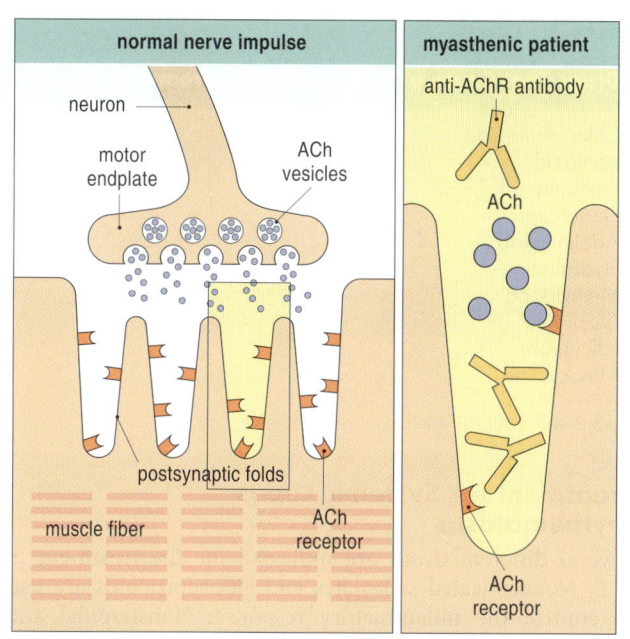

Figure 16-6

Normally, a nerve impulse passing down a neuron arrives at a motor endplate and causes the release of acetylcholine (ACh). This diffuses across the neuromuscular junction, binds ACh receptors (AChR) on the muscle, and causes ion channels in the muscle membrane to open, which, in turn, triggers muscular contraction. In myasthenia gravis, antibodies to the receptor block the binding of the ACh transmitter. The effect of the released vesicle is therefore reduced, and the muscle can become very weak. Antibody blocking receptors are only one of the factors operating in the disease. (From Roitt I, Brostoff J, Male D, et al: Immunology, ed 7, Philadelphia, 2006, Mosby.)

acetylcholine fixed to the functional motor plate receptors. In the treatment of more severe or difficult cases, immunosuppressive agents such as cyclosporine are used (see Chapter 7 for a discussion on the mechanism of action and adverse health effects of immunosuppressive agents).

SYSTEMIC LUPUS ERYTHEMATOSUS

SLE is a multiple-organ disease occurring primarily in women of child-bearing age. It is characterized by multiple-organ inflammation. Almost any organ system can be involved, but the central nervous system (CNS), the renal system, and the pulmonary organs are common targets. Clinical manifestations include arthritis, glomerulonephritis, hemolytic anemia, neurologic disorders, and rashes. The classic SLE rash is a macular butterfly-shaped rash on the bridge of the nose and the cheeks or a discoid rash with red, raised patches on the face, scalp, and body (Figure 16-8).

SLE is considered an autoimmune disease because of the presence of autoantibodies directed at double-stranded deoxyribonucleic acid (anti-dsDNA) and core proteins of small nuclear ribonucleoproteins (anti-Sm). The presence of these antibodies is associated exclusively with SLE and is therefore included in the diagnostic criteria for the disease. Circulating immune complexes often settle out in the small vessels in the joints and kidneys causing arthritis, glomerulonephritis, and inflammatory vasculitis (Figure 16-9).

The pathophysiology of the disease is complex and may involve two immunologic defects. Evidence indicates that individuals with SLE have a defect in the innate killing Fas mechanism that normally destroys auto-reactive T and B cells. Hence, auto-reactive lymphocytes persist in the circulation. Individuals with SLE also have reduced synthesis of C1q, C2, and C4a and defective complement receptors on macrophages. Reduction in complement synthesis reduces the release of chemotactic factors and the influx of phagocytic cells, which normally remove immune complexes. Since immune complexes are not removed, they are deposited in the capillary bed and the glomeruli of the kidneys.

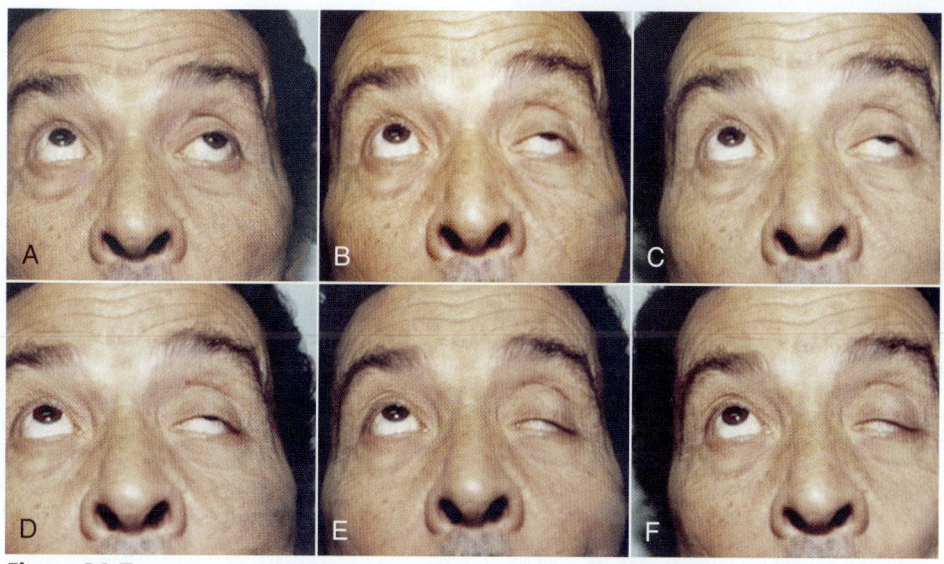

Figure 16-7

Ptosis observed in a patient with myasthenia gravis. (From Awwad S, Ma'luf R, Hamush N: Myasthenia gravis. Emedicine multimedia, 2010: Available at http://emedicine.medscape.com/article/1216417-overview. Accessed September 2010.)

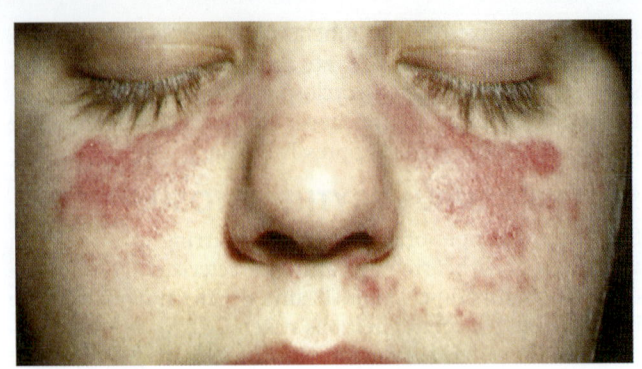

CHAPTER 16 AUTOIMMUNITY

Figure 16-8
The characteristic facial rash of systemic lupus erythematosus. Although this butterfly-shaped rash was first used to recognize the disease, it is only seen in a proportion of patients who have the disease when defined immunologically. (From Parham P: The immune system, ed 2, New York, 2005. Photograph courtesy of M. Walport.)

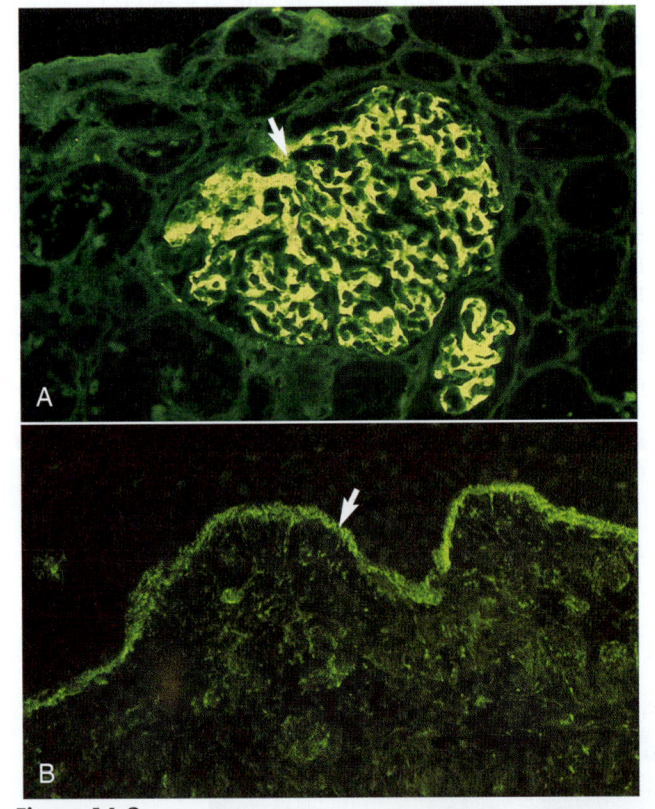

Figure 16-9
Deposition of immunoglobulin G (IgG) in the kidney and skin of persons with systemic lupus erythematosus (SLE). These photographs of tissue were obtained from persons with SLE and stained with fluorescent anti-IgG. **A,** Section from a kidney showing a glomerulus with deposits of IgG (*arrow indicating bright areas of staining*). **B,** Section of the skin showing deposition of IgG along the dermal–epidermal junction (*arrow indicating bright green staining*). (**A,** From McCance KL, Huether SE: Pathophysiology: The biological basis for disease in adults and children, ed 5, St Louis, 2006, Mosby. Courtesy of Dr. Helmut Rennke, Department of Pathology, Brigham and Women's Hospital, Boston, MA. **B,** Courtesy of Dr. Richard Sontheimer, Department of Dermatology, University of Texas Southwestern Medical School, Dallas, TX. Modified from Kumar V, Abbas A, Fausto N: Robbins and Cotran pathologic basis of disease, ed 7, Philadelphia, 2005, Saunders.)

BOX 16-1
Drugs That Cause a "Lupus-Like" Syndrome

Chlorpromazine
Isoniazid
Procainamide*
Etanercept
Adalimumab
Hydralazine*
Methyldopa
Quinidine*
Infliximab
Minocycline*

*Drugs with high risk for "lupus-like" syndrome.

Treatment for Systemic Lupus Erythematosus

Several different drugs are indicated for the treatment for SLE. Nonacetylated salicylates and glucocorticoids are used to control the inflammatory response. Nonsteroidal antiinflammatory drugs (NSAIDs) are indicated for the management of mild to moderate pain.

DRUG-INDUCED "LUPUS-LIKE" DISEASE

Drugs often cause a transient "lupus-like" syndrome. This syndrome differs from classic SLE in several ways. In the lupus-like syndrome, anti-DNA antibody production is transient, and memory cells are not generated. When the drug is discontinued, symptoms abate, and the patient returns to a normal state. Pharmaceuticals commonly associated with drug induced lupus-like syndrome are listed in Box 16-1.

The mechanisms involved in drug-induced lupus-like syndrome are unclear. However, agents inhibiting the methylation of T cell DNA (e.g., procainamide and hydralazine) cause the overexpression of eukocyte function–associated antigen 1 (LFA-1) or CD11a/CD18. T cells overexpressing LFA-1 adhere to the vascular cells and become auto-reactive. Clinical symptoms are dependent on cumulative drug dosage and liver CYA P-450 genotypes. For example, 30% to 60% of procainamide is excreted as N-acetylprocainamide, and the rate of metabolism is genetically determined. Slow metabolism of the drug is associated with the autoimmune response.

GOODPASTURE SYNDROME

Goodpasture syndrome is characterized by pulmonary hemorrhage and a rapidly progressing glomerulonephritis. Patients present to the physicians with hemoptysis, dyspnea, and generalized weakness. The syndrome is characterized by antibodies directed at noncollagenous domains (NC1) of the alpha 3 chains of type IV collagen in the basement membranes of the lungs and kidneys (Figure 16-10).

These epitopes are normally sequestered from immune recognition. Injury to the basement membrane from smoking, inhaled hydrocarbons, or viral infections may expose these antigens. Additional genetic and immunologic factors may be necessary for the autoimmune response. Goodpasture syndrome has a strong genetic component, and a positive association with HLA DRB1*1501 is necessary for the presentation of collagen epitopes to auto-reactive T cells. In addition, individuals lack a critical B cell Fc receptor (FcγRIIB), which normally inhibits B cell activation, proliferation, and autoantibody production.

CHAPTER 16 AUTOIMMUNITY   133

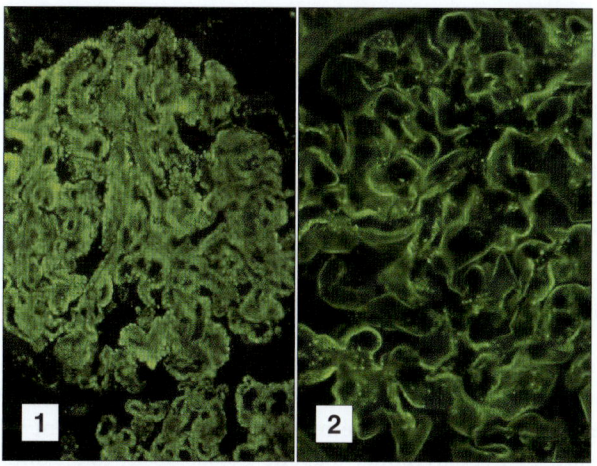

Figure 16-10

These renal sections compare the effect of systemic lupus erythematosus. (type III hypersensitivity) **(1)** and Goodpasture syndrome (type II hypersensitivity) **(2)**. In each case, the antibody is detected with fluorescent anti-IgG. Complexes, formed in blood and deposited in the kidney, form characteristic "lumpy bumpy" deposits **(1)**. The anti–basement membrane antibody in Goodpasture syndrome forms an even layer on the glomerular basement membrane **(2)**. (From From Roitt I, Brostoff J, Male D, et al: Immunology, ed 7, Philadelphia, 2006, Mosby. Courtesy of Dr. S. Thiru.)

Treatment for Goodpasture Syndrome

Treatment for Goodpasture syndrome is focused on removal of circulating autoantibodies and downregulating the immune response. Autoantibodies are removed by plasmapheresis. To diminish the immune response, pulse-dosed glucocorticoids and cytotoxic alkylating agents are used. Auto-reactive B cells can also be reduced by treatment with anti-CD20 (rituximab). CD20 is present on immature B cells, but not antibody-producing plasma cells. Anti-CD20 selectively depletes the immature B cells and prevents the repopulation of antibody-producing plasma cells.

MOLECULAR MIMICRY

Microbial infections have been postulated as triggers for many autoimmune diseases. In theory, a genetically susceptible host is infected with a microbe that expresses antigens that are similar, but not identical, to the host's self-markers (Figure 16-11).

The immune response to the microbe generates antibodies that react with both the pathogen and the host tissue. Molecular mimicry may play a role in type 1a diabetes, ankylosing spondylitis, rheumatoid arthritis, reactive arthritis, and acute rheumatic fever.

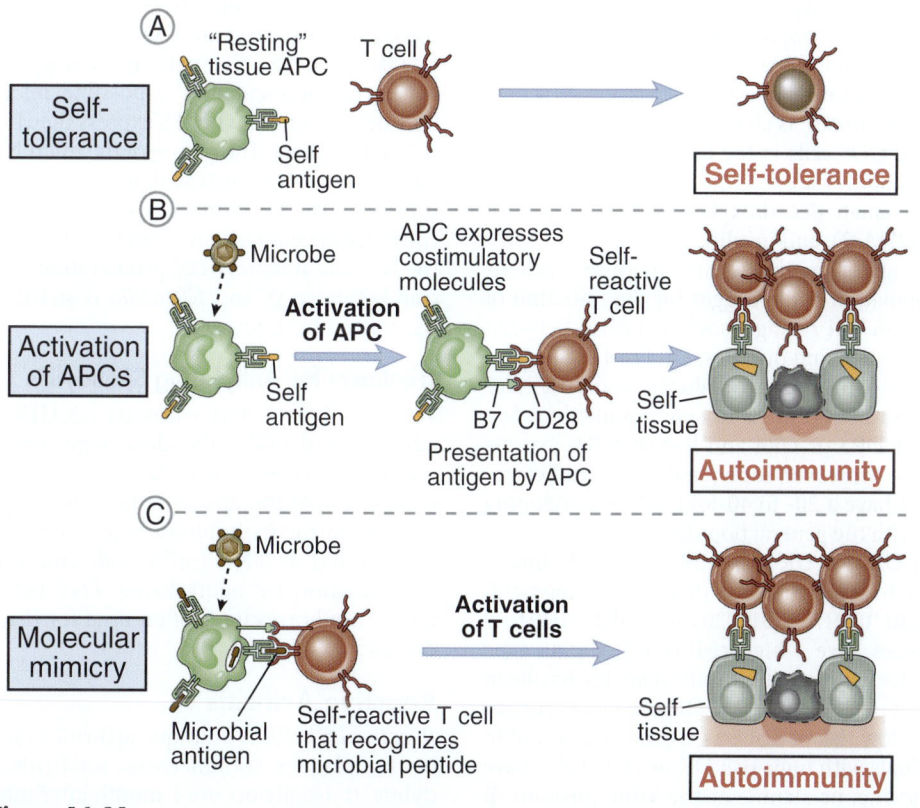

Figure 16-11

Role of infections in the development of autoimmunity. **A,** Normally, the encountering of a mature self-reactive T cell with a self-antigen presented by a co-stimulator–deficient resting tissue antigen-presenting cell (APC) results in peripheral tolerance by anergy. (Other possible mechanisms of self-tolerance are not shown.) **B,** Microbes may activate the APCs to express co-stimulators, and when these APCs present self-antigens, the self-reactive T cells are activated, rather than rendered tolerant. **C,** Some microbial antigens may cross-react with self-antigens (molecular mimicry). Therefore, immune responses initiated by microbes may activate T cells specific for self-antigens. (From Abbas AK, Lichtman AH, Pillai S: Cellular and molecular immunology, ed 6 [updated edition], Philadelphia, 2010, Saunders.)

Diabetes (Type 1a)

The pancreas functions both as an endocrine organ and an exocrine organ. As an exocrine organ, it produces digestive enzymes that are secreted into the small intestine. These enzymes include trypsin, chymotrypsin, lipases, and amylases. Pancreatic endocrine function is facilitated by three different pancreatic cell types found in the islets of Langerhans. These cells produce glucagon (α cells), insulin (β cells), and somatostatin and gastrin (δ cells).

Type 1a diabetes is a disease characterized by the destruction of the β cells and low or absent insulin in blood. Insulin is an anabolic hormone that reduces the levels of circulating glucose by allowing its entrance into muscle cells and conversion to a storage molecule called *glycogen*. When insulin is unavailable, glucose cannot be stored as glycogen and begins to accumulate in blood. Osmotic diuresis occurs when glucose enters the kidneys and changes the osmotic pressure in the renal tubule. The increase in osmotic pressure also causes water accumulation in the lumen and prevents water re-adsorption. This results in increased thirst, increased urinary output, and dehydration. In addition, individuals with type 1a diabetes have excessive weight loss despite an adequate caloric intake. Weight loss occurs because patients with diabetes cannot process many of the calories in their food.

The type 1a autoimmune form of diabetes has several synonyms, including *insulin-dependent diabetes mellitus (IDDM)*, *juvenile diabetes*, and *insulin-dependent diabetes*. Autoimmune diabetes affects 0.3% of the population by puberty, making it the third most prevalent disease among children. After puberty, the incidence declines rapidly.

The onset of clinical disease is characterized by an infiltration of both CD4 and CD8 cells in the pancreas and by β cell destruction. Autoantibodies are also produced and directed at small forms of glutamate decarboxylase (GAD65), protein tyrosine phosphatase (IA-2), and insulin.

The pathophysiology of the disease may require a genetically susceptible population and a trigger for the initiation of the autoimmune response. A strong association exists between HLA-DR3, DR-4, and DQ1 and diabetes. DR3 or DR4 is present in 95% of patients with type 1a diabetes, and 30% have inherited both DR3 and DR4. In Caucasian populations, less than 50% have either DR3 or DR4 and less than 3% express both class II markers. Moreover, individuals who are heterozygous for DR3/DR4 have a 20- to 40-fold risk of developing diabetes compared with the general population.

Individuals with DR3 or DR4 also inherit closely linked DQ1 β alleles, which are critical to disease development. In Caucasians, DRB1*0301/DQB1*0201 or DRB1*040101/DRB1*0302 haplotypes have a high risk of developing type 1a diabetes. Resistance or susceptibility to diabetes has been mapped to residues at position 57 in the DR and DQ β-chains. In individuals with a low risk of diabetes, aspartate is found in position 57. Individuals with high-risk DR or DQ alleles have uncharged valine, serine, or alanine at the same position. It is speculated that pancreatic autoantigens are presented to T cells in the context of these DQ and DR molecules.

The trigger for fulminating diabetes may be a viral infection. In humans, these viruses include cytomegalovirus (CMV), EBV, Coxsackie virus, rubella virus, mumps virus, varicella zoster virus, and rotavirus. CMV may lyse β cells, releasing glutamate decarboxylase 65 (GAD65) from the cell surface. GAD65 binds to DQβ1 susceptibility alleles and is presented to the CD4Th2 cell, which stimulates B cells to produce autoantibodies.

Diabetes may also be triggered by molecular mimicry between viruses and β cell autoantigens. For example, EBV expresses a five-amino-acid sequence that is shared with high-risk DR and DQ alleles suggesting that the HLA alleles alone can act as antigens. Coxsackie virus capsid proteins and GAD65 share sequence homologies and cross-reactive antigens. Rotavirus, which is the most common cause of childhood diarrhea, also shares homologous amino acid sequences with GAD65 and IA-2.

Treatment for Diabetes

Insulin is the mainstay of treatment to control diabetes. The treatment depends on the medical status of the patient with regard to hypoglycemia, diabetic ketoacidosis, and complications such as macrovascular disease leading to myocardial ischemia.

Ankylosing Spondylitis

Ankylosing spondylitis (AS) is a chronic inflammatory disease of the spinal sacroiliac region, which connects spine to the pelvis. The disease appears to be mediated by CD8 cells. Constant inflammation causes fusion of the vertebrae, which results in chronic back pain and limited mobility. Occasionally, inflammation of the shoulders, hips, and knees occurs. In rare instances, the disease is associated with inflammation of the heart, lungs, and kidneys.

Like diabetes, the pathophysiology of AS has a strong genetic component and a possible microbial trigger. Over 90% of individuals with AS express the HLA B*2704 and HLA B*2705 markers. The nature of the microbial trigger is unclear. Early studies demonstrated an association between *Klebsiella* infections and the clinical onset of AS. Two *Klebsiella* proteins (nitrogenase enzyme and pulD secretion protein) can bind to the B27 and initiate T cell proliferation. However, the association between AS and *Klebsiella* is strictly circumstantial and has not yet been proven.

Treatment for Ankylosing Spondylitis

To control pain and stiffness, NSAIDs and analgesics are administered under the close supervision of a physician. If the disease is present in the peripheral joints, sulfasalazine is an effective therapy to reduce inflammation. TNF plays a key role in the pathophysiology of AS. Monoclonal antibodies directed at TNF (infliximab and golimumab) decrease inflammation by neutralizing TNF before it can reach its target. Methotrexate is often used for the treatment of severe disease.

Reactive Arthritis

Reactive arthritis is a unique arthritic condition characterized by skin plaques, conjunctivitis, urethritis, arthritis, and spondylitis. It usually occurs 1 month after infection with sexually transmitted microbes (*Chlamydia* or *Neisseria gonorrhoeae*) or select enteric organisms (*Yersinia*, *Salmonella*, *Shigella*, *Campylobacter*, and *Clostridium*). It is a classic example of a disease caused by molecular mimicry with the generation of auto antigen-specific CD8 cells. In the case of *Chlamydia*, evidence suggests that the microbe shares epitopes with HLA B*2704 and HLA B*2705. These B27 alleles bind a specific arthritogenic peptide that is recognized by CD8 cells. The evidence for molecular mimicry is much clearer with regard to the enterics. Extensive cross-reactivity occurs between B27 alleles and the molecules expressed by *Yersinia, Salmonella,* and *Shigella.* Cross-reactive antigens are usually outer membrane proteins (e.g., YadD), which are virulence factors or cationic membrane pore proteins (e.g., OmpH).

Acute Rheumatic Fever

Infection with group A *Streptococcus* species can progress from pharyngitis to acute rheumatic fever and permanent heart damage. Antibodies produced in response to the streptococcal infection cross-react with the myocardial heart valves. Acute interstitial valvulitis may cause edema. If untreated, destruction of the valves may cause valvular insufficiency.

Treatment for Rheumatic Fever

Therapy is directed at elimination of the streptococcal pharyngitis before it progresses to rheumatic fever and at downregulating the autoimmune inflammatory response. Penicillin or other cell wall inhibitors are used to eliminate the organism. NSAIDs or prednisone rapidly reduce the inflammatory response.

Rheumatoid Arthritis

Rheumatoid arthritis (RA) is a chronic disease characterized by inflammatory responses involving the synovial membranes and articular joint structures. However, often remote inflammatory responses occur in the heart, lung, liver, skin, and vasculature. While the disease onset can occur in the second decade of life, normal onset is between the fourth and fifth decades of life.

Genetics influences both the incidence and severity of the disease. A strong association exists between HLA-DR4 subsets and RA. Over 70% of patients with RA express the DR4 marker compared with 28% of normal controls. The risk of developing the disease increases in persons expressing DRB*0401 and DRB*0404. Disease severity is increased in individuals expressing DRB*0402 or BRB*0403. A skewed HLA pattern on lymphocytes in the synovium strongly suggests a genetic susceptibility related to the expression of class II DR alleles. A feature of these alleles is that they share a common five-amino-acid motif (QKRAA) in the β-chain of the DR molecule. These HLA alleles may bind auto-reactive antigens or act as cross-reactive antigens in the response to viral infections.

A viral etiology for RA has been suspected for many years. Parvovirus 19, human T cell leukemia virus (HTLV), herpes types 6 and 8, human endogenous virus 5, and EBV have all been implicated as causative agents of RA. EBV has attracted much attention because EBV-encoded protein gp-110 has a sequence homology with (QKRAA) epitopes.

Although the trigger is unknown, activated macrophages play a role in the initiation of RA lesions by secreting TNF and IL-2, which stimulate fibroblasts. In turn, fibroblasts produce a number of factors that act directly or indirectly to cause tissue damage. One of the major factors produced by fibroblasts is receptor-activated NF-κB ligand (RANKL), which stimulates osteoclasts to destroy bone tissue. Other fibroblast-produced factors are prostaglandin E_2 (PGE_2) and the cytokines IL-6 and IL-8. These cytokines stimulate polymorphonuclear leukocytes to produce additional proteases and oxygen-derived free radicals (ODFRs). ODFRs degrade hyaluronic acid, which acts as a lubricant in joints. In the absence of hyaluronic acid, inflammation causes articular nerve hyperexcitablity and pain.

Immune complexes, known as *rheumatoid factors (RFs)*, are found in both the serum and synovial fluids of patients with RA. RF is an autoantibody against the Fc portion of another antibody. The production of RF by B cells is accelerated by macrophage-produced IL-6. Immunoglobulin M (IgM) antibodies are the predominant RFs, but IgG and IgA RFs are also found in the synovium. RFs are present in 70% to 80% of adults with RA but occur at a much lower frequency in juvenile rheumatoid arthritis.

The mechanism by which the Fc portion of antibodies becomes antigenic has recently been defined. Under normal conditions, antibodies are heavily glycosylated to sequester potential auto-reactive antigens in the Fc region. However, proteases in the synovial fluid of patients with RA remove sugars from the Fc portion of the IgG molecule, exposing

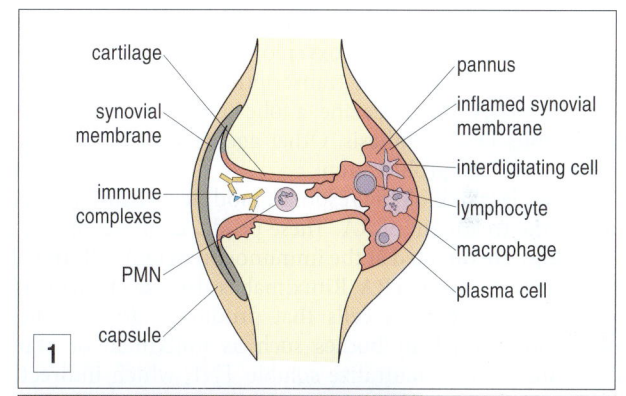

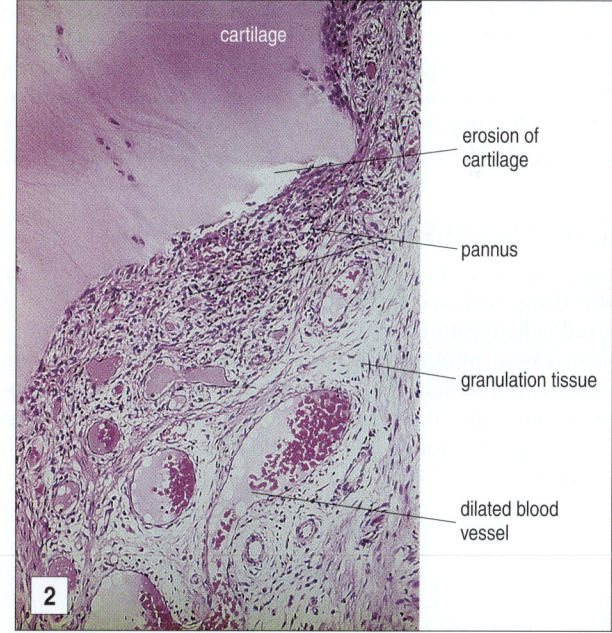

Figure 16-12

In the joint affected by rheumatoid arthritis, an inflammatory infiltrate is found in the synovial membrane, which hypertrophies forming a "pannus" (**1** and **2**). This covers and eventually erodes the synovial cartilage and bone. Immune complexes and neutrophils (polymorphonuclear leukocytes [PMNs]) are detectable in the joint space and in extra-articular tissue, where they may give rise to vasculitic lesions and subcutaneous nodules. (From Roitt I, Brostoff J, Male D, et al: Immunology, ed 7, Philadelphia, 2006, Mosby. Histologic section reproduced from Woolf N: Pathology: basic and systemic. London, 1998, W.B. Saunders.)

auto-reactive antigens. RFs bind to the agalactosyl Fc domains, creating immune complexes. Deposition of these immune complexes in small blood vessels activates complement, which leads to joint destruction and pannus formation. Pannus is a layer of granulation tissue consisting of proliferating fibroblasts and inflammatory cells (Figure 16-12).

In the pannus, inflammatory cells secrete IL-1, PGA_2 and PGE_2, platelet-derived growth factor, and plasminogen activators, all of which accelerate the destruction of cartilage and synovial cells.

Treatment for Rheumatoid Arthritis

Multiple therapies are used for the treatment of RA. Early in the disease process, disease-modifying antirheumatic drugs (DMARDs) are used to prevent irreversible damage to joints. DMARDs include methotrexate, azathioprine, hydroxychloroquine sulfate, sulfasalazine, cyclosporine, and monoclonal antibodies. The therapy is designed to reduce the proliferation of auto-reactive cells and decrease inflammation. Methotrexate, azathioprine, and hydroxychloroquine sulfate interfere with DNA synthesis or the transcription of DNA to ribonucleic acid (RNA). Sulfasalazine, a folic acid pathway inhibitor, also inhibits DNA synthesis. Other agents such as cyclosporine inhibit T cell proliferation.

A new class of biologic response modifiers (BRMs) is also used in the treatment of RA. These products of recombinant technology are directed at the immunocompetent cells or soluble factors involved in RA. Rituximab is also used to decrease the number of plasma cells that produce autoantibodies. Other monoclonal antibodies such as infliximab or etanercept are used to neutralize soluble TNF, which indirectly plays a role in bone destruction. Anakinera, a nonglycosylated form of the human IL-1 receptor antagonist (IL-1Ra) is effective in reducing inflammation. In more advanced cases, NSAIDs are indicated for reduction of pain and inflammation. NSAIDs may be used in concert with COX-2 inhibitors which are also anti-inflammatory, analgesic, and anti-pyretic agents.

AUTOIMMUNE HEMOLYTIC ANEMIA

Drugs can induce anemias by direct and indirect means. Some drugs such as α–methyldopa interact with Rh molecules on red cells creating a "neoantigen." Penicillin and cephalosporin cause autoimmune hemolytic anemia by a different mechanism. At high doses, haptenic penicillin and cephalosporin molecules coat red blood cells, creating an antigen that elicits the production of IgG. Complement activation lyses red blood cells.

Treatment for Autoimmune Hemolytic Anemia

Mild autoimmune hemolytic anemia is treated with corticosteroids to slow red blood cell lysis. More severe forms are treated with immunosuppressive drugs (e.g., cyclophosphamide, azathioprine) and plasmapheresis.

SUMMARY

- Autoimmune diseases affect a significant proportion of the population in the United States, and the incidence is heavily skewed toward females.
- The immune response can be mediated by antibodies, macrophages, or lymphocytes.
- An autoimmune response is directed at specific organs or multiple organs, tissues, or soluble factors.
- The risk of developing autoimmune diseases is associated with single nuclear polymorphisms within a specific allele of the human leukocyte molecule.
- Environmental factors, viral infections, and bacterial infections may trigger active disease in genetically susceptible individuals.

REFERENCES

Arbuckle MR, McClain MT, Rubertone MV, et al: Development of autoantibodies before the clinical onset of systemic lupus erythematosus, N Engl J Med 349(16):1526, 2003.

Bach JF: Infections and autoimmune diseases, J Autoimmun 25(Suppl):74, 2005.

Bahn RS: Clinical review 157: Pathophysiology of Graves' ophthalmopathy: The cycle of disease, J Clin Endocrinol Metab 88(5):2003, 1939.

Burke WJ: Myasthenia gravis: A clinical review, Clin Exp Neurol 17:1, 1981.

Davidson A, Diamond B: Autoimmune diseases, N Engl J Med 345(5):340, 2001.

Edwards JC, Szczepanski L, Szechinski J, et al: Efficacy of B-cell-targeted therapy with rituximab in patients with rheumatoid arthritis, N Engl J Med 350(25):2572, 2004.

Maxfield DL, Boyd WC: Pernicious anemia: A review, an update, and an illustrative case, J Am Osteopath Assoc 83(2):133, 1983.

Mazzaferri EL, Skillman TG: Thyroid storm. A review of 22 episodes with special emphasis on the use of guanethidine, Arch Intern Med 124(6):684, 1969.

McKenzie JM: Review: Pathogenesis of Graves' Disease: Role of the long-acting thyroid stimulator, J Clin Endocrinol Metab 25:424, 1965.

Spesivtseva VG: Etiology, pathogenesis, and diagnosis of diffuse toxic goiter and Hashimoto's thyroiditis [translation], Ter Arkh 53(10):147, 1981.

Von Herrath MG, Fujinami RS, Whitton JL: Microorganisms and autoimmunity: Making the barren field fertile? Nat Rev Microbiol 1(2):151, 2003.

ASSESSMENT QUESTIONS

1. In Graves' disease, the autoantibody acts as a surrogate for:
   A. Thyrotropin-releasing hormone
   B. Thyroid-stimulating hormone
   C. Thyrotropin
   D. Anterior pituitary–stimulating hormone

2. Hashimoto's thyroiditis is characterized by:
   A. Rapid heartbeats
   B. Tremors
   C. Sweating
   D. Fatigue

3. Myasthenia gravis is characterized by:
   I.   Antibodies to acetylcholine
   II. Antibodies to acetylcholinesterase
   III. Antibodies to the acetylcholine receptor
   A. I
   B. III
   C. I and II
   D. II and III
   E. I, II, and III

4. Which of the following antibodies is associated with systemic lupus erythematosus?
   I.   Anti–single-stranded DNA
   II. Anti–double-stranded DNA
   III. Anti–small nuclear ribonucleoprotein
   A. I
   B. III
   C. I and II
   D. II and III
   E. I, II, and III

5. Which of the following is *not* a synonym for type 1a diabetes?
   A. Diabetes mellitus
   B. Type II diabetes
   C. Insulin-dependent diabetes
   D. Juvenile diabetes

6. Patients with ankylosing spondylitis have:
   I.   Chronic inflammation of the spinal sacroiliac
   II. HLA B*2704 and HLA B*2705 alleles
   III. DRB*0401 and DRB*0404 alleles
   A. I
   B. III
   C. I and II
   D. II and III
   E. I, II, and III

7. Rheumatoid factors are:
   A. Antibody DNA complexes
   B. Antibody RNA complexes
   C. Antibody complexes
   D. Antibody thyroglobulin complexes

8. Which of the following is *not* produced by fibroblasts?
   A. RANKL
   B. PGE_2
   C. Cytokines IL-6 and IL-8
   D. IL-2

CHAPTER 17

Transplantation

LEARNING OBJECTIVES

- List three human leukocyte antigen (HLA) class I loci
- List the three HLA class II loci
- Compare and contrast the two antibody tests that are used to determine tissue compatibility
- Compare and contrast the three tests used to identify HLA antigens on the donor and recipient cells
- Differentiate between the serial summation or high determinant model and the multiple determinant model for T cell activation
- Define autograft, isograft, allograft, and xenograft
- Discuss the major impediments to successful use of xenografts
- Discuss the advantages of transgenic pigs as a source of organs for transplantation
- Compare and contrast the immunologic mechanisms active in hyperacute rejection and acute rejection
- Discuss the immunologic mechanisms active in chronic rejection
- Identify the role of minor HLA molecules in long-term transplant survival
- List the five families of drugs that are used to prevent graft rejection
- Discuss the mechanism of action (MOA) of corticosteroids
- Recognize the MOA of calcineurin inhibitors used to prevent graft rejection
- Identify the MOA of lymphocyte proliferation inhibitors used to prevent graft rejection
- List the monoclonal antibodies use to prevent graft prevention
- Identify the target cells and receptors for the monoclonal antibodies used to prevent graft rejection
- Identify the role of polyclonal antibodies in graft prevention
- Compare and contrast induction immunosuppression, maintenance immunosuppression, and rescue immunosuppression
- Recognize surface molecules that are unique to hematopoietic stem cells
- Identify the three sources of hematopoietic stem cells
- Explain the advantages and disadvantages of using the three sources of stem cells
- Compare and contrast myeloablative and nonmyeloablative conditioning of the host bone marrow prior to transplantation
- Define graft-versus-host disease (GVHD)
- List the target organs involved in acute GVHD reactions
- Explain the immunologic mechanisms active in acute GVHD
- Identify the drugs used to treat acute GVHD
- Explain the immunologic mechanisms active in chronic GVHD
- Identify the drugs that are used to treat chronic GVHD

KEY TERMS

Acute rejection
Allogeneic graft
Antibody cross-matching
Autograft
Chronic rejection
Graft-versus-host disease
Hyperacute rejection
Induction immunosuppression
Isograft
Maintenance immunosuppression
Polymerase chain reaction
Rescue immunosuppression
Sequence-based oligonucleotides
Sequence-based typing
Sequence-specific primers
Xenograft

INTRODUCTION

The transplantation era began in 1944 when Peter Medawar demonstrated that human skin grafts between unrelated donors were rejected, but the rejection rate decreased when a graft was obtained from a related donor. He suggested that the immune system recognized the skin from unrelated donors as foreign and mounted a vigorous immune response. In 1958, Jean Dausset described the first human leukocyte-specific antigen (HLA-A2) and demonstrated that these antigens were important in the recognition of foreign tissue. Between 1962 and 1980, immunologists and geneticists identified different HLA loci and determined that HLAs on donated organs were the targets of an immune response to transplanted tissue or organs. Matching donor and recipient HLAs prior to transplantation greatly increased graft survival. Introduction of anti-rejection drugs such as azathioprine, cyclosporine, and tacrolimus has significantly lessened the risk of organ rejection over time.

Between 28,000 and 36,000 organ transplantations are performed in the United States yearly. The most commonly transplanted organs are kidney, heart, and liver. But other organs, including cornea, lung, liver, pancreas, intestine, bone, skin, and bone marrow, can be transplanted. Organ transplantation has been hampered by a scarcity of available organs and bone marrow donors. Currently, over 85,000 individuals in the United States are awaiting organ transplantation.

TYPES OF TRANSPLANTATIONS

The four types of transplantations are as follows: (1) When the same individual serves as the donor and the recipient of the transplanted tissue, the graft is termed an *autologous graft*, or an *autograft*. (2) Tissue transplanted between genetically identical twins is called an *isograft*, or a *syngeneic transplant*. (3) A graft between unrelated or mismatched individuals is an *allogeneic transplant*. (4) When organs are transplanted across species barriers from animals to humans, the grafts are termed *xenografts* (Figure 17-1).

XENOGRAFTS

Xenografts merit more discussion because they solve the problem of organ shortages and long waiting times for transplants. Pigs are useful for transplantation purposes because of the similarity of organ size, weight, and physiology between pigs and humans. However, xenotransplantation has proved impractical because humans have pre-existing immunoglobulin M (IgM) antibodies directed at porcine carbohydrate antigens containing α-galactosyl residues that are expressed on porcine cells. When porcine organs are transplanted into humans, hyperacute rejection occurs within hours.

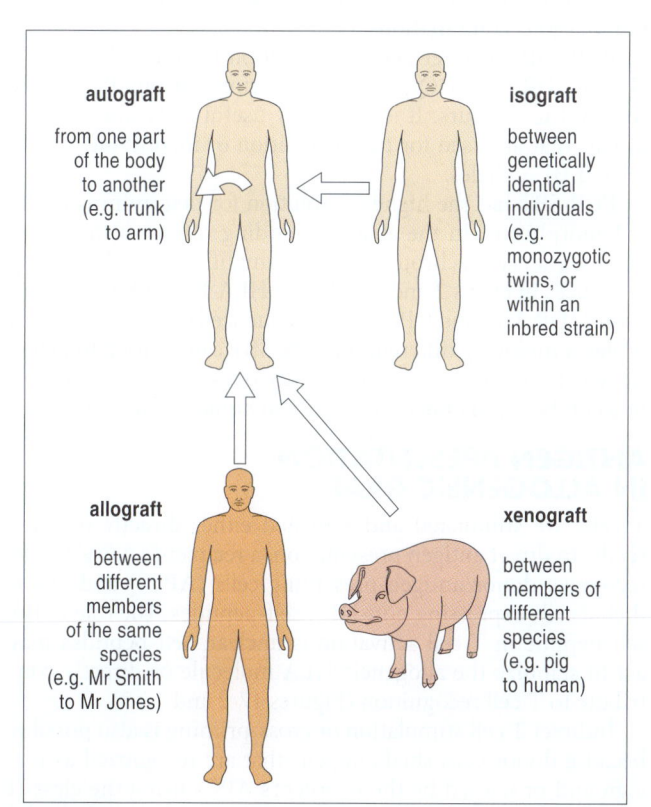

To prevent xenograft rejection, recombinant deoxyribonucleic acid (DNA) technology has been used to create transgenic pigs that can be used as a source of tissue and organs. Cells from these pigs do not express the carbohydrate antigens that elicit the IgM response. Moreover, cells express molecules that downregulate natural killer (NK) cells (ecto-5′-nucleotidase) or prevent complement activation (CD55 and CD59).

Before xenotransplantation can be implemented in clinical practice, questions concerning the risk of microbial and viral transmission from pigs to humans must be addressed and resolved. Although pigs and humans have been in close contact for centuries and xenografts are unlikely to harbor new or novel infectious agents, little is known about exogenous and endogenous retroviruses in pigs. In vitro, endogenous porcine retroviruses can infect human cell lines.

HUMAN LEUKOCYTE ANTIGEN MARKERS AND TRANSPLANTATION

Major histocompatibility complex (MHC) antigens in animals and HLAs are considered "self-molecules" and determine acceptance or rejection of transplanted tissue (see Chapter 4). The three class I loci (HLA-A, HLA-B, and HLA-C) and the three class II loci (HLA-DR, HLA-DQ, and HLA-DP) molecules in humans are important in transplantation.

Each individual has two complete sets of the six HLA molecules. One set is inherited from the father and another set from the mother. Each set of HLA molecules is called a *haplotype*. Since extensive polymorphism and multiple alleles exist in each locus, individuals may have homozygous or heterozygous alleles at each locus.

TEST FOR TISSUE COMPATIBILITY IN SYNGENEIC AND ALLOGENEIC GRAFTS

Antibody Cross-Matching

As a consequence of blood or platelet transfusion, a previous organ transplantation, or multiple pregnancies, many individuals have antibodies directed at major (classes I and II) or minor (class III) HLA antigens. For example, approximately 20% of patients on the kidney transplantation list have high levels of anti-HLA antibodies in serum. The presence of pre-existing antibodies limits the population of potential donors and extends the waiting time for a kidney. Individuals with no pre-existing HLA antibodies usually receive a kidney within 500 days from the date their name appears on the transplantation registry. If high levels of pre-existing antibodies are present, the waiting time is 2300 days.

An initial test determines the presence of anti-HLA–specific antibodies in the recipient's serum. In a lymphocytotoxicity assay, serum from the recipient is made to react with ethidium bromide–stained T and B cells from the donor. In the presence of antibodies and complement, dead cells stain red, and live cells stain green. Cytotoxicity is reported as a percentage of the donor's cells killed in the assay. This means that the higher the concentration of cells that register as dead, the higher the antibody concentration. The presence of preformed antibodies to the HLA molecules on the donor tissue precludes the possibility of successful transplantation.

The recipient's serum is also tested for non-HLA–specific antibodies directed at the donor's endothelial cells. Endothelial cells are the initial contact point between the graft and host tissue, and rejection begins at this interface. The presence of

Figure 17-1
The genetic relationship between the donor and the recipient determines whether or not rejection will occur. Autografts or isografts are usually accepted, whereas allografts and xenografts are not. (From Roitt I, Brostoff J, Male D, et al: Immunology, ed 7, Philadelphia, 2006, Mosby.)

CHAPTER 17 TRANSPLANTATION

A Normal

T cell receptor — Foreign peptide — Self MHC

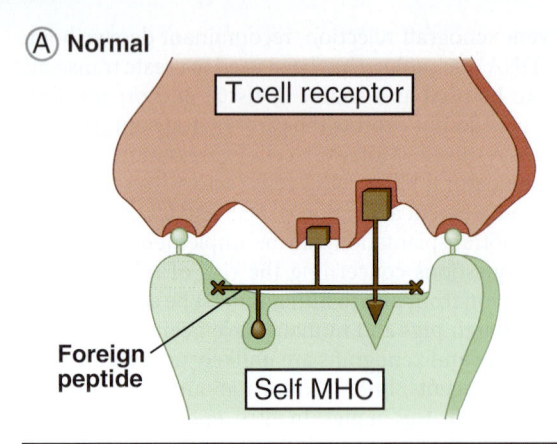

Self MHC molecule presents foreign peptide to T cell selected to recognize self MHC weakly, but may recognize self MHC–foreign peptide complexes well

B Allorecognition

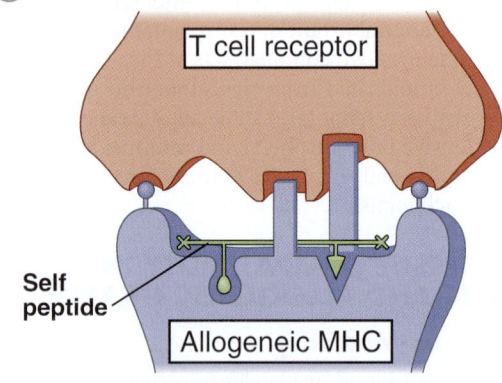

T cell receptor — Self peptide — Allogeneic MHC

The self MHC–restricted T cell recognizes the allogeneic MHC molecule whose structure resembles a self MHC–foreign peptide complex

C Allorecognition

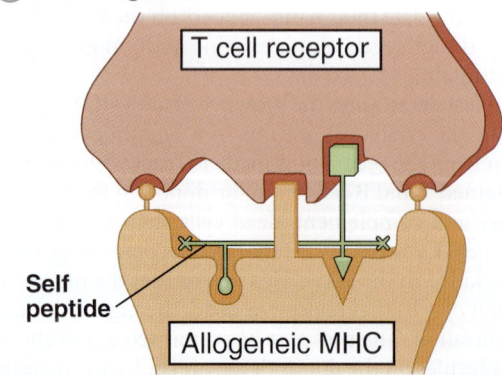

T cell receptor — Self peptide — Allogeneic MHC

The self MHC–restricted T cell recognizes a structure formed by both the allogeneic MHC molecule and the bound peptide

Figure 17-2

Molecular basis of direct recognition of allogeneic major histocompatibility complex (MHC) molecules. Direct recognition of allogeneic MHC molecules may be thought of as a cross-reaction, in which a T cell specific for a self–MHC molecule–foreign peptide complex (**A**) also recognizes an allogeneic MHC molecule (**B, C**). Nonpolymorphic donor peptides, labeled "self-peptide," may not contribute to allorecognition (**B**), or they may (**C**). (From Abbas AK, Lichtman AH, Pillai S: Cellular and molecular immunology, ed 6 [updated edition], Philadelphia, 2010, Saunders.)

anti–endothelial cell antibodies increases the risk of antibody-mediated organ rejection.

Tissue Cross-Matching

Several DNA-based molecular diagnostic techniques are used to type and cross-match tissue for transplantation. Polymerase chain reactions (PCRs) are used to amplify stretches of genomic DNA encoding HLA molecules. Allelic polymorphism within each locus is identified through hybridization with sequence-specific primers (SSP) or sequence-specific oligonucleotides (SSO) or sequence-based typing (SBT). The choice of assays depends on the clinician's requirements with regard to resolution, sensitivity, and speed.

The PCR-SSO is a low-cost, high-volume assay that can screen a large number of potential donors with low or intermediate HLA resolution. Each probe is complementary to different motifs within an allelic hypervariable region of HLA molecules. Thus, the technique can identify heterozygous or homozygous combinations.

PCR-SSP has intermediate resolution for HLA-A, HLA-B, HLA-C, DR, and DQ and can be performed rapidly usually within 3 to 4 hours. It is especially useful in typing cadaver organs that are used for transplantation or identifying closely related HLA alleles.

PCR-SBT has the highest resolution for determining allelic polymorphisms. In the assay, the coding region of the entire HLA sequence on chromosome 6 is amplified by PCR. Coding sequences in exons 2 and 3 (HLA-A, HLA-B, and HLA-C) and exon 2 (DR, DQ, and DP) are then sequenced to determine HLA alleles. Employing different formats, SBT can be used to determine heterozygous sequences at each locus, haploid sequences, or a combination of heterozygous and homozygous sequences.

ANTIGEN PRESENTATION IN ALLOGENEIC GRAFTS

T cells are stimulated and activated either directly or indirectly. In direct antigen presentation, a recipient's naïve T cells recognize donor antigen-presenting cells (APCs) and endothelial cells expressing non-HLA self-peptides. The role of the self-peptide in T cell activation is unclear. Self-peptides may act to stabilize the allogeneic HLA molecule or directly contribute to T cell recognition (Figures 17-2 and 17-3).

Indirect T cell stimulation or cross-priming is also possible because donor cells shed antigens that are recognized as foreign and processed by the recipient's APCs using the class II antigen-presentation pathway. Some antigen escapes from the phagosome and is processed in the class I pathway for presentation to CD8 cells. Indirect antigen presentation and cross-priming contribute to chronic rejection of liver or heart and to defense against intracellular bacteria, viruses, and tumor cells.

HIGH FREQUENCY OF ALLO-REACTIVE T CELLS

The response to alloantigens is vigorous. The percentage of T cells responding to alloantigens is much higher than the percentage of T cells responding to microbes or foreign peptides. In a normal response to microbes or viruses, 1 per 100,000 T cells is activated. When exposed to allogeneic cells, 1 per 100 to 1 per 1000 T cells are activated.

The rapid response to alloantigens suggests the presence of primed T cells directed at allogeneic cells. Although the exact mechanism is not fully delineated, two mechanisms have been proposed. The *serial summation* or *high determinant model* postulates that donor HLA molecules plus self-antigens are presented on recipients' APCs. Allo-reactive T cells engage the donor's HLA complex with a low affinity, which partially activates the cell and makes it more likely to trigger the proliferation of cytotoxic T cells on subsequent interactions with the peptide–MHC complex. Engagement of multiple HLA complexes expressed on the APC fully activates the allo-reactive T cell. In the *multiple determinant model*, allo-reactive T cells react with the HLA–self-antigen complex with moderate affinity and immediately begin to proliferate.

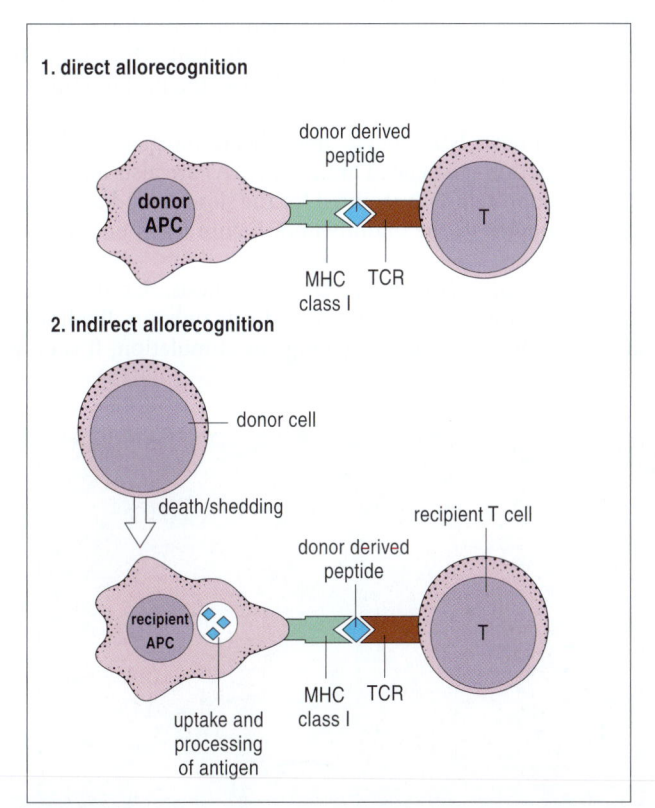

Figure 17-3

1, In direct allorecognition, the T cell directly recognizes the donor antigen-presenting cell (APC), with the T cell receptor (TCR) binding donor major histocompatibility complex (MHC) molecules that bear the donor peptide. **2,** Indirect allorecognition is more similar to conventional T cell recognition in that recipient T cells recognize the foreign (donor-derived) antigen that has been taken up and processed by recipient APCs. The TCR therefore recognizes the recipient MHC-bearing donor peptide. Although the frequency of the direct pathway allorecognition is high, the frequency for the indirect pathway is no higher than that seen for normal antigens. (From Roitt I, Brostoff J, Male D, et al: Immunology, ed 7, Philadelphia, 2006, Mosby.)

REJECTION OF SOLID ORGANS

Hyperacute Rejection

When the recipient has pre-existing IgM antibodies to the donor's HLA antigens (Figure 17-4), a hyperacute rejection occurs within minutes. Heart and kidney transplants are highly susceptible to hyperacute rejection, whereas liver transplants are resistant.

In hyperacute rejection, antibodies bind to the endothelial cells of blood vessels and activate the complement cascade. Complement-damaged endothelial cells release surface heparin sulfate, which exposes platelet-activating molecules. Endothelial cells also secrete high-molecular-weight von Willebrand factor, which accelerates platelet aggregation and thrombosis. If the graft survives the hyperacute rejection, delayed vascular rejection occurs within 36 to 48 hours. This reaction is mediated by cytolytic NK cells engaging the Fc receptors on cell-bound IgG (antibody-dependent cellular cytotoxicity). This increases the destruction of endothelial cells and extends the vascular thrombosis. In practice, hyperacute rejection is a rare event because the recipient is screened for antibodies directed at the donor's tissue.

Acute Rejection

Acute rejection begins within a week of transplantation and is mediated by allo-reactive T cells that have been directly and indirectly stimulated. The response is initiated by the presence of donor dendritic cells (passenger leukocytes) expressing HLA and co-stimulatory molecules necessary to activate T cells. Donor dendritic cells migrate to the recipient's lymph nodes and generate a CD8 alloimmune response, which targets endothelial cells in the graft. CD8 cells infiltrate the subendothelium and disrupt or lift the endothelial cells of blood vessels from the underlying connective tissue causing vascular endotheliitis or intimal arteritis in the microvasculature and medium-sized arteries (Figure 17-5).

In addition, CD4Th1 cells secrete cytokines that activate an inflammatory response, which culminates in a cellular response composed of macrophages and lymphocytes.

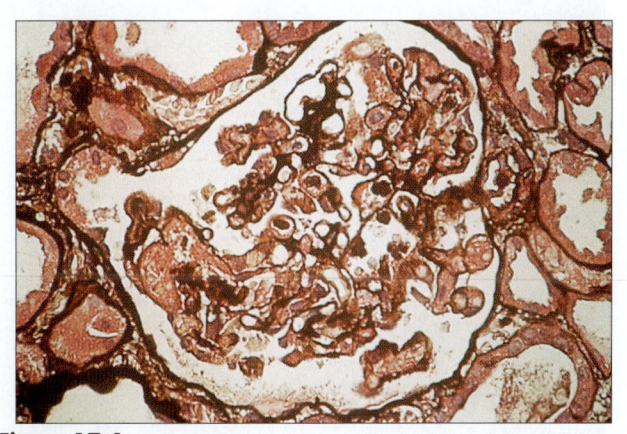

Figure 17-4

Extensive necrosis of the glomerular capillary associated with massive interstitial hemorrhage. This extensive necrosis is preceded by an intense polymorphonuclear infiltration, which occurs within the first hour of the graft's revascularization. The changes shown here occurred 24 to 48 hours after this. (H&E stain: ×200.) (From Roitt I, Brostoff J, Male D, et al: Immunology, ed 7, Philadelphia, 2006, Mosby.)

Chronic Rejection

Chronic graft rejection occurs after 6 months to a year and involves both cell-mediated and antibody-mediated responses. The pathophysiology of rejection differs according to the nature of the transplanted organ. In heart transplants, accelerated atherosclerosis or hardening of the arteries is the major cellular change. Over time, the vessel parenchyma is replaced with fibrous tissue, and blood flow is compromised. This affects cardiac output and venous return. In turn, the defective cardiac output causes ventricular fibrillation and death. Chronic rejection of transplanted kidneys causes damage and scarring of the blood vessels that is characterized by smooth muscle proliferation, tubular atrophy, and thickening of the intima of blood vessels (Figure 17-6). These changes cause glomerular hypertension and retention of fluids, which ultimately lead to kidney failure.

The lung and the liver undergo different pathologic changes. In the lung, eosinophilic scarring of the terminal and respiratory bronchioles partially or totally obliterates the airway lumen to create a pathologic condition called *bronchiolitis obliterans*. Livers undergoing chronic rejection have a reduced number of bile ducts, which is known as *vanishing bile duct syndrome*.

SURVIVAL RATES

Although the 5-year survival rate for all transplanted organs is above 80%, survival falls to 54% at 10 years (Figure 17-7).

The reduced survival rate may be attributed to immune reactions directed at minor histocompatibility, antigens, self-antigens, or both. H-Y molecules, which are expressed only on male cells, are an example of minor histocompatibility antigens. In murine transplantation studies, syngeneic females have been seen to reject male skin grafts via an immune response to H-Y antigens. The nature of the self-antigens involved in graft rejection is unclear, but they are believed to be normal polymorphic peptides that bind to host MHC molecules to elicit an allogeneic response.

Treatment to Prevent Rejection

To reduce the likelihood of transplant rejection, patients are placed on a lifelong regimen of immunosuppression therapy. Five different agents are used, individually or in combinations, to prevent graft rejection. These agents are (1) corticosteroids, (2) calcineurin inhibitors, (3) anti-proliferative agents, (4) monoclonal antibodies, and (5) polyclonal antibodies.

Corticosteroids exert multiple effects on the immune system. They cause a lymphopenia that removes CD4 cells from the peripheral circulation and redistributes them to the spleen and bone marrow. T cell proliferation and B cell maturation also are impacted by corticosteroids. Th1 and Th2 lymphocytes do not respond to interleukin 1 (IL-1) and cannot synthesize a number of proinflammatory cytokines that include IL-2, IL-6, interferon gamma (IFN-γ), and tumor necrosis factor alpha (TNF-α).

Calcineurin inhibitors (cyclosporine and tacrolimus) bind to intracellular proteins called *cyclophilin* or *immunophilin* and inhibit the transcription of IL-2. The lack of IL-2 prevents autocrine and paracrine stimulation of T cells.

Mycophenolate mofetil was introduced to overcome the often severe side effects of calcineurin inhibitors. Mycophenolate is metabolized to mycophenolic acid, which inhibits the de novo DNA biosynthesis and blocks the proliferation of T and B cells.

The synthesis lymphocyte alpha4beta1 integrins and leukocyte function–associated antigens (LFA) are also inhibited. These glycoproteins are required for the slowing and tethering of lymphocytes to the endothelium before trans-endothelial migration.

Azathioprine also blocks DNA synthesis. Unlike other agents, azathioprine is cytostatic and acts only on dividing T and B lymphocytes following antigenic stimulation. It is only

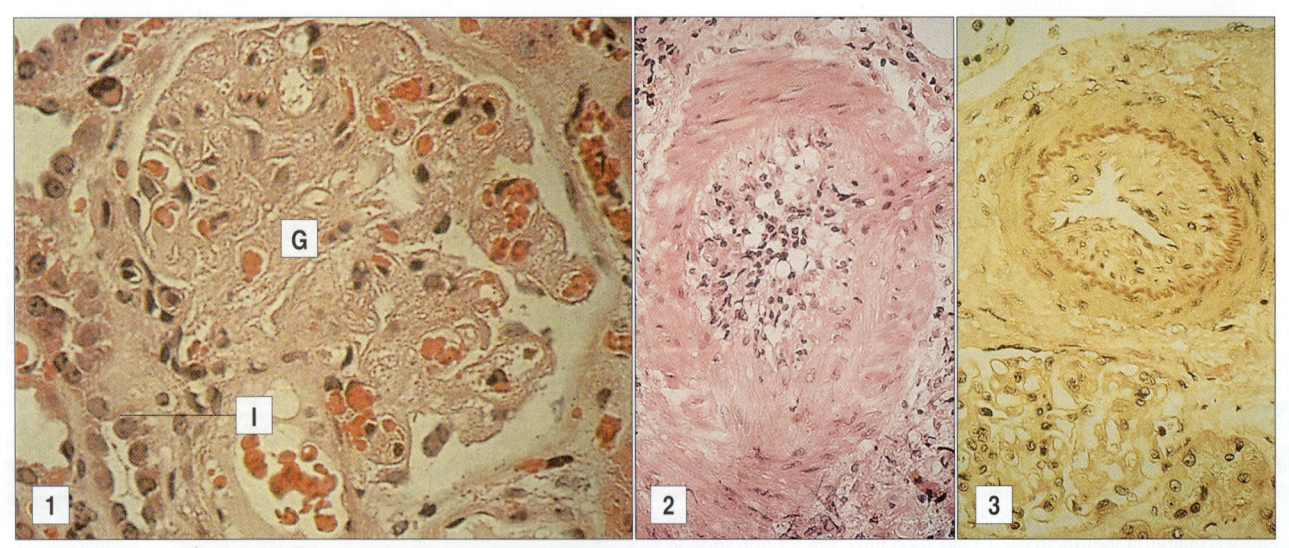

Figure 17-5

1, Small lymphocytes and other cells are accumulating in the interstitium of the graft. Such infiltration (*I*) is characteristic of acute rejection and occurs before the appearance of any clinical signs. (H&E stain.) **2**, H&E stain of acutely rejecting kidney showing vascular obstruction. **3**, van Gieson's stain of acutely rejecting kidney showing the end stage of this process. (*G*, Glomerulus.) (From Roitt I, Brostoff J, Male D, et al: Immunology, ed 7, Philadelphia, 2006, Mosby.)

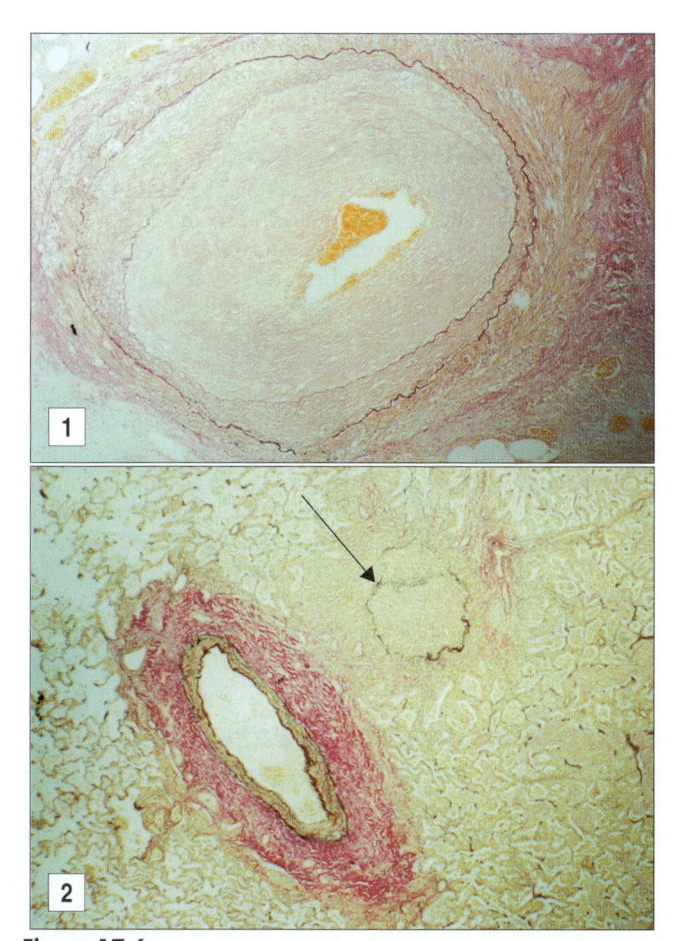

moderately immunosuppressive and does not affect antibody synthesis or inflammatory cell responses.

Monoclonal and polyclonal antibodies are effective in preventing early organ rejection. Monoclonal antibodies are designed to inhibit T cell activation (muromonab-CD3) or to block IL-2 receptor interactions (basiliximab and daclizumab) and are useful in induction immunosuppression. Polyclonal antibodies are directed at multiple epitopes that include CD2, CD3, CD4, CD8, CD11a, and CD18. Polyclonal antibodies include anti-thymocyte globulin–equine and anti-thymocyte globulin–rabbit. The anti–T cell serum depletes the allo-reactive T cell population.

Treatment regimens are usually divided into induction, maintenance, and rescue therapies. Induction therapy is used at the time of transplantation and is designed for short-term use when the risk of transplantation rejection is the highest. Induction immunosuppression varies with the type of transplant. An intense course of antibody therapy is used in patients receiving heart, lung, and kidney transplants. In contrast, inductive immunotherapy is not used in patients receiving liver transplants.

Maintenance immunosuppression uses less toxic therapeutic doses that can be administered for long periods. Dosages are tailored to the needs of each individual, maintaining a careful balance to ensure immunosuppression without predisposing the recipient to infections. Maintenance immunosuppression usually consists of a corticosteroid, a calcineurin inhibitor, and a lymphocyte proliferation inhibitor. Corticosteroids are prescribed for the majority of patients, but therapies that avoid steroids are being developed. With the exception of heart transplant recipients, most recipients receive tacrolimus. Mycophenolate mofetil is now used in place of azathioprine. Unlike maintenance therapy, rescue immunosuppression is used during an episode of graft rejection. It uses intense, short-term therapy that varies according to the nature of the transplant.

HEMATOPOIETIC STEM CELL TRANSPLANTATION

Patients with leukemia and lymphoma are usually treated with a combination of chemotherapy and irradiation designed to destroy the rapidly dividing cancer cells (Box 17-1).

Figure 17-6
Grafts that survive acute rejection are still capable of undergoing chronic rejection. **1,** Section taken from a patient with chronic rejection of the heart graft. The lumen of the blood vessel in the heart has been narrowed as a result of thickening of the wall of the vessel, limiting the blood supply to the heart. **2,** Section taken from a patient with chronic rejection of the lung, showing obliterative bronchiolitis (*arrow*) blocking the airways. (From Roitt I, Brostoff J, Male D, et al: Immunology, ed 7, Philadelphia, 2006, Mosby. Kindly supplied by Professor Marlene Rose, Imperial College London, Harefield Hospital, and Dr. Margaret Burke, Pathology Department, Royal Brompton Hospital and Harefield Hospital.)

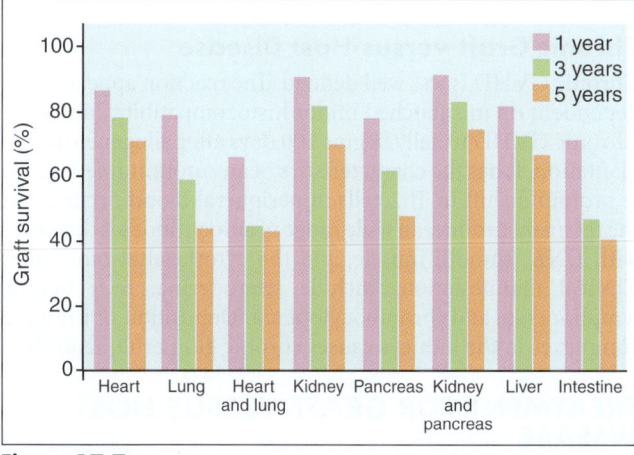

Figure 17-7
Graft survival rates of transplants for primary transplantations performed between 1995 and 2002 in the United States. Survival rates for repeat transplantations are generally somewhat lower.

BOX 17-1
Diseases Treated by Autologous and Allogeneic Bone Marrow Transplantations

Autologous Transplants

Multiple myeloma
Neuroblastoma
Non-Hodgkin's lymphoma
Hodgkin's disease
Acute myeloid leukemia (AML)
Medulloblastoma
Germ-cell tumors

Allogeneic Transplants

Acute myelogenous leukemia
Non-Hodgkin's lymphoma
Hodgkin's disease
Acute lymphoblastic leukemia (ALL)
Chronic myeloid leukemia (CML)
Myelodysplastic syndromes
Multiple myeloma
Chronic lymphocytic leukemia

Bone marrow, which contains proliferating cells, is often severely damaged or destroyed by high-dose cancer treatments. Bone marrow is critical to the survival of the host because it contains three types of multi-potential stem cells that give rise to red and white blood cells, osteoblasts, chondrocytes, myocytes, and endothelial cells. Bone marrow function can be restored by bone marrow transplantation (BMT), peripheral blood stem cell transplantation (PBSCT), or umbilical cord blood stem cell transplantation (UBSCT).

Characteristics of Human Stem Cells

In 1998, hematopoietic stem cells were identified on the basis of CD markers (CD34+, CD31–, CD59+, thy 1+, and CD38–) expressed on the cell surface. On the basis of CD expression, stem cells can be easily purified by using the fluorescence-activated cell sorter (FACS). Purification of CD34+ cells eliminates donor lymphocytes that can attack the recipient's tissue.

Bone Marrow Stem Cells

Bone marrow stem cells are used in syngeneic and allogeneic transplantations. To release stem cells from stroma, the recipient is primed with granulocyte colony-stimulating factor (G-CSF). Free stem cells are aspirated from the posterior iliac crests of the hip. Aspirated marrow contains a large stem cell population (1 stem cell per 100,000 cells). However, the use of bone marrow stem cells has several disadvantages. Aspirations are surgical procedures usually performed under general anesthesia. Multiple aspirations may be required over time to acquire enough stem cells for transplantation. The effective therapeutic dose of marrow stem cells is 5×10^6/kg.

Peripheral Blood Stem Cells

Peripheral blood is now the primary source for stem cells. Although small numbers normally circulate in blood, administration of G-CSF and a chemokine receptor inhibitor (plerixafor) causes an influx of marrow stem cells into peripheral blood. It is approved for mobilization of stem cells in patients with non-Hodgkin's lymphoma and multiple myeloma. Because small numbers of stem cells (20–50 cells/mL) are found in blood under the best of circumstances, repeated cell recovery is necessary. A minimum of 1×10^6 cells/kg of body weight is necessary for successful stem cell engraftment, but the preferred number is 2 to 2.5×10^6 cells/kg.

The use of peripheral blood stem cells has several advantages. The cells are easy to collect, and multiple collections are possible. Peripheral blood stem cells also engraft rapidly, and they quickly restore bone marrow function, especially platelet function. Rapid engraftment contributes to higher graft survival rates compared with bone marrow stem cell transplants. A disadvantage is that blood contains 10-fold more T cells that often attack the recipient's tissue, causing a unique situation where the graft rejects the host tissue.

Umbilical Cord Blood Stem Cells

Placenta and umbilical cord blood are rich sources of stem cells. Cord blood contains hematopoietic stem cells and pluripotential stem cells that are capable of developing into multiple germ cell lineages. Use of cord blood is advantageous because collection poses no risks to mother and infant. Moreover, the stem cell population has reduced expression of HLA markers and are not considered foreign by any recipient. During delivery, only 50 to 90 mL of cord blood can be collected. Cord blood for transplantation is therefore reserved only for small children because of the low number of stem cells and the finite nature of the preparation. The minimum cell dose used in reconstitution is 2.5×10^7 cells/kg.

TRANSPLANTATION PROTOCOL

Bone marrow from autologous and allogeneic donors can be used in transplantations. Autologous transplants are preferred because transplantation morbidity and mortality are greatly reduced. Allogeneic transplantation still requires careful attention to HLA typing. Complete matching at all loci is considered ideal for transplantation. However, a single mismatch in any loci is considered acceptable in most transplantation protocols.

For successful transplantation, the recipient's immune system must be ablated to ensure that the recipient does not reject the graft. In myeloablative protocols, high-dose chemotherapy and radiation are administered before transplantation. Myeloablative regimens are extremely toxic, resulting in high peritransplantation morbidity from kidney, liver, and gastrointestinal toxicity. To reduce the risks associated with myeloablation, irradiation and chemotherapeutic agents with less toxicity are used in a nonmyeloablative or low-dose marrow preparation. This approach reduces peritransplantation morbidity and mortality, but GVHD remains a major clinical problem.

GRAFT-VERSUS-HOST DISEASE

GVHD occurs when allo-reactive T cells from the donor attack the recipient's tissue. The reaction develops when cells or tissue containing lymphocytes or lymphocyte progenitors are infused into immunosuppressed individuals.

Acute Graft-versus-Host Disease

Acute GVSD usually occurs within the first 100 days of engraftment. The primary organs affected by acute GVHD are the skin, liver, and intestinal tract. Rejection is characterized by a rash with erythema, liver damage, and moderate diarrhea. In acute GVHD, donor cells release proinflammatory cytokines, which upregulate the expression of major and minor HLA molecules and T cell co-stimulatory molecules on recipient cells. Donor CD4Th2 cells react with class II molecules on the surface of recipient macrophages and dendritic cells. In turn, the Th2 cells produce IFN-γ and IL-2, which activate both cytotoxic CD8 T cells and NK cells. Effector cells damage tissue, and the production of TNF-α augments tissue destruction.

Chronic Graft-versus-Host Disease

Chronic GVHD is less well defined. The reaction appears to be dependent on mismatched minor histocompatibility antigens. Chronic GVHD usually begins 100 days after allogeneic transplantation. It has the characteristics of an autoimmune disease. A profound shift to Th2 cells in peripheral blood occurs, and the recipient produces a wide range of autoantibodies that react with DNA, smooth muscle, and the cytoskeletal molecules. Clinical manifestations include scleroderma, liver failure, lymphopenia, and thrombocytopenia. Deposition of immune complexes in the kidneys causes chronic glomerulonephritis.

TREATMENT FOR GRAFT-VERSUS-HOST DISEASE

Acute Rejection

Methotrexate is the primary drug used to treat acute GVHD. Methotrexate, however, has been replaced by mycophenolate, which has less toxicity and can be used in combination with calcineurin inhibitors (cyclosporine and tacrolimus). Alemtuzumab or anti-thymocyte globulin (ATG) can also be used to reduce the number of allo-reactive T cells. Alemtuzumab targets CD52 molecules expressed on mature lymphocytes.

Chronic Rejection

Chronic rejection is an uncommon event and may resolve spontaneously without treatment. Extensive chronic GVHD is treated with oral prednisone in combination with cyclosporine.

SUMMARY

- It is possible to transplant organs, tissue, and stem cells from donors related or unrelated to the recipient.
- Recognition of donor human leukocyte antigens (HLAs) and self-antigens cause graft rejection.
- HLAs on donor and recipient tissues are usually matched before transplantation.
- Different immune mechanisms are active in hyperacute, acute, and chronic graft rejections.
- Survival of grafts is extended by the use of induction immunosuppression, maintenance immunosuppression, and rescue immunosuppression.
- Bone marrow function can be re-established by hematopoietic stem cell transplantation using bone marrow, peripheral blood, and umbilical stem cells.
- Reconstituted bone marrow contains the lymphocyte progenitors that can mount an immune response against host tissue, resulting in graft-versus-host disease (GVHD).

REFERENCES

Allan JS: Public health concerns take center stage in Nuffield Council on Bioethics: A review of animal-to-human transplants: The ethics of xenotransplantation, Sci Eng Ethics 2(4):486, 1996.

Barrett AJ: Graft-versus-host disease: A review, J R Soc Med 80(6):368, 1987.

Greenstein JL, White-Scharf M: Xenotransplantation: A review of current issues, J Biolaw Bus 2(1):46, 1998.

Heeger PS: T-cell allorecognition and transplant rejection: A summary and update, Am J Transplant 3(5):525, 2003.

Iannone R, Davies SM: Tissue typing for hematopoietic cell transplantation: Newer techniques and newer antigens for which cross-matching is helpful, Pediatr Transplant 9(Suppl 7):76, 2005.

Jiang S, Herrera O, Lechler RI: New spectrum of allorecognition pathways: Implications for graft rejection and transplantation tolerance, Curr Opin Immunol 16(5):550, 2004.

Lechler RI, Sykes M, Thomson AW, Turka LA: Organ transplantation—how much of the promise has been realized? Nat Med 11(6):605, 2005.

Martins AA, Paiva A, Morgado JM, et al: Quantification and immunophenotypic characterization of bone marrow and umbilical cord blood mesenchymal stem cells by multicolor flow cytometry, Transplant Proc 41(3):943, 2009.

Patience C, Takeuchi Y, Weiss RA: Infection of human cells by an endogenous retrovirus of pigs, Nat Med 3(3):282, 1997.

Rocha PN, Plumb TJ, Crowley SD, et al: Effector mechanisms in transplant rejection, Immunol Rev 196:51, 2003.

Rogers NJ, Lechler RI: Allorecognition, Am J Transplant 1(2):97, 2001.

Sayegh MH, Carpenter CB: Transplantation 50 years later—progress, challenges, and promises, N Engl J Med 351(26):2761, 2004.

Steels E, Meuleman N, Vereecken P, et al: Graft-versus-host disease: Review of 22 cases, Acta Clin Belg 59(4):182, 2004.

ASSESSMENT QUESTIONS

1. An organ transplanted between genetically identical twins is known as a(n):
   A. Xenograft
   B. Autograft
   C. Isograft
   D. Allogenic graft

2. Hyperacute rejection of transplants is caused by:
   A. Pre-existing antibodies to the donors' HLA antigens
   B. Passenger leukocytes
   C. Cytotoxic T cells
   D. CD4Th1 cells

3. Which of the following is the most common source of stem cells used in an autologous transplantation?
   A. Bone marrow
   B. Peripheral blood
   C. Umbilical cord blood
   D. Placental cord blood

4. Reduced survival of transplants at 5 and 10 years is caused by:
   I. Recognition of the donors' minor HLA antigens
   II. Recognition of the donors' self-antigens
   III. Tolerance to maintenance immunosuppression
   A. III
   B. I and II
   C. II and III
   D. I, II, and III

5. The major impediment to xenotransplantation is:
   A. The presence of pre-existing anti-HLA antibodies
   B. The presence of pre-existing antibodies to porcine endothelial cells
   C. The presence of pre-existing antibodies to carbohydrate antigens containing alpha galactosyl residues
   D. A rapid graft-versus-host reaction

6. A graft-versus-host reaction is most commonly associated with:
   A. Kidney transplantations
   B. Heart transplantations
   C. Lung transplantations
   D. Hematopoietic stem cell transplantations

CHAPTER 18

Antigen Presentation for Cell-Mediated Response

LEARNING OBJECTIVES

- Draw the structure of a class I antigen-presenting molecule
- Explain antigen processing and presentation to CD8 T cells
- Recognize the role of ubiquitin in antigen processing
- Identify the role of heat shock protein 70 (HSP70) in antigen processing
- Discuss the roles of transporter-associated antigen processing (TAP) protein, tapasin, and calreticulin in antigen processing
- Compare and contrast the function of class I and CD1 molecules
- Explain cross-priming

KEY TERMS

Calreticulin
Cell-mediated immunity
CD1
Class I molecules
Class II molecules
Cross-priming
Endogenous antigen
Exogenous antigen
Proteasome
Transporter-associated antigen processing (TAP) protein
Tapasin
Ubiquitination

INTRODUCTION

Previous chapters in this text focused on antibody responses initiated by class II molecule antigen presentation to CD4Th2 cells. Although antibodies are efficient in dealing with exogenous antigens or extracellular microbes, they are ineffective in eradicating intracellular microbes, viruses, and tumor cells. A cell-mediated response, which is usually mounted in response to these endogenous antigens, consists of lymphocytes, activated macrophages, and natural killer (NK) cells. The nature of the cellular response is a reflection of antigen presentation. If antigens are presented in the context of class II or CD1 molecules, CD4Th1 cells promote an inflammatory response that involves macrophages, lymphocytes, and fibroblasts. When antigens are presented by class I molecules, cytotoxic T cells are activated. These cells are able to lyse target cells following cell-to-cell contact.

CLASS I PROTEINS

Class I molecules are found on all the nucleated cells in the body and present antigen to CD8 T cells. They consist of a single, α-chain transmembrane protein that is stabilized by a second protein known as β_2-*microglobulin* (see Chapter 4).

Because the processed antigens are bound to class I molecules at the ends, the length of the antigen is restricted to 9 to 11 amino acids (Figure 18-1).

CLASS I MOLECULES AND ANTIGEN PRESENTATION

Endogenous antigens are generally large molecules that must be digested and fragmented before presentation to lymphocytes. Antigens are marked for enzymatic degradation by a process known as *ubiquitination*. In the process, molecules of ubiquitin are attached to the antigen by covalent bonding between amino groups of ubiquitin and lysine amino acids in the antigen. When four or more ubiquitin molecules bind to the antigen, the complex is shuttled to a series of proteasomes for fragmentation. During transport through the cytoplasm, heat shock protein 70 (HSP70) interacts with the ubiquitinated protein and protects it from enzymatic digestion. Initial digestion takes place in a 20S proteasome. The low-activity 20S proteasome consists of two α-subunits and two β-subunits, each having seven globular protein subsets. Only three β-subunits (MB1, delta, and zeta) are enzymatically active. Antigen fragments produced by the 20S proteasome vary widely in length (Figure 18-2).

To increase the rate of antigen fragmentation and to generate more homogeneous antigen fragments, the three β-proteasome subsets are replaced with high-activity enzymes (LMP2, LMP7, and MECL1). Additional subunits, which accelerate antigen processing, are also added to create a 26S proteasome. Digestion in the 26S proteasome produces 9 to 11 amino acid sequences, which are suitable for class I loading.

Antigens fragmented in the cytosol must be transported to the endoplasmic reticulum (ER) before they can be loaded onto class I molecules. Transporter-associated antigen processing (TAP) proteins are used to move antigenic fragments from the cytoplasm into the ER. TAP is actually a heterodimer of TAP1 and TAP2. Both isoforms are required for antigen transport and for the stabilization of class I molecules. With the exception of fragments with C-terminal proline and glycine, all peptides will bind to TAPs. Peptide fragments are loaded onto class I molecules in the ER.

Prior to antigen loading, the class I molecule forms complexes with three proteins: (1) a transmembrane-associated protein, called the *TAP-binding protein*, or *tapasin*, (2) a chaperone protein

148 CHAPTER 18 ANTIGEN PRESENTATION FOR CELL MEDIATED RESPONSE

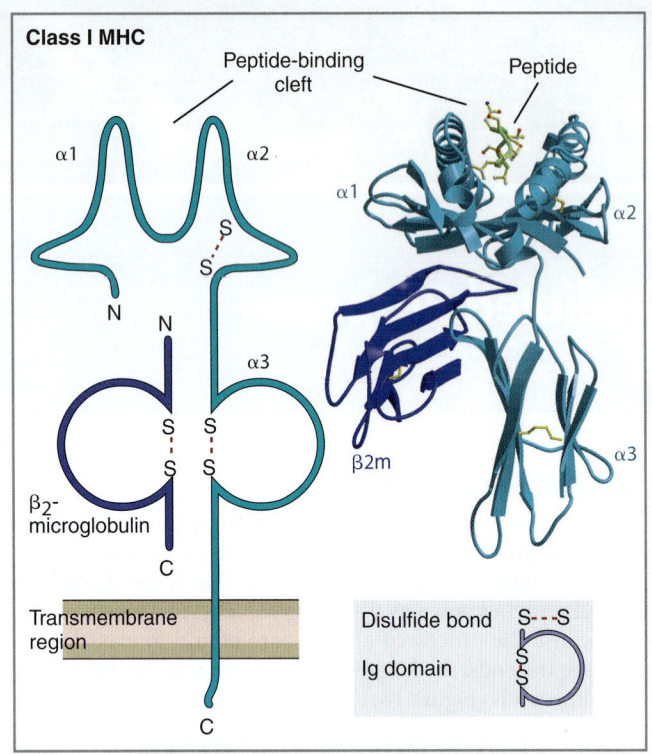

Figure 18-1

The structure of class I major histocompatibility complex (MHC) molecules in animals. This structure is identical to HLA class I molecules found in man. The schematic diagram and model of the crystal structure of class I MHC illustrates the domains of the molecules. The class I molecule contains peptide-binding clefts and invariant portions that bind CD8 (the β_3-domain of class I). (From Abbas AK, Lichtman AH: Basic immunology: functions and disorders of the immune system, ed 2 [updated edition], Philadelphia, 2006, Saunders. Crystal structures courtesy of Dr. P. Bjorkman, California Institute of Technology, Pasadena, CA.)

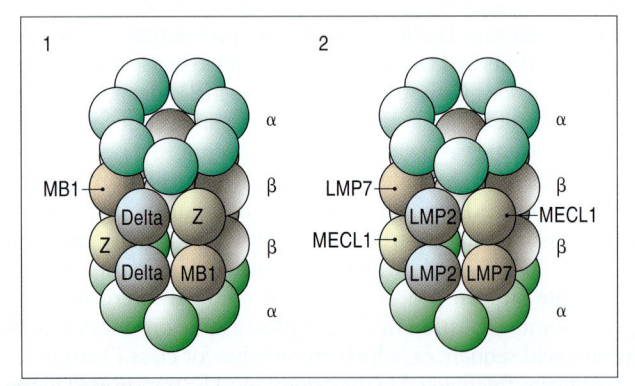

Figure 18-2

The 20S proteasome, shown in cartoon form, is composed of four stacked discs, two identical outer discs of α-subunits, and two similar inner disks comprising β-subunits. Each disc has seven different subunits. Peptides enter the body of the proteasome for cleavage into peptides. **1,** Only three of the β-subunits are active. In normal proteasomes, these are called MB1, delta, and Z. **2,** Interferon gamma (IFN-γ) treatment of cells results in replacement of these three subunits by the two major histocompatibility complex (MHC)-encoded proteins, LMP2 and LMP7, as well as a third inducible protein, MECL1. These subunits are shown adjacent to each other here, whereas they are actually in separate parts of the β-ring and some would be hidden at the back of the structure shown. (From Roitt I, Brostoff J, Male D, et al: Immunology, ed 7, Philadelphia, 2006, Mosby.)

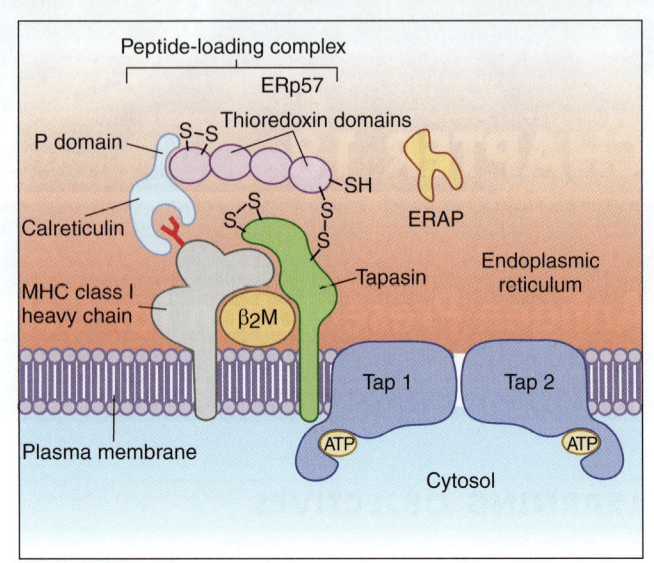

Figure 18-3

Major histocompatibility complex (MHC) class I peptide-loading complex. A single tapasin molecule is associated with the TAP heterodimer here, although data suggest that four may be present. The peptide-loading complex, plus endoplasmic reticulum aminopeptidase (ERAP), is found in macrophage and dendritic cell (DC) phagosomes. (Ackerman A, Cresswell P: Cellular mechanisms governing cross presentation of exogenous antigens, Nat Immunol 5(7):678, 2004.)

called *calreticulin,* and (3) a thiol oxidoreductase (ERp57). The oxidoreductase attaches to calreticulin and covalently links to tapasin by using disulfide bonds (Figure 18-3). In addition to stabilizing the class I–β_2-microglobulin complex, tapasin may encourage the binding of high-affinity antigens to the class I molecule. Antigenic fragments are loaded onto the class I molecule after it is stabilized.

If the antigenic fragments are longer than 9 to 11 amino acids, an ER aminopeptidase (ERp57) trims the antigen's hydrophobic N-terminus so that the overall length is between 9 and 11 amino acids. The peptide-loaded class I molecules are transferred to the Golgi apparatus, which functions to package proteins for secretion. From the Golgi apparatus, specialized vesicles transport the antigen-loaded class I molecules to the cell surface.

CD1 PROTEINS

The CD1 family is unrelated to class I and II molecules and represents a third lineage of antigen-presenting molecules that are expressed by B cells, monocytes, and dendritic cells (see Chapter 4). They differ in intracellular trafficking, antigen processing, and antigen loading. Peptides binding to CD1 are much longer than the typical 9 to 11 amino acids found in class I binding clefts because CD1 has three anchor positions, one at each end and one in the middle.

CD1 binds lipid molecules from bacteria, self-antigens, and synthetic antigens. Bacterial antigens are highly conserved mycolyl, diacylglycerols, and lipopeptides from pathogenic *Mycobacterium*, *Plasmodium*, and *Leishmania* species. CD1-restricted T cells play a critical role in resolution of infections by these organisms. Autoimmune disease may occur when CD1s are loaded with self-antigens such as phospholipids, phosphatidylinositol, or phosphatidylethanolamine.

CD1 AND ANTIGEN PRESENTATION

Antigen processing is similar to that described for exogenous antigens, but antigen loading differs significantly. CD1s are synthesized in the ER and most move directly to the cell surface

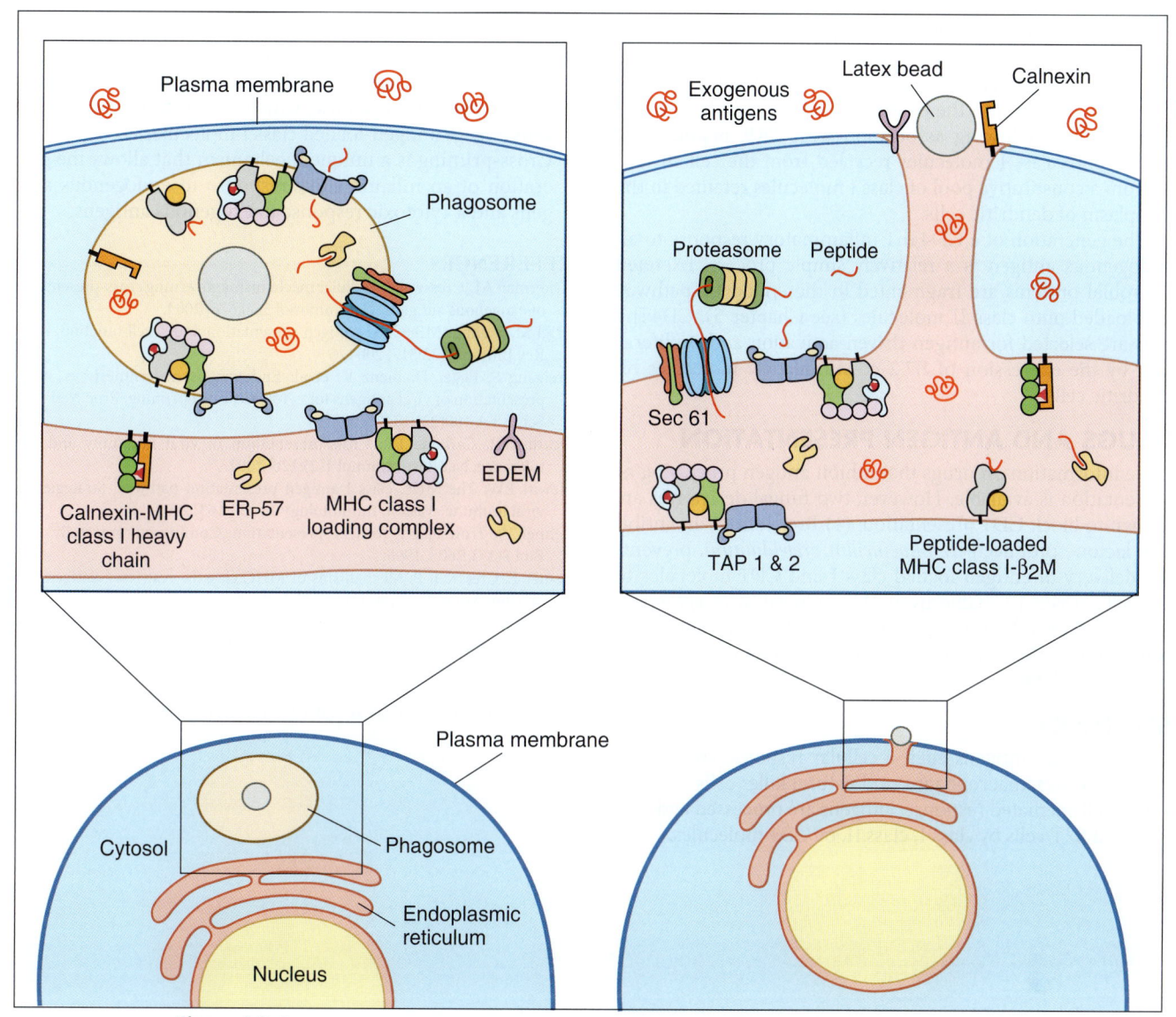

Figure 18-4

Two models of cross-presentation. **A,** The phagosome is self-contained, incorporating Sec61, associated proteasomes, and the peptide-loading complex. A concerted mechanism functioning in the phagosome is responsible for the generation of major histocompatibility complex (MHC) class I–peptide complexes from proteins internalized into the same phagosome. **B,** External proteins have direct access to the endoplasmic reticulum (ER) by transiently available continuities or by a regulated mechanism. In this case, cross-presentation could occur in the ER itself. This mechanism may be more important for antigens internalized by pinocytosis or receptor-mediated endocytosis. (Ackerman A, Cresswell P: Cellular mechanisms governing cross presentation of exogenous antigens, Nat Immunol 5(7):678, 2004.)

without being antigen loaded. Antigens are captured by mannose receptors and internalized into endosomes. The endosomal pathway is necessary for efficient T cell stimulation by all known bacterial lipid antigens. In the endosome, the presence of saposon lipid transfer proteins and a low pH allow transfer of the lipid antigens to CD1 molecules that have been recycled from the cell membrane to the endosome. Following stabilization, the antigen-loaded CD1 enters the secretory pathway and is redistributed to the cell surface.

Antigen presentation by CD1 group I and group II family members elicits different immune responses. For example, antigen presentation by CD1a, CD1b, and CD1c initiate a cellular inflammatory response that culminates in granulomatous lung disease. Conversely, antigen presented by C1d drives the response toward T helper cell (CD4Th2)–driven B cell–mediated responses.

CROSS-PRIMING AND ANTIGEN PRESENTATION

The fundamental paradigm of antigen presentation is that exogenously derived peptides are presented to Th2 cells by class II molecules, and CD8 cytotoxic T cells are activated after presentation of endogenous peptides by class I molecules. However, the paradigm fails to explain the generation of CD4Th1 cellular inflammatory responses to endogenously derived antigens or the CD8 cytotoxic response to exogenous antigens.

Both mechanisms can be explained by the concept of cross-priming by dendritic cells. As a consequence of normal microbial metabolism, endogenous proteins are excreted from infected cells and become exogenous antigens. Intact tumor cells are also considered exogenous antigens. Following ingestion, cells and excreted proteins are placed in phagosomes (Figure 18-4).

In the generation of cytotoxic T cells, the early phagocytic vesicles or phagosomes fuse with the ER membrane and use the protein translocation channel Sec61 to funnel partially degraded antigen into the cytoplasm, where it is digested by proteasomes. Following association with TAP, peptides are loaded onto class I molecules recycled from the cell surface or from a constitutive pool of class I molecules retained in the cytoplasm of dendritic cells.

The generation of a CD4Th1 inflammatory response to an endogenous antigen is a relatively simple process. Excreted microbial proteins are fragmented in the endocytic pathway and loaded onto class II molecules (see Chapter 5). CD4Th1 cells are selected for antigen-driven activation and proliferation by the expression of B7.2 co-stimulatory molecules on dendritic cells.

DRUGS AND ANTIGEN PRESENTATION

Little information on drugs that inhibit antigen processing or presentation is available. However, two fungal derivatives are known to block CD1 presentation: (1) Brefeldin A, an antibiotic lactone produced by *Eupenicillin brefeldianum*, prevents the delivery of antigen-loaded class I and CD1 molecules to the cell surface. (2) Bafilomycin A, produced by *Streptomyces griseus*, inhibits the transport of antigens from the late endosomes to the ER. As a consequence, the immune system cannot be stimulated.

SUMMARY

- Endogenous antigens elicit a cellular response comprising lymphocytes, macrophages, and natural killer cells.
- In a cell-mediated response, antigens are processed and presented to T cells by class I, class II, or CD1 molecules.
- The two types of cellular responses are (1) inflammatory response, which is generated following interactions between antigen-loaded class II or CD1 molecules and CD4Th1 cells; and (2) cytotoxic response, which is engendered when CD8 cells engage antigen-loaded class I molecules.
- Cross-priming is a unique mechanism that allows the generation of an inflammatory response to endogenous antigens and a cytotoxic response to exogenous antigens.

REFERENCES

Ackerman AL, Cresswell P: Cellular mechanisms governing cross-presentation of exogenous antigens, Nat Immunol 5(7):678, 2004.

Brigl M, Brenner MB: CD1: Antigen presentation and T cell function, Annu Rev Immunol 22:817, 2004.

Freigang S, Egger D, Bienz K, et al: Endogenous neosynthesis vs. cross-presentation of viral antigens for cytotoxic T cell priming, Proc Natl Acad Sci U S A 100(23):13477, 2003.

Heath WR, Carbone FR: Cross-presentation in viral immunity and self-tolerance, Nat Rev Immunol 1(2):126, 2001.

Hewitt EW: The MHC class I antigen presentation pathway: Strategies for viral immune evasion, Immunology 110(2):163, 2003.

Lehner PJ, Trowsdale J: Antigen presentation: Coming out gracefully, Curr Biol 8(17):R605, 1998.

Pamer E, Cresswell P: Mechanisms of MHC class I—restricted antigen processing, Annu Rev Immunol 16:323, 1998.

Rock KL, York IA, Goldberg AL: Post-proteasomal antigen processing for major histocompatibility complex class I presentation, Nat Immunol 5(7):670, 2004.

Watts C: The exogenous pathway for antigen presentation on major histocompatibility complex class II and CD1 molecules, Nat Immunol 5(7):685, 2004.

ASSESSMENT QUESTIONS

1. CD1 molecules usually bind:
   I. Highly conserved microbial lipids
   II. Highly conserved self-antigens
   III. Highly conserved viral proteins
   A. I
   B. III
   C. I and II
   D. II and III
   E. I, II, and III

2. Cross-priming explains:
   I. The generation of CD4Th2 cells to endogenous antigens
   II. The generation of CD8 cells to exogenous antigens
   III. The generation of CD4Th1 cells to endogenous antigens
   A. I
   B. III
   C. I and II
   D. II and III
   E. I, II, and III

3. In an inflammatory response, the selection and activation of CD4Th1 cells by antigen-loaded class II molecules are determined by the:
   A. Expression of CD28 on T cells
   B. Expression of CTLA4 on T cells
   C. Expression of B7.1 on dendritic cells
   D. Expression of B7.2 on dendritic cells

4. Which of the following is *not* associated with a cell-mediated response?
   A. B cells
   B. T cells
   C. Macrophages
   D. Natural killer (NK) cells

5. Antigen-presenting CD1 molecules are expressed on:
   I. B cells
   II. Monocytes
   III. Dendritic cells
   A. I
   B. III
   C. I and II
   D. II and III
   E. I, II, and III

6. The protein that transports endogenous antigens from the cytosol to the endoplasmic reticulum is known as:
   A. Tapasin
   B. Calreticulin
   C. Oxidoreductase
   D. Transporter-associated antigen processing (TAP) protein

CHAPTER 19

Delayed-Type Hypersensitivity Reactions

LEARNING OBJECTIVES

- Identify the definition of delayed-type hypersensitivity (DTH)
- Compare and contrast immediate and cell-mediated hypersensitivities
- List the six *Mycobacterium* species that are human pathogens
- Recognize the components of an acid-fast cell wall
- Explain the role of the natural resistance–associated macrophage protein (NRAMP) and intracellular survival of the tuberculosis bacterium
- Explain the relationship between interferon gamma (IFN-γ) and DTH
- Explain the relationship between vitamin D and leprosy
- Compare and contrast the three histologic stages of tuberculosis
- Recognize the cellular components in a granuloma
- Describe the Mantoux test
- Compare and contrast *Mycobacterium tuberculosis* and Bacille Calmette-Guérin (BCG)
- Explain the mechanism involved in the QuantiFERON-Gold test
- Recognize the four front-line drugs used to treat active tuberculosis and their mechanisms of action
- Recognize the second-line drugs used to treat active tuberculosis and their mechanisms of action
- Identify the definition of multidrug-resistant–tuberculosis (MDR–TB)
- Define extensively drug-resistant–tuberculosis (XDR–TB)
- Identify the dimorphic phases of histoplasmosis
- Compare the role of macroconidia and the yeast form in the pathogenesis of histoplasmosis
- Recognize regions of the United States where histoplasmosis is endemic
- Compare and contrast granuloma formation in histoplasmosis and tuberculosis
- Identify the groups at risk for progressive disseminated histoplasmosis
- Identify the dimorphic forms of *Coccidioides immitis*
- Identify regions of the United States where *Coccidioides* is endemic
- Recognize the role of arthroconidia in the pathogenesis of coccidioidomycosis
- Differentiate between spherules and endospores in the pathogenesis of coccidioidomycosis
- Recognize the drugs used to treat histoplasmosis and coccidioidomycosis and their mechanisms of action
- Compare and contrast contact dermatitis, irritant dermatitis, and photocontact dermatitis
- Recognize the drugs that are used to treat contact dermatitis
- Explain the immunologic skin response to nickel
- Identify the role(s) of Th17 cells in metal hypersensitivity
- Recognize the drugs that are used to treat nickel hypersensitivity
- List the three members of the *Toxicodendron* genus that cause skin reactions
- Identify the haptenic substance produced by the *Toxicodendron* species
- Explain the immunologic response to urushiol
- List the drugs that are used to treat poison ivy reaction
- Explain the immunologic and biologic responses active in celiac sprue

KEY TERMS

Allergic contact dermatitis
Arthroconidia
Bacille Calmette-Guérin (BCG)
Conidia
Cord factor
Extensively drug-resistant tuberculosis
Gliadin
Granuloma
Interferon gamma (IFN-γ)
Lysosomes
Mantoux test
Multidrug-resistant tuberculosis
Mycolic acids
Natural resistance–associated macrophage protein (NRAMP)
Photocontact dermatitis
T17 cells
Tumor necrosis factor
Urushiol
Vitamin D receptor

INTRODUCTION

Delayed-type hypersensitivity (DTH) is a unique type of cell-mediated immunity. The name originated from the skin test used in the diagnosis of tuberculosis and denotes cellular infiltrates causing induration and erythema at the skin test site within 24 to 72 hours. DTH was coined to describe the reaction to the tuberculosis skin test and to differentiate between delayed cellular skin test results and antibody-mediated immediate skin test results. The term has been expanded to include cell-mediated reactions to bacteria or fungi infecting lungs and skin responses to chemicals and plants. In the lung, cellular responses to tuberculosis, histoplasmosis, and coccidioidomycosis are considered DTH reactions. Skin reactions to nickel and poison ivy also are DTH reactions.

The principal effectors of DTH reactions are CD4Th1 lymphocytes, monocytes or macrophages, CD8Tc1 cells, and natural killer (NK) cells. The histopathology of DTH lesions varies with the nature of the antigen, the type of effector cells, and the anatomic location.

DELAYED-TYPE HYPERSENSITIVITY RESPONSES IN THE LUNG

Tuberculosis

The family Mycobacteriaceae contains the *Mycobacterium* genus. Within the genus are six different human pathogens (Table 19-1). (1) *M. tuberculosis* causes most of the 9.1 million cases of pulmonary tuberculosis in the world. (2) *M. leprae*, which is also known as *Hansen's bacillus*, is commonly found in tropical countries and is the etiological agent of leprosy. (3&4) *Mycobacterium avium* and *M. intracellulare* are found in soil, water systems, birds, and other domestic animals. Because the two species are difficult to identify in the laboratory, they are designated as the *Mycobacterium avium* complex (MAC). Patients with acquired immunodeficiency syndrome (AIDS) and therapeutically immunosuppressed individuals are frequently infected by MAC organisms. (5) *M. bovis* is a cattle-adapted species of tuberculosis that is also found in wild and domestic animals, but it causes less than 1% of all tuberculosis infections. Human infection is caused by inhalation of droplets containing live organisms or by ingestion of unpasteurized milk. Ingestion leads to extrapulmonary tuberculosis in lymph nodes and skeletal bones. (6) *Mycobacterium africanum* is commonly found in West Africa, where it accounts for 25% of tuberculosis cases.

Tuberculosis: Virulence Factors

In the lung, survival of the tuberculosis bacterium is determined, in part, by cell-wall mycolic acids and a lipoarabinomannan known as the *cord factor*. Mycolic acids, which are 50% of the dry weight of the cell wall (Figure 19-1), form a hydrophobic barrier that prevents the entry of drugs, disinfectants, and other harsh chemicals. Cord factor inhibits the interferon (IFN)–induced activation of macrophages and stimulates the production of tumor necrosis factor alpha (TNF-α).

Laboratory Identification of *Mycobacterium* Species

Laboratory identification of mycobacteria is difficult because conventional stains do not penetrate the cell wall. However, mycobacteria can be identified by the Ziehl Neelsen stain, which uses a combination of heat and carbolfuchsin to drive the stain into the cell wall. Only the *Mycobacterium* and *Nocardia* species retain the dye following harsh treatment with an acid–alcohol mixture. Thus, these species are designated *acid-fast organisms*.

Pathophysiology of Tuberculosis

Exposure to tuberculosis occurs by inhalation of droplets containing live organisms. Because of their small size, the organisms are usually deposited in the distal areas of the lung. In

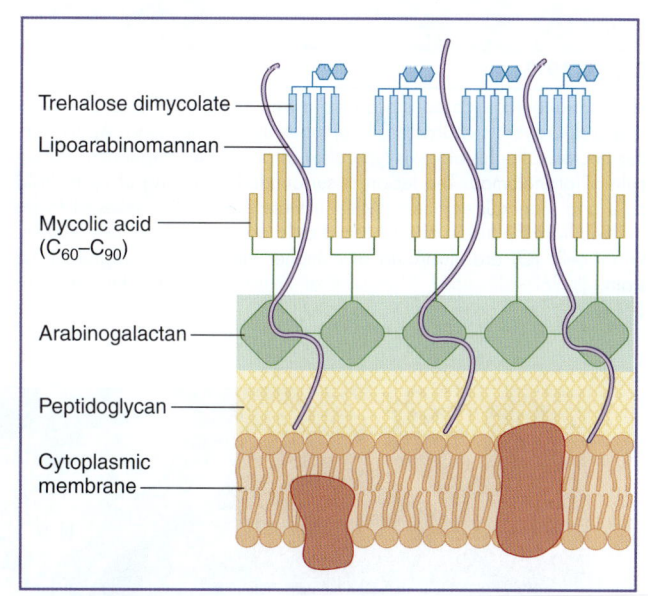

Table 19-1	Species of Tuberculosis Infecting Humans
Pathogen	**Infection/Transmission**
Mycobacterium tuberculosis	Human tuberculosis. Transmitted by inhalation route
Mycobacterium leprae	Hansen's disease, or leprosy. Transmitted by inhalation route
Mycobacterium avium-intracellulare	Group of closely related opportunistic pathogens that infect immunosuppressed patients with human immunodeficiency virus (HIV). Transmitted by inhalation and oral routes
Mycobacterium bovis	Tuberculosis in cattle. Can be transmitted to humans via infected milk or aerosols
Mycobacterium africanum	Commonly found in West Africa. Spread by the airborne route

Figure 19-1
Mycobacterial cell wall. The mycobacterial cell envelope is rich in waxes and lipids, especially mycolic acids, which are covalently linked to arabinogalactans. The unique long-chain mycolic acid trehalose 6,6′-dimycolate (C_{60}–C_{90}) is responsible for the "cording" seen with virulent strains, giving colonies a serpentine morphology. Mycolic acids form an asymmetric lipid bilayer with shorter-chain glycerophospholipids. The cell envelope also contains peptidoglycan and has a complex glycolipid structure forming the outermost layer, which sits atop the peptidoglycan and lipid bilayer of the cytoplasmic membrane. Other important components include lipoarabinomannan and arabinogalactan. (From Actor JK: Elsevier's integrated immunology and microbiology, Philadelphia, 2007, Mosby.)

the first stage of the disease, mycobacteria take up residence in phagosomes within alveolar macrophages and prevent intracellular killing by inhibiting maturation of the phagosome and fusion with endosomes and lysosomes which contain antimicrobial proteins and enzymes. Rapid logarithmic multiplication of mycobacteria in macrophages eventually causes the death of the cells and creates a small necrotic area in the lung. Free mycobacteria are ingested by circulating monocytes and transported to the mediastinal lymph node. Antigen stimulation in the lymph node generates CD4Th1, CD8, and long-lived memory cells.

In the second stage, which occurs 3 weeks after infection, CD4Th1 cells migrate from the lymph node to the infection site and undergo rapid proliferation. CD4Th1 and CD8 cells secrete TNF-α and IFN-γ. TNF-α is responsible for most of the lung damage noted in mycobacteria infections. IFN-γ–stimulated macrophages produce nitric oxide by oxidation of L-citrulline. Additional interactions between nitric oxide and singlet oxygen form peroxynitrite (ONOO−), which is microcidal. The role of CD8 cells in tuberculosis is unclear. They may contribute to the lesion by producing IFN-γ, by directly killing infected cells, or by both mechanisms (Figure 19-2).

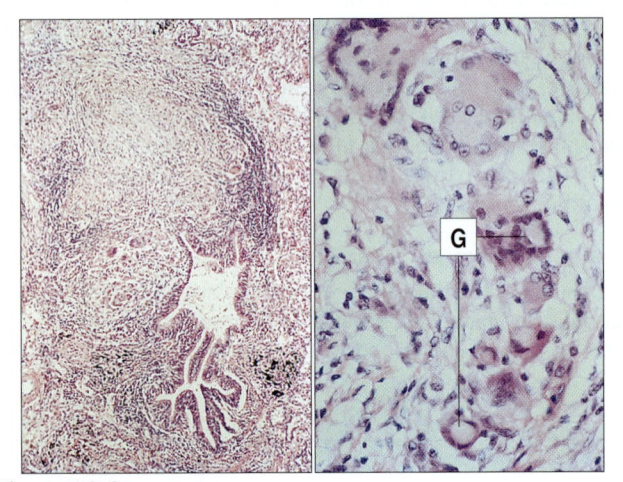

In the third phase of the disease, macrophage-derived reactive oxygen species cause necrosis of lung tissue. The production of chemotactic factors causes an influx of activated monocytes into the area. In an attempt to destroy the bacteria, activated monocytes surround the caseous center and release additional cytotoxic molecules. Some monocytes become flattened and are known as *epithelioid cells* (Figure 19-3). Fusion of macrophage membranes often creates giant cells with multiple nuclei.

In a final attempt to contain the infection, fibroblasts are called into the area and produce collagen, which encapsulates the inflammatory cells surrounding the lesion. The accumulation of macrophages, lymphocytes, and fibroblasts is called a *granuloma*. Constant production of TNF and IFN-γ is required for the maintenance of the granuloma; if the granuloma is not maintained, it becomes unstable, liquefies, and creates a permissible environment for bacterial growth. As a consequence of rapid bacterial growth, the infection erodes into blood vessels and small airways. Dissemination in blood allows the organism to establish secondary infections in other organs and bone. This form of the disease is known as *miliary tuberculosis*. Mycobacteria in the airways also rapidly proliferate in the highly aerobic environment and are expelled from the lung by coughing or sneezing.

Genetics and *Mycobacterium* Infections

The role of host genetics in *Mycobacterium* infection was suggested by an accidental administration of virulent *M. tuberculosis* to 249 babies in Lubeck, Germany, in 1926. Although 76 babies died of the disease, 123 had lung lesions that healed, and another 50 babies had no signs of infection. This suggested that genetics influences susceptibility to tuberculosis. Subsequent studies indicated that persons at risk for active

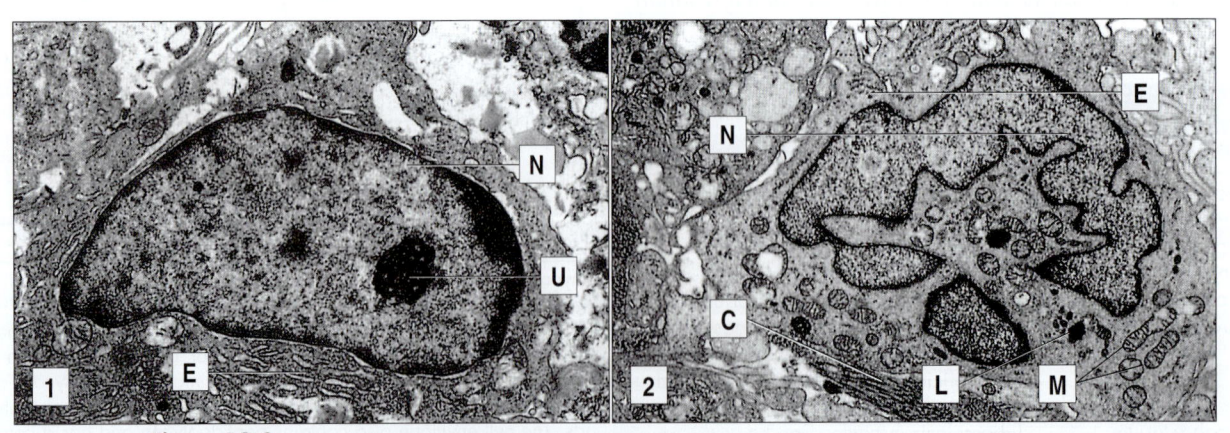

Figure 19-2
The central area of caseous necrosis in which much of the cellular structure is destroyed is characteristic of tuberculosis in the lung. Apart from this necrosis, the histology is typical of chronic T cell–dependent "tuberculoid" granulomas. The lesion is surrounded by a ring of epithelioid cells and mononuclear cells. Multinucleate giant cells, believed to be derived from the fusion of epithelioid cells, are also present (*left*: ×170). Giant cells *(G)* are illustrated at a higher magnification (*right*). (H&E stain.) (In Roitt I, Brostoff J, Male D, et al: Immunology, ed 7, Philadelphia, 2006, Mosby. Courtesy of Dr. G. Boyd.)

Figure 19-3
The epithelioid cell is the characteristic cell of granulomatous hypersensitivity. The extent of the endoplasmic reticulum *(E)* is compared. **1,** In the epithelioid cell (×4800). **2,** In a tissue macrophage (×4800). (*C*, Collagen; *L*, lysosome; *M*, mitochondria; *N*, nucleus; *U*, nucleolus.) (In Roitt I, Brostoff J, Male D, et al: Immunology, ed 7, Philadelphia, 2006, Mosby. Courtesy of M.J. Spencer.)

tuberculosis have dysfunctional receptors for IFN-γ or vitamin D. Some individuals also have a defect in the production of natural resistance–associated macrophage proteins (NRAMPs).

Interferon Gamma Receptor Deficiency. IFN-γ is a CD4Th1-produced cytokine that activates IFN-γ receptors expressed by other T cells, NK cells, and macrophages or monocytes. IFN increases bacterial killing by monocytes and alveolar macrophages. Individuals with an IFN-γ receptor deficiency are at risk for infection with *M. tuberculosis*, *M. africanum*, and *M. bovis*.

Vitamin D Receptor Deficiency. Lymphocytes, dendritic cells, and macrophages have intracellular receptors for the active form to 1 alpha, 25-dihydroxyvitamin D3 [1,25(OH)$_2$D$_3$]. Association of vitamin D with the vitamin D receptor (VDR) initiates transcription and translation of gene products that activate macrophages and Th1 cells while suppressing the activity of Th2 cells.

Failure to express the VDR increases the risk for *M. leprae* infection and determines whether the patient develops the lepromatous form or the tuberculoid form of the disease. In individuals with VDR deficiency, a CD4Th2 response with antibody production occurs. The Th2 response results in lepromatous leprosy characterized by numerous intracellular bacterial growth and severe tissue damage. In contrast, patients with functional VDRs mount a vigorous Th1 inflammatory response, which isolates the bacteria in granuloma and minimizes tissue damage. This type of response is called *tuberculoid leprosy*.

Natural Resistance–Associated Macrophage Protein (NRAMP) Deficiency. Early in the infection, two NRAMPs play a role in the destruction of mycobacteria: (1) NRAMP1 is localized in endosomal vesicles that fuse with phagosomes. NRAMP1 reduces the pH of the phagosome to levels that are toxic to the bacteria. (2) NRAMP2 is an efflux pump that exports iron and other cations from the phagosome. Mutations in NRAMP1 and NRAMP2 genes influence the phagosomal function of alveolar macrophages. In patients with an NRAMP1 deficiency, the pH of the phagolysosomes is near pH 6.8, which fosters bacterial growth. As a consequence of defective NRAMP2 production, iron accumulates in the phagosome and is used in the synthesis of bacterial heme–containing cytochromes during bacterial replication.

In Vivo Tuberculin Skin Test

Exposure to tuberculosis generates a population of long-lived memory cells. The Mantoux, or PPD (purified protein derivative of tuberculosis), skin test is now the standard test to determine previous exposure to tuberculosis bacilli. In the Mantoux test, PPD is injected intradermally, and the reaction site is viewed at 48 and 72 hours. If memory cells are present, an influx of macrophages and lymphocytes around the injection site causes a hard, raised indurated area with clearly defined margins (Figure 19-4). The cellular development of a positive skin test response to tuberculosis is shown in Figure 19-5.

The interpretation of skin test reactions is difficult. A positive skin test only indicates previous exposure to tuberculosis or vaccination with an attenuated strain of *M. bovis* called *Bacille Calmette-Guérin* (BCG). However, a significant false-negative rate in the Mantoux test does occur. Between 20% and 25% of patients with active tuberculosis have a negative skin test. Clinical history, radiologic studies, and sputum

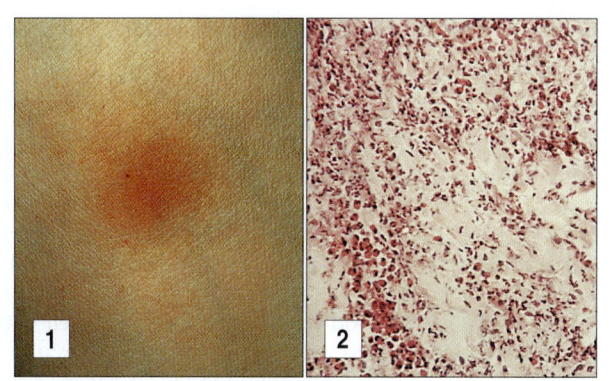

Figure 19-4

The response to an injection of the leprosy bacillus into a sensitized individual is known as the *Fernandez reaction*. **1**, The reaction is characterized by an area of firm red swelling of the skin and is maximal 48 to 72 hours after challenge. **2**, Histologically, a dense dermal infiltrate of leukocytes is seen. (H&E stain: ×80.) (From Roitt I, Brostoff J, Male D, et al: Immunology, ed 7, Philadelphia, 2006, Mosby.)

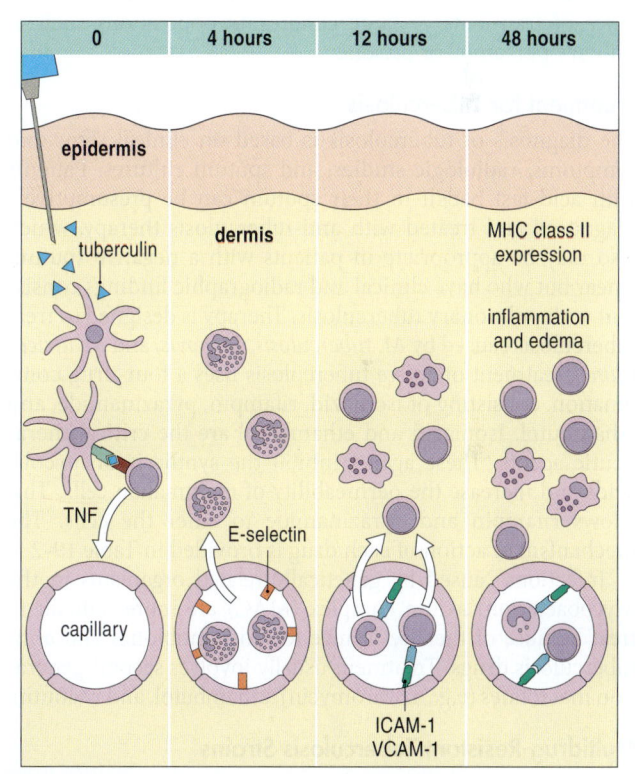

Figure 19-5

This diagram illustrates cellular movements following intradermal injection of tuberculin. Within 1 to 2 hours, expression of E-selectin occurs on the capillary endothelium, leading to a brief influx of neutrophil leukocytes. By 12 hours intercellular adhesion molecule 1 (ICAM-1) and vascular cell adhesion molecule 1 (VCAM-1) on endothelium bind the integrins LFA-1 and VLA-4 on monocytes and lymphocytes, leading to the accumulation of both cell types in the dermis. This peaks at 48 hours and is followed by expression of the major histocompatibility complex (MHC) class II molecules on keratinocytes. Edema of the epidermis is not present. (From Roitt I, Brostoff J, Male D, et al: Immunology, ed 7, Philadelphia, 2006, Mosby.)

cultures are used to support a tentative diagnosis of active tuberculosis.

In Vitro Tests for Exposure to Tuberculosis

The T-SPOT.TB and the QuantiFERON Gold test (GFT-G) are two in vitro tests that detect memory cells and identify tuberculosis or latent tuberculosis. The former is being evaluated by the U.S. Food and Drug Administration (FDA) for clinical use, and the latter test has been approved and is commercially available.

In the GFT-G test, blood lymphocytes are incubated with tuberculosis antigens not found in environmental tuberculosis species, PPD, or BCG vaccines. If an individual has memory cells to tuberculosis or a latent tuberculosis infection, T cells will produce INF-γ, which is measured in the laboratory using enzyme-linked immunosorbent assay (ELISA).

In vitro tests have many advantages. The test can be completed in 1 day with no need for a second patient visit. It is more accurate than the skin test, and the interpretation of results is not affected by a reader's bias or capability. Moreover, previous BCG immunizations do not influence the results. In vitro testing has great usefulness for tuberculosis surveillance of transients or large congregate populations such as military personnel or prisoners.

Treatment for Tuberculosis

The diagnosis of tuberculosis is based on clinical signs and symptoms, radiologic studies, and sputum cultures. Patients with acid-fast bacilli in their sputum can be presumptively diagnosed and treated with anti-tuberculosis therapy, which also may be appropriate in patients with a negative sputum smear but who have clinical and radiographic findings consistent with pulmonary tuberculosis. Therapy is designed to treat tuberculosis caused by *M. tuberculosis*, *M. bovis*, and *M. africanum*. Treatment of active tuberculosis uses a four-drug combination, consisting of isoniazid, rifampin, pyrazinamide, and ethambutol. Isoniazid and ethambutol are the critical therapeutic agents. These agents inhibit the synthesis of mycolic acids and increase the permeability of mammalian cells. This allows rifampin and pyrazinamide to enter the cells. The mechanism of action of each drug is provided in Table 19-2.

Infections caused by genetically related organisms in the Mycobacterium avium complex (MAC) are more difficult to treat because of their resistance to most antibiotics and anti-tuberculosis drugs. Treatment usually involves second-generation macrolides (e.g., azithromycin), ethambutol, and rifabutin.

Multidrug-Resistant Tuberculosis Strains

Over the past 16 years, two forms of drug resistance have emerged. Multidrug-resistant tuberculosis (MDR-TB) is defined as a tuberculosis strain that is resistant to, at least, isoniazid and rifampin. Resistance is associated with random mutations that alter the structure or quantity of intracellular drug targets. In 2005, the overall rate of MDR-TB with resistance to isoniazid and rifampin was 1.2%, with the rates for individual states varying from 0 to 3.7%. Worldwide, the number of new MDR-TB cases in 2005 was estimated at 480,000. When second-line drugs for tuberculosis (Table 19-3) are mismanaged or misused, extensively drug-resistant tuberculosis (XDR-TB) strains develop. These strains are resistant to isoniazid and rifampin as well as any of the fluoroquinolones and any of the second-line drugs. An estimated 40,000 new cases of XDR-TB are reported yearly in the developing countries. Between 1993 and 2006, only 49 cases of XDR-TB were reported in the United States.

Table 19-2 First-Line Drugs Used to Treat Tuberculosis

Drug	Action	Type
Isoniazid	Inhibits mycolic acid synthesis	Bactericidal
Pyrazinamide	Analog of nicotinamide	Bactericidal or bacteriostatic, depending on concentration
Rifampin	Rifampin inhibits prokaryotic ribonucleic acid (RNA) polymerase. Inhibits the translation of proteins	Bactericidal
Ethambutol	Inhibits mycolic acid synthesis	Bacteriostatic

Table 19-3 Second-Line Drugs Used to Treat Tuberculosis

Drug	Action	Type
Para-amino-salicylic acid (Sodium PAS)	Competitive inhibitor of folic acid	Bacteriostatic
Capreomycin	Believed to inhibit protein synthesis by binding to 70S ribosome	Bactericidal
Cycloserine	Structural analog of D-alanine in cell walls. Inhibits cell wall synthesis	Bacteriostatic
Avlosulfon	Competitive inhibitor of folic acid	Bacteriostatic (experimental)
Levofloxacin	Inhibits deoxyribonucleic acid (DNA) gyrase and causes DNA breakage	Bactericidal
Amikacin	Irreversibly binds to 30S subunit of bacterial ribosomes and blocks protein synthesis	Bactericidal
Rifabutin	Inhibits ribonucleic acid (RNA) polymerase	Bactericidal
Azithromycin	Inhibits transfer RNA (tRNA) peptidase	Bactericidal

Histoplasmosis

Histoplasma capsulatum is a dimorphic saprophytic fungus that grows rapidly in damp, acidic soil contaminated with bird or bat guano. The fungus is endemic in the Ohio and Mississippi River valleys (Figure 19-6). Over 80% of persons living in these areas have been exposed to the organism and have a positive skin test to histoplasmin. Over 40 million people are currently infected with *Histoplasma*. In the majority of cases, the infection is asymptomatic and resolves in several months.

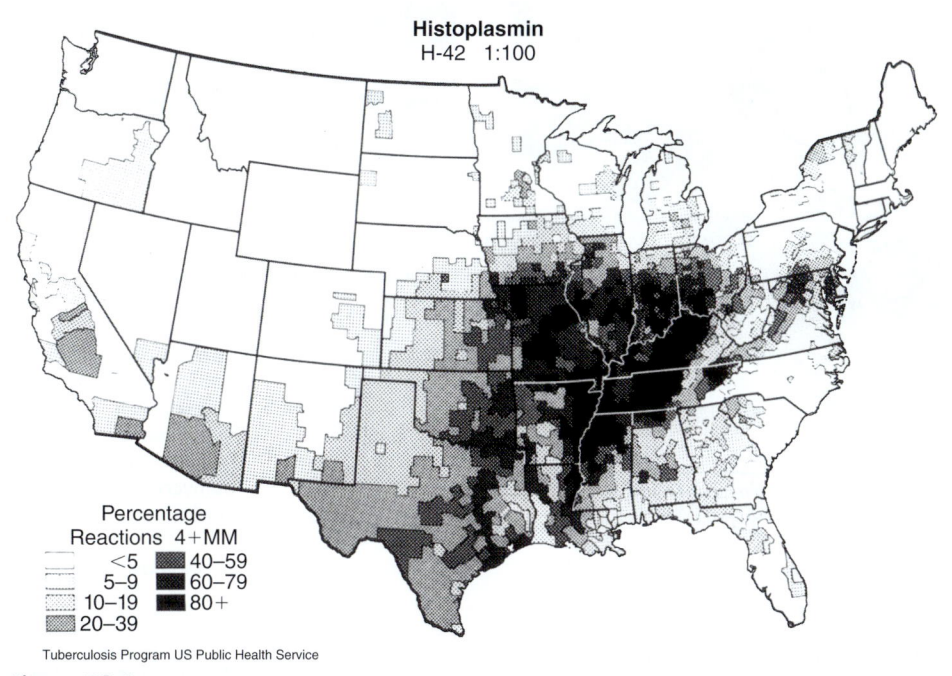

CHAPTER 19   DELAYED-TYPE HYPERSENSITIVITY REACTIONS   157

Figure 19-6
Map of United States showing geographic variations in the frequency of reactors to histoplasmin among Navy recruits, 1958–1965. (From CDC Public Health Image Library Photo ID #452. Courtesy of Dr. Errol Reiss.)

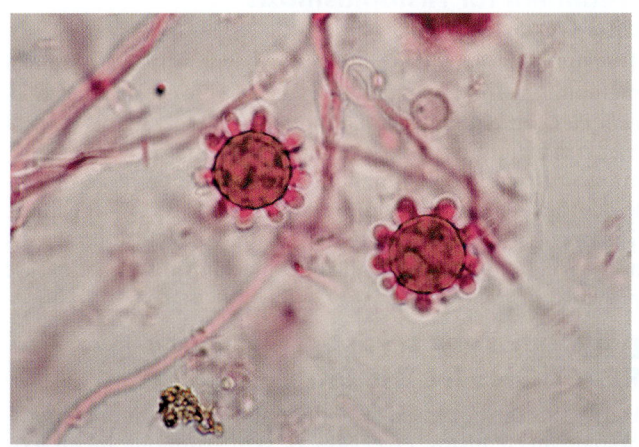

Figure 19-7
This photomicrograph shows two tuberculate macroconida of the Jamaican isolate of *Histoplasma capsulatum*. (From CDC Public Health Image Library Photo ID #4023. Courtesy of Libero Ajello.)

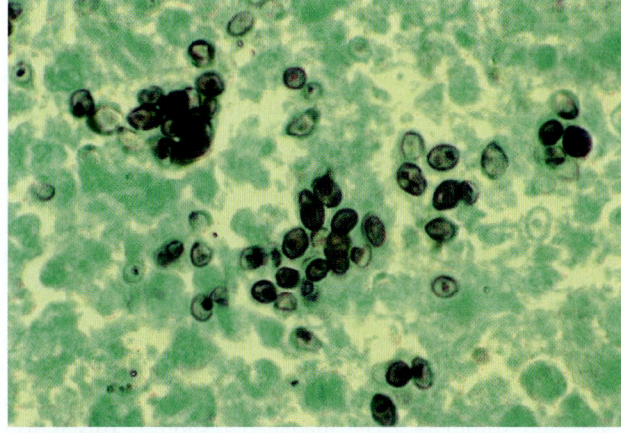

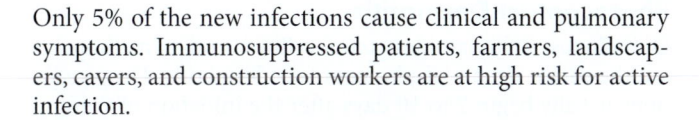

Figure 19-8
Methenamine silver stain of *Histoplasma capsulatum* yeast form in the human lung. (From CDC Public Health Image Library Photo ID #867. Courtesy of Dr. Edwin P. Ewing, Jr.)

Only 5% of the new infections cause clinical and pulmonary symptoms. Immunosuppressed patients, farmers, landscapers, cavers, and construction workers are at high risk for active infection.

Pathophysiology of Histoplasmosis

At ambient temperatures in the soil, the fungus grows as a mycelium with hyphae that produce macroconidia and microconidia (Figure 19-7). When soil is disturbed by occupational or recreational activities, conidia are easily aerosolized and inhaled. Conidia are ingested by alveolar macrophages and germinate into a single-cell yeast form (Figure 19-8).

The pathophysiology of the disease is similar to that of tuberculosis. The yeast form survives in alveolar macrophages by preventing NRAMP1 acidification of phagosomes. Some of the infected macrophages migrate to the hilar or mediastinal lymph, where they stimulate a cell-mediated response.

A cell-mediated response is mounted 10 to 14 days after infection. IFN-γ and TNF-α produced by CD4Th1 memory cells activate the fungistatic activities of the resident alveolar macrophages and peripheral blood monocytes. To contain the infection, lesions are ultimately encapsulated with collagen. Over a period of several years, calcium is deposited around the capsule, and the lesion becomes totally calcified.

A progressive form of histoplasmosis is an emerging problem in patients with secondary or therapy-induced immunodeficiencies. Individuals with AIDS have a high risk of

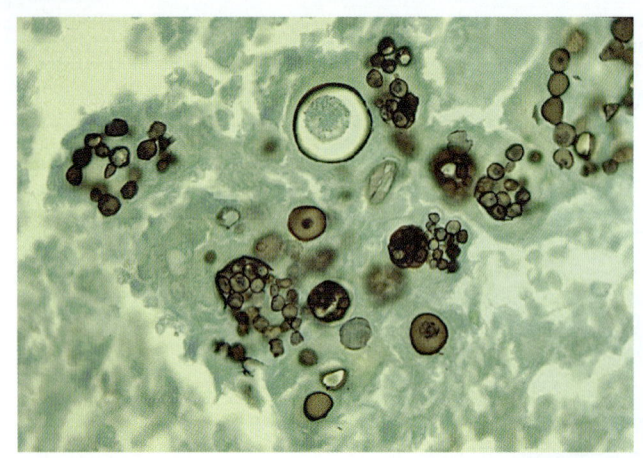

Figure 19-9

Methenamine silver stain showing spherule and endospore forms of *Coccidioides immitis* in the human lung. (From CDC Public Health Image Library Photo ID #578. Courtesy of Dr. Edwin P. Ewing, Jr.)

developing progressive disease, in which the fungus or its toxic products disseminate throughout the body and cause septic shock and kidney and liver failure.

Coccidioidomycosis or Valley Fever

Coccidioides immitis is a saprophytic, dimorphic fungus that is restricted to the San Joaquin valley in California, southern Arizona, New Mexico, west Texas, and the Sonoran desert regions of Mexico. In the soil, the fungus grows as a mold with septate hyphae or arthroconidia. Alternate arthroconidia undergo autolysis creating a fragile, segmented hyphal structure.

Pathophysiology of Coccidioidomycosis

When the soil is disturbed, segmented hyphae rupture and release arthroconidia into the atmosphere. Arthroconidia are easily inhaled and localize in the alveoli, where they transform into multi-nucleated spherules that contain hundreds of endospores (Figure 19-9).

Rupture of the spherule releases the endospores into the lung alveoli. Some of the endospores are ingested by alveolar macrophages and monocytes, which migrate to local lymph nodes and stimulate a cell-mediated response. This is followed by an influx of monocytes, neutrophils, and CD4Th1 lymphocytes into the infected area. The evolution of the granuloma is similar to that described for tuberculosis. The granuloma, however, is unique in that B lymphocytes are found in the lesion, and antibodies to coccidioidal antigens are generated. Complement activation may also play a role in the immune response by generating neutrophil chemotactic factors.

Over 60% of infections are asymptomatic. Most active infections are confined to the lung and lung-associated lymph nodes. Less than 1% of individuals with clinical symptoms develop disseminated disease that spreads to the lungs, liver, brain, skin, heart, and pericardium. African Americans, Filipino Americans, and Hispanic Americans have a 10-fold higher risk for disseminated coccidioidomycosis compared with the general population. Disseminated disease is also found in individuals with secondary immunodeficiencies as a result of disease or therapeutic immunosuppression.

Table 19-4 Drugs Used to Treat Histoplasmosis and Coccidioidomycosis

Drug	Used to Treat	Action
Amphotericin B	Histoplasmosis and coccidioidomycosis	Binds to sterols, and ergosterol in the cell membrane causing leakage of cytoplasmic fluids
Itraconazole	Histoplasmosis and coccidioidomycosis	Inhibits the synthesis of ergosterol
Ketoconazole	Histoplasmosis and coccidioidomycosis	Inhibits the synthesis of ergosterol
Fluconazole	Histoplasmosis and coccidioidomycosis	Prevents the conversion of lanosterol to ergosterol
Posaconazole	Histoplasmosis	Blocks ergosterol synthesis in membrane
Naproxen	Histoplasmosis	Decreases leukotriene synthesis, lysosomal enzyme release, neutrophil aggregation
Ibuprofen	Histoplasmosis	Decreased prostaglandin synthesis

Treatment for Histoplasmosis and Coccidioidomycosis

Therapy is designed to inhibit sterol synthesis in the fungal membranes. The plasma membranes of *Histoplasma* and *Coccidioides* contain ergosterol, a nonpolar sterol. Sterols control membrane fluidity, passage of material in and out of the fungi, and some physiologic functions. Inhibition of ergosterol synthesis causes membrane failure, and osmotic lyses of the fungi. Therapeutic agents used in the treatment of histoplasmosis and coccidioidomycosis and their mechanisms of action are provided in Table 19-4.

DELAYED-TYPE HYPERSENSITIVITY REACTIONS IN THE SKIN

Dermatitis can be caused by both nonimmunologic and immunologic mechanisms. Over 80% of skin eruptions are an irritant dermatitis caused by exposure to acids, alkalis, solvents, soaps, and metals. These skin eruptions have no immunologic basis. Only photocontact dermatitis and allergic contact dermatitis are believed to be immunologically mediated.

Photocontact Dermatitis

Quinolones, sulfonamides, tetracyclines, and trimethoprim are the major agents of photocontact dermatitis. Drug reactions usually begin 7 to 10 days after the initiation of therapy and usually occur in the sun-exposed areas of the skin. Lesions are usually pruritic, erythematous, and vesicular and resemble severe sunburn. Symptoms subside rapidly following cessation of the drug therapy.

Photocontact dermatitis is a cell-mediated response to drugs or drug metabolites that act as haptens. Photohaptenic drugs bind to class II molecules on Langerhans cells. Exposure to sunlight induces structural changes in the bound hapten and the class II molecule creating an antigen that is recognized by CD4Th1 cells. Cytokines released from the T cells induce changes in skin cells.

Contact Dermatitis

Twenty-five chemicals and one plant species cause the majority of DTH reactions in the skin. The agents include nickel, paraphenylenediamine (permanent hair dyes), formaldehyde releasers (quaternium-15 and isothiazolinones), neomycin, latex manufacturing process contaminants, and poison ivy. With the exception of nickel and poison ivy, the nature of the cell-mediated responses to the other irritants is unclear.

Nickel Hypersensitivity

Nickel is a major component of studded earrings, costume jewelry, watches, belt buckles, dental appliances, and orthopedic prosthetics. Usually, the nickel is covered by an outer layer of gold or silver alloy. With normal wear, the outer coat erodes, liberating nickel ions. Animal models suggest that nickel sensitivity differs from classic DTH reactions. In the nickel reaction, Langerhans cells transport nickel to the lymph node, where it stimulates a specialized T cell population known as *Th17 cells*. These T cells produce a specialized cytokine known as *interleukin 17A* (IL-17A). Activated Th17 cells migrate to the skin, where they release IL-17A, which upregulates cellular adhesion factors on keratinocytes and promotes localization of the inflammatory cells in the skin.

A genetic component associated with nickel sensitivity does exist. When compared with the normal population, a significant increase is seen in the frequency of HLA-DRw6 in individuals with nickel contact dermatitis.

Treatment of Contact Dermatitis

Topical and systemic corticosteroids are the mainstays of contact dermatitis treatment modalities. However, other topical immunomodulators (TIMs) and immunosuppressive agents are used to treat dermatitis as well. The full spectrum of available drugs are listed in Table 19-5.

PLANTS AND HYPERSENSITIVITY REACTIONS

Members of the plant genus *Toxicodendron* cause contact dermatitis. This genus includes poison ivy, poison oak, and poison sumac. Poison ivy usually grows east of the Rocky Mountains and in Canada. Poison oak usually grows in the western and southeastern parts of the United States, in Canada, and in Mexico. Sumac is also found in the eastern parts of the United States and in southern Canada.

Sap from these *Toxicodendron* species contains a mixture of saturated and unsaturated catechols known as *urushiol*. The immunologic response to haptenic urushiol is unique. Langerhans cells ingest free urushiol and use cross-priming to load haptens onto class I molecules. Unlike classic DTH reactions, urushiol-specific cytotoxic CD8 T cells proliferate in the lymph node and enter the peripheral circulation. The CD8 cells attack any cell that has urushiol on its surface. Lysis of skin cells allows fluid to enter the skin, creating the characteristic weeping poison ivy lesions.

Treatment for Poison Ivy Dermatitis

Drugs used to treat poison ivy dermatitis are similar to those used for treating contact dermatitis. Nonprescription topical products such as hydrocortisone, antihistamines, astringents, and anesthetics are useful in alleviating the pruritus and inflammation associated with poison ivy skin reactions. A list of other drugs used to treat poison ivy and their mechanisms of action is provided in Table 19-6.

Table 19-5 Drugs Used to Treat Contact Dermatitis

Drug	Action
Prednisone	Anti-inflammatory drug that prevents diapedesis and suppresses polymorphonuclear (PMN) functions
Pimecrolimus	Binds to cytostolic immunophilin receptor 2 and inhibits production of proinflammatory cytokines
Tacrolimus	Inhibits transcription of interleukin 3 (IL-3), IL-4, IL-5, and tumor necrosis factor alpha (TNF-α)
Triamcinolone	Inhibits migration of PMNs and decreases capillary permeability

Table 19-6 Drugs Used to Treat Poison Ivy

Drug	Action
Prednisone	Anti-inflammatory that prevents diapedesis and suppresses polymorphonuclear (PMN) functions
Diphenhydramine	Prevents the release of mediators from basophils and mast cells
Hydroxyzine	Antagonizes H1 receptors in the skin
Cimetidine	Antagonizes H2 receptors in the skin

DELAYED-TYPE HYPERSENSITIVITY REACTIONS IN THE INTESTINE

Celiac Sprue or Gluten-Sensitive Enteropathy

Celiac sprue is a chronic autoimmune inflammatory response which damages the intestinal mucosa and impedes normal digestion and absorption of foods. Patients with the classic form of celiac sprue present with moderate to severe diarrhea and failure to thrive.

The etiologic agent of the disease is gliadin, a component of gluten found in wheat, rye, barley, and oats. In the intestine, gliadin is deaminated by a transaminase to create two negatively charged proteins. A large protein fragment remains complexed with catalytic transaminase and is processed and presented to T cells in the context of class II molecules. Within the lamina propria, antigen presentation stimulates proliferation of CD4Th1 cells and IFN-γ production. IFN activates macrophages that release enzymes and cytokines, which increase mucosal permeability and damage the mucosa.

The second protein, a small negatively charged molecule, stimulates the enteric epithelial cells to secrete IL-15, which upregulates the expression of antigenic proteins on mucosal cells. These proteins are the target of both CD8 and NK cells.

A genetic component to celiac sprue does exist. Approximately 95% of individuals with celiac sprue have a DQ2 heterodimer composed of DQB1*02 and DQA1*05. These class II molecules avidly and selectively bind negatively charged proteins.

Treatment for Celiac Sprue

The primary treatment is the removal of gluten from the diet. In patients undergoing an acute clinical episode, a combination of corticosteroids and gluten elimination bring the disease into remission. At this point, diet control is sufficient to control the disease.

SUMMARY

- Delayed-type hypersensitivity (DTH) reactions denote cell-mediated responses that occur in the lung, skin, or intestine.
- Bacteria, fungi, chemicals, and plant products can cause DTH in the lung or skin.
- Tuberculosis is the prototypic DTH response in the lung.
- Genetics and immunologic defects increase the risk for tuberculosis.
- Antibiotics and nickel are the major causes of allergic contact dermatitis.
- Contact dermatitis, which is a DTH response, has different histologic characteristics compared with antibody-mediated atopic dermatitis.
- Gliadin, a component of gluten, is found in wheat, rye, barley, and oats and is the etiologic agent that causes celiac sprue.

REFERENCES

Ampel NM: Coccidioidomycosis: A review of recent advances, Clin Chest Med 30(2):241, 2009.

Britton WJ, Lockwood DN: Leprosy, Lancet 363(9416):1209, 2004.

Cano MV, Hajjeh RA: The epidemiology of histoplasmosis: A review, Semin Respir Infect 16(2):109, 2001.

Casanova JL, Abel L: Genetic dissection of immunity to mycobacteria: The human model, Annu Rev Immunol 20:581, 2002.

Ciclitira PJ, King AL, Fraser JS: AGA technical review on Celiac Sprue. American Gastroenterological Association, Gastroenterology 120(6):1526, 2001.

Cohen J: Nickel sensitivity, JAMA 222(5):585, 1972.

Enk AH, Katz SI: Contact sensitivity as a model for T-cell activation in skin, J Invest Dermatol 105(Suppl 1):80S, 1995.

Flynn JL, Chan J, Triebold KJ, et al: An essential role for interferon gamma in resistance to *Mycobacterium tuberculosis* infection, J Exp Med 178(6):2249, 1993.

Girolomoni G, Sebastiani S, Albanesi C, et al: T-cell subpopulations in the development of atopic and contact allergy, Curr Opin Immunol 13(6):733, 2001.

Kalish RS, Wood JA, LaPorte A: Processing of urushiol (poison ivy) hapten by both endogenous and exogenous pathways for presentation to T cells in vitro, J Clin Invest 93(5):2039, 1994.

Mozzanica N, Rizzolo L, Veneroni G, et al: HLA-A, B, C and DR antigens in nickel contact sensitivity, Br J Dermatol 122(3):309, 1990.

North RJ, Jung YJ: Immunity to tuberculosis, Annu Rev Immunol 22:599, 2004.

Romani L: Immunity to fungal infections, Nat Rev Immunol 4(1):1, 2004.

Toubiana R, Berlan J, Sato H, et al: Three types of mycolic acid from Mycobacterium tuberculosis Brevanne: Implications for structure-function relationships in pathogenesis, J Bacteriol 139(1):205, 1979.

Wallis RS, Broder MS, Wong JY, et al: Granulomatous infectious diseases associated with tumor necrosis factor antagonists, Clin Infect Dis 38(9):1261, 2004.

Wheat LJ: Histoplasmosis: A review for clinicians from non-endemic areas, Mycoses 49(4):274, 2006.

ASSESSMENT QUESTIONS

1. Which of the following is *not* a genetic defect that increases the risk of tuberculosis infections?
   I. Defective natural resistance–associated macrophage proteins (NRAMPs)
   II. Defective vitamin D receptor
   III. Defective complement receptor
   A. I
   B. III
   C. I and II
   D. II and III
   E. I, II, and III

2. Which of the following is a component of an acid-fast cell wall?
   I. Peptidoglycan
   II. Mycolic acids
   III. Cord factor
   A. I
   B. III
   C. I and II
   D. II and III
   E. I, II, and III

3. Histoplasmosis is endemic in:
   A. The Sonoran desert
   B. The Ohio and Mississippi river basins
   C. The Missouri river basin
   D. Southern California

4. Multidrug-resistant strains of tuberculosis are resistant to:
   A. Fluoroquinolones
   B. Avolsulfon
   C. Cycloserine
   D. Isoniazid

5. Which of the following antibiotics is *not* a cause of photocontact dermatitis?
   A. Quinolones
   B. Sulfonamides
   C. Penicillin
   D. Tetracyclines

6. Which of the following cells is unique in the delayed-type hypersensitivity (DTH) response to nickel ions?
   A. T cells
   B. Th17 cells
   C. Monocytes
   D. Langerhans cells

CHAPTER 20

Cytotoxic T Cells

LEARNING OBJECTIVES

- Identify the role of dendritic cells in cytotoxic T cell activation
- Identify the two signals necessary to activate cytotoxic T cells
- Identify the molecules that stabilize the interaction between cytotoxic T cells and target cells
- Identify the three different mechanisms that cytotoxic T cells use to kill target cells
- Identify the role of perforin in the lysis of target cells
- Identify the role of granulysin in the lysis of target cells
- Understand the mechanism of perforin-granzyme–induced cell death
- Identify the cellular location of CD95L (FasL) and CD95R (FasR)
- Understand the mechanism of FasL-FasR–induced cell death
- Compare and contrast the biologic functions of tumor necrosis factor alpha (TNF-α) and TNF-β
- Compare and contrast the immunologic functions of CD8 populations
- Identify the characteristics of a tumor infiltrating lymphocyte (TIL)
- Identify two factors that may inhibit the function of TILs
- Speculate on the role of CD4 cytotoxic cells in microbial and tumor immunity
- Identify the four different mechanisms that tumor cells use to evade cytotoxic T cells
- Identify the two mechanisms that influenza viruses use to evade cytotoxic T cells
- Identify the mechanisms used by latent viruses to evade the immune system
- Recognize the immunologic defect in familial erythrophagocytic lymphohistiocytosis type 2 (FHLH2)
- Identify the therapeutic agents used to treat FHLH2
- Identify the immunologic defect in autoimmune lymphoproliferative syndrome type 2 (APLS2)
- Recognize the therapeutic agents used to treat APLS2
- Identify the immunologic defect in Papillon–Lefèvre syndrome (PLS)
- Recognize the therapeutic agents used to treat PLS

KEY TERMS

Antigen drift
Antigen shift
Cathepsin C
Cytotoxic T cells
Fas-associated protein with death domains (FADD)
Granulysin
Granzyme
Fas ligand (FasL)
Fas receptor (FasR)
Perforin
Serglycin
Tumor necrosis factor receptor–associated protein with death domains (TRADD)
Trail protein
Tumor necrosis factor-β
Tumor infiltrating lymphocyte (TIL)

INTRODUCTION

Evolutionary pressures resulted in the development of efficient cell-based methods to kill infected or abnormal cells. CD8, CD4, and natural killer (NK) cells (see Chapter 21) are the major effector cells involved in this cell-mediated response. Cytotoxic CD8 and CD4 cells are antigen specific and genetically restricted. In contrast, NK cells can kill a wide variety of target cells without the need for antigen presentation on class I proteins. Lysis of target cells follows cell-to-cell contact between effector and target cells. Other cells such as monocytes and eosinophils also have the ability to kill cells. However, killing by these cells is facilitated by the secretion of cytolytic cytokines or proteins and does not require cell-to-cell contact or antigen presentation by class I or II molecules.

CD8 CYTOTOXIC CELLS

Cytotoxic T cells are activated by dendritic cells that express antigen-loaded class I molecules. Dendritic cells ingest intact cells (cross-priming) or free antigens. After processing, antigens are presented in the context of class I or class II molecules. Three signals are required for T cell activation and proliferation. The initial signal is provided by the interaction between the CD8 T cell receptor (TCR) and antigen-loaded class I molecules on dendritic cells (Figure 20-1). The second signal is provided by CD28 on T cells interacting with B7-1 on antigen-presenting cells. Proliferation of activated cytotoxic T cells requires the production of interleukin 12 (IL-12) by dendritic cells and autocrine production of IL-2.

CD8 Subpopulations

Two subpopulations of CD8 cells can be differentiated by patterns of cytokine production. For example, CD8Tc1 cells, which provide defense against tumors and viral infections, secrete IL-2, interferon gamma (IFN-γ), and TNF-β. Conversely, CD8Tc2 cells secrete IL-4, IL-5, and IL-10. Within the CD8Tc2 population are two other populations known as *Tc2a* and *Tc2b*. The biologic function of CD8Tc2a cells is ill defined. They are strongly cytotoxic and may play a role in neurologic and autoimmune diseases. CD8Tc2b cells are only weakly cytotoxic but secrete proteins that prevent intracellular viral replication. In organs that are critical to survival (e.g., brain), CD8Tc2b cells resolve viral infections without destroying the organs.

CD4 CYTOTOXIC CELLS

One of the basic paradigms of immunology is that CD4 cells are involved in inflammatory reactions or antibody production and that CD8 cells are cytotoxic cells. This paradigm has been challenged by recent findings of cytotoxic CD4 cells in peripheral blood. Normally, this population represents less than 2% of the total CD4 population but can expand rapidly during some infections. Although the total numbers of CD4 cells is low in patients with acquired immuno deficiency syndrome (AIDS), 50% of circulating CD4 cells phenotype as cytotoxic CD4 memory cells. These cells have granules containing perforin and granzymes and toxicity is restricted to class II protein–expressing cells. Like CD8 cytotoxic cells, CD4 lysis of infected cells occurs via the perforin, FasL–FasR, and TNF pathways.

The physiologic role of CD4 cytotoxic cells in immunity is not fully delineated. It is tempting to speculate, however, that these cells are involved in the containment of viral infections of B cells and macrophages (Epstein-Barr virus [EBV]–infected B cells or human immunodeficiency virus [HIV]–infected CD4 cells).

LYSIS OF TARGET CELLS

Target cells can be lysed in three ways: (1) One mechanism involves cytoplasmic granules containing perforin and granzymes. (2) A second mechanism involves the interaction between a *Fas ligand (FasL)* molecule expressed on cytotoxic T cells and a *Fas receptor (FasR)* molecule expressed on most target cells. (3) The third mechanism involves ligation of TNF-β receptors (TNFR) expressed on target cells.

Perforin–Granzyme Cytolysis

In perforin–granzyme–target cell lysis, cytotoxic T cells bind antigen-loaded class I antigens on the target cell. The initial reaction is stabilized by CD8, CD2, and leukocyte function–associated antigen 1 (LFA-1) (see Figure 20-1), which creates a small immunologic synapse between the two cells.

Following synapse formation, microtubules within the T cell align themselves so that unidirectional movement of intracellular granules occurs toward the synapse.

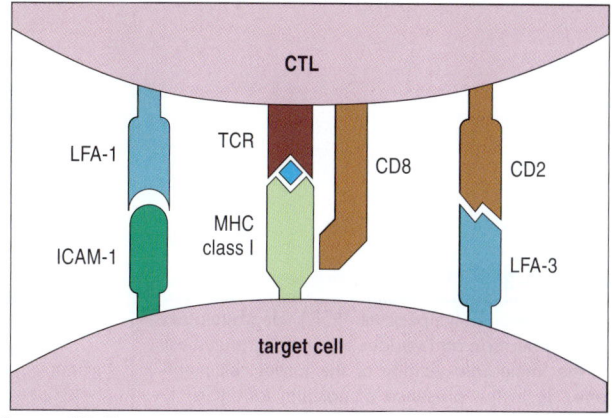

Figure 20-1

Some of the ligands involved in the interaction between cytotoxic T lymphocytes (CTLs) and their targets. (*ICAM-1*, intercellular adhesion molecule-1; *TCR*, T cell receptor; *LFA-3*, leukocyte functional antigen-1.) (From Roitt I, Brostoff J, Male D, et al: Immunology, ed 7, Philadelphia, 2006, Mosby.)

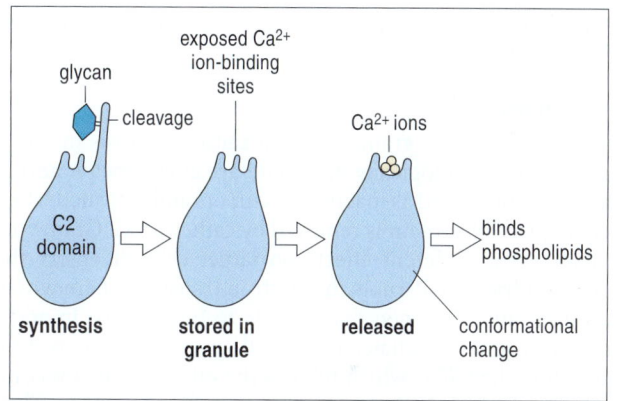

Figure 20-2

Perforin is synthesized with a tailpiece of 20 amino acid residues with a large glycan residue attached. In this form, it is inactive. Cleavage of the tailpiece within the granules allows calcium ions (Ca^{2+}) to access a site associated with the C2 domain of the molecule, but the molecule is thought to be maintained in an inactive state by low Ca^{2+} concentrations in the granules. Following secretion, the increased Ca^{2+} concentration permits a conformational change, which exposes a phospholipid-binding site, allowing the perforin to bind to the target membrane as a precursor to polymerization. (From Roitt I, Brostoff J, Male D, et al: Immunology, ed 7, Philadelphia, 2006, Mosby.)

Granules containing granulysin, perforin, granzymes, and cathepsin C move along the microtubules and fuse with the target cell plasma membrane (Figure 20-2).

Perforin may contribute to cytolysis by two different mechanisms: (1) In one mechanism, granulysin alters membrane permeability and facilitates the insertion of perforin into target cell membranes. Perforin forms homopolymeric pores, through which granzymes are injected into the target cell. (2) In an alternative method, a protein known as *serglycin* assembles a complex of granulysin, perforin, and granzymes in the small gap between effector and target cells. The complex is ingested by target cells by using receptor-mediated endocytosis and is placed into a cytoplasmic endosome. Granulysin and perforin create pores in the endosomal membrane and release several granzymes into the cytoplasm.

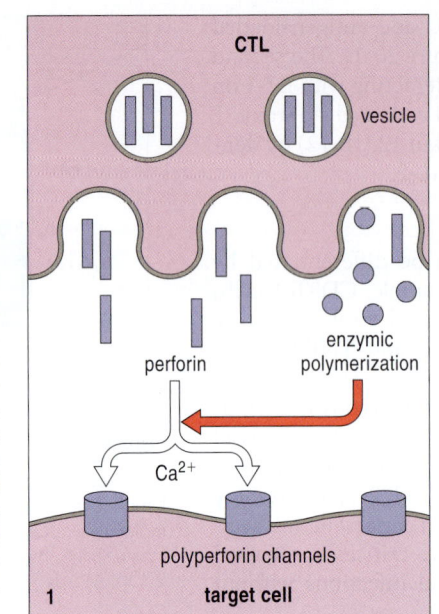

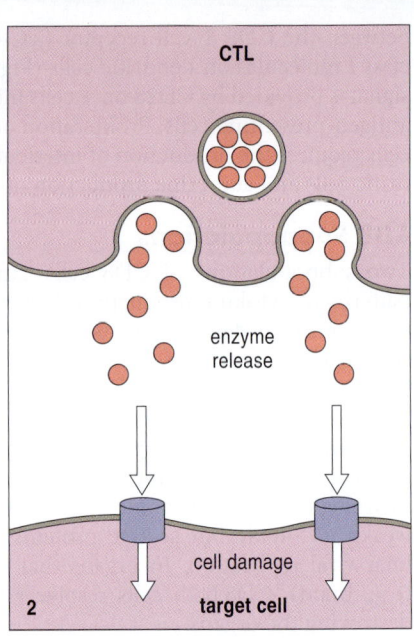

Figure 20-3

The cytotoxic T lymphocyte (CTL) degranulates, releasing perforin and various enzymes (granzymes) into the immediate vicinity of the target cell membrane. **1,** In the presence of calcium ions (Ca^{2+}), perforin binds to the target cell membrane and forms polyperforin channels. **2,** Enzymes that activate the apoptosis pathways, degradative enzymes, and other toxic substances released from the cytotoxic cell may pass through the channels in the target cell membrane and cause cell damage or killing. (From Roitt I, Brostoff J, Male D, et al: Immunology, ed 7, Philadelphia, 2006, Mosby.)

A summary of the perforin–granzyme pathway is provided in Figure 20-3.

Granzymes

Of the five different granzymes that cause apoptosis in target cells, the most biologically important are granzymes A and B. They are synthesized as inactive precursors and activated when a small piece of protein is removed by cathepsin C. Granzyme A has several different effects on target cells. It enters the mitochondria and disrupts the electron transport chain which produces singlet oxygen that is toxic to target cells. In addition, granzyme A initiates target cell apoptosis by activating a protein called *SET*, which relieves the inhibition of a second protein called *NME-1*, an enzyme that destroys deoxyribonucleic acid (DNA) (Figure 20-4). Granzyme B has a more limited biologic function and causes apoptosis by activating a caspase-dependent cascade, which cleaves procaspases to activate caspases 10, 3, and 7.

FasL–FasR Cytolysis

FasL, or CD95L, is expressed on the surface of activated CD8 cells. Ligation of a homotrimeric FasR (CD95) on target cells activates death domains, which bind to an adaptor protein called Fas-associated protein with death domains (FADD). In turn, FADD activate caspases 8 and 10. When high calcium concentrations are present, additional caspases (3, 6, and 7) activate endonucleases, which fragment DNA (Figure 20-5).

Tumor Necrosis Factor Beta–Tumor Necrosis Factor Receptor 1 Cytolysis

TNF-β belongs to the TNF superfamily that also includes TNF-α. TNF-β, or lymphotoxin, is produced by activated T and B cells. It has many of the proinflammatory properties of TNF-α, but it also is involved in biologic processes that include cell proliferation and apoptosis (see Figure 20-5). Ligation of TNF-β and the TNF receptor 1 (TNFR-1) on the target cell activates one of two apoptotic pathways: (1) In one pathway, receptor trimerization creates a binding site for the TNFR-associated proteins with death domains (TRADD). TRADD complexes with proteins known as *RIP* and *RAIDD* and activates caspase 2 of the apoptotic pathway. In the TNF-related apoptosis-inducing ligand (TRAIL) pathway, TRADD complexes with FADD and activates caspase 8 and 10 that are critical to the induction of apoptosis.

TUMOR-INFILTRATING LYMPHOCYTES

Tumor-infiltrating lymphocytes (TILs) are often found in melanomas and solid tumors of the kidney, colon, and lung. TILs comprise CD8 cells and a small population of cytotoxic CD4 cells and are the result of antigen-driven recruitment and proliferation of oligoclonal T cells within the tumor. The presence of inflammatory cells and CD8 TILs in tumors is considered evidence of a vigorous anti-tumor response and is associated with a favorable clinical prognosis in some forms of cancer.

EVASION OF T KILLER CELLS BY TUMOR CELLS

Tumor cells have well-developed active mechanisms to evade lymphocyte killer cells. Downregulation of class I molecule expression occurs in every solid tumor, but the frequency varies with tumor types. Other tumors lack B7 co-stimulatory molecules (CD80) necessary to activate T cells. High levels of FasL (CD95L) are also expressed by NK lymphomas, large granular lymphocytic leukemia cells, melanomas, hepatocellular carcinomas, and astrocytomas. Activated T cells express both Fas and FasL. Engagement of FasL on the tumor cell and FasR on the T cell initiates the apoptotic sequence, which results in the death of the T cell and downregulation of the immune response. Some tumors also produce transforming growth factor beta (TGF-β), which inhibits IL-2–dependent proliferation of T and B cells.

EVASION OF THE IMMUNE RESPONSE BY VIRUSES

Viruses have well-developed strategies to evade the immune system and promote their replication. Influenza viruses express hemagglutinins and neuraminidase, which are recognized by the immune system. Over time, mutations result in slight changes in the protein structure and formation of new antigenic

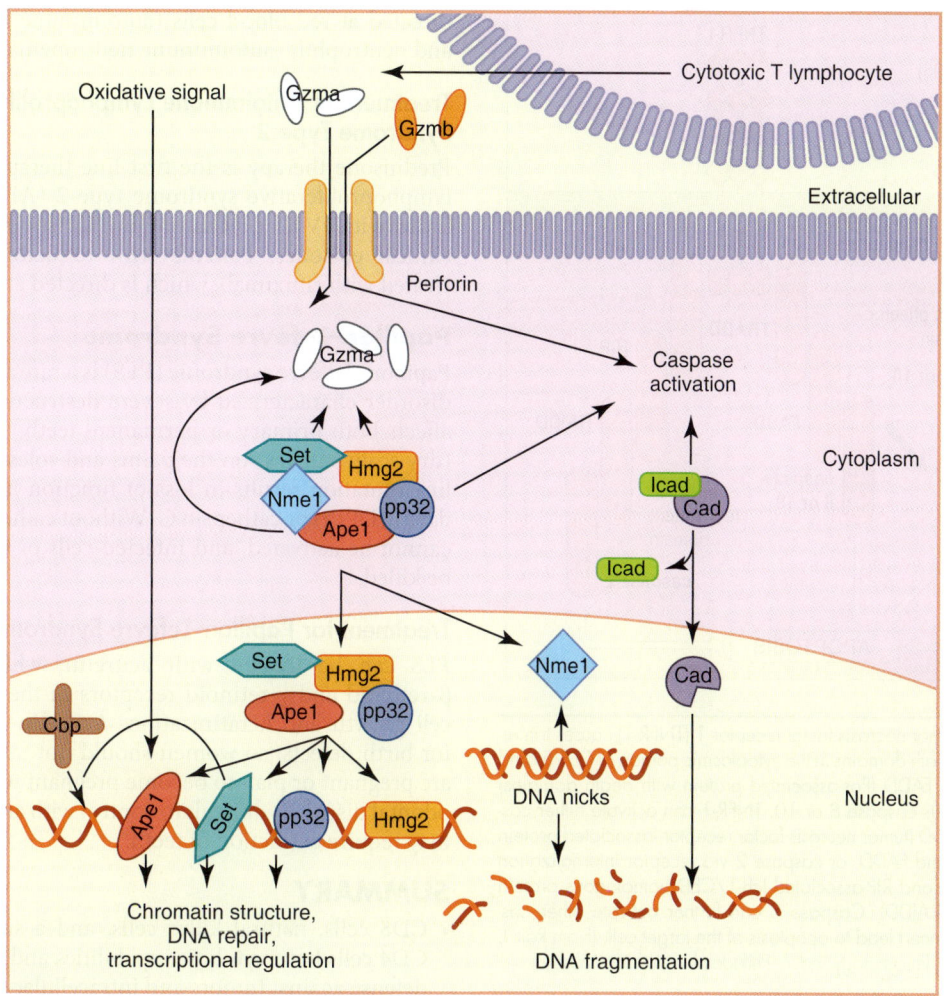

Figure 20-4

SET protein complex activation by granzyme A. (From www.biocarta.com/pathfiles/m_set Pathway.asp)

epitopes. This phenomenon is known as *antigenic drift*. Yearly influenza epidemics are a reflection of antigenic drift. During yearly epidemics, the immune system creates memory cells that recognize hemagglutinin and neuraminidase antigens. Because of selection and environmental pressures, influenza antigens drift over the next 12 months. In the next influenza season, the new epitopes that are distinct from previous virus strains are not recognized by the influenza memory cells. By the time the immune response is mounted (7–10 days), the virus has been transmitted to another susceptible individual.

A more problematic change in hemagglutinins is *antigenic shift*, which results from genetic recombination of animal and human influenza viruses. For example, the great influenza pandemic of 1918 occurred when swine and human influenza strains exchanged genetic material to create major changes in hemagglutinins and neuraminidase. Unlike normal influenza strains, which only infect the lung, the recombinant influenza infected many organs in the body. The vigorous Tc1 killer cell response caused the destruction of many organs. The pandemic strain killed 10 to 38 million people within 18 months.

Viruses use a number of different mechanisms that prevent the expression of antigen-loaded class I molecules on the cell surface. For example, proteins produced by herpes virus inhibit the function of transporter-associated antigen processing (TAP), preventing the transfer of antigenic fragments from the cytosol to the endoplasmic reticulum (ER). Adenoviruses, which infect the respiratory tract, eyes, and intestine, produce a number of different proteins that prevent the transfer of the class I molecules from the ER to the Golgi apparatus.

IMMUNODEFICIENCY AND T KILLER CELLS

Familial Erythrophagocytic Lymphohistiocytosis Type 2

Familial erythrophagocytic lymphohistiocytosis type 2 (FHLH2) is a potentially fatal disease caused by the nonmalignant proliferation of macrophages and T lymphocytes. The term denotes the fact that activated, proliferating tissue macrophages (histiocytes) ingest red blood cells, white blood cells, and platelets. Unless the patient is rescued by bone marrow transplantation, the disease is invariably fatal.

The major immunologic defect is impaired perforin and granzyme secretion from CD8 cells and NK cells. The defect is compounded by the uncontrolled release of proinflammatory (e.g., IL-1, IL-6, and TNF-α) cytokines. A positive feedback loop amplifies cytokine production, resulting in a cytokine storm that causes significant tissue damage in the liver, spleen, central nervous system, and bone marrow.

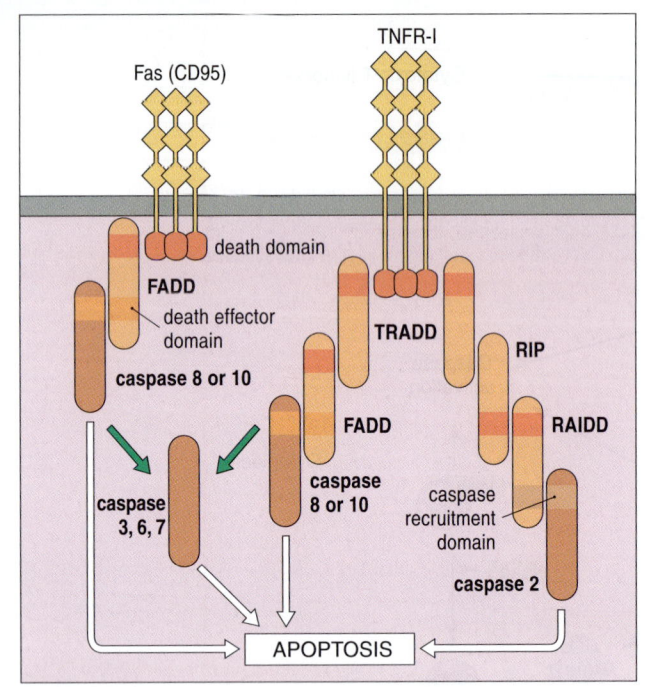

Figure 20-5

Ligation of CD95 or tumor necrosis factor receptor 1 (TNFR-1) causes trimerization of receptors. Death domains in the cytoplasmic portion of CD95 bind to the adapter protein FADD (Fas-associated protein with death domains) (MORT1), which recruits caspase 8 or 10. TNFR-1 can activate either caspase 8 or 10, via TRADD (tumor necrosis factor receptor–associated protein with death domains) and FADD, or caspase 2 via receptor internalization and degradation (RIP) and RIP-associated Ich-1/CED homologous protein with death domains (RAIDD). Caspase 8 can further activate other caspases, and these in concert lead to apoptosis of the target cell. (From Roitt I, Brostoff J, Male D, et al: Immunology, ed 7, Philadelphia, 2006, Mosby.)

Treatment for Familial Erythrophagocytic Lymphohistiocytosis Type 2

Several forms of FHLH2 exist. The low-risk, non–life-threatening FHLH2 is usually treated with cyclosporine A, steroids, and pooled intravenous immunoglobulin (IVIG). As stated in previous chapters, IVIG downregulates the production of proinflammatory cytokines and blocks the Fc receptors on macrophages. Severe and aggressive FHLH2 caused by EBV infections requires etoposide and dexamethasone therapy for 8 weeks. Etoposide is a topoisomerase II inhibitor that arrests cell division in the S or G2 phases of cell division. Intrathecal administration of methotrexate also effectively controls neurologic involvement. Long-term remission greater than 2 years is possible with combined therapy of anti-thymocyte globulin (ATG), steroids followed by cyclosporine A, and intrathecal methotrexate.

Autoimmune Lymphoproliferative Syndrome Type 2

Autoimmune lymphoproliferative syndrome type 2 (APLS2), or Canale-Smith syndrome, is characterized aberrant lymphocyte proliferation, which results in splenomegaly and lymphadenopathy in the neck. Individuals with ALPS2 have germ-line mutations in the FasR, which prevent intracellular signaling and apoptosis. The defective FasR allows the accumulation of activated lymphocytes, which produce antibodies directed at red blood cells (autoimmune hemolytic anemia) and neutrophils (autoimmune neutropenia).

Treatment of Autoimmune Lymphoproliferative Syndrome Type 2

Prednisone therapy is the first-line therapy for autoimmune lymphoproliferative syndrome type 2 (APLS2). When combined with IVIG, prednisone is effective in controlling acute clinical episodes. Patients with refractory disease can be treated with rituximab, which is directed at CD20 on B cells.

Papillon–Lefèvre Syndrome

Papillon–Lefèvre syndrome (PFS) is a rare autosomal recessive disorder characterized by severe destruction of bone, which affects both primary or permanent teeth, and hyperkeratosis (dry scaly patches) on the palms and soles of the feet. Germline mutation results in loss of function in dipeptidyl peptidase I (DPPI) or cathepsin C. Without cathepsin C, granzymes cannot be activated, and infected cells or tumor cells cannot be killed.

Treatment for Papillon–Lefèvre Syndrome

PLS can be treated with acitretin, which interacts with β-retinoid and γ-retinoid receptors in the skin and prevents cell growth and keratinization. Acitretin poses a slight risk for birth defects, so women should not take the drug if they are pregnant or plan to become pregnant within 3 years. Periodontal disease is difficult to control with antibiotics alone and may require extraction of teeth.

SUMMARY

- CD8 cells, natural killer cells, and a small population of CD4 cells have cytolytic capabilities and are the first line of defense against tumors and intracellular microbes.
- A subpopulation of CD8 cells, known as *CD8Tc2b*, can control viral infections without lysis of infected cells. These CD8 cells are especially important in controlling infections in organs that have no capacity for regeneration.
- Target cells can be lysed by perforin–granzymes, FasL–FasR interactions, and TNF-β ligation with its receptor.
- CD8 cells often infiltrate solid tumors and are therefore known as *tumor-infiltrating lymphocytes*. The presence of these cells in a tumor usually increases patient survival.
- The inability to produce perforin–granzymes or the presence of dysfunctional Fas molecules is associated with increased risk of viral infections and autoimmune diseases.

REFERENCES

Aggarwal BB: Comparative analysis of the structure and function of TNF-alpha and TNF-beta, Immunol Ser 56:6, 1992.

Catalfamo M, Henkart PA: Perforin and the granule exocytosis cytotoxicity pathway, Curr Opin Immunol 15(5):522, 2003.

Dhanrajani PJ: Papillon-Lefevre syndrome: Clinical presentation and a brief review, Oral Surg Oral Med Oral Pathol Oral Radiol Endod 108(1):1, 2009.

Dorothee G, Ameyar M, Bettaieb A, et al: Role of Fas and granule exocytosis pathways in tumor-infiltrating T lymphocyte-induced apoptosis of autologous human lung-carcinoma cells, Int J Cancer 91(6):772, 2001.

Finke JH, Rayman P, Hart L, et al: Characterization of tumor-infiltrating lymphocyte subsets from human renal cell carcinoma: Specific reactivity defined by cytotoxicity, interferon-gamma secretion, and proliferation, J Immunother Emphasis Tumor Immunol 15(2):91, 1994.

Horn M, Stutte HJ, Schlote W: Familial erythrophagocytic lymphohistiocytosis (Farquhar's disease): Involvement of the central nervous system, Clin Neuropathol 21(4):139, 2002.

Lieberman J: The ABCs of granule-mediated cytotoxicity: New weapons in the arsenal, Nat Rev Immunol 3(5):361, 2003.

Lord SJ, Rajotte RV, Korbutt GS, et al: Granzyme B: A natural born killer, Immunol Rev 193:31, 2003.

Lowin B, Peitsch MC, Tschopp J: Perforin and granzymes: Crucial effector molecules in cytolytic T lymphocyte and natural killer cell-mediated cytotoxicity, Curr Top Microbiol Immunol 198:1, 1995.

Loy TS, Diaz-Arias AA, Perry MC: Familial erythrophagocytic lymphohistiocytosis, Semin Oncol 18(1):34, 1991.

MacArthur GJ, Wilson AD, Birchall MA, et al: Primary CD4+ T-cell responses provide both helper and cytotoxic functions during Epstein-Barr virus infection and transformation of fetal cord blood B cells, J Virol 81(9):4766, 2007.

Melief CJ: Mini-review: Regulation of cytotoxic T lymphocyte responses by dendritic cells: Peaceful coexistence of cross-priming and direct priming? Eur J Immunol 33(10):2645, 2003.

Merlo A, Turrini R, Bobisse S, et al: Virus-specific cytotoxic CD4+ T cells for the treatment of EBV-related tumors, J Immunol 184(10):5895–5902, 2004.

Oren H, Ozkal S, Gülen H, et al: Autoimmune lymphoproliferative syndrome: Report of two cases and review of the literature, Ann Hematol 81(11):651, 2002.

Peters PJ, Borst J, Oorschot V, et al: Cytotoxic T lymphocyte granules are secretory lysosomes, containing both perforin and granzymes, J Exp Med 173(5):1099, 1991.

Revell PA, Grossman WJ, Thomas DA, et al: Granzyme B and the downstream granzymes C and/or F are important for cytotoxic lymphocyte functions, J Immunol 174(4):2124, 2005.

Ruddle NH: Tumor necrosis factor (TNF-alpha) and lymphotoxin (TNF-beta), Curr Opin Immunol 4(3):327, 1992.

Wong P, Pamer EG: CD8 T cell responses to infectious pathogens, Annu Rev Immunol 21:29, 2003.

Zaidi N, Kalbacher H, Cathepsin E: A mini review, Biochem Biophys Res Commun 367(3):517, 2008.

ASSESSMENT QUESTIONS

1. Papillon–Lefèvre syndrome is associated with a defect in:
   A. Cathepsin C
   B. TAP function
   C. Fas receptor (FasR) function
   D. Defective Fas ligand (FasL)

2. Autoimmune lymphoproliferative syndrome type 2 (APLS2) is caused by:
   A. Defective interleukin 2 (IL-2) production
   B. Defective tumor necrosis factor alpha (TNF-α) production
   C. Defective transforming growth factor beta (TGF-β) production
   D. Defective Fas receptors (FasR)

3. In cell-mediated lysis of target cells, cathepsin C activates:
   A. Granzyme
   B. Perforin
   C. TNF-α
   D. Fas-associated protein with death domains (FADD)

4. Which of the following is required to fully activate CD8Tc1 cells?
   A. Interaction between CD8 and antigen-loaded class I molecules
   B. Interaction between CD28 and B7.1 molecules
   C. Autocrine stimulation by IL-2
   D. All of the above

5. Which of the following is *not* a mediator of target cell lysis?
   A. Perforin
   B. Fas
   C. TNF
   D. TAP

6. Which of the following is a mechanism by which tumor cells evade the immune system?
   A. Upregulation of class I molecules
   B. Upregulation of class II molecules
   C. Upregulation of B7-2 molecules
   D. Downregulation of TAP proteins

CHAPTER 21

Natural Killer Cells

LEARNING OBJECTIVES

- Identify the phenotypic characteristics of natural killer (NK) cells
- Recognize the mechanism by which NK cells recognize aberrant or infected cells
- Differentiate between the two major classes of activation and inhibition molecules of NK cells
- Compare and contrast immunoreceptor tyrosine-based activation motif (ITAM) and immuno-receptor tyrosine-based inhibitory motif (ITIM) signaling pathways in NK cell activation or inhibition
- Identify the major ligand CD94–NKG2 complex
- Understand the roles of human leukocyte antigen C (HLA-C) and HLA-G in NK cell activation or inhibition
- Compare and contrast the physiologic roles of the subpopulations of NK cells
- Contrast the roles of NK cells in viral infections and tumor surveillance
- Explain the mechanism involved in antibody-dependent cellular cytotoxicity (ADCC)
- Differentiate between NK cells, lymphokine-activated killer (LAK) cells and natural killer T cells (NKT cells)
- Compare and contrast the physiologic roles of NK cells and NKT cells
- Recognize the phenotypic characteristics of NKT cells
- Recognize the two major subsets of NKT cells
- Discuss the role of alpha galactosyl ceramide (α-GalCer) in NKT cell stimulation
- Compare the roles of IL-12 and IL-13 in tumor immunity
- Explain the relationship between type I NKT cells and asthma
- Identify the roles of type II NKT cells in viral and autoimmune diseases
- Identify the nature of the genetic defect in Chediak-Higashi syndrome (CHS)

INTRODUCTION

Natural killer (NK) cells are defined by the expression of CD16 and CD56 surface molecules. In peripheral blood, two populations of NK cells are present. One population comprises large granular lymphocytes that are phenotyped as CD3−, CD16+, CD56+, and CD94+ cells. Since they do not express T or B cell markers, they are considered to be of a third lymphocyte lineage. The second population of NK cells comprises T cells that express both T cell and NK cell markers (CD3+, CD16+, CD56+ or CD3+, CD16−, CD56+). These cells are known as *natural killer T cells* (NKT cells) to differentiate them from large granular lymphocytes.

NK and NKT cells have different functions. NK cells are part of the innate cell-mediated response to infected or tumor cells. They recognize and lyse cells with downregulated human leukocyte antigen (HLA) class I molecules. In contrast to classic NK cells, NKT cells have limited cytolytic capability and require antigen presentation. Emerging evidence also suggests that NKT cells are involved in immediate allergic reactions, suppression of auto-reactive lymphocytes, and tumor immunity. Activation or inhibition of NK and NKT cells is dictated by interactions between cell receptors and HLA class IB molecules or CD1 molecules on target cells.

NATURAL KILLER CELL RECEPTORS

CD94–NKG2 Receptors

The most studied NK cell receptor is CD94—a type 2 "lectin-like" receptor expressed on both NK cells and cytotoxic T cells (CTLs). To create an active receptor, CD94 pairs with NKG2A, B, C, E, or F. NK cell function is dictated by different pairings between CD94 and NKG family members. For example, NKG2A and NKG2B dimerize with CD94 and inhibit NK cell function. Conversely, CD94–NKG2C dimers activate NK cells (Figure 21-1).

Killer Cell Immunoglobulin-Like Receptors

Killer cell immunoglobulin-like receptors (KIRs) are encoded by a family of 15 polymorphic genes and two pseudogenes on chromosome 19. KIRs are membrane anchor proteins that possess either two (KIR2DS) or three (KIR3DS) immunoglobulin domains (Figure 21-2).

Within each subfamily, KIRs that inhibit or activate NK cells are present (Table 21-1).

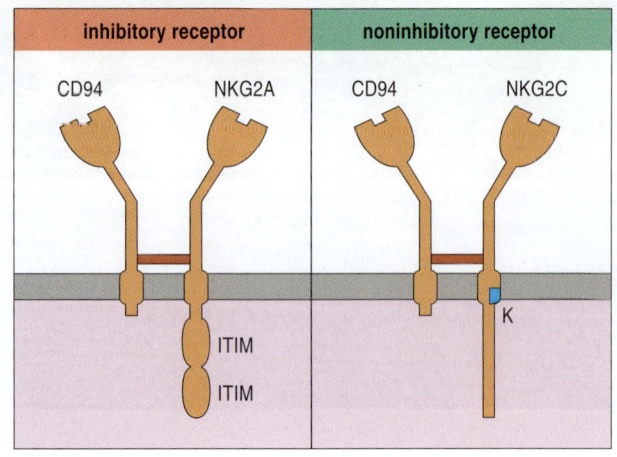

Figure 21-1

Inhibitory receptors consist of CD94 disulfide-bonded (red) to peptides from the NKG2 locus, such as NKG2A, which have intracellular domains carrying ITIMs (immunoreceptor tyrosine-based inhibitory motifs). Noninhibitory receptors (such as CD94/NKG2C) lack ITIMs but have a charged lysine residue (K) in the transmembrane segment that allows them to interact with signal-transducing molecules. (From Roitt I, Brostoff J, Male D, et al: Immunology, ed 7, Philadelphia, 2006, Mosby.)

Table 21-1 Immune Receptors Encoded by Genes in the Leukocyte Receptor Complex Region

Names	CD	Function	Signaling	Ligand
KIR3DL3	CD158z	Inhibition	ITIM	
KIR2DL3	CD158b2	Inhibition	ITIM	HLA-C S77/N80
KIR2DL2	CD158b1	Inhibition	ITIM	HLA-C S77/N80
KIR2DL1	CD158a	Inhibition	ITIM	HLA-C N77/K80
KIR2DS1	CD158h	Activation	DAP12	HLA-C, weakly
KIR2DS2	CD158j	Activation	DAP12	
KIR2DS4	CD158i	Activation	DAP12	HLA-C, weakly
KIR3DL2	CD158k	Inhibition	ITIM	HLA-A
KIR2DL3	CD158i	Inhibition	ITIM	HLA-C

HLA, Human leukocyte antigen; ITIM, immunoreceptor tyrosine-based inhibitory motifs; KIR, killer cell immunoglobulin-like receptor.
Modified from Cooper MD, Lewis LL, Conley, ME, et al: Immunodeficiency disorders. American Society of Hematology Education Program, pp. 314–330, 2003. Hematology 2003, The American Society of Hematology.

Figure 21-2

Killer cell immunoglobulin-like receptors (KIRs) consist of either two or three extracellular immunoglobulin superfamily domains. The inhibitory forms are longer and have intracellular ITIMs (immunoreceptor tyrosine-based inhibitory motifs), whereas the noninhibitory forms have the charged residue in the membrane comparable with the noninhibitory forms of CD94–NKG2. (From Roitt I, Brostoff J, Male D, et al: Immunology, ed 7, Philadelphia, 2006, Mosby.)

TARGET CELL RECOGNITION MOLECULES

NK cells do not detect aberrant or infected cells. Rather, they recognize cells that lack HLA class I molecules. This observation has led to the development of the "missing self" hypothesis of NK cell activation. The hypothesis suggests that NK cells can kill normal cells but are prevented from doing so by the presence of inhibitory factors such as HLA class I markers. Downregulation of class I molecules allows NK cells to engage other molecules that either activate or inhibit the NK cell.

HLA-E, a nonclassic HLA locus, is the natural ligand for CD94–NKG2A and B complexes. HLA-E binds the peptide leader sequence from HLA-G. The HLA-G sequence is encoded upstream of the open reading frame for the α-chain. In the cytoplasm, the N-terminal fragment of the leader sequence is released after cleavage by signal peptidases and endoplasmic reticulum (ER) proteases. The small leader peptide is loaded into the binding groove in the ER and transported to the cell surface (Figure 21-3).

KIRs also interact with HLA-C alleles to activate or inhibit NK cell function. Alleles that inhibit NK cell function have dimorphic polymorphisms at positions 77 and 80 of the binding cleft. The HLA-C1 group variants with serine at position 77 and asparagines at position 80 are HLA-Cw*102, *304, *0702, and Cw*0801. HLA-C alleles with these polymorphisms bind to the NK inhibitory receptors KIR2DL2 and KIR2DL3 and occasionally to the activating factor KIR2DS2. A second variant or HLA-C2 type 2 has asparagine at position 77 and lysine at position 80 (HLA-Cw*0201, *0401, *0501, *0601, and *1503) and binds KIR2DL1, which inhibits the NK response.

INTRACELLULAR SIGNALING BY NATURAL KILLER CELLS

Inhibition or activation of NK cells depends on the presence or absence of long cytoplasmic tails containing immunoreceptor tyrosine-based inhibitory motifs (ITIMs). Receptors with ITIMs are usually phosphorylated and recruit phosphatases such as SHIP-1 (SH2 [Src homology 2]-containing inositol phosphatase-1) and SHIP-2 that inhibit intracellular signaling. In contrast, receptors that lack long cytoplasmic tails associate with DNAX-activating protein of 10Kda (DAP10) and DAP12 proteins, which act as immunoreceptor tyrosine-based activation motifs (ITAM). Phosphorylation of zeta-chain-associated protein kinase (ZAP) initiates a signaling cascade, which activates NK cells (Figure 21-4).

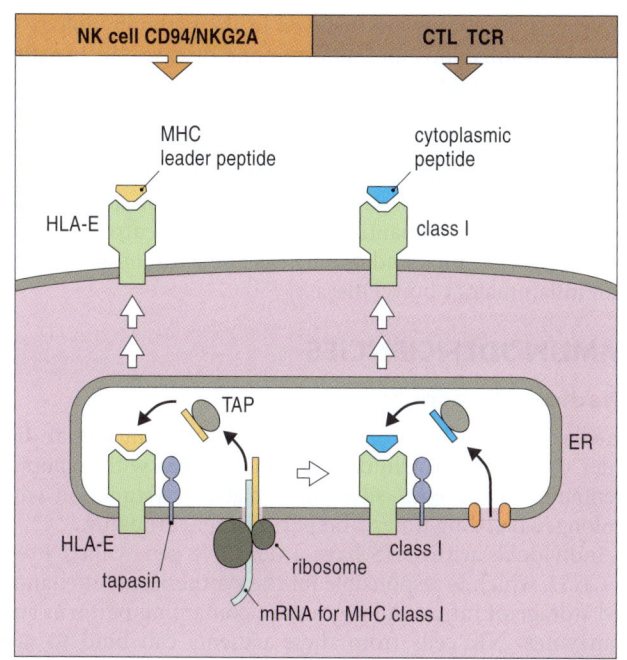

Figure 21-3

Leader peptides from major histocompatibility complex (MHC) class I molecules are loaded onto human leukocyte antigen E (HLA-E) molecules in the endoplasmic reticulum (ER), a process that requires transporter associated with antigen processing (TAP) and tapasin to assemble functional HLA-E molecules. These are presented at the cell surface for review by the CD94 series of receptors on NK cells (*left*). The MHC class I molecules, meanwhile, present antigenic peptides from cytoplasmic proteins that have been transported into the ER. These complexes are presented to the T cell receptor (TCR) on CD8+ CTLs. (From Roitt I, Brostoff J, Male D, et al: Immunology, ed 7, Philadelphia, 2006, Mosby.)

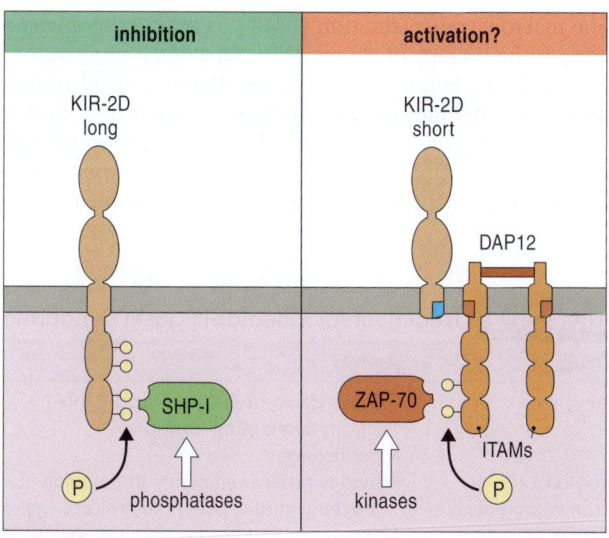

Figure 21-4

Following phosphorylation of its ITIMs (immunoreceptor tyrosine-based inhibitory motifs), the inhibitory receptors of natural killer (NK) cells can bind to phosphatases, including SHP-1 and SHP-2, which inhibit killing. The noninhibitory forms of the receptor associate with a dimeric molecule DAP12, via the complementarity-charged residues in their membranes. DAP12 has immunoreceptor tyrosine-based activation motifs (ITAMs). When phosphorylated, this recruits kinases of the Syk family or ZAP-70. Whether this leads to NK cell activation or whether it modulates the inhibitory signals is not known. (From Roitt I, Brostoff J, Male D, et al: Immunology, ed 7, Philadelphia, 2006, Mosby.)

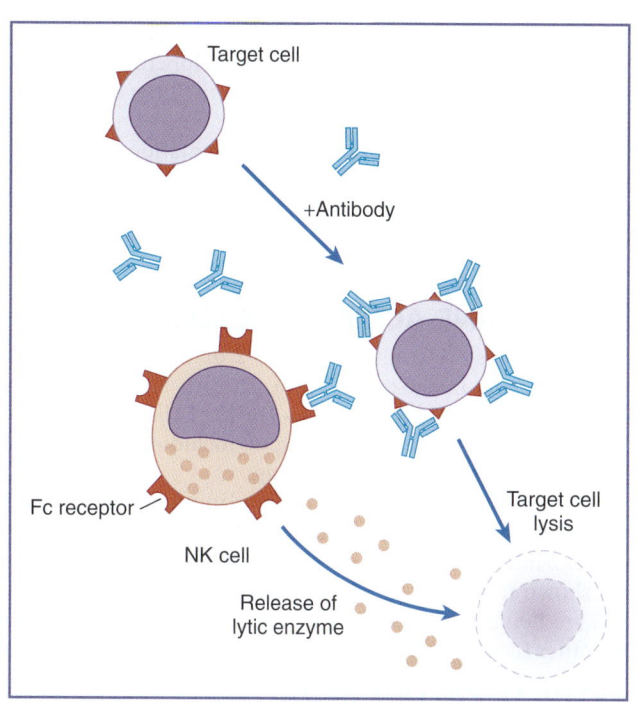

Figure 21-5

Antibody-dependent cell-mediated cytotoxicity (ADCC). ADCC is a phenomenon by which target cells coated with antibodies are destroyed by specialized killer cells. Among the cells that mediate ADCC are natural killer (NK) cells, neutrophils, and eosinophils. The killing cells express receptors for the Fc portion of antibodies that coat the targets. Recognition of antibody-coated targets leads to the release of lytic enzymes at the site of Fc-mediated contact. Target cell killing may also involve perforin-mediated membrane damage. Eosinophils can function in a similar manner to kill large parasites. (From Actor JK: Elsevier's integrated immunology and microbiology, Philadelphia, 2007, Mosby.)

SUBPOPULATIONS OF NATURAL KILLER CELLS AND TARGET CELL LYSIS

Using flow cytometry, NK cell subpopulations can be indentified on the basis of the numbers of CD56 glycoproteins on the cell surface. Approximately 95% of NK cells express low numbers of CD56 and are termed *CD56^{dim}*. These cells lyse target cells by using perforin and granzymes. CD56^{dim} cells also express CD16, which is a low-affinity Fc gamma (Fc-γ) receptor. Engagement of the NK cell Fc receptor by antibodies bound to target cells initiates the release of perforin and granzymes. This mechanism is known as *antibody-dependent cellular cytotoxicity (ADCC)* or *killer (K) cell cytotoxicity* (Figure 21-5).

Five percent of NK cells express large numbers of CD56 (*CD56^{bright}*). This population does not contain perforin granules and is not cytotoxic. The CD56^{bright} cells secrete interferon gamma (IFN-γ) and other proinflammatory cytokines such as IL-5, IL-13, and TNF-α.

FUNCTION OF NATURAL KILLER CELLS

NK cells play a critical role in the innate response to viruses, tumors, and fungal infections. During the early stages of a viral infection, NK cells are the primary effector cells. In some instances, NK cells may supplant the T cell response during infections by viruses that downregulate the HLA class I marker expression.

NK cells also play a critical role in the defense against tumors. Because of their presence in peripheral blood, NK cells intercept and kill cancer cells before they can metastasize to distant sites in the body.

NK cells play an indirect role in the termination of opportunistic *Candida albicans* and *Aspergillus* infections in immunosuppressed individuals. Production of INF-γ by noncytotoxic NK cells activates macrophage and effector lymphocytes and recruits neutrophils to kill the fungi.

LYMPHOKINE-ACTIVATED KILLER CELLS

When NK cells are stimulated by IL-2 or INF-γ, a dramatic increase occurs in the synthesis of perforin and granzymes. These cells, known as *lymphokine-activated killer (LAK) cells*, can lyse a broad range of tumor types, including those which are normally resistant to NK cell lysis.

LAK cells have been used in tumor immunotherapy with varying degrees of success. Infusion of autologous LAK cells and IL-2 into patients with some end-stage metastatic cancers was shown to reduce or eradicate the tumor. Currently, LAK cells are being evaluated for the treatment of neuroblastoma and other recurrent brain tumors.

NATURAL KILLER T CELLS

On the basis of the structure of the T cell receptor, NKT cells are subdivided into type I and type II cells. Type I NKT (CD3+, CD16+, CD56+) cells have an invariant T cell receptor alpha (TCR-α) chain rearrangement (Valpha24:Jalpha18 chains). These cells recognize a self-glycolipid antigen called *alpha galactosylceramide* (α-GalCer) presented by CD1 molecules. Antigen-activated type I NKT cells release proinflammatory cytokines such as INF-γ, IL-2, IL-4, IL-12, and IL-13, which can modulate Th1 and Th2 response.

Type II NKT (CD3+, CD16–, CD56+) cells lack the TCR invariant TCR (Valpha24–) α-chain rearrangement but still recognize antigens presented by CD1. The self-antigens, presented by CD1, however, differ from those recognized by type I NKT cells. The physiologic role of type II NKT cells has not been well studied. In animal models, type II NKT cells can augment or inhibit an immune response.

NATURAL KILLER T CELLS IN DISEASE

In the immune response to tumors, type I NKT cells can be protective or suppress the immune response. α-GalCer–stimulated type I NKT cells are indirectly involved in the defense against tumors. Type I NKT cells produce INF-γ, which increases CD8 and NK cell lysis of target cells. Cytokines from type I NKT cells also stimulate dendritic cells to produce IL-12, which is important in tumor immunity. IL-12 confers migratory properties to T cells and prepares tumor masses to accept the migrating T cells. In contrast, the production of IL-13 from type I NKT cells has been implicated in the suppression of the anti-tumor response.

Type I NKT cells may also play a critical role in immediate allergic reactions. Patients with severe asthma or uncontrolled asthma have elevated numbers of type I NKT cells in bronchial and alveolar fluids. These cells produce high levels of IL-4, IL-13, and INF-γ. IL-4 production by type I NKT cells may direct the Th2 response and the production of immunoglobulin E (IgE). Although the mechanism is unknown, IL-13 plays a critical role in the development of airway hyperresponsiveness, airway remodeling, mucus secretion, and recruitment of eosinophils.

Type II NKT cells are involved in the pathophysiology of some viral infections and autoimmune diseases. In hepatitis C infections, type NKT II cells produce cytokines that stimulate a Th1 response required for resolution of the infection. In ulcerative colitis, type II NKT cells produce IL-13, which shifts the response to Th2 cells and antibody production. IL-13 acts directly on B cells, stimulating proliferation and isotypic switching to IgG. Autoantibodies directed at neutrophil granules, the portal tract, and colon cells are common in patients with inflammatory bowel disease.

IMMUNODEFICIENCIES

Chediak-Higashi Syndrome

Chediak-Higashi syndrome (CHS) is a rare autosomal disorder of childhood. Children usually present with hypopigmentation of the eyes, silver hair, platelet dysfunction with prolonged bleeding times, and peripheral neuropathy.

Individuals with CHS have a defective gene called *LYST* or *CHS1*, which is responsible for the synthesis, maintenance, and storage of intracellular granules containing perforin and granzymes. NK cells from these patients can bind to target cells but cannot kill cells using the perforin–granzyme pathway.

The inability to form granules is not restricted to NK cells. Neutrophils (azurophilic granules), leukocytes (lysosomes), and melanocytes (melanosomes) also have defective granules. Most patients have a high risk for Epstein-Barr virus (EBV) infections and exhibit a life-threatening, nonmalignant lymphoma-like infiltration of multiple organs. Most patients die from repeated bacterial infections by *Staphylococcus aureus*, *Streptococcus pyogenes*, or *Pneumococcus* species.

Treatment for Chediak-Higashi Syndrome

Bone marrow transplantation (BMT) from an HLA-matched sibling is the therapy of choice. Without a BMT, most individuals usually die before 10 years of age. Before transplantation, patients are maintained on a therapy regimen that controls infections and prevents the spread of viral infections (Table 21-2). Although BMT resolves the immunologic issue, it has no effect on the neurologic and pigmentation problems.

Table 21-2	Treatment for Chediak-Higashi Syndrome
Drug	**Action**
Acyclovir	Causes deoxyribonucleic acid (DNA) chain termination during viral replication
Pooled immunoglobulin	Provides passive immunity to common bacteria and viruses. Neutralizes anti-myelin antibodies involved in peripheral neuropathy
Interferon alpha-2a and -2b	Prevents spread of viral infections, inhibits proliferation of lymphocytes, and downregulates immune responses
Vincristine	Decreases reticuloendothelial function
Vinblastine	Disrupts the formation of the mitotic spindle and arrests cell proliferation at metaphase
Colchicine	Decreases leukocyte motility and phagocytosis in inflammatory responses

SUMMARY

- Natural killer (NK) cells are large granular lymphocytes that are neither T cells nor B cells.
- NK cells are part of the innate immune response and are involved in the resolution of viral and fungal infections. They also prevent tumor metastases.
- NK cells recognize aberrant or infected cells with downregulated HLA class I molecules and engage other nonclassic HLA antigens that activate or inhibit NK cells.
- NK cells lyse target cells by using perforin and granzymes or antibody-dependent cellular cytotoxicity.
- Lymphokine-activated killer (LAK) cells are NK cells that have been stimulated with interferon gamma (IFN-γ) or interleukin 2 (IL-2). These cells can kill a wide range of tumor cells, including those normally resistant to NK cell lysis.
- Small populations of T cells also act as NK cells and are designated as NKT cells.
- NKT cells recognize self-antigens presented by CD1 molecules.
- NKT cells are involved in the pathophysiology of asthma, hepatitis C, and ulcerative colitis.

REFERENCES

Chung KF: Individual cytokines contributing to asthma pathophysiology: Valid targets for asthma therapy? Curr Opin Investig Drugs 4(11):1320, 2003.

Colonna M, Borsellino G, Falco M, et al: HLA-C is the inhibitory ligand that determines dominant resistance to lysis by NK1- and NK2-specific natural killer cells, Proc Natl Acad Sci U S A 90(24):12000, 1993.

Dorak MT: Role of natural killer cells and killer immunoglobulin-like receptor polymorphisms: Association of HLA and KIRs, Methods Mol Med 134:123, 2007.

Falk CS, Steinle A, Schendel DJ: Expression of HLA-C molecules confers target cell resistance to some non-major histocompatibility complex-restricted T cells in a manner analogous to allospecific natural killer cells, J Exp Med 182(4):1005, 1995.

Katz P, Zaytoun AM, Fauci AS: Deficiency of active natural killer cells in the Chediak-Higashi syndrome. Localization of the defect using a single cell cytotoxicity assay, J Clin Invest 69(6):1231, 1982.

Kawano T, Cui J, Koezuka Y, et al: Natural killer-like nonspecific tumor cell lysis mediated by specific ligand-activated Valpha14 NKT cells, Proc Natl Acad Sci U S A 95(10):5690, 1998.

O'Callaghan CA: Molecular basis of human natural killer cell recognition of HLA-E (human leucocyte antigen-E) and its relevance to clearance of pathogen-infected and tumour cells, Clin Sci (Lond) 99(1):9, 2000.

Perussia B: Lymphokine-activated killer cells, natural killer cells and cytokines, Curr Opin Immunol 3(1):49, 1991.

Sankhla SK, Nadkarni JS, Bhagwati SN: Adoptive immunotherapy using lymphokine-activated killer (LAK) cells and interleukin-2 for recurrent malignant primary brain tumors, J Neurooncol 27(2):133, 1996.

Sullivan LC, Clements CS, Beddoe T: The heterodimeric assembly of the CD94-NKG2 receptor family and implications for human leukocyte antigen-E recognition, Immunity 27(6):900, 2007.

Valteau-Couanet D, Leboulaire C, Maincent K, et al: Dendritic cells for NK/LAK activation: Rationale for multicellular immunotherapy in neuroblastoma patients, Blood 100(7):2554, 2002.

Wingender G, Kronenberg M: Role of NKT cells in the digestive system. IV. The role of canonical natural killer T cells in mucosal immunity and inflammation, Am J Physiol Gastrointest Liver Physiol 294(1):1, 2008.

Winter CC, Long EO: A single amino acid in the p58 killer cell inhibitory receptor controls the ability of natural killer cells to discriminate between the two groups of HLA-C allotypes, J Immunol 158(9):4026, 1997.

Yang G, Volk A, Petley T, et al: Anti-IL-13 monoclonal antibody inhibits airway hyperresponsiveness, inflammation and airway remodeling, Cytokine 28(6):224, 2004.

ASSESSMENT QUESTIONS

1. Which of the following is the ligand for CD94-NKG2 receptors?
   I. Human leukocyte antigen E (HLA-E)
   II. HLA C
   III. HLA-B
   A. I
   B. III
   C. I and II
   D. II and III
   E. I, II, and III

2. Natural killer (NK) cells recognize aberrant or infected cells that have:
   A. Downregulated HLA class I molecules
   B. Downregulated HLA class II molecules
   C. Upregulated HLA-G molecules
   D. Upregulated HLA-E molecules

3. Which of following cytokines is necessary for the generation of lymphokine-activated killer (LAK) cells?
   I. Interferon gamma (IFN-γ)
   II. Interleukin 2 (IL-2)
   III. Tumor necrosis factor alpha (TNF-α)
   A. I
   B. III
   C. I and II
   D. II and III
   E. I, II, and III

4. Type I NKT cells recognize self-antigens presented by:
   A. HLA-E
   B. HLA-B
   C. HLA-C
   D. CD1

5. Type I NKT cells are involved in:
   A. Asthma
   B. Ulcerative colitis
   C. Chediak-Higashi syndrome
   D. Hepatitis C

6. The ligand for the killer cell immunoglobulin-like receptors (KIRs) is:
   A. HLA-A
   B. HLA-G
   C. HLA-C
   D. HLA-B

CHAPTER 22

Factors That Influence the Immune Response

LEARNING OBJECTIVES

- Compare and contrast the determinant selection and hole in the T cell repertoire models
- Recognize how the physical form of the antigen influences the immune response
- Compare and contrast the roles of immature and mature dendritic cells in the activation or inhibition of an immune response
- Compare the effects of low-dose and high-dose antigens on T and B cells
- Recognize the two mechanisms by which passively administered immunoglobulin downregulates the immune response
- Compare and contrast the three different CD4 regulator cells
- Identify the role of FOXp3 in the downregulation of an immune response
- Identify the disease caused by mutations in FOXp3
- Compare and contrast the characteristics of antigen-stimulated CD4 regulator cells
- Recognize the role of Qa-1 in immune regulation by CD8 cells
- Explain activation-induced cell death (AICD)
- Compare and contrast the AICD mechanisms involved in the downregulation and termination of an immune response
- Identify the defects or alterations in AICD in individuals with systemic lupus erythematosus (SLE)
- Differentiate between an idiotope and an idiotype
- Explain idiotype network theory
- Recognize the two mechanisms by which anti-idiotype antibodies can downregulate an immune response

KEY TERMS

Anergy
FOXp3
Idiotope
Idiotype
NTreg cell
Qa-1
Regulator cells
Treg1 cell
TH3 cell

INTRODUCTION

The generation of an immune response is determined by genetic factors related to the nature of the antigen, dose, and route of administration. Once a response is mounted, it must be carefully controlled to ensure that it is not directed at normal host tissue. A response must also be easily downregulated when no more antigen is present to drive the immune response.

The immune system has multiple control mechanisms available to damper an immune response after the antigen has been reduced or eliminated. A network of CD4 and CD8 regulatory cells (Tregs) suppresses the function of the lymphocytes involved in autoimmune diseases, allergies, and transplant rejection but without disrupting the function of lymphocytes involved in normal adaptive immune responses. Responses are dampered by two different mechanisms: (1) Some responses are terminated by the killing of CD4 effector cells by a mechanism called *activation-induced cell death (AICD)*. (2) Other responses may be terminated by a perforin and granzymes, anti-inflammatory cytokines, or an anti-idiotypic network.

GENETICS AND THE IMMUNE RESPONSE

Human Leukocyte Antigen Glycoproteins and the Immune Response

Some individuals are genetically restricted and are unable to respond to specific antigens. Failure to respond to a specific antigen can be explained by the *determinant selection* and *hole in the T cell repertoire* models. The determinant selection model proposes that class II molecules differ in their ability to bind processed antigens. In essence, individuals lack human leukocyte antigen (HLA) molecules that present a specific antigen to T cells. Conversely, the hole in the T cell repertoire model proposes that class II antigen presentation is normal but that some individuals lack a lymphocyte with a T cell receptor (TCR) that recognizes the specific antigen. In both cases, T cell activation fails to occur.

PHYSICAL AND BIOLOGIC FACTORS INFLUENCING THE IMMUNE RESPONSE

Form of Antigen and Route of Administration

The physical form of the antigen is important in the generation of an immune response. Because insoluble antigens are easily processed by macrophages, large aggregates favor the

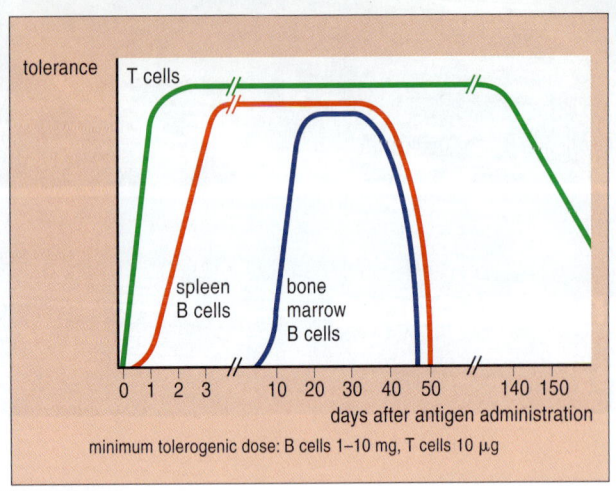

Figure 22-1

A mouse was given a T-dependent antigen (human γ-globulin) at tolerance-inducing doses, and the duration of tolerance was measured. T cell tolerance was more rapidly induced and more persistent than B cell tolerance. Bone marrow B cells may take considerably longer to tolerize than splenic B cells. Typically, much less antigen is needed to tolerize T cells—10 μg as opposed to 1 to 10 mg, a 1000-fold difference. (From Roitt I, Brostoff J, Male D, et al: Immunology, ed 7, Philadelphia, 2006, Mosby.)

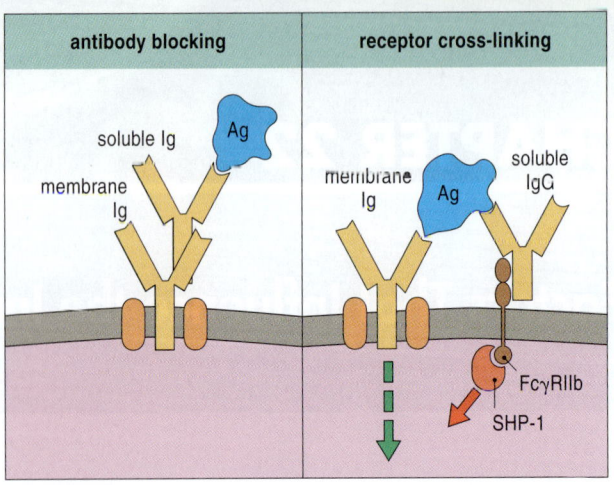

Figure 22-2

In antibody blocking, high doses of soluble immunoglobulin (Ig) block the interaction between an antigenic determinant (epitope) and membrane immunoglobulin on B cells. In effect, the B cell is then unable to recognize the antigen. This receptor-blocking mechanism also prevents B cell priming, but only antibodies that bind to the same epitope to which the B cell's receptors bind can do this. In receptor cross-linking, low doses of antibody allow cross-linking by the antigen of a B cell's Fc receptors and its antigen receptors. The FcγRIIB receptor associates with a tyrosine phosphatase (SHP-1), which interferes with cell activation by tyrosine kinases associated with the antigen receptor. This allows B cell priming but inhibits antibody synthesis. Antibodies against different epitopes on the antigen can all act by this mechanism. (From Roitt I, Brostoff J, Male D, et al: Immunology, ed 7, Philadelphia, 2006, Mosby.)

generation of an immune response. In contrast, small, soluble antigens cannot be processed by antigen-presenting cells and generate a tolerogenic effect.

The route of administration also determines whether the host mounts an immune response or becomes tolerogenic. Intramuscular and subcutaneous administration of antigens usually elicits an immune response by favoring antigen uptake and presentation by Langerhans cells. In contrast, inhalation, oral, or intravenous administration often fails to generate an immune response.

Maturity of the Antigen-Presenting Cell

Dendritic cells (DCs) are the major antigen-presenting cells in the body. They originate in bone marrow and are released into peripheral blood before migration to lymph nodes. In tissues and lymph nodes, DCs are present as "immature," partially differentiated cells. These cells can capture and present the antigen in the context of class II molecules but lack the co-stimulatory molecules B7-1 and B7-2, which normally engage CD28 receptors on T cells (see Chapter 6). T cells interacting with immature DCs become anergic. Anergic T cells cannot proliferate or respond to antigen stimulation. In contrast, mature DCs in tissue express class I or class II molecules as well as co-stimulatory molecules. They are efficient in presenting antigens to T cells within the lymph node.

Antigen Concentration

When the antigen is administered over a wide concentration range, only intermediate concentrations induce an immune response. High doses paralyze the immune system by inactivating B cells. Low doses or subimmunogenic doses administered over an extended period inactivate T cells (Figure 22-1).

Passively Administered Immunoglobulin

High doses of passively administered immunoglobulin can suppress the immune response. Pooled immunoglobulin contains antibodies to common bacterial and viral pathogens. Interaction between antibodies in pooled serum and microbial antigens creates immune complexes that block B cell receptor (BCR) activation. Pooled immunoglobulin also suppresses an immune response by engaging the FcγRIIB receptors expressed by monocytes, macrophages, and lymphocytes. FcγRIIB has a cytoplasmic immuno-receptor tyrosine-based inhibitory motif (ITIM), which associates with a tyrosine phosphatase (SHP-1) and downregulates intracellular signaling (Figure 22-2).

REGULATOR CELLS

The concept of suppressor cells was introduced by Gershon and Kondo in 1971. They demonstrated that the transfer of immunocompetent cells from an immunized mouse to a naïve mouse downregulated an immune response to the same antigen. Because of an inability to identify suppressor cells in lymphoid organs, the concept of regulator cells was largely discarded. The advent of flow cytometry and cell sorting made it possible to identify and isolate CD4 and CD8 regulator cell populations. Regulator cells play a role in downregulating auto-reactive lymphocytes, reducing inflammation, mediating tolerance to superantigens, and maintaining self-tolerance.

CD4 Regulator Cells

A population of CD3+, CD4+, and CD25+ cells in peripheral blood suppresses autoimmune reactions and response to infectious disease. These cells have been designated T regulator (Treg) cells. Three subpopulations of CD4 Tregs have been identified and are known as *natural Tregs*, *Treg1*, and *TH3*.

Figure 22-3

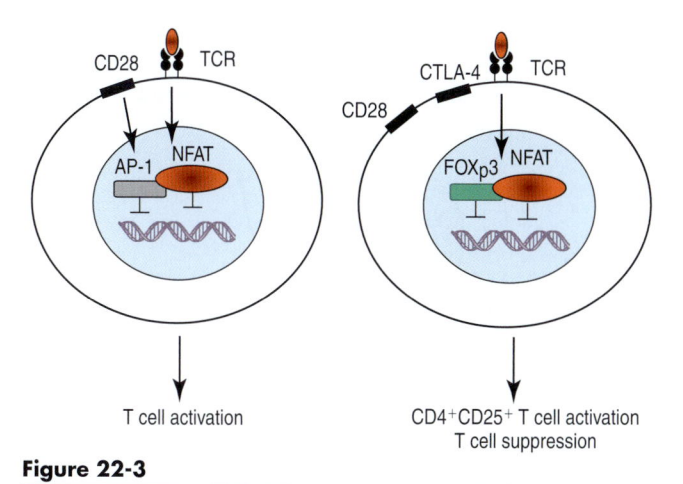

FOXp3 regulates nuclear factor of activated T cell (NFAT)–mediated gene transcription in CD4+CD25+ regulatory T cells. In both conventional T cells (*left*) and CD4+CD25+ regulatory T cells (*right*), T cell receptor (TCR)–mediated activation upregulates the expression of the transcription factor NFAT. On TCR stimulation and CD28-mediated co-stimulation, NFAT binds to AP-1 in conventional T cells but to FOXp3 in CD4+CD25+ regulatory T cells. As a consequence, activation results in the transcription of a different set of genes in both cell types. (From Vliet J, Nieuwenhaus E: IPEX as a result of mutations in FOXp3, Clin Dev Immunol 2007.)

Natural CD4 Tregs

Natural Tregs (NTregs) are educated in the thymus during the negative selection process (see Chapter 1). In the thymus, naïve cells bind to macrophages and dendritic cells, expressing high levels of HLA self-peptides. Thymocytes binding to the HLA molecules with intermediate affinity are considered NTregs that exit the thymus and circulate in peripheral blood. NTregs require antigen presentation by class II molecules, the presence of co-stimulatory molecules, stimulation of the high-affinity interleukin 2 (IL-2) receptor by exogenous IL-2, and cell-to-cell contact.

Stimulation of the high-affinity IL-2 receptor activates the JAK1–JAK3 pathway, which phosphorylates STAT3 and STAT5. The STATs, which are translocated to the nucleus, upregulate the synthesis of intracellular forehead helix or winged transcription factor (FOXp3). Binding of FOXp3 to NFAT (nuclear factor of activated T cells) alters the translocation within the nucleus and upregulates the expression of CD25 (the α-chain of the high-affinity IL-2 receptor), CTLA-4, and a glucocorticoid-induced tumor necrosis receptor (GITR). The mechanism is shown in Figure 22-3.

NTregs downregulate an immune response by two different mechanisms: (1) Using CTLA-4 ligation with B7 molecules on dendritic cells, NTregs downregulate dendritic cells and damper the activation of T cells. Activated NTregs also produce IL-10 and transforming growth factor beta (TGF-β). Both cytokines have immuno-regulatory functions. A summary of the possible interactions between NTregs and conventional T cells is shown in Figure 22-4.

FOXp3 Deficiency. Mutations in the FOXp3 gene occur in the forkhead domain that is critical to NFAT binding. Impaired FOXp3 function results in an immune polyendocrinopathy, enteropathy, and X-linked disorder (IPEX). Symptoms include cachexia and growth retardation. Patients present with severe watery diarrhea, type I insulin-dependent diabetes, thyroid disorders, or eczema. Without treatment, affected children usually die within the first 2 years of life. Severe enteric infections associated with catheters or diarrhea contribute to mortality.

Treatment for X-Linked Disorder. Little information on the treatment of IPEX is available. Immunosuppressive therapy and bone marrow transplantation have shown variable results. Immunosuppressive therapy is difficult because of toxicity and infectious complications.

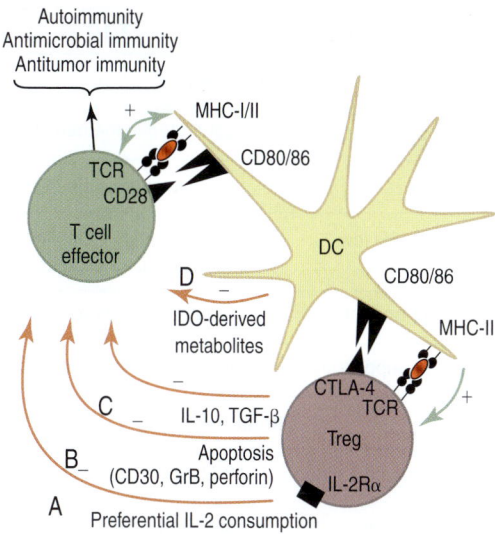

Figure 22-4

Schematic representation of the regulation of the function of effector T cells by CD4+CD25+ regulatory T cells. On antigen-specific activation by dendritic cells (DCs), CD4+CD25+ regulatory T (Treg) cells can suppress immune responses through the following mechanisms: **A,** preferential consumption of IL-2 by CD4+CD25+ regulatory T cells instead of effector T cells. **B,** Induction of effector T cell apoptosis via CD30/CD30L interactions or perforin/granzyme B (GrB). **C,** Production of immunosuppressive cytokines interleukin 10 (IL-10) and transforming growth factor beta (TGF-β) by CD4+CD25+ regulatory T cells. **D,** Production of immunosuppressive tryptophane metabolites as a result of upregulation of indoleamine-2, 3-dioxygenase (IDO) in dendritic cells (DCs). (From Vliet J, Nieuwenhaus E: IPEX as a result of mutations in FOXp3, Clin Dev Immunol 2007.)

Treg1 Cells

A small population of circulating CD4+, CD25−, and IL-10+ cells have regulatory activity and have been designated *T regulatory cells type 1 (Treg1)*. These cells have variable expression of FOXp3, require antigen stimulation, and do not need IL-2 stimulation or cell-cell contact for activation. Treg1 cells lyse effector cells using the classical perforin-granzyme lytic pathway.

TH3 Regulator Cells

Another population of regulator cells (TH3) is found in the intestinal mucosa and is important in establishing oral tolerance or in downregulating the immune response to ingested antigens. The similarities and differences between Treg cells are shown in Figure 22-5.

CD8 Regulator Cells

CD8 regulator cells kill CD4 cells by a unique mechanism. Activated CD4 cells express Qa-1, a nonclassic HLA glycoprotein that presents a small hydrophobic peptide (AMAPRTLLL)

CD4+CD25+ Treg	Tr1/TH3
Differences	
generated in the thymus	generated in the periphery
express FOXp3	variable expression of FOXp3
CD25 high, CD45R low	CD45R0 high, CD45RB low, variable CD25 expression
cell contact dependent	cell contact independent
require IL-2 for suppression	IL-2-independent suppression
Similarities	
triggered by specific antigen	triggered by specific antigen
secrete IL-10/TGF-β	secrete IL-10/TGF-β
unresponsive to anti-CD3 in vitro	unresponsive to anti-CD3 in vitro

Figure 22-5
The similarities and differences in the generation and function of the subsets of naturally occurring thymic and peripherally induced CD4+ regulatory T cells. (From Roitt I, Brostoff J, Male D, et al: Immunology, ed 7, Philadelphia, 2006, Mosby.)

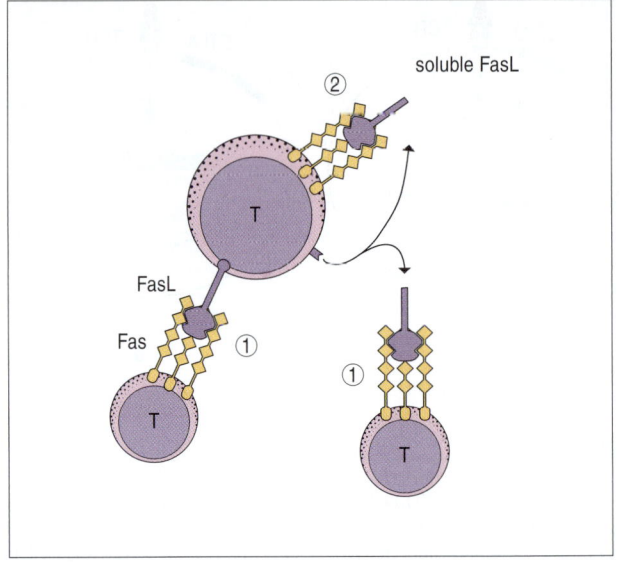

Figure 22-6
Activated T cells express both FasR (CD95) and the ligand for this molecule (FasL). **1,** Fratricide can result either from direct cell contact or from cleavage of FasL and the ligation of FasR by soluble FasL. **2,** Autocrine suicide can result from the interaction of soluble FasL with FasR. (From Roitt I, Brostoff J, Male D, et al: Immunology, ed 7, Philadelphia, 2006, Mosby.)

derived from the leader sequences of other HLA class I molecules. Engagement of the Qa-1 and CD8 TCR activates a population of CD8 suppressor cells, which differentiate into CD8 Tc1 cells with high levels of FOXp3. Using the perforin–granzymes lytic pathway, activated CD8 suppressor cells kill any antigen-driven, activated CD4 cells expressing the Qa-1 self-peptide.

Mucosal CD8 cells may play a role in the downregulation of an allergic response. Initial exposure to allergen-naïve T cells default to a Th2 cytokine pattern and production of immunoglobulin E (IgE). Repeated exposure to TGF-β produced by antigen-driven CD4 regulator cells generates a population of CD8 regulatory cells. These cells react with Qa-1 markers on activated CD4Th2 cells and downregulate IgE synthesis.

ACTIVATION-INDUCED CELL DEATH

Antigen-driven expansion of T cells and B cells can be inhibited by a process called *activation-induced cell death (AICD)*. Cell death is mediated by FasL–FasR engagement. Fas ligand (FasL) is a homotrimeric membrane molecule on the regulator cells that bind three Fas molecules on target cells. Clustering of Fas receptor (FasR) molecules brings intracellular death domains and adaptor proteins close to create a death-inducing signal complex (DISC). Engagement of FasL and FasR activates the DISC complex and triggers downstream endonucleases that degrade deoxyribonucleic acid (DNA).

CD4 regulator cells express FasL, and activated T cells express both FasR and FasL. FasL–FasR interactions between the regulatory and effector cells is often fatal to the activated T cell. Reduction in activated T cells downregulates the immune response. However, termination of an immune response also requires "suicide" by any remaining activated T cells. Autologous killing is achieved by the cleavage of the membrane-bound FasL by a zinc-dependent metalloprotease called *matrilysin*. Soluble FasL binds to FasR on the same cell in an autocrine manner to kill the T cell and terminate the response (Figure 22-6).

FasL–FasR Engagement and Disease

Defective FasL–FasR engagement plays a role in select autoimmune diseases. In animal models of systemic lupus erythematosus (SLE), auto-reactive cells persist in the host because of defective FasL–FasR interactions. FasR-induced apoptosis may also play a role in the termination of viral diseases. Human immunodeficiency virus (HIV)–infected CD4 cells express high numbers of FasR. It has been proposed that the destruction of HIV-infected CD4 cells may be the result of FasL–FasR interactions. In the case of HIV infections, the mechanism may serve as an alternative to classic cytotoxic T cell killing mediated by perforin and granzymes.

IDIOTYPE NETWORK THEORY

The idiotype network theory was proposed by Jerne in 1974 as a means for explaining immune modulation. The amino acid sequences in the complementarity-determining regions (CDRs) of antibodies that make contact with the antigen are a mirror image of the antigen that stimulated its production. Each CDR amino acid sequence is called an *idiotope*. Although most idiotopes are associated with the antigen-binding region of the antibody, they can be associated with other sites on the antibody. Collectively, clusters of idiotopes in and around the CDR are called the *antibody idiotype*.

Idiotopes are considered foreign to the host, and antibodies directed at the idiotype can be generated. Mechanistically, the initial antibody idiotype (Ab1) is the three-dimensional mirror image of the antigen that elicited its production. To interact with Ab1, the anti-idiotype antibody (Ab2) would have a CDR that is consistent with the three-dimensional structure

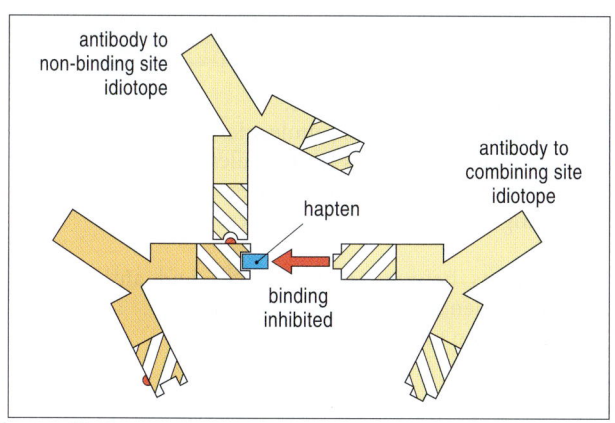

Figure 22-7

An anti-idiotype serum may contain antibodies directed at various sites on the immunoglobulin molecule. The sites associated with the combining site are site-associated idiotopes. Binding to these can be inhibited by haptens. Antibodies to non-binding site idiotopes (non–site associated) are not inhibited by haptens. (From Roitt I, Brostoff J, Male D, et al: Immunology, ed 7, Philadelphia, 2006, Mosby.)

of the antigen that stimulated the production of Ab1. Since Ab2 has the structure of a specific antigenic epitope, it can react with the TCR or BCR of the lymphocyte clone that is specific for the antigen and block the engagement of the TCR and antigen-loaded class I or II glycoproteins (Figure 22-7) on dendritic cells.

The immune response to idiotypes located outside the CDRs facilitates the formation of large immune complexes. Interactions between the immune complexes and FcγRIIB activate a cytoplasmic ITIM that downregulates auto-reactive B cells.

SUMMARY

- The generation of an immune response is influenced by host genetics, the physical characteristics of the antigen, the route of administration, and the maturity of the antigen-presenting cell.
- The immune response is controlled by CD4 and CD8 regulator cells.
- Immune responses are downregulated by anti-inflammatory cytokines, lysis of activated CD4 cells, and anti-idiotypic antibodies.

REFERENCES

Bennett CL, Ochs HD: IPEX is a unique X-linked syndrome characterized by immune dysfunction, polyendocrinopathy, enteropathy, and a variety of autoimmune phenomena, Curr Opin Pediatr 13(6):533, 2001.

Chess L, Jiang H: Resurrecting CD8+ suppressor T cells, Nat Immunol 5(5):469, 2004.

Cohn M: The concept of functional idiotype network for immune regulation mocks all and comforts none, Ann Inst Pasteur Immunol 137(1):64, 1986.

Cottrez F, Groux H: Specialization in tolerance: Innate CD(4+)CD(25+) versus acquired TR1 and TH3 regulatory T cells, Transplantation 77(Suppl 1):S12, 2004.

Fehervari Z, Sakaguchi S: CD4+ Tregs and immune control, J Clin Invest 114(9):1209, 2004.

Hamad AR, Schneck JP: Activation-induced T cell death is regulated by CD4 expression, Int Rev Immunol 20(5):535, 2001.

Hori S, Sakaguchi S: Foxp3: A critical regulator of the development and function of regulatory T cells, Microbes Infect 6(8):745, 2004.

Jiang H, Chess L: An integrated view of suppressor T cell subsets in immunoregulation, J Clin Invest 114(9):1198, 2004.

Papiernik M: Natural CD4+ CD25+ regulatory T cells. Their role in the control of superantigen responses, Immunol Rev 182:180, 2001.

Sattaporn S, Eremin O: Dendritic cells (I): Biological functions, J R Coll Surg Edinb 46(1):9, 2001.

Tung KS: Human sperm antigens and antisperm antibodies I, Studies on vasectomy patients, Clin Exp Immunol 20(1):93, 1975.

ASSESSMENT QUESTIONS

1. Low concentrations of antigen administered to the host usually inactivate:
   A. T cells
   B. B cells
   C. Macrophages
   D. Dendritic cells

2. Pooled immunoglobulin downregulates the immune system by:
   I. Formation of immune complexes that block interaction with the B cell receptor (BCR)
   II. Interaction with Fc receptors on monocytes or macrophages, which downregulates antigen processing and human leukocyte antigen (HLA) class II expression
   III. Expression of the Fas ligand (FasL) on activated T cells

   A. I
   B. III
   C. I and II
   D. II and III
   E. I, II, and III

3. Which of the following regulator cells are interleukin and contact dependent?
   A. NTregs
   B. Treg1
   C. TH3
   D. CD8

4. CD8 regulator cells recognize:
   A. Antigen-loaded class I molecules
   B. Antigen loaded class II molecules
   C. Antigen-loaded CD1 molecules
   D. Antigen-loaded Qa-1 molecules

5. Interactions between naïve T cells and antigen-pulsed immature dendritic cells usually result in:
   A. Activation of the T cell
   B. Lysis of the T cell
   C. T cell anergy
   D. Downregulation of class II molecules on the dendritic cell

6. The FOXp3 transcription factor is only found in:
   A. Activated CD8 regulator cells
   B. Activated CD4 regulator cells
   C. All T cells
   D. Mature dendritic cells

CHAPTER 23

Cytokines and Biologic Modifiers

LEARNING OBJECTIVES

- Differentiate between a cytokine and an interleukin (IL)
- List the cells that produce IL-1
- Identify the three biologic functions of IL-1
- Identify the immunologic and genetic defects in patients with cryopyrin-associated periodic syndrome (CAPS)
- Design a treatment regimen for CAPS
- List the cells that produce IL-2
- Compare and contrast IL-2 receptors on activated and naïve T cells
- Compare the roles of IL-2 in autocrine and paracrine signaling
- Explain the relationship between natural killer (NK) cells, IL-2, and lymphokine-activated killer (LAK) cells
- Recognize the biologic role of aldesleukin
- Identify the biologic role(s) of IL-11 and the clinical usefulness of oprelvekin
- Compare and contrast type I and type II interferons (IFNs) and their biologic functions
- List the cellular sources of type I and type II IFNs
- Describe the role of IFNs in viral infections
- List the commercially available natural and synthetic IFNs
- Define tumor necrosis factor (TNF)
- Compare the functions of TNF at low and high concentrations
- Discuss the role of TNF in the pathophysiology of rheumatoid arthritis (RA)
- Identify the two monoclonal antibodies used in the treatment of RA
- Recognize the biologic target of etanercept
- Identify the biologic roles of IL-3, macrophage–colony-stimulating factor (M-CSF), granulocyte-macrophage–CSF (GM-CSF), and granulocyte-CSF (G-CSF)
- Differentiate between tumor-specific antigen (TSA) and tumor-associated antigen (TAA)
- Compare and contrast the structure of heat shock proteins (HSPs) from normal and malignant cells
- Compare and contrast normal and malignant carbohydrate tumor antigens
- Identify the two antigens present on germ-line tumor cells
- Discuss the advantages and disadvantages of whole-cell tumor vaccines
- Discuss the advantages and disadvantages of dendritic cell vaccines
- Identify the advantages and disadvantages of viral vector vaccines
- Explain the relationship between B cell receptors (BCRs), B cell malignancies, and idiotype vaccines

KEY TERMS

Colony-stimulating factor (CSF)
Cryopyrin-associated periodic syndrome (CAPS)
Cytokines
Dendritic cell cancer vaccine
Idiotypic cancer vaccine
Interferon (IFN)
Interleukin 1 (L-1)
Interleukin 2 (L-2)
Interleukin 11 (L-11)
Tumor-associated antigen (TAA)
Tumor necrosis factor (TNF)
Tumor-specific antigen (TSA)
Whole-cell cancer vaccine

INTRODUCTION

Biologic response modifiers (BRMs) are natural or synthetic substances that stimulate the immune system or restore normal numbers of immunocompetent cells in peripheral blood. BRMs include cytokines, interleukins (ILs), interferons (IFNs), and colony-stimulating factors (CSFs). In the broadest sense, human cancer vaccines are considered BRMs, since they modify the immune response to tumors.

CYTOKINES AND INTERLEUKINS

Cytokines are a family of small-molecular-weight, soluble proteins that activate or inhibit the function of cells. Within the cytokine family are ILs, IFNs, and other factors that stimulate the differentiation of stem cells in bone marrow. ILs and IFNs facilitate cross-talk between immunocompetent cells, which results in an alteration of biologic function. Bone marrow–stimulating factors induce the differentiation of macrophages and granulocytes and their release into peripheral blood.

Table 23-1	Gene Abnormalities in Cryopyrin-Associated Periodic Syndrome (CAPS)		
Syndrome	Gene and Locus	Protein	Mode of Inheritance
MWS	NLRP3 (CIAS1), 1q44	Cryopyrin (NALP3/PYPAF1)	Autosomal dominant
FCAS	NLRP3 (CIAS1), 1q44	Cryopyrin (NALP3/PYPAF1)	Autosomal dominant
NOMID	NLRP3 (CIAS1), 1q44	Cryopyrin (NALP3/PYPAF1)	Autosomal dominant

Modified from Hereditary periodic fever syndromes. Available at www.emedicine.medscape.com/article/952254-overview. Accessed 11/01/10.

Interleukin 1

IL-1 is synthesized by macrophages, monocytes, dendritic cells, and keratinocytes. It comprises two different polypeptides (IL-1α and IL-1β), each having a molecular weight of 17 kilodaltons (kDa). The effects of IL-1 are wide ranging and concentration dependent. At low concentrations, IL-1 upregulates leukocyte adhesion factors, which facilitates the tethering of immunocompetent cells before their transmigration into tissue. As part of an innate immune response, IL-1 acts as an endogenous pyrogen, which raises the body temperature above 100.4° F (see Chapter 2). The temperature increase prevents microbial growth and accelerates lymphocyte division and the onset of an adaptive immune response.

Interleukin 1 and Disease

Cryopyrin-associated periodic syndrome (CAPS) comprises a group of inherited diseases that are characterized by the overproduction of IL-1β. CAPS is characterized by short, intense inflammatory reactions with rashes, fever or chills, redness of eyes, joint pain, and adolescent deafness. Included in the CAPS family are:
- Familial cold auto-inflammatory syndrome (FCAS)
- Muckle-Wells syndrome (MWS)
- Neonatal-onset multisystem inflammatory disease (NOMID)

Individuals with CAPS have an autosomal dominant mutation in the *NLRP3* gene that prevents the synthesis of cryopyrin (Table 23-1). Under normal conditions, cryopyrin interacts with apoptosis-associated Speck-like protein and caspase 1 to increase the synthesis of IL-1β (see Table 23-1).

IL-1 as a Biologic Response Modifier

Fusion proteins, receptor antagonists, and monoclonal antibodies are used to neutralize the physiologic effects of soluble IL-1 or block the interactions with the receptor. Rilonacept is a fusion protein that contains the IL-1 receptor coupled with the Fc portion of immunoglobulin G (IgG). It binds and neutralizes soluble IL-1 before it can interact with its receptor. Canakinumab is a humanized monoclonal antibody directed at IL-1β. It blocks the effects of IL-1β and has no cross-reactivity with IL-1α or the IL-1 receptor. Anakinra is an IL-1 receptor antagonist that downregulates or blocks intracellular signaling. Many of these BRMs are used to treat patients with CAPS (Table 23-2).

Interleukin 2

Interleukin 2 (or T cell growth factor) is a glycosylated protein synthesized by activated T cells. Synthesis is transient, with peak activity occurring 4 hours after T cell activation. Autocrine IL-2 stimulation of activated T cells is necessary for the activation and proliferation of CD8+ and CD4+ cells (see Chapter 7). By increasing the synthesis of perforin and granzymes, IL-2 transforms natural killer (NK) cells into lymphokine-activated killer (LAK) cells.

Table 23-2	Treatment for Cryopyrin-Associated Periodic Syndrome (CAPS)	
Product	Description	Disease
Rilonacept	Fusion product of the interleukin 1 (IL-1) receptor and the Fc portion of immunoglobulin G (IgG)	Familial cold auto-inflammatory syndrome (FCAS) Muckle-Wells syndrome (MWS)
Canakinumab	Fully humanized monoclonal antibody directed at IL-1β	Neonatal-onset multisystem inflammatory disease (NOMID)
Anakinra	Nonglycosylated form of the human IL-1 receptor antagonist (IL-1Ra)	Neonatal-onset multisystem inflammatory disease (NOMID)

IL-2 as a Biologic Response Modifier

Administration of IL-2 can augment or inhibit immune function. Blocking the interaction between IL-2 and the high-affinity IL-2 receptor prevents autocrine stimulation of T cells and the initiation of an immune response. Two commercially available monoclonal antibodies block autocrine stimulation. Daclizumab is a humanized IgG$_1$, and basiliximab is a chimeric (murine–human) antibody. Both antibodies are directed at the α-chain of the human high-affinity IL-2 receptor. They are administered in concert with cyclosporine and corticosteroid therapy to prevent the rejection of allografts.

Recombinant IL-2 is also used to stimulate the immune system. Aldesleukin is a recombinant human IL-2 produced in *Escherichia coli*. It is indicated for the treatment of metastatic renal cell carcinoma in adults.

Aldesleukin has serious side effects. In some patients, it induces capillary leak syndrome (CLS), which is characterized by leakage of fluid into tissue and the loss of vascular tone. The rapid drop in blood pressure results in reduced organ perfusion, hypotension, and death.

Interleukin 11

IL-11 is one of several uncharacterized proteins that stimulate the proliferation and differentiation of platelet progenitors.

IL-11 as a Biologic Response Modifier

Oprelvekin is a recombinant IL-11 produced in *E. coli*. It is indicated for the prevention of severe thrombocytopenia following immunosuppressive therapy in patients with nonmyeloid malignancies.

INTERFERONS

IFNs, a group of proteins usually produced in response to viral infections, are divided into two broad groups: type I and type II. The two subclasses of type I interferons are known as *IFN-α* and *IFN-β*. Type I IFN-α is produced by lymphocytes. Type I IFN-β is produced by fibroblasts. IFN-γ is also produced by lymphocytes and is the only known type II IFN. IFN-γ has a unique role in immune responses. It directs immune responses by recruiting Th1 cells to the inflammatory site and by downregulating the activity of Th2 cells. At the site of the inflammatory reaction, IFN-γ upregulates the expression of vascular adhesion factors that tether immunocompetent cells to the vascular endothelium before diapedesis.

Interferons and Viral Infections

Containment of viral infections is the primary biologic role of type I IFNs. Infected cells secrete IFNs, which warn adjacent cells of the infection risk. Uninfected, IFN-stimulated cells produce a unique 2'5' oligoadenylate synthetase that activates several nucleases and kinases. Nucleases cleave viral ribonucleic acid (RNA) preventing transcription and translation of viral proteins and the synthesis of new viral RNA. Kinases also inhibit the synthesis of viral proteins by downregulating protein elongation factors (ELF-2).

Synthetic and Natural Interferons and Biologic Modifiers

A number of synthetic and natural IFN-α, IFN-β, and IFN-γ are used in immunotherapy for viral infections, melanoma, and various lymphocyte malignancies. A list of commercially available interferons is provided in Table 23-3.

Table 23-3 Commercially Available Natural and Synthetic Interferons

Product	Description	Disease
Roferon-A	Recombinant interferon alpha (IFN-α)-2a Produced in *Escherichia coli*	Hepatitis C Hairy cell leukemia Chronic myelogenous leukemia
Intron A	Recombinant IFN-α-2b Produced in *E. coli*	Chronic hepatitis C Kaposi sarcoma Condylomata acuminata Follicular lymphoma Malignant melanoma Hairy cell leukemia
Alferon N	INF-α-n3 Natural IFN Produced by human leukocytes	Condylomata acuminata
Avonex	Recombinant IFN-β-1a Produced in Chinese hamster ovary cells	Relapsing forms of multiple sclerosis
Betaseron	Recombinant IFN-β-1b Produced in *E. coli*	Relapsing forms of multiple sclerosis
Actimmune	Recombinant IFN-γ-1b Produced in *E. coli*	Chronic granulomatous disease Severe malignant osteoporosis

TUMOR NECROSIS FACTOR

Tumor necrosis factor (TNF) is a 17-kDal protein produced by monocytes, macrophages, and T cells after exposure to bacterial endotoxins. The name is derived from in vitro studies, which showed that nonphysiologic TNF levels killed tumor cells. At low physiologic concentrations, TNF activates macrophages, which release endogenous pyrogens and proinflammatory prostaglandins that increase phagocytosis, chemotaxis of neutrophils, and the expression of vascular adhesion factors.

At high concentrations, TNF causes tissue injury, intravascular coagulation, shock, and circulatory collapse. TNF perpetuates coagulation by downregulating activated protein C (aPC) expressed on endothelial cells. aPC acts as an anticoagulant by degrading clotting factors Va and VIIIa. In the absence of aPC, excessive coagulation causes disseminated intravascular coagulopathy (DIC). Microthrombi localize in the small capillaries of the hands and feet, blocking blood flow and creating gangrenous lesions.

TNF contributes to vascular collapse by activating nitric oxide (NO) synthetase, which catalyzes the formation of NO. NO decreases myocardial contractibility and relaxes smooth muscle in the vasculature, which depresses blood pressure and tissue perfusion. The clinical endpoints are hypovolemic shock and death.

Tumor Necrosis Factor and Disease

TNF plays a major role in the pathogenesis of rheumatoid arthritis (RA) (see Chapter 16). Synovial macrophages secrete high concentrations of TNF and IL-2, which interact with receptors on fibroblasts. Bone matrix degrading proteases, prostaglandin E_2 (PGE_2), IL-6, and IL-8 are secreted by activated fibroblasts. The ILs stimulate polymorphonuclear leukocytes (PMNs) to produce additional bone-degrading proteases and B cells to produce rheumatoid factor (RF).

Tumor Necrosis Factor as a Biologic Response Modifier

In addition to standard anti-inflammatory agents, three biologic response modifiers are often used to treat RA, psoriatic and juvenile arthritis, Crohn's disease, ulcerative colitis, and ankylosing spondylitis. Biologic response modifiers (BRMs) neutralize the activity of TNF by preventing interactions with transmembrane receptors. Infliximab and adalimumab are monoclonal antibodies that bind to soluble TNF with high affinity (10^{-11}M). Etanercept is a fusion protein that consists of the TNF receptor linked to the Fc portion of human IgG_1.

COLONY-STIMULATING FACTORS

Colony-stimulating factors (CSFs) are a diverse group of glycoproteins that induce differentiation of white blood cells in bone marrow. The CSF family includes:

- Multiple-colony-stimulating factor, or interleukin 3 (IL-3)
- Macrophage–colony-stimulating factor (M-CSF)
- Granulocyte-macrophage–colony-stimulating factor (GM-CSF)
- Granulocyte–colony-stimulating factor (G-CSF)

Multiple-Colony-Stimulating Factors or Interleukin 3

IL-3 stimulates bone marrow stem cells to differentiate into myeloid progenitor cells. It also stimulates the proliferation of mature granulocytes, monocytes, and dendritic cells. IL-3 is secreted by lymphocytes, epithelial cells, and astrocytes. The role of IL-3 in disease is unclear.

Macrophage–Colony-Stimulating Factor

M-CSF is a nonglycosylated protein that induces the mobilization and differentiation of macrophage precursors. When used in conjunction with G-CSF, it also mobilizes endothelial cell precursors and revascularizes ischemic tissue.

Granulocyte-Macrophage–Colony-Stimulating Factor

GM-CSF is secreted by a wide variety of lymphoid and non-lymphoid cells. Stimulation of stem cells induces maturation and differentiation of granulocytes (e.g., polymorphonuclear leukocytes [PMNs], eosinophils, and basophils) and monocytes.

Granulocyte–Colony-Stimulating Factor

G-CSF stimulates the production of PMNs, which are necessary for the ingestion and intracellular destruction of bacteria. It is often used to increase neutrophil numbers and decrease infections in patients with nonmyeloid malignancies. It is also indicated in patients with acute myeloid leukemia, bone marrow transplants, and severe, chronic neutropenia.

Colony-Stimulating Factors as Biologic Response Modifiers

A number of commercially available CSFs are indicated for the treatment of diseases ranging from malignancies, viral infections, and autoimmune diseases. A list of commercially available CSFs is provided in Table 23-4.

TUMOR ANTIGENS

Two different tumor antigens are used in the preparation of cancer vaccines. Tumor-specific transplantation antigens (TSTAs) are unique to tumor cells and are not expressed on normal cells. Tumor-associated transplantation antigens (TATAs) are expressed on both normal and cancer cells.

TUMOR-SPECIFIC TRANSPLANTATION ANTIGENS

Tyrosinase

Tyrosinase catalyzes the oxidation of tyrosine to produce melanin and is considered a specific marker for melanoma. In mutant melanoma cells, a misfolded tyrosinase variant is not subject to normal controls or proteolysis. Therefore, increased production of melanin characteristic of melanoma occurs.

MAGE-A3

MAGE-A3 is a large-molecular-weight protein expressed on melanoma, breast, and glial tumors and non–small-cell lung cancers (NSCLC). Because MAGE-A3 preferentially stimulates cytotoxic (CD8+) T cells, it is an excellent candidate for inclusion in a vaccine. However, CD8 responses are elicited when antigens are presented by human leukocyte antigen (HLA)-A1, -A2, -A24, -B37, and -B44. An experimental MAGE-A3 vaccine has been shown to reduce the re-emergence of NSCLC after conventional surgery.

Carcinoembryonic Antigen

Carcinoembryonic antigen (CEA) is an 180-kDal polypeptide produced during fetal development and functions as a cellular adhesion factor during organ formation. Individuals with colorectal cancers have elevated levels of CEA in the blood. CEA is immunogenic and causes a vigorous T cell response.

Alpha Fetal Protein

Alpha fetal protein (AFP) is the major protein produced by the liver during fetal development. Levels decrease rapidly after birth, reaching steady state levels at 8 to 12 months. AFP is elevated in the serum of individuals with hepatocellular carcinoma, germ-cell tumors, and metastatic cancers.

Heat Shock Proteins

Most tumor antigens belong to a family of heat shock proteins (HSPs) present in the cytosol, endoplasmic reticulum (ER), and mitochondria. HSPs are produced in response to environmental stress (e.g., heat or cold) or cellular stress and act as molecular chaperones that assist in the proper folding of proteins or mark proteins for degradation. On the basis of molecular size, HSPs are subdivided into HSP90 (gp96), HSP70 (HSP/c70), calreticulin, and HSP170 (grp170). Tumor-specific proteins are bound in the binding cleft of the HSPs from tumor cells. Only the peptide–HSP complex is immunogenic. Neither the HSP nor the tumor protein alone stimulates the immune system (Figure 23-1).

The HSP tumor protein complex binds to macrophages and dendritic cells (DCs) using a CD91 receptor. Once internalized, the peptide is processed in both the endogenous and exogenous pathways and presented to lymphocytes using class I and class II molecules (Figure 23-2). HSPs are currently being tested for efficacy in the treatment of patients with recurrent or progressive glioma.

Melanoma Antigen Recognized by T Cells

Melanoma antigen recognized by T cells (MART-1) is a 180-amino-acid protein antigen found on cells in the skin, retina, and melanocytes. This marker is overexpressed in melanoma cells and stimulates a vigorous T cell response.

Table 23-4 Commercially Available Colony-Stimulating Factors

Product	Description	Function	Treatment
Neupogen	G-CSF	Stimulates production of granulocytes	Nonmyeloid malignancies; Acute myelogenous leukemia; Severe chronic neutropenia
Neulasta	Polyethylene glycol conjugated G-CSF	Stimulates long-term production of granulocytes	Nonmyeloid malignancies; Acute myelogenous leukemia; Severe chronic neutropenia
Leukine	GM-CSF	Stimulates production of both granulocytes and macrophages	Acute myelogenous leukemia in older adults

G-CSF, Granulocyte–colony-stimulating factor; *GM-CSF*, granulocyte-macrophage–colony-stimulating factor.

NY-ESO-1

NY-ESO-1 is a 180-amino-acid protein, which is expressed in many different tumors. It is unique in that it stimulates both CD4 and CD8 cells. However, the CD4 response is genetically restricted to antigens presented by DRB1 and DRB4.

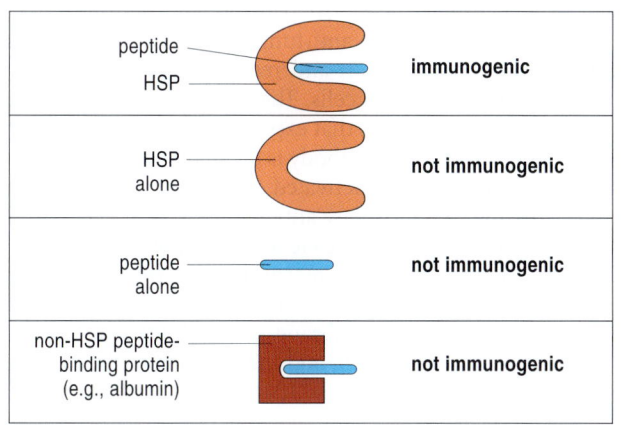

Figure 23-1

Heat shock protein (HSP) molecules chaperone peptides in a peptide-binding pocket. The specificity of immunogenicity derives from the peptides rather than the HSP itself—dissociation of HSP-associated peptides from HSPs abrogate the tumor rejection activity. (From Roitt I, Brostoff J, Male D, et al: Immunology, ed 7, Philadelphia, 2006, Mosby.)

Mucins

Mucins (MUCs) are a family of large-molecular-weight glycoproteins found on epithelial cells. MUC-1 is expressed in almost all solid tumors and some leukemia, lymphoma, multiple myeloma, and breast cancer cells. Over 80% of tumor cells express an underglycosylated, truncated MUC-1 that exposes a neoantigen.

Sialyl Tn Antigen

Some mucins have increased sialylation of terminal structures and are known as *sialyl Tn (sTn) antigens*. The mucin core contributes to tumor cell aggregation and protects metastatic tumor cells from degradation in blood. Tn antigens are overexpressed in gastric, colorectal, ovarian, breast, and pancreatic carcinomas.

CANCER VACCINES

With the exception of the viral vaccines used to prevent cervical and liver cancers, most vaccines are designed to stop cancer tumor growth or eliminate cancer cells remaining after chemotherapy. Vaccines administered to the host can consist of tumor-specific proteins or tumor-associated proteins or carbohydrates, modified autologous or allogeneic tumor cells, antigen-pulsed dendritic cells, idiotypic antigens, viral vectors, or DNA.

Whole-Cell Vaccines

Whole-cell vaccines are prepared using irradiated autologous or allogeneic tumor cells. Autologous vaccines are prepared from a patient's tumor cells and reinjected into the same

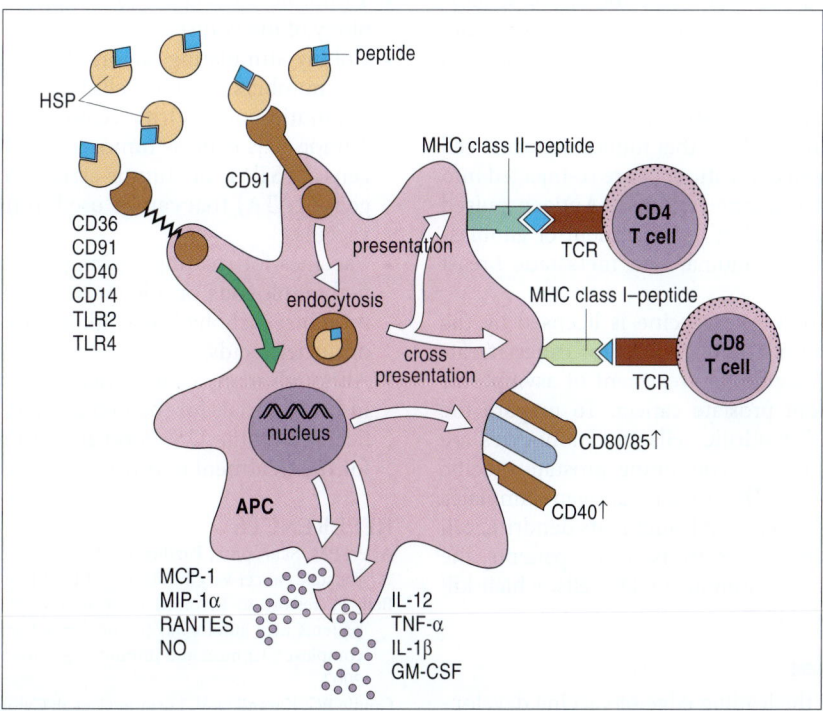

Figure 23-2

Once introduced into the antigen-presenting cell (APC), the heat shock protein (HSP)–chaperoned peptides follow the endogenous class I pathway as well as the exogenous class II pathway of antigen presentation and are processed and represented by the major histocompatibility complex (MHC) class I and MHC class II molecules of the APCs. HSP ligation induces the production of chemokines and cytokines and the upregulation of CD40 and CD80/85. (*MCP-1*, monocyte chemotactic protein-1; *MIP-1α*, macrophage inflammatory protein-1α.) (From Roitt I, Brostoff J, Male D, et al: Immunology, ed 7, Philadelphia, 2006, Mosby. Redrawn from Srivastava P: Nat Rev Immunol 2:185, 2002. Copyright 2002, Nature Reviews Immunology, www.nature.com/reviews.)

patient. These vaccines have limited usefulness because tumor cells rarely express co-stimulatory molecules (e.g., B7-1 or B7-2) necessary to stimulate the immune system. Allogeneic vaccines are prepared from cells grown in the laboratory. Often, these vaccines contain a mixture of cells obtained from several different individuals. To increase immunogenicity, whole-cell vaccines are genetically modified to express co-stimulatory molecules or combined with an adjuvant. Adjuvants create an insoluble depot of antigens, which are slowly released over time and continually stimulate the immune system.

Idiotypic Antigen Vaccines

Idiotypic vaccines are a therapeutic target for treatment of B cell malignancies. Since the malignant cells are derived from a single B cell clone, each B cell in the malignant population has a B cell receptor (a monomeric IgM) with a homogeneous idiotope. Isolation and purification of idiotypic molecules form the basis for the vaccine. Idiotypic vaccines have several limitations. First, the B cell receptor idiotype differs with each patient, and each vaccine must be patient specific. Second, the idiotypic molecules are haptens that must be coupled with an immunogenic protein such as keyhole limpet hemocyanin (KLH) to stimulate the immune system. Idiotypic vaccines produce strong anti-tumor effects and improved clinical outcomes in patients with follicular lymphoma.

Dendritic Cell Vaccines

To prepare the vaccine, intact tumor cells or tumor-specific antigens are reacted with mature dendritic cells isolated from peripheral blood. Tumor cells are ingested and processed and presented in context with class I and class II molecules. In vitro, dendritic cells are often stimulated with GM-CSF, IL-4, and interferon gamma (IFN-γ) that induce dendritic cell maturation. Antigen-pulsed dendritic cells are re-injected into the host to stimulate an immune response. Antigen-pulsed dendritic cell vaccines are used in the treatment of glioblastoma, glioma, ductal cell carcinoma, and metastatic breast cancer.

At the present time, only one vaccine is licensed by the U.S. Food and Drug Administration (FDA) for cancer treatment. Sipuleucel-T is a vaccine for treatment of asymptomatic, hormone-independent prostate cancer. To prepare the vaccine, peripheral blood dendritic cells and monocytes are incubated with a fusion protein containing prostate-specific antigen (PSA) and GM-CSF. The prostate antigen stimulates the immune system, and the GM-CSF augments dendritic cell development and longevity. When infused into patients, the antigen-pulsed dendritic cells stimulate CD8 cells, which kill the tumor cells that express PSAs.

Viral Vector Vaccines

Viral vector vaccines are the leading edge of vaccine development. To prepare the vaccine, tumor antigen genes (transgenes) are inserted into a gene-depleted adenovirus or modified vaccinia Ankara virus that can infect, but not replicate in, human cells.

Continued transcription and translation of transgene DNA results in the production of tumor antigens. Modified adenovirus-containing CEA and GM-CSF genes are being evaluated for the treatment of CEA-expressing tumors.

DNA VACCINES

In the preparation of DNA vaccines, tumor antigen genes are inserted into a small circular, extrachromosomal DNA fragment called a *plasmid*. When injected into the patient, the plasmid begins the transcription and translation of tumor antigens and cytokines.

A plasmid vaccine is currently in clinical trials for the treatment of melanoma. The SCIB1 plasmid vaccine uses a novel mechanism to generate an anti-tumor response, which causes inhibition of tumor growth and regression of both primary and metastatic melanoma cells. The plasmid genes code for a human antibody molecule that expresses a tyrosinase and two helper cell epitopes. The antibody is taken up by dendritic cells and presented to T cells. Activated cells attack any melanoma cells expressing the tyrosinase antigen.

A major limitation of nucleic acid vaccines is that only a small fraction of the injected plasmids reach the nucleus. The application of an electrical pulse to the cell membrane (electroporation) increases membrane permeability, the number of plasmids entering the cell, and the strength of the immune response.

SUMMARY

- Cytokines, interleukins (ILs), and growth factors are small-molecular-weight messengers that activate or inhibit the function of leukocytes and accelerate the maturation of precursor cells.
- Interferons (IFNs) are important in the defense against the spread of viral infections in the host.
- Tumor necrosis factor (TNF) plays a role in the pathophysiology of many diseases.
- Colony-stimulating factors (CSFs) are used to restore normal numbers of white cells in peripheral blood or to induce maturation of dendritic cells and monocytes.
- Tumor cells express tumor-associated transplantation antigens (TSTA) or tumor-associated transplantation antigens (TATA) that can be used in the preparation of cancer vaccines.
- Vaccines for treating existing cancers can consist of modified autologous or allogeneic tumor cells, proteins, fusion proteins, carbohydrates, idiotypic molecules, viral vectors, or nucleic acids.
- Although many cancer treatment vaccines are being tested in clinical trials for their efficacy, only Sipuleucel-T has been licensed by the U.S. Food and Drug Administration (FDA) for the treatment of prostate cancer.

REFERENCES

Arlen PM, Skarupa L, Pazdur M, et al: Clinical safety of a viral vector based prostate cancer vaccine strategy, J Urol 178(4 Pt 1):1515, 2007.

Belli F, Testori A, Rivoltini L, et al: Vaccination of metastatic melanoma patients with autologous tumor-derived heat shock protein gp96-peptide complexes: Clinical and immunologic findings, J Clin Oncol 20(20):4169, 2002.

Coulie PG, Karanikas V, Lurquin C, et al: Cytolytic T-cell responses of cancer patients vaccinated with a MAGE antigen, Immunol Rev 188:33, 2002.

de Gruijl TD, van den Eertwegh AJ, Pinedo HM, et al: Whole-cell cancer vaccination: From autologous to allogeneic tumor- and dendritic cell-based vaccines, Cancer Immunol Immunother 57(10):1569, 2008.

Kao JY, Zhang M, Chen CM, et al: Superior efficacy of dendritic cell-tumor fusion vaccine compared with tumor lysate-pulsed dendritic cell vaccine in colon cancer, Immunol Lett 101(2):154, 2005.

Klein G: The strange road to the tumor-specific transplantation antigens (TSTAs), Cancer Immun 1:6, 2001.

Murthy V, Moiyadi A, Sawant R, et al: Clinical considerations in developing dendritic cell vaccine based immunotherapy protocols in cancer, Curr Mol Med 9(6):725, 2009.

Nesslinger NJ, Ng A, Tsang KY, et al: A viral vaccine encoding prostate-specific antigen induces antigen spreading to a common set of self-proteins in prostate cancer patients, Clin Cancer Res 16(15):4046, 2009.

Ovali E, Dikmen T, Sonmez M, et al: Active immunotherapy for cancer patients using tumor lysate pulsed dendritic cell vaccine: A safety study, J Exp Clin Cancer Res 26(2):209, 2007.

Patel PH, Kockler DR, Sipuleucel T: A vaccine for metastatic, asymptomatic, androgen-independent prostate cancer, Ann Pharmacother 42(1):91, 2008.

Ruffini PA, Neelapu SS, Kwak LW, et al: Idiotypic vaccination for B-cell malignancies as a model for therapeutic cancer vaccines: From prototype protein to second generation vaccines, Haematologica 87(9):989, 2002.

Saenz-Badillos J, Amin SP, Granstein RD: RNA as a tumor vaccine: A review of the literature, Exp Dermatol 10(3):143, 2001.

Scanlan MJ, Gordon CM, Williamson B, et al: Identification of cancer/testis genes by database mining and mRNA expression analysis, Int J Cancer 98(4):485, 2002.

Srivastava P: Interaction of heat shock proteins with peptides and antigen presenting cells: Chaperoning of the innate and adaptive immune responses, Annu Rev Immunol 20:395, 2002.

Toh HC, Wang WW, Chia WK, et al: Clinical benefit of allogeneic melanoma cell lysate-pulsed autologous dendritic cell vaccine in MAGE-positive colorectal cancer patients, Clin Cancer Res 15(24):7726, 2009.

ASSESSMENT QUESTIONS

1. The only FDA-approved vaccine for the treatment of tumors is indicated for treatment of:
   A. Breast cancer
   B. Melanoma
   C. Prostate cancer
   D. Glioma

2. In the development of viral vaccines for treatment of cancer, which of the following viruses are used?
   I.   Adenoviruses
   II. Vaccinia virus
   III. Cytomegalovirus
   A. I
   B. III
   C. I and II
   D. II and III
   E. I, II, and II

3. Idiotypic vaccines are small fragments of the:
   I.   B cell receptor
   II. T cell receptor
   III. Immunoglobulin G (IgG) antibody
   A. I
   B. III
   C. I and II
   D. II and III
   E. I, II, and III

4. Which of the following neutralizes the physiologic effects of interleukin 1 (IL-1)?
   A. Anakinra
   B. Daclizumab
   C. Basiliximab
   D. Oprelvekin

5. Autologous whole-cell tumor cells are ineffective as vaccines because they lack:
   A. T cell receptors
   B. Class I molecules
   C. Co-stimulatory molecules
   D. Killer cell immunoglobulin-like receptors (KIRs)

6. Which of the following is *not* a tumor-specific transplantation antigen?
   A. Tyrosinase
   B. MAGE-A3
   C. NY-ESO-1
   D. Heat shock protein

CHAPTER 24

Vaccines in Theory and Practice

LEARNING OBJECTIVES

- Define virulence factors
- Compare and contrast exotoxins, endotoxins, and enterotoxins
- Identify mucosal-associated lymphoid tissue (MALT) inductive and effector sites
- Compare the anatomic features of nasal-associated lymphoid tissue (NALT), bronchial-associated lymphoid tissue (BALT), and gut-associated lymphoid tissue (GALT)
- List the seven different types of vaccines
- Define attenuation
- Identify the five live attenuated viral vaccines
- Recognize the three live attenuated bacterial vaccines
- Compare and contrast the advantages and disadvantages of live attenuated vaccines
- Define inactivated vaccine
- List the advantages and disadvantages of inactivated vaccines
- Define subunit vaccine
- Compare and contrast toxins and toxoids
- Define conjugate vaccine
- Identify the usefulness of a conjugate vaccine
- Recognize reassortment vaccines
- Define recombinant vaccine
- Compare and contrast the advantages and disadvantages of bacterial or fungal expression vectors
- Identify the two viral vectors used in recombinant vaccines
- Understand the method used to create plant vaccines
- Define adjuvants
- Compare and contrast systemic and mucosal adjuvants
- Identify the mechanisms by which aluminum salts stimulate the immune system
- Compare and contrast Freund's complete adjuvant (FCA) and Freund's incomplete adjuvant (FIA)
- Identify the impediments to using FCA in humans
- Discuss the relationship between muramyl dipeptide and mycobacterial cell walls
- Compare and contrast monophosphoryl lipid (MPL) and muramyl dipeptide (MDP)
- Define oligonucleotide
- Recognize the three different oligodeoxynucleotide (ODN) classes and their functions
- Relate the structural and biologic functions of liposomes
- Define excipient

KEY TERMS

Adjuvant
Attenuation
Endotoxin
Enterotoxin
Exotoxin
Fimbriae
Freund's adjuvant
Liposomes
Oligonucleotide
Pili
Squalene
Toxoids
Vaccine

INTRODUCTION

Vaccination began with Lady Mary Wortley Montagu, the wife of the English Ambassador to Turkey. In 1723, she popularized the Turkish practice of variolation, in which small amounts of dried smallpox were scratched into the skin of healthy people. In fact, the term *variola* comes from the Latin word *varus*, meaning "mark on the skin." Variolation proved to be protective against smallpox infection. In 1796, Edward Jenner heard stories that dairymaids were immune to smallpox if they had previously been infected with cowpox. Jenner showed that infections with cowpox provided protection from smallpox and that cowpox could be transmitted from dairymaid to dairymaid as a deliberate protection mechanism. Using the Latin word *vacca*, meaning "cow," Jenner coined the name for the new procedure *vaccination*.

Louis Pasteur recognized the value of Jenner's work and believed that vaccines could prevent many infectious diseases. During his lifetime, Pasteur developed vaccines for chicken cholera, rabies, and anthrax by using weakened organisms. In the twentieth century, microbiologists came to understand the differences between innocuous and infectious microbes. Highly infectious bacteria were termed *virulent organisms* and infectivity was determined by the presence of virulence factors.

VIRULENCE FACTORS

Virulence factors include molecules that allow bacterial attachment to mammalian cells such as bacterial pili and fimbriae; polysaccharide capsules that surround pneumococcus and

Pseudomonas and prevent phagocytosis; and toxins produced or released from gram-positive and gram-negative bacteria, respectively.

Three types of toxins are produced by bacteria: (1) *Exotoxins* are proteins synthesized and secreted by gram-positive bacteria. Exotoxins destroy mammalian cells or disrupt cellular function. For example, diphtheria toxin inhibits ribosome function and protein translation in mammalian cells, which ultimately kills the cells. Tetanus toxin accelerates the production of neurotransmitters that promote muscle contraction in the face (lockjaw) or in the long muscles in the back (opistothenosis). (2) *Endotoxins* are lipopolysaccharide components of the gram-negative cell wall. They consist of a long antigenic polysaccharide and a lipid A fragment that interacts with mammalian cells and contributes to septic or endotoxic shock. Unlike exotoxins, endotoxins are only released on the death of the bacteria. (3) *Enterotoxins* are secreted molecules that cause food poisoning and diarrhea. Staphylococcal, cholera, and clostridia enterotoxins produce transient effects in humans. *Escherichia coli* O157:H7 produces a potent enterotoxin that causes severe diarrhea, dehydration, and death.

TYPES OF VACCINES

Vaccines are administered by subcutaneous, intramuscular, or mucosal routes. Administration by the intramuscular or subcutaneous route stimulates systemic immunity in the spleen, lymph nodes, and peripheral blood. The vaccines interrupt person-to-person transmission and prevent the spread of infectious agents to the critical organs in the body. Mucosal vaccines stimulate local immune responses to microbes at the point of entry into the body. Moreover, antigen-stimulated lymphocytes from the initial site travel to other mucosal surfaces conferring immunity at multiple mucosal sites (see Chapter 1). Mucosal vaccines are advantageous because they prevent both infection and dissemination to critical organs and are easy to administer.

ROUTE OF ADMINISTRATION AND MUCOSAL IMMUNITY

The route of administration determines which mucosal surface is stimulated by microbial agents. Oral administration induces antibody responses in the small intestine, ascending colon, and mammary and salivary glands. In contrast, nasal administration protects the upper airways and the lungs but has no effect on the lymphoid tissue in the gut (Figure 24-1).

Mucosal-Associated Lymphoid Tissue

Mucosal-associated lymphoid tissue (MALT) is a generic name for collections of lymphoid cells, small lymphoid nodes, and organs found in the gastrointestinal, urogenital, and respiratory tracts (see Chapter 1). MALT has both inductive and effector sites in the mucosa. Inductive sites include mucosal lymphoid nodules as well as M cells that transport foreign material to the lymphocytes in the submucosa. In the lymphoid nodes, T and B cells interact to produce immunoglobulin A (sIgA). Following antigen stimulation, T and B cells migrate to multiple effector sites throughout the submucosa. MALT is divided into segments on the basis of anatomic location: nasal-associated lymphoid tissue (NALT), bronchial-associated lymphoid tissue (BALT), and gut-associated lymphoid tissue (GALT).

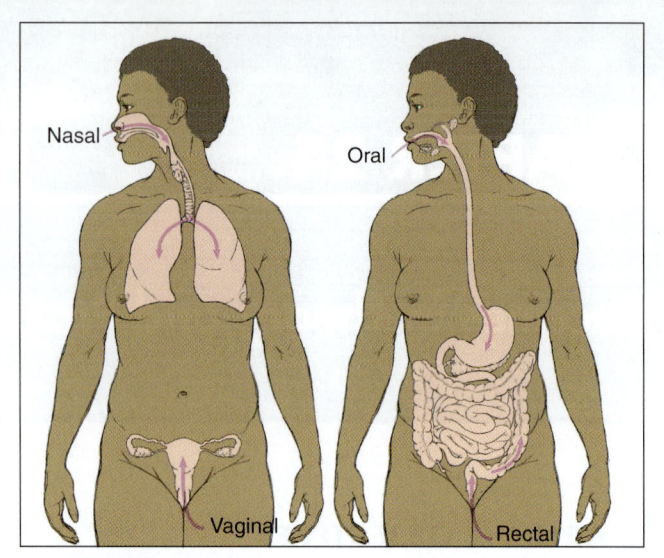

Figure 24-1

Vaccination routes and protection of organs and tissue. (From van Ginkel FW, Nguyen HH, McGhee JR: Vaccines for mucosal immunity to combat emerging infectious diseases, Emerg Infect Dis 6(2):1, 2000.)

Nasal-Associated Lymphoid Tissue

NALT is found in the salivary glands and the Waldeyer's ring, including the palatine, tubal, pharyngeal, and lingual tonsils. Tonsillar anatomy is similar to that of lymph nodes in that it contains T and B cells in follicular germinal centers and mantle zones. B cells in tonsillar germinal centers produce a predominance of IgG antibodies rather than sIgA antibodies.

Bronchial-Associated Lymphoid Tissue

BALT comprises lymphocyte aggregations located randomly along the bronchial tree. More defined aggregations are found around the bifurcations of the bronchi and bronchioli. Both T and B cells are found in the aggregates. B cells are heavily skewed toward the production of sIgA.

Gut-Associated Lymphoid Tissue

Lymphocytes are scattered beneath the epithelium along the entire gastrointestinal tract. Organized lymphocyte clusters in Peyer's patches contain CD4+ T helper cells, mature B cells, macrophages, and dendritic cells (see Chapter 1). GALT functions to protect mucous membranes from colonization and infections by pathogenic organisms.

TYPES OF VACCINES

- Live, attenuated vaccines
- Inactivated vaccines
- Subunit vaccines
- Toxoid vaccines
- Conjugate vaccines
- Recombinant vector vaccines
- Virosomes
- Plant vaccines

Live Attenuated Vaccines

Before a live organism can be used in a vaccine, it must undergo a process known as *attenuation*, which reduces virulence while maintaining immunogenicity. In the classic attenuation process, microbes are passed through unnatural hosts, grown on unusual media, or exposed to harsh chemicals for extended periods. As a consequence, microbes usually lose the critical genes necessary to produce virulence factors.

A new approach known as *rationale attenuation* inactivates or removes virulence genes by targeted mutation or gene deletion. Because of their small genome, viruses are relatively easy to attenuate. The Sabin polio, measles–mumps–rubella (MMR), chickenpox, herpes zoster, and hepatitis A vaccines contain live attenuated viruses. Bacteria, which have a larger genome, are more difficult to attenuate. Only three bacteria have been attenuated and used in vaccines. Live attenuated vaccines for typhoid fever and cholera are used in some parts of the world. Attenuated *Mycobacterium bovis*, known as *Bacille Calmette-Guérin (BCG)*, is used as a vaccine in Europe and other countries. In veterinary medicine, a live attenuated *Bacillus anthracis* Sterne strain is used to vaccinate cows and horses against anthrax.

The use of live attenuated vaccines has advantages as well as disadvantages. A major advantage is that the body does not differentiate between an attenuated microbe and a wild-type microbe, and both elicit a vigorous, long-lasting immune response. Moreover, only one immunization is required for lasting protection.

However, attenuated viral and bacterial vaccines have some disadvantages. Viruses used in vaccines can mutate and revert to being virulent organisms. For example, it is estimated that 1 case per 2.5 million doses of the attenuated, oral Sabin vaccine results in vaccine-associated poliomyelitis. Live attenuated viruses are also shed by the respiratory route and pose a health risk to immunosuppressed individuals. Conversely, live attenuated bacterial vaccines often fail to stimulate MALT. For example, attenuated cholera bacteria fail to express a molecule necessary for M cell attachment and transport the bacteria to MALT located in the submucosa. Attenuated *Salmonella* bacteria are better immunogens, but three to four immunizations are necessary to stimulate MALT, and protection is achieved in only 66% of vaccinated individuals.

Unlike other live attenuated vaccines, the BCG vaccine is highly successful in preventing person-to-person transmission of tuberculosis and has few side effects. When children are vaccinated, the vaccine elicits a cell-mediated response that is highly protective in 80% to 90% of children. The BCG vaccine is used in countries that have a high incidence of tuberculosis, tuberculomeningitis, and blood-borne tuberculosis. More than one billion individuals have been vaccinated since 1921 with few side effects. The vaccine is not used in the United States because of the low incidence of tuberculosis and the vaccine's interference with tuberculosis skin tests. Individuals vaccinated with BCG will have false-positive skin tests, and this often complicates or delays decisions concerning treatment.

Inactivated Vaccines

Inactivated vaccines consist of organisms killed by physical or chemical means. Killed bacteria are advantageous because they do not revert to the virulent state and pose little health risk to immunosuppressed subjects. However, they have several disadvantages. When administered intramuscularly, subcutaneously, or by both routes, inactivated vaccines are only weakly immunogenic and often require booster immunizations to achieve lasting protection. The Salk polio and some seasonal influenza vaccines contain inactivated viruses.

Subunit Vaccines

Whole-cell vaccines often contain nonantigenic molecules that can cause rare systemic and frequent local adverse health effects. Toxicity is reduced by eliminating all nonantigenic molecules while retaining the antigenic molecules or critical epitopes that are necessary for protection against infection. For example, the pertussis component of the diphtheria–pertussis–tetanus (DPT) vaccine comprises inactivated pertussis toxin, purified filamentous hemagglutinin, fimbriae, and pertactin. Subunit vaccines are advantageous because they do not cause infections and pose little risk to immunosuppressed individuals.

Toxoid Vaccines

Modified bacterial exotoxins known as *toxoids* are used in vaccines. Toxins are treated with iodine, pepsin, ascorbic acid, or formalin (a mixture of formaldehyde and sterile water) to reduce toxicity while retaining the ability to stimulate an immune response. Antibodies directed at the toxoid neutralize exotoxins before they reach the target cell. Diphtheria and tetanus vaccines contain toxoids which stimulate an immune response.

Conjugate Vaccines

Polysaccharide capsules are the major virulence factors for pneumococcus and *Pseudomonas* but have limited usefulness in vaccines because they are poor immunogens and type II T cell–independent antigens (see Chapter 8). To elicit a T cell–dependent response and the generation of memory cells, capsular polysaccharides are usually conjugated to tetanus toxoid (*Haemophilus* vaccine), diphtheria protein (*Pneumococcus*), or an outer membrane complex from *Neisseria meningitidis* serogroup B. Conjugate vaccines against *Haemophilus* and pneumococcus are included in the routine pediatric immunization schedules.

Reassortment Vaccines

Reassortment vaccines usually contain a noninfective virus that expresses antigens from multiple human and animal strains of the same virus. For example, a chicken egg can be infected with two different viruses. One strain can infect humans, while the other strain is noninfective but grows well in eggs. One of the genetic reassortments in the egg produces a virus that expresses the antigens from the infective virus but is noninfective and grows well in eggs. This reassortment virus would be used in a vaccine. Another example of reassortment is the rotavirus vaccine. Rhesus monkey or bovine rotavirus strains (which do not infect humans) and three human–rhesus reassortment rotavirus strains are mixed together. The reassortment rotavirus, which expresses antigens from all four strains and does not infect or replicate in humans, is used in the vaccine.

Recombinant Bacterial Vaccines

Plasmids containing antigen genes from virulent organisms are inserted into nonpathogenic commensal organisms such as *Lactobacillus, Lactococcus,* or *Streptococcus gordonii*. When transcribed and translated, the antigens and virulence factors are expressed on the surface of the nonpathogenic organism. When administered as a vaccine, a strong immune response is generated to the virulence factors.

Recombinant Viral Vaccines

Genes from pathogenic microbes can also be added to attenuated viruses. Members of the poxvirus family (e.g., vaccinia, fowlpox, canarypox) and adenoviruses are common viral vectors. The most common vector is an attenuated vaccinia Ankara virus (MVA), which has lost 15% to 20% of the genes required for viral replication. It cannot replicate in human cells, but antigenic proteins are continually transcribed and translated.

Antigen-expressing, replication-deficient adenovirus vectors are also used in vaccines. In vivo adenovirus vectors stimulate dendritic cell maturation and strong immune response. The usefulness of adenovirus vaccine vectors is limited because most people have pre-existing antibodies to adenoviruses and the vector is neutralized before it can infect target tissue.

Heterologous Recombinant Proteins

Plasmids with microbial or viral genes coding for virulence factors are inserted into commensal *E. coli* or baker's yeast. These expression vectors synthesize and secrete antigenic proteins from pathogenic bacteria or microbes. Antigens are purified from growth media. The hepatitis B vaccine contains purified antigens produced by yeast expression vectors.

Although yeast expression systems provide a low-cost, high-volume method for antigen production, they have limitations. Secreted proteins are often misfolded, truncated, or lack the three-dimensional structure of the target antigen. Aberrant proteins generate a weak immune response.

PLANT VACCINES

Experimental edible vaccines, which offer protection against diarrheal disease, have been developed by using potatoes, rice, and bananas as vaccinating agents. To prepare a vaccine, microbial antigen genes are inserted into a Ti plasmid isolated from *Agrobacterium tumefaciens*. A modified Ti plasmid is capable of integrating into the plant cell genome and transforming the plant. The mature, transformed plant produces glycosylated microbial proteins in the edible parts of the plant. After the plant part is ingested, antigens stimulate local immunity, systemic immunity, or both. The benefits of edible vaccines are enormous. Inexpensive vaccines can be grown locally and administration of these vaccines does not require invasive medical procedures.

ADJUVANTS

When used with vaccinating agents, adjuvants augment systemic or mucosal immunity. Adjuvants in vaccines designed to elicit systemic immunity (intramuscular or subcutaneous administration) create an insoluble antigen depot at the vaccination site. Slow release of the antigen from the depot stimulates the immune system over an extended period. A different strategy is used to stimulate MALT. Mucosal adjuvants complex with the antigen and deliver it to M cells, which transport the antigen to submucosal lymphocytes. Mucosal adjuvants are usually proteins from pathogenic enteric bacteria, enterotoxins, or deoxyribonucleic acid (DNA). Attachment to M cells requires that the adjuvant have the same size, charge, and hydrophobicity as the native molecule.

Adjuvants and Systemic Immunity
Aluminum Salts
Aluminum hydroxide, aluminum phosphate, and potassium aluminum sulfate (alum) are used as adjuvants in vaccines designed to stimulate systemic immunity. Aluminum salts are used in DPT, pneumoccal conjugate, hepatitis A, papilloma, anthrax, and rabies vaccines. Like other systemic adjuvants, they form an insoluble depot and slowly release the antigen, which stimulates an antibody response.

Although adjuvants containing aluminum salts are safe, they do induce granulomas at the vaccination site. In some individuals, an increased risk of immunoglobulin E (IgE) production and neurotoxicity exists.

Squalene Adjuvants
Squalene is a naturally occurring molecule found in plants and some foods. MF59 and ASO3 adjuvants consist of a small concentration of squalene (4.3%) and Tween 80 surfactant. Squalene is a weak adjuvant and other immunogenic molecules (e.g., mycobacterial cord factor or lipid A) are usually added to increase immunogenicity. Squalene adjuvants have been a component of influenza vaccines in Europe since 1997, and over 22 million individuals have been vaccinated with few adverse effects. Squalene adjuvants are not used in vaccines licensed in the United States.

Freund's Adjuvants
Freund's complete adjuvant (FCA) was the first adjuvant used to enhance immune responses. FCA is composed of killed *Mycobacterium tuberculosis* or *M. butyricum* suspended in mineral oil, water, and a surfactant called *mannide monooleate*. Although FCA is highly effective in stimulating a cell-mediated inflammatory response, it cannot be used in humans because it causes inflammatory reactions, ulcerations, and granulomas at the injection site. Oil and water emulsions without killed mycobacteria are known as *Freund's incomplete adjuvant (FIA)*, which stimulates only an antibody response. FIA is occasionally used in vaccines.

Muramyl Peptides
N-Acetylmuramyl-L-alanyl-D-isoglutamine, or muramyl dipeptide (MDP), is a *Mycobacterium* cell wall fragment, which is a nontoxic adjuvant. The adjuvant effect varies with the route of administration. When administered in saline, it induces an antibody response. A strong cellular immune response is induced when MDP is mixed with glycerol. Mifamurtide, a synthetic derivative of MDP, is licensed in Europe for augmenting the immune response in patients with nonmetastasizing, resectable osteosarcoma.

Liposomes
Liposomes are synthetic phosphatidylcholine lipid bilayers similar to those found in mammalian membranes. Under proper conditions, antigens can be incorporated into spherical liposomes. To stimulate the systemic immune system, liposomes fuse with macrophage membranes, and antigens are internalized and processed for presentation to lymphocytes. Liposomes are ineffective in stimulating mucosal immunity because they become trapped in the intestinal mucosal layer and never reach the M cells.

Adjuvants and Mucosal Immunity
Monophosphoryl Lipid A
Monophosphoryl lipid A (MPL) is a detoxified endotoxin lipid A fraction, which lacks a saccharide and a phosphate group. The detoxified MPL has no physiologic toxicity but retains the adjuvant effect of the parental endotoxin. The mechanism of action is unclear. Evidence indicates that MPL upregulates co-stimulatory molecules (B7-1 and B7-2) on monocytes,

Table 24-1 ISS Class and Stimulation of Immunocompetent Cells

ISS Class	Sequence and Structural Elements	Plasmacytoid Dendritic Cell INF-α Production	Plasmacytoid Dendritic Cell Maturation	B Cell Activation
CpG-A	Phosphodiester CpG motifs flanked by phosphorothioate polyguanosine	++++	±	±
CpG-B	CgG motifs phosphorothioate monomers	±	+++	+++
CpG-C	5' TCG and >12-nucleotide palindromic sequences and phosphorothioate monomers	+++	+++	+++

Modified from Higgins D, Marshall JD, Traquina P, et al: Immunostimulatory DNA as a vaccine adjuvant, Expert Rev Vaccines 6(5):747, 2007.

macrophages, and dendritic cells. It may also stimulate the maturation of CD4Th1 and CD4Th2 cytokines. MPL is used as an adjuvant in hepatitis B vaccines licensed in select European countries. Ceravix, a vaccine for papilloma-induced cervical cancer, also uses MPL and aluminum hydroxide as adjuvants.

Bacterial Enterotoxins

Cholera toxins (CTs) and heat labile (LT) *E. coli*–associated enterotoxins are closely related and cause cholera and traveler's diarrhea, respectively. Enterotoxins are useful adjuvants that increase antigen presentation and B cell differentiation into plasma cells producing sIgA. Both have limited usefulness because of the generation of a strong immune response to the enterotoxins. Significant safety issues are related to the use of intact enterotoxins as adjuvants. Both are highly toxic and cause diarrhea, Bell's palsy, and other neurologic effects.

A novel fusion-protein adjuvant reduces the toxicity associated with enterotoxins. The fusion protein consists of the α_1-subunit of the cholera toxin (CTA) fused with a B cell targeting molecule (D) from *Staphylococcus aureus* protein A. The CTA1-DD adjuvant is nontoxic when administered intranasally or parenterally. It acts by increasing the production of secretory IgA and IgG.

Oligodeoxynucleotides

Unlike mammalian DNA, bacterial DNA contains islands with a high percentage of unmethylated CpG dinucleotides. The term *CpG* refers to a cytosine connected to a guanine by a phosphate group. These sequences, known as *CpG motifs* or *immunostimulatory sequences (ISSs)*, are divided into three different classes (Table 24-1).

CpG-A oligodeoxynucleotides (ODNs) are large-molecular-weight aggregates with 200 to 600 base pairs (bps). CpG-A motifs induce the synthesis of interferon alpha (IFN-α) from human peripheral blood mononuclear and plasmacytoid dendritic cells. In turn, the IFN activates natural killer cells to become lymphokine-activated killer (LAK) cells. CpG-B has a phosphothionate DNA backbone and few CpGs. The B class ODNs activate B cells and upregulate class II molecules. Recently, a third class of ODNs (CpG-C) has been described. CpG-C blends the properties of both A and B classes and drives the differentiation of CD8 cytotoxic T lymphocytes (CTLs).

EXCIPIENTS IN VACCINES

Excipients are additives found in vaccines. Some are purposefully added to prevent microbial contamination or to stabilize the vaccines. Other excipients are remnants of the manufacturing process that are carried over into the final product. Excipients found in vaccines include antibiotics, egg protein, monosodium glutamate, gelatin, yeast, and latex.

Antibiotics

Antibiotics are commonly used in the production of bacterial and viral vaccines to prevent contamination. Antibiotics such as neomycin, polymyxin B, gentamicin, or streptomycin are carried over into the final vaccine. Although these antibiotics are generally regarded as safe, the risk of antibiotic-induced contact dermatitis at the injection site does exist. A history of contact dermatitis is not a contraindication for the administration of vaccines containing antibiotics. However, persons with more serious reactions to these antibiotics should be cognizant of the risk. Vaccines containing antibiotics are listed in Tables 24-2 and 24-3.

Egg Protein

Several viruses used in vaccines are grown in embryonated chicken eggs (e.g., influenza vaccines) or tissue culture–adapted chicken embryo fibroblasts (e.g., measles and mumps vaccines). Egg albumin from eggs or tissue culture media is often carried over into influenza vaccines. Although anaphylaxis is a theoretical risk in individuals with egg allergy, those with a history of nonfatal egg-induced anaphylaxis tolerate exposure to vaccines with 1.2 µg/mL or 0.6 µg/dose of egg protein. However, individuals highly sensitive to egg protein should consult their physicians before receiving vaccination. Vaccines containing egg protein are listed in Table 24-4.

Monosodium Glutamate

Monosodium glutamate (MSG) causes a syndrome commonly referred to as *Chinese restaurant syndrome*, or *MSG symptom complex*. The most common symptoms are hives, abdominal cramps, nausea, vomiting, and diarrhea. The mechanism is unclear, and evidence does not support an IgE-mediated reaction. The incidence of adverse effects caused by MSG in vaccines is unknown. Vaccines containing MSG are listed in Table 24-5.

Gelatin

Gelatin is found in MMR, varicella, shingles, and rabies vaccines and protects the vaccine from the effects of heat and cold. Gelatin produced by boiling the bones and connective tissue of cows and pigs or poorly hydrolyzed gelatin in vaccines increase the risk for allergic reactions and anaphylaxis. The incidence of gelatin anaphylaxis in the United States is

Table 24-2	Vaccines Containing Neomycin	
Vaccine	**Target Microbe**	**Neomycin Concentration**
Afluria (CSL)	Influenza	≤0.2 pg
Attenuvax (Merck)	Measles	25 µg
Dryvax (W)	Smallpox	100 µg/mL
Fluvirin (Novartis)	Influenza	≤2.5 µg
H1N1 (CSL)	H1N1 influenza	≤0.2 pg
H1N1 (Novartis)	H1N1 influenza	≤2.5 µg
Havrix (GSK)	Hepatitis A	≤40 ng/mL
Imovax Rabies (sp)	Rabies	<150 µg
IPOL (sp)	Polio	<5 ng
Kinrix (GSK)	Diphtheria–tetanus–acellular pertussis (DTaP)/inactivated polio virus (IPV)	≤0.05 ng
Meruvax II (Merck)	Rubella	25 µg
MMR II (Merck)	Measles–mumps–rubella (MMR)	25 µg
Mumpsvax (Merck)	Mumps	25 µg
Pediarix (GSK)	Diphtheria–tetanus–acellular pertussis (DTaP)–hepatitis B–inactivated polio virus (IPV)	≤0.05 ng
Pentacel (sp)	DTaP–IPV–*Haemophilus influenzae* type B (Hib)	<4 pg
ProQuad (Merck)	MMR + Varicella	<16 µg
RabAvert (Chiron)	Rabies	<1 µg
Twinrix (GSK)	Hepatitis AB	≤20 ng
Varivax (Merck)	Varicella	Trace amounts
Zostavax (Merck)	Varicella zoster	Trace amounts

Modified from the Institute for Vaccine Safety. Johns Hopkins Bloomberg School of Public Health: www.vaccinesafety.edu. Accessed 12/01/10.

Table 24-4	Vaccines Containing Hen Egg Albumin	
Vaccine	**Target Molecule**	**Egg Albumin Concentration**
Afluvia (CSL)	Influenza	≤1 µg
Fluarix (GSK)	Influenza	≤0.1 µg
FluLaval (GSK)	Influenza	≤1 µg
Fluvirin (Novartis)	Influenza	Residual
Fluzone (sp)	Influenza	Residual
H1N1 (CSL)	H1N1 Influenza	≤1 µg
H1N1 (Novartis)	H1N1 Influenza	≤1 µg

Modified from the Institute for Vaccine Safety. Johns Hopkins Bloomberg School of Public Health: www.vaccinesafety.edu. Accessed 12/01/10.

Table 24-5	Vaccines Containing Monosodium Glutamate	
Vaccine	**Target Microbe**	**MSG Concentration**
Flumist (MedImmune)	Influenza	0.188 mg/dose
H1N1-nasal (MedImmune)	H1N1 Influenza	0.188 mg/dose
ProQuad (Merck)	MMR + Varicella	0.4 mg
Varivax (Merck)	Varicella	0.5 mg
Zostavax (Merck)	Varicella zoster	0.62 mg

Modified from the Institute for Vaccine Safety. Johns Hopkins Bloomberg School of Public Health: www.vaccinesafety.edu. Accessed 12/01/10.

Table 24-3	Vaccines Containing Polymyxin B, Gentamicin, or Streptomycin		
Antibiotic	**Vaccine**	**Target Microbe**	
Polymyxin B	Dryvax (W)	Smallpox	
	Fluvirin (Novartis)	Influenza	
	H1N1 (Novartis)	H1N1 Influenza	
	IPOL (sp)	Polio	
	Kinrix (GSK)	Diphtheria–tetanus–acellular pertussis (DTaP)/inactivated polio virus (IPV)	
	Pediarix (GSK)	DTaP–hepatitisB–IPV	
	Pentacel (sp)	DTaP–IPV–*Haemophilus influenzae* type B (Hib)	
Gentamicin	Flumist (MedImmune)	Influenza	
	Fluarix (GSK)	Influenza	
	H1N1-nasal (MedImmune)	H1N1 Influenza	
Streptomycin	Dryvax (W)	Smallpox	

Modified from the Institute for Vaccine Safety. Johns Hopkins Bloomberg School of Public Health: www.vaccinesafety.edu. Accessed 12/01/10.

reported to be 1.8 cases per one million doses after the introduction of gelatin-containing vaccines. Gelatin-containing vaccines are listed in Table 24-6.

Latex

Natural rubber is used in the manufacture of syringe plungers, vial stoppers, and injection ports. Because rubber is obtained and processed in countries other than the United States, some rubber contains allergens or allergenic products carried over from the manufacturing process. Although rare, injection-associated allergic reactions to latex have been reported. A case was reported of a patient with severe latex allergy who suffered an anaphylactic reaction following the administration of the hepatitis B vaccine.

SUMMARY

- Vaccines are necessary to prevent person-to-person transmission of infectious diseases.
- Vaccines contain virulence factors from bacteria and viruses.
- Vaccines stimulate systemic or mucosal immunity.
- Killed, attenuated, subunit, conjugate, and reassortment vaccines are licensed in the United States.
- Adjuvants are added to vaccines to enhance the immune response to microbial and viral virulence factors.
- Additives or excipients such as antibiotics, egg protein, monosodium glutamate, gelatin, and latex are found in vaccines.

Table 24-6 Vaccines Containing Porcine Gelatin

Vaccine	Target Microbe	Gelatin Concentration
Attenuvax (Merck)	Measles	Hydrolyzed gelatin, 14.5 mg
Flumist (MedImmune)	Influenza	Hydrolyzed gelatin, 2.00 mg
Fluzone (Sanofi Pasteur)	Influenza	0.05% (added as a stabilizer)
H1N1 (Sanofi Pasteur)	H1N1 Influenza	0.05% (added as a stabilizer)
H1N1-nasal (MedImmune)	H1N1 Influenza	Hydrolyzed gelatin, 2.00 mg
JE-Vax (RIMD/BIKEN)	Japanese encephalitis	<500 µg
Meruvax II (Merck)	Rubella	Hydrolyzed gelatin, 14.5 mg
MMR II (Merck)	Measles–mumps–rubella (MMR)	Hydrolyzed gelatin, 11 mg
Mumpsvax (Merck)	Mumps	Hydrolyzed gelatin, 14.5 mg
ProQuad (Merck)	MMR + Varicella	Hydrolyzed gelatin, 14.5 mg
Varivax (Merck)	Varicella	Hydrolyzed gelatin, 12.5 mg/dose
YF-Vax (Sanofi Pasteur)	Yellow fever	0.05% as a stabilizer
Zostavax (Merck)	Varicella zoster	Hydrolyzed gelatin, 15.58 mg

Modified from the Institute for Vaccine Safety. Johns Hopkins Bloomberg School of Public Health: www.vaccinesafety.edu. Accessed 12/01/10.

REFERENCES

Agren L, Lowenadler B, Lycke N: A novel concept in mucosal adjuvanticity: The CTA1-DD adjuvant is a B cell-targeted fusion protein that incorporates the enzymatically active cholera toxin A1 subunit, Immunol Cell Biol 76(3):280, 1998.

Audibert FM, Lise LD: Adjuvants: Current status, clinical perspectives and future prospects, Immunol Today 14(6):281, 1993.

Curtiss R III: Bacterial infectious disease control by vaccine development, J Clin Invest 110(8):1061, 2002.

Eldridge JH, Staas JK, Meulbroek JA, et al: Biodegradable microspheres as a vaccine delivery system, Mol Immunol 28(3):287, 1991.

Fine PE: Herd immunity: History, theory, practice, Epidemiol Rev 15(2):265, 1993.

Gagnon R, Primeau MN, Des Roches A, et al: Safe vaccination of patients with egg allergy with an adjuvanted pandemic H1N1 vaccine, J Allergy Clin Immunol 126(2):317, 2007.

Herman JJ, Radin R, Schneiderman R: Allergic reactions to measles (rubeola) vaccine in patients hypersensitive to egg protein, J Pediatr 102(2):196, 1983.

James JM, Zeiger RS, Lester MR, et al: Safe administration of influenza vaccine to patients with egg allergy, J Pediatr 133(5):624, 1998.

Kelso JM, Jones RT, Yunginger AW: Anaphylaxis to measles, mumps, and rubella vaccine mediated by IgE to gelatin, J Allergy Clin Immunol 91(4):867, 1993.

Kotani S, Watanabe Y, Kinoshita F, et al: Immunoadjuvant activities of synthetic N-acetyl-muramyl-peptides or -amino acids, Biken J 18(2):105, 1975.

Neutra MR, Kozlowski PA: Mucosal vaccines: The promise and the challenge, Nat Rev Immunol 6(2):148, 2006.

Petrovsky N, Aguilar JC: Vaccine adjuvants: Current state and future trends, Immunol Cell Biol 82(5):488, 2004.

Pichichero ME, Badgett JT, Rodgers GC Jr, et al: Acellular pertussis vaccine: Immunogenicity and safety of an acellular pertussis vs. a whole cell pertussis vaccine combined with diphtheria and tetanus toxoids as a booster in 18- to 24-month old children, Pediatr Infect Dis J 6(4):352, 1987.

Russell M, Pool V, Kelso JM, et al: Vaccination of persons allergic to latex: A review of safety data in the Vaccine Adverse Event Reporting System (VAERS), Vaccine 23(5):664, 2004.

Singer S, Johnson CE, Mohr R, et al: Urticaria following varicella vaccine associated with gelatin allergy, Vaccine 17(4):327, 2004.

Snider DP: The mucosal adjuvant activities of ADP-ribosylating bacterial enterotoxins, Crit Rev Immunol 15(3–4):317, 1995.

Souza AR, Braga JA, de Paiva TM, et al: Immunogenicity and tolerability of a virosome influenza vaccine compared to split influenza vaccine in patients with sickle cell anemia, Vaccine 28(4):1117, 2010.

Storm G: Liposome advances. Sixth International Conference. Progress in drug and vaccine delivery, IDrugs 7(2):122, 2004.

van der Lubben IM, Verhoef JC, Borchard G, et al: Chitosan and its derivatives in mucosal drug and vaccine delivery, Eur J Pharm Sci 14(3):201, 2001.

Walker RI: New strategies for using mucosal vaccination to achieve more effective immunization 12(5):387, 1994.

Williams AN, Woessner KM: Monosodium glutamate "allergy": Menace or myth? Clin Exp Allergy 39(5):640, 2009.

Worm M, Sterry W, Zuberbier T: Gelatin-induced urticaria and anaphylaxis after tick-borne encephalitis vaccine, Acta Derm Venereol 80(3):232, 2000.

Zinkernagel RM: On natural and artificial vaccinations, Annu Rev Immunol 21:515, 2003.

ASSESSMENT QUESTIONS

1. Which of the following is *not* a live attenuated vaccine?
   A. *Salmonella* vaccine
   B. Cholera vaccine
   C. Bacille Calmette-Guérin (BCG) vaccine
   D. Salk polio vaccine

2. Chemically altered exotoxins are known as:
   A. Endotoxins
   B. Toxoids
   C. Enterotoxins
   D. Excipients

3. Which of the following adjuvants is used to stimulate systemic immunity?
   A. Aluminum salts
   B. Monophosphoryl A
   C. Bacterial endotoxins
   D. Liposomes

4. Which of the following is *not* a characteristic of vaccines containing carbohydrates?
   A. Immunoglobulin M (IgM) antibody production
   B. T cell–independent antigen
   C. Memory cell formation
   D. Repeating epitopes

5. Which of the following are considered virulence factors?
   A. Capsular polysaccharides
   B. Fimbriae
   C. Pili
   D. All of the above

6. Which of the following is a toxin associated with food poisoning and diarrhea?
   A. Exotoxin
   B. Endotoxin
   C. Enterotoxin
   D. Toxoid

CHAPTER 25

Vaccine-Preventable Diseases

LEARNING OBJECTIVES

- Identify the etiologic agent of diphtheria
- Recognize the most virulent strain of diphtheria
- Explain the relationship between iron and diphtheria exotoxin production
- Restate the diphtheria exotoxin mechanism of action
- Design a therapeutic regimen to treat diphtheria
- Define toxoid
- Identify the etiologic agent of whooping cough
- Restate the pertussis toxin mechanism of action
- Design a therapeutic regimen to treat whooping cough
- Compare and contrast whole-cell and acellular pertussis vaccines
- Identify the etiologic agent of tetanus
- Restate the tetanus exotoxin mechanism of action
- Identify the four different types of tetanus
- Design a therapeutic regimen to treat tetanus
- Identify the most common etiologic strain of *Haemophilus* infections
- Identify the major *Haemophilus* virulence factors
- Identify the factors that increase the risk of *Haemophilus* infections in children
- Explain the difference between T cell–dependent antigens and T cell–independent antigens
- Compare and contrast type I and II T cell–independent antigens
- Explain the rationale for conjugating capsular antigens to proteins
- Design a therapeutic regimen to treat *Haemophilus* infections
- Identify the major virulence factor associated with *Streptococcus pneumoniae*
- Identify the four different diseases caused by pneumococcus
- Identify therapeutic agents used to treat pneumococcal diseases
- Discuss the advantages and disadvantages of the licensed pneumococcal vaccines
- Define meningitis
- Identify the major strains of *Neisseria meningitidis* that causes infections in the United States
- Identify the major virulence factors associated with *N. meningitidis*
- Identify the three sequelae associated with meningitis
- Identify the role of lipo-oligosaccharide (LOS) in the pathophysiology of meningitis
- Explain the relationship between *N. meningitidis* and the formation of microthrombi, petechiae, and purpura
- Understand the advantages and disadvantages of the three meningitis vaccines
- Recognize the four different types of polio infections and the three types of paralytic polio
- Discuss the mechanisms involved in post-polio syndrome (PPS)
- Compare and contrast the Sabin vaccine and the Salk vaccine for polio
- Identify the complications of rubeola infections
- Identify the two types of rubeola vaccines
- Compare and contrast rubeola and rubella infections
- Discuss congenital rubella syndrome
- Identify the five complications of mumps infections
- Compare and contrast the pathophysiology of varicella infection and varicella zoster infection
- Identify the four sequelae of chickenpox infections
- Explain the mechanism involved in post-herpetic neuralgia
- Design a therapeutic regimen to treat herpes zoster
- Compare and contrast the varicella vaccine and the varicella zoster vaccine
- Compare the transmission routes of hepatitis A and B
- Design a therapeutic regimen to treat hepatitis
- Compare and contrast the vaccines for hepatitis A and B
- Identify the host range for influenza types A, B, and C
- Explain the roles of hemagglutinins and neuraminidase in influenza infectivity
- Compare and contrast antigenic drift and antigenic shift
- Compare and contrast the pathophysiology of seasonal influenza and pandemic influenza
- Design a therapeutic regimen to treat influenza
- Identify the two types of influenza vaccines
- Compare and contrast inactivated and attenuated influenza vaccines
- Identify the disease caused by rotavirus
- Identify the rotavirus strains endemic in the United States
- Explain the pathophysiology of rotavirus infections
- Compare and contrast the three rotavirus vaccines
- Identify the diseases and syndromes caused by papilloma virus
- Identify the papilloma serotypes that cause skin and genital warts
- Identify the papilloma serotypes that cause 70% of cervical cancers

- Identify the therapeutic agents used to treat papilloma virus infections
- Identify the two papilloma vaccines
- Identify the advantages and limitations of papilloma vaccines

KEY TERMS

Antigenic drift
Antigenic shift
Bacteremia
Bacteriophage
Congenital rubella syndrome
Cytokine storm
Disseminated intravascular coagulopathy (DIC)
Elongation factor 2
Fimbriae
Gamma amino butyric acid
Hemagglutinin
Herd immunity
Intussusceptions
Koplik spots
Lipooligosaccharide
Neuraminidase
Nosocomial infections
Opisthotonos
Orchitis
Osteomyelitis
Otitis media
Pertactin
Post-herpetic neuralgia
Ramsay Hunt syndrome
Reye syndrome
Sabin vaccine
Salk vaccine
Tetanospasmin
Trismus
Vaccine-associated paralytic poliomyelitis (VAPP)

INTRODUCTION

Mass vaccination programs have been highly successful in reducing the 57 million deaths caused by infectious diseases in the world each year. The World Health Organization's (WHO) global initiatives have eradicated smallpox and reduced the incidence of measles and polio deaths. In the last 7 years, vaccination reduced the incidence of measles-related deaths by 74%. Polio is now endemic only in four countries, as opposed to 185 countries in 1988.

In the United States, the success of mass vaccination programs may be one of the greatest public health achievements of the twentieth century. Prior to the institution of mass vaccination programs, 100,000 cases of diphtheria, whooping cough, and tetanus occurred each year. After the institution of vaccination programs, the incidence of these diseases is between 1 and 5000 cases per year. Vaccines against measles, mumps, rubella, and *Haemophilus* have also reduced annual disease incidence to less than 500 cases per year.

Mass vaccination programs are based on the concept of *herd immunity*. When a high proportion of a population is vaccinated, person-to-person disease transmission is interrupted by surrounding the infected person with vaccinated individuals. The percentage of vaccinated individuals necessary to disrupt transmission depends on the infectivity of the microbe and the number of secondary infections that are transmitted by a single index case in a susceptible population. Using these data, crude herd immunity thresholds for potentially vaccine-preventable diseases can be calculated mathematically. The threshold of herd immunity is the minimum percentage of the population that must be immunized to prevent person-to-person transmission. When the minimum threshold is reached, disease transmission is stopped, and the epidemic or pandemic is halted. Herd immunity thresholds for childhood diseases are provided in Table 25-1.

Table 25-1 Herd Immunity Thresholds for Common Childhood Diseases

Infection	No. of Individuals Infected from an Index Case	Herd Immunity Threshold (%)
Diphtheria	6–7	85
Measles	12–18	83–94
Mumps	4–7	75–86
Pertussis	12–17	92–94
Polio	5–7	80–86
Rubella	6–7	83–85

Modified from Fine P: Herd immunity: History, theory, practice, Epidemiol Rev 15(2):265, 1993.

The previous chapter discussed the general nature of vaccines, additives, and adjuvants. This chapter explores the natures of vaccine-preventable diseases and vaccines licensed for use in the United States.

DIPHTHERIA

Diphtheria is a multiple-organ disease caused by gram-positive *Corynebacterium diphtheriae*. The three strains of corynebacteria are *gravis*, *intermedius*, and *mitis*. The gravis strain is the most virulent because it divides every 60 minutes and produces large amounts of exotoxin.

Diphtheria Exotoxin

The exotoxin-producing diphtheria bacteria carries a bacteriophage (bacterial virus) gene (*Dtox*) that codes for the exotoxin. Expression of the *Dtox* gene is controlled by a diphtheria iron-dependent repressor gene (*DtoxR*). If sufficient iron is available, the *DtoxR* gene synthesizes a repressor protein that inhibits the transcription and translation of the *Dtox* gene. When iron stores are exhausted, the repressor protein is not synthesized and the toxin gene is transcribed and translated.

The diphtheria exotoxin is a classic two component A+B protein subunit toxin. Using the B subunit, the intact toxin binds to epidermal growth factor (EGF) receptors on epithelial cells. Protease activity associated with the EGF receptor cleaves the toxin into A and B fragments. The A fragments undergo endocytosis and target nicotinamide adenine dinucleotide (NAD), a coenzyme involved in redox reactions in the cytochrome system. The A subunit has both glycohydrolase and ribosyl transferase activities. Glycohydrolase splits the NAD molecule into nicotinamide and adenosine diphosphate (ADP) ribose. Using the ribosyl transferase function, the A subunit attaches ADP-ribose to histidine (diphthamide) found in the elongation factor 2 (EF-2) protein, which assists in joining of amino acids during protein synthesis (Figure 25-1).

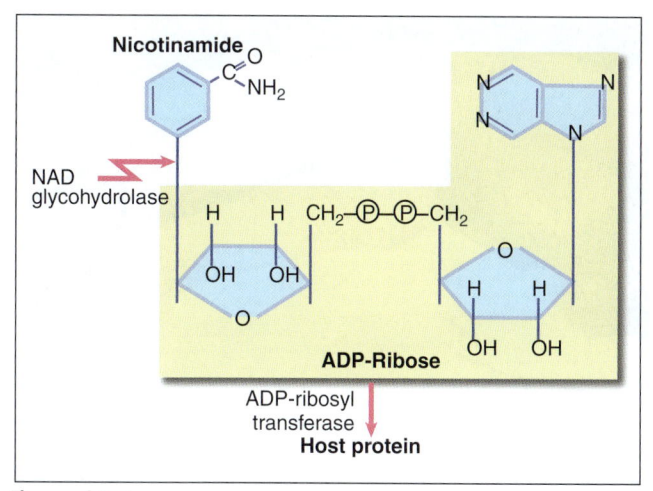

Figure 25-1
Enzymatic activity of adenosine diphosphate (ADP)—ribosylating toxins. These toxins catalyse two processes: (1) the cleavage of nicotinamide from the substrate NAD+ (glycohydrolase) and (2) the transfer of the ADP-ribose moiety to the host target protein (ADP-ribosyl transferase). (From Herderson B, Wilson M, McNab R, et al: Cellular microbiology: Bacteria host interactions in health and disease, Oxford, 1999, Wiley, John & Sons, Inc.)

Exotoxin inactivation of EF-2 prevents peptide elongation. The reaction is as follows:

$$EF\text{-}2 + NAD + Toxin \longrightarrow EF\text{-}2 - ADP\text{ ribose} + NADH$$

Diphtheria Pathophysiology

Diphtheria organisms colonize the tonsils and the pharynx. The secreted exotoxin destroys surrounding tissue, and leakage of blood and plasma in the necrotic tissue activates fibrin, which creates a pseudomembrane at the back of the throat. If untreated, the membrane ultimately obstructs airflow and causes death.

The exotoxin is also transported to the heart, muscle, adrenal glands, kidneys, liver, and spleen. The most frequent diphtheria complications are myocarditis and neuritis. Abnormal heart rhythms occur early in the infection, and necrosis of heart muscle often leads to heart failure.

Treatment

Treatment for active disease usually entails a combination of antitoxin and antibiotics. Equine diphtheria antitoxin is available from the Centers for Disease Control and Prevention (CDC). Antitoxin is most effective in the early stages of the infection because it neutralizes free diphtheria. A 14-day regimen of erythromycin or intramuscular procaine penicillin G also is recommended to treat active cases. Since the bacterium is transmitted by respiratory aerosols, persons coming in contact with the infected patient are given a course of benzathine penicillin G or oral erythromycin. Therapeutics used to treat diphtheria are listed in Table 25-2.

Diphtheria Vaccine

Diphtheria toxoid is usually included with other antigens in combination vaccines of varying strengths. In the description of diphtheria vaccines, uppercase letters (D, P, or T) denote full strength diphtheria, pertussis, and tetanus. Lowercase letters (d and p) indicate reduced concentrations of diphtheria and pertussis in the vaccine. Acellular components of a vaccine are represented by the lowercase "a" (DTaP).

DTaP and DT vaccines are used through 6 years of age. The DTaP also is formulated with inactivated polio–hepatitis B (Pediarix). Adult Td can be used to vaccinate individuals 7 years and older. Tdap vaccines are available for children between 10 and 18 years of age (Boostrix), and Adacel is approved for individuals 11 to 64 years of age.

Following a four-vaccination series over 8 months, the clinical efficacy is 97%. However, diphtheria immunity wanes with age, and children and adults are at risk for contracting the disease. To maintain protective immunity, children vaccinated with DTaP should receive booster doses at 4 to 6 years of age and every 10 years thereafter. Older children vaccinated with adult Td or Tap should receive a booster shot every 10 years.

PERTUSSIS (WHOOPING COUGH)

The etiologic agent of whooping cough is *Bordetella pertussis*, an aerobic, gram-negative rod. The term *whooping cough* is derived from the unique paroxysmal coughing pattern associated with the disease. As a consequence of prolonged coughing, the individual is unable take air into the lungs. When the coughing stops, a protracted inspiratory effort with an associated high-pitched "whoop" occurs. Coughing begins 1 to 2 weeks after infection and lasts for 6 to 10 weeks.

B. pertussis produces a number of virulence factors that include filamentous hemagglutinin (FHA), fimbriae, adenylate cyclase, pertactin, and toxin production. *B. pertussis* attaches itself to cells in the respiratory tract using the FHA. Secondary attachment points are facilitated by fimbriae and pertactins. The pathology of the disease is caused by a pertussis toxin, a tracheal cytotoxin, and a dermonecrotic toxin.

Pertussis Toxin

The *B. pertussis* toxin (PTx) is an A+B subunit toxin. Attachment to the cell is facilitated by the B units, and the A unit is responsible for the toxicity. PTx is a ribosyl transferase, which binds ADP-ribose to a membrane-bound regulatory G1 molecule. Inactivation of the G1 protein allows uncontrolled conversion of adenosine triphosphate (ATP) to cyclic adenosine monophosphate (cAMP). Accumulating cAMP disrupts normal cellular function and alters hormone activity. For example, increased cAMP levels increase sensitivity to histamine, which results in increased capillary permeability, hypotension, and shock. PTx also downregulates both cellular and antibody-mediated immune responses, increasing the risk for secondary infections.

Tracheal Cytotoxin

The tracheal cytotoxin is a cell wall peptidoglycan fragment and cannot be classified as an exotoxin or an endotoxin. The toxin kills ciliated epithelial cells in the respiratory tract and

Table 25-2 Therapeutic Agents Used to Treat Diphtheria

Penicillin G	Arrests bacterial cell wall synthesis by inhibiting cross-linking cell wall polymers
Erythromycin	Binds to 50S ribosomal subunits and prevents ribosomal translocation
Diphtheria antitoxin	Provides passive protection against circulating toxin. It has no effect on bound toxin

Table 25-3	Agents Used to Treat Whooping Cough
Erythromycin	Binds to 50S ribosomal subunits and prevents ribosomal translocation
Azithromycin	Same as above
Clarithromycin	Same as above
Trimethoprim/Sulfamethoxazole	Inhibits bacterial synthesis of folic acid

Table 25-4 Composition of Acellular Pertussis Vaccines

Product	Target Population	Pertussis Toxin	FHA	PERT	FIM
Daptacel	Infant	10	5	3	5
Infantrix	Infant	25	25	8	
Tripedia	Infant	23	23		
Boostrix	Adult	8	8	2.5	
Adacel	Adult	2.5	5	3	5

FHA, Filamentous hemagglutinin; *FIM*, fimbriae; *PERT*, pertactin.
Modified from Centers for Disease Control and Prevention. Atkinson W, Hamborsky J, McIntyre S, editors: Epidemiology and prevention of vaccine preventable diseases, ed 10, Washington, DC, 2007, Public Health Foundation.

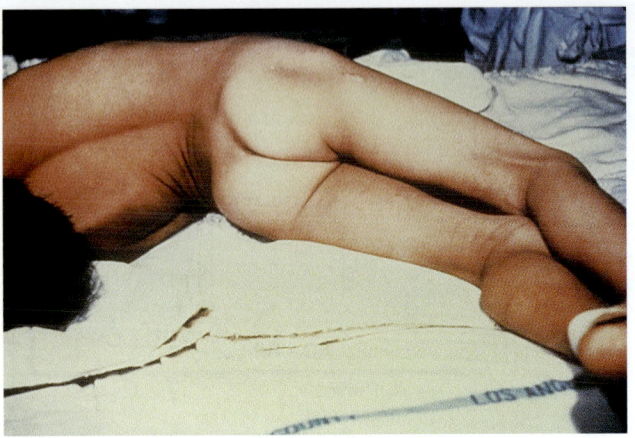

Figure 25-2
Opisthotonos. (From the CDC Public Health Image Library, Photo ID#6373.)

stimulates the release of interleukin 1 (IL-1), which acts as an endogenous pyrogen.

Dermonecrotic Lethal Toxin
Dermonecrotic lethal toxin is an exotoxin that causes local necrosis of tissue adjacent to areas colonized by pertussis. The role of the lethal toxin in the pathophysiology of whooping cough is unknown.

Treatment
The treatment of choice is erythromycin, which reduces transmission and the number of organisms in the respiratory tract. Other drugs such as clarithromycin or trimethoprim-sulfamethoxazole can also be used in treatment (Table 25-3).

Vaccine
The original whole-cell, inactivated pertussis (wBP) vaccine was developed in the 1930s. Although the vaccine was effective, it contained small amounts of the lipopolysaccharide endotoxin. The endotoxin caused significant adverse health effects, including acute encephalopathy, febrile seizures, and hypotonic or hypertonic episodes. The vaccine has been discontinued in the United States.

Acellular subunit pertussis (aBP) vaccines were introduced in 1996 for pediatric use and for adolescent and adult use in 2005. All aBP vaccines contain a pertussis toxoid. However, the concentrations of the filamentous hemagglutinin, fimbriae, and pertactin in vaccines vary considerably (Table 25-4). None of the vaccines contain the pertussis endotoxin.

Following the standard four-dose immunization regimen, between 70% and 90% of the patients are protected from pertussis infection for 5 to 10 years.

TETANUS
Clostridium tetani is a gram-positive, anaerobic organism that is a common inhabitant in the intestines of horses, sheep, cattle, dogs, cats, rats, and guinea pigs. In soils contaminated with animal manure, the vegetative microbe derives nutrients from dead or decaying organic material. When nutrients become limited, the bacteria form spores, which are impervious to heat, chemicals, and other environmental toxins. Viable spores can persist in soil for decades.

Tetanus Toxin
C. tetani spores infect humans by accident, through a deep puncture wound. A deep wound ensures an oxygen-depleted (anaerobic) environment, which allows spores to germinate into vegetative bacteria. Vegetative bacteria release two protein exotoxins—tetanolysin and tetanospasmin. Tetanolysin lyses red blood cells but has no other physiologic function. Tetanospasmin is responsible for the recognized pathophysiology of tetanus.

Tetanospasmin is a 150-kiloDalton (kDal) A+B toxin. The B subunit binds to membrane gangliosides on neural pathways, and the complete toxin is transported to peripheral nerve end plates, the sympathetic nervous system, the spinal cord, and the brain. In the nerve endings, the A subunit inactivates synaptobrevin and prevents the release of gamma amino butyric acid (GABA) and glycine, which normally control the release of acetylcholine. Uncontrolled acetylcholine synthesis and increased nerve firing cause unpredictable muscle contractions, spasms, and seizures characteristic of tetanus.

Clostridium tetani and Disease
Four clinical forms of tetanus have been described: (1) generalized (most common), (2) local (common), (3) cephalic (rare), and (4) neonatal (common in the developing countries).

Generalized Tetanus
Trismus, or lockjaw, is the first sign of generalized tetanus. This is usually followed by a stiff neck, difficulty in swallowing or breathing, and abdominal muscle rigidity. Severe muscular contractions are frequent and last 5 to 10 minutes. Contractions in the long muscles of the back often arch the back in a characteristic form called *opisthotonos*, which often results in fractures of the spine (Figure 25-2). If the toxin reaches the lung, paralysis of respiratory muscles causes death.

Table 25-5	Agents Used in the Treatment of Tetanus
Tetanus immunoglobulin	Provides passive immunity by neutralizing free toxin
Metronidazole	Is considered a prodrug, which results in the production of cytotoxic radicals
Penicillin G	Arrests bacterial cell wall synthesis by inhibiting cross-linking cell wall polymers
Erythromycin	Binds to 50S ribosomal subunits and prevents ribosomal translocation
Clindamycin	Bacteriostatic agent that binds to 50S ribosomal subunit
Tetracycline	Blocks binding of aminoacyl transfer ribonucleic acid (tRNA) to the ribosomal A site

Table 25-6	Agents Used to Treat *Haemophilus* Infections
Ceftriaxone	Arrests bacterial cell wall synthesis by cross-linking cell wall polymers
Cefotaxime	Same as above
Meropenem	Arrests bacterial cell wall synthesis in a manner similar to penicillin
Chloramphenicol	Inhibits the ribosomal peptidyl transferase which elongates polypeptides
Ampicillin	Interferes with transpeptidation step of peptidoglycan biosynthesis
Dexamethasone	Suppresses migration of polymorphonuclear leukocytes into inflamed areas
Rifampin	Binds to β-prime subunit of deoxyribonucleic acid (DNA)-dependent ribonucleic acid (RNA) polymerase and inhibits the transcription of messenger RNA (mRNA)

Under the best of circumstances, the mortality rate from tetanus in unvaccinated individuals ranges between 40% and 78%.

Localized Tetanus

Localized tetanus is characterized by muscle contraction near the injury site. The contractions are self-limiting and seldom result in long-term complications.

Cephalic Tetanus

Cephalic tetanus occurs when the organism is present in the flora of the middle ear. Paralysis of facial muscles occurs when nerve transmission is inhibited in the branches of the fifth cranial nerve.

Neonatal Tetanus

Neonatal tetanus is a form of generalized tetanus that occurs in infants when spores infect the unhealed umbilical cord stump. Neonatal tetanus is rare in the United States but common in other countries when contaminated instruments are used to cut the umbilical cord. Globally, an estimated 257,000 deaths occur from neonatal tetanus each year.

Treatment

Tetanus immune globulin (TIG) or equine tetanus antitoxin is usually administered to persons with active tetanus. If TIG is unavailable, intravenous immunoglobulin (IVIG) containing anti-tetanus toxin antibodies is used. Both preparations neutralize and remove free toxins but have no effect on neuronal-bound toxin. To provide active immunity, immunization with the tetanus toxoid should begin as soon as the patient's condition permits. Common therapeutic agents used to treat tetanus are listed in Table 25-5.

Tetanus Vaccine

Like the diphtheria toxin, tetanus toxin is treated with formalin to create a toxoid. It is offered as a fluid toxoid or absorbed to aluminum hydroxide. Although both formulations induce antibodies, a higher antibody response and duration of protection is induced by the adsorbed toxoid. Tetanus toxoid is available as a stand-alone vaccine or combined with diphtheria toxoid and acellular pertussis to form the DTaP vaccine. Three doses of tetanus toxoid in children 7 years of age and older or four doses in infants confer immunity in 100% of individuals. Without booster doses, immunity wanes, and antibody levels fall below the protective levels after 10 years.

HAEMOPHILUS INFLUENZAE TYPE B

Haemophilus influenzae is an encapsulated gram-negative coccobacillus. It is the etiologic agent of meningitis, otitis media, epiglottitis, pneumonia, arthritis, occult febrile bacteremia, septic arthritis, cellulitis, and purulent pericarditis.

A polyribosyl phosphate (PRP) capsule appears to be the major *Haemophilus* virulence factor. It protects the organism from phagocytosis and the effects of complement. There are different capsular serotypes (A–F), however, *H. influenzae* type b (Hib) serotype accounts for 95% of all infections. *Haemophilus* is endemic in the United States, with epidemics occurring every 3 to 5 years. Most epidemics originate in nurseries or daycare centers, and a single index case can infect 90% of contacts with 48 hours.

Treatment

Children with Hib respiratory infections usually require hospitalization and treatment with cephalosporin or chloramphenicol and ampicillin. Since many Hib strains produce a β-lactamase and are resistant to ampicillin, these medications are not used as monotherapy for severe disease. Third-generation cephalosporins are the drugs of choice to treat invasive *Haemophilus* infections and meningitis. Glucocorticoids are also useful for reducing the risk of deafness associated with meningitis (Table 25-6).

Vaccines

To convert the capsules to a T cell–dependent antigen, *Haemophilus* capsular polysaccharides are conjugated to proteins such as the diphtheria toxoid, the tetanus toxoid, or meningococcal outer membrane proteins (Table 25-7). Three conjugate vaccines are licensed in the United States for the vaccination of infants as young as 6 weeks of age. Each conjugate vaccine uses a different protein carrier.

PNEUMOCOCCUS

Streptococcus pneumoniae is a gram-positive bacterium that is most commonly found in the nasopharynx in children and adults. In high density populations such as military installations or prisons, 50% to 60% of the population may be asymptomatic

Table 25-7	Conjugate Vaccines Licensed by the U.S. Food and Drug Administration
Vaccine	**Carrier Protein**
HbOC (Hib TITER)	Diphtheria protein
PRT-T ActHIB	Tetanus toxoid
PRP-OMP (Pedvax HIB)	Meningococcal protein

From Centers for Disease Control and Prevention. Atkinson W, Hamborsky J, McIntyre S, editors: Epidemiology and prevention of vaccine preventable diseases, ed 10, Washington, DC, 2007, Public Health Foundation.

carriers. Pneumococci are the most common cause of community-acquired pneumonia (CAP), meningitis, and bacteremia.

A polysaccharide capsule surrounding the bacterium is the major virulence factor. It prevents phagocytosis and inhibits the deposition of the complement fragment C3b.

Capsules form the basis for pneumococcal serotyping. More than 90 different serotypes have been reported, and 23 to 25 pneumococcal serotypes infect humans. Two different numbering systems are used to identify pneumococcal serotypes. In the American system, serotypes are numbered in the order in which they were discovered and associated with disease. A Danish numbering system, which is more accepted by clinicians and microbiologists, groups serotypes with similar antigenicity. Predominant serotypes vary by geographic area, socioeconomic status, and age of the patient. Ten common serotypes account for 65% of invasive diseases in adults. Other serotypes (4 and 14) and serogroups (6, 7, 8, 9, 18, 19, and 23) are associated with pneumococcal infections in children younger than 6 years of age.

Pneumococcal Diseases

From the initial colonization in the respiratory tract, the organism spreads into the paranasal sinuses, the middle ear, the lung, and the brain. In children and older adults, pneumococci also cause osteomyelitis, endocarditis, cellulitis and brain abscesses.

Pneumonia

S. pneumoniae is the major cause of community-acquired lobar pneumonia. In lobar pneumonia, an entire lung lobe is infected and filled with serous fluid. A subsequent inflammatory response creates a purulent exudate in the infected lobe. A lobe containing fluid or exudates is commonly termed a *consolidated lung*. Pneumonia is a leading cause of death in children. Each year 1.8 million children under the age of 6 years die from pneumonia worldwide.

Otitis Media

In some individuals, the organism migrates up the eustachian tube to the middle ear. Inflammatory cells occlude the eustachian tubes and create negative pressure in the middle ear. If the pressure is not equalized by normal ventilation, serous fluid accumulates in the ear. Increased fluid pressure on the tympanic membrane causes pain and difficulty hearing. Severe infections may result in damage to the auditory nerve or perforation of the eardrum.

Bacteremia

In 25% to 30% of pneumonia cases, bacteria enter the blood. More than 50,000 pneumococcal bacteremia cases are reported each year, with the highest incidences in older adults and in infants. Most adults have evidence of a focal infection and frank bacteremia. In children 2 years of age or younger, occult bacteremia may occur in a healthy, febrile child without focal lung lesions. The fatality rate is 20% to 60% in patients with pneumonia and bacteremia.

Pneumococcal Meningitis

Streptococcus pneumoniae is the leading cause of bacterial meningitis among children under 5 years of age. In the United States, an estimated 3000 to 6000 cases are reported each year. The symptoms and sequelae are similar to those described for *Haemophilus* infection. The mortality rate is approximately 30% in younger individuals and 80% in older adults.

Treatment

Third-generation cephalosporins (ceftriaxone or cefotaxime) and vancomycin comprise the antibiotic regimen of choice. Evidence suggests that administration of corticosteroids such as dexamethasone also reduces the mortality rate and neurologic sequelae.

Vaccines

Pneumococcal vaccines are unique in that they do not prevent infection. However, they are highly effective in preventing invasive or systemic diseases in patients who develop pneumonia.

Capsular Polysaccharide Vaccines

The polyvalent vaccine (Pneumovax), or PPV23, contains capsular antigens from 23 different pneumococcal serotypes. These serotypes cause 96% of pneumonias and invasive disease in the developed countries. The vaccine also includes six serotypes that most frequently cause invasive drug-resistant pneumococcal infections in children. Over 80% of adults vaccinated form antibodies within 2 to 3 weeks, and antibodies may persist for 5 to 10 years. The vaccine is recommended for individuals over 50 years of age and for individuals aged 2 to 64 years who have a high risk of pneumococcal disease. Individuals at risk for developing severe disease include those with chronic conditions such as chronic cardiovascular disease, chronic pulmonary disease, diabetes, alcoholism, or liver cirrhosis.

The Pneumovax vaccine has several limitations. Capsular polysaccharides are T cell–independent type II antigens, which produce only transient immunoglobulin M (IgM) antibodies. Some children under 2 years of age may not respond to the PPV23 vaccine because of a developmental block in the production of IgG_2 protective antibodies.

Pneumococcal Conjugate Vaccines

In 2000, the U.S. Food and Drug Administration (FDA) licensed the first conjugate pneumococcal vaccine (PCV7). Prevnar comprises capsular polysaccharides from seven pneumococcal serotypes (4, 9V, 14, 19F, 23F, 18C, and 6B). These serotypes account for 86% of bacteremia, 83% of meningitis, and 65% of otitis media cases in the United States. The conjugate vaccine acts as a T cell–dependent antigen that generates a primary and anamnestic response in both adults and young children.

Prevnar. Prevnar is recommended for children younger than 12 months and for children between the ages of 24 and 59 months who have underlying medical conditions. Over 90% of vaccinated individuals develop antibodies after completion of the four-dose immunization series.

Prevnar 13. Prevnar 13 is indicated for active immunization for the prevention of invasive disease caused by *S. pneumoniae* serotypes 1, 3, 4, 5, 6A, 6B, 7F, 9V, 14, 18C, 19A, 19F, and 23F and otitis media caused by serotypes 4, 6B, 9V, 14, 18C, 19F, and 23F. It is approved for use in children aged 6 weeks to 5 years.

NEISSERIA MENINGITIDIS

N. meningitidis is a gram-negative organism with a specialized endotoxin referred to as a *lipooligosaccharide (LOS)*. An anti-phagocytic capsule and the LOS are the major neisserial virulence factors. Thirteen different capsular serotypes have been reported. However, only five serogroups (A, B, C, Y, and W135) infect humans. As with other pathogenic bacteria, the major serotype causing disease differs by geographic region. For example, serotype A is a common cause of disease in Africa, but it is rarely found in the United States.

Humans are the only reservoir, and the organism is commonly found in the posterior nasal pharynx. At any point in time, 10% of the adolescent population are asymptomatic carriers. During an epidemic, the carrier rate may exceed 80%. Infection is transmitted from carriers to nonimmune individuals through respiratory droplets.

Meningococcal Diseases

N. meningitidis is the etiologic agent of meningitis and pneumonia. When disseminated by blood (bacteremia), bacteria can infect multiple organs. The onset of disease is rapid, and patients become symptomatic within 24 hours of exposure. Under the best of circumstances and appropriate antimicrobial therapy, the case fatality rate is 10% to 15%. In cases of fulminating bacteremia, the case fatality rate is 40%. Approximately 20% of patients surviving meningitis have sequelae such as neurologic deficits or loss of hearing, skin, digits, or limbs because of gangrene.

Neisserial Meningitis

Meningitis is an inflammation of the meninges and infection of the subarachnoid cerebrospinal fluid (CSF). Rapid bacterial growth, an inflammatory response, and release of LOS are responsible for both the pathophysiology and disease sequelae such as deafness and gangrene in hands and feet.

Bacterial growth causes obstruction of normal CSF flow, increased cranial pressure, and destruction of brain tissue. The inflammatory response to the organism often damages cranial nerve VIII, which controls hearing.

LOS enters the bloodstream and binds to a lipid-binding protein (LBP). In turn, the complex is transferred to a CD14 and Toll-like receptor 4 (TLR4) expressed by monocyte and endothelial cell membranes. CD14 intracellular signaling triggers three major physiologic events that include activation of the coagulation complement pathways and septic shock.

Activation of the Coagulation Pathway. Disseminated intravascular coagulopathy (DIC) and gangrene are caused by activation of the coagulation pathway. LOS stimulates endothelial cells to express tissue factor (TF). Interactions between clotting factor VII (FVIIa) and TF activate the coagulation cascade and the formation of microthrombi. These small blood clots circulate in peripheral blood until they are trapped in the small capillaries of the hands and feet. Occlusion of capillary blood flow results in tissue necrosis and gangrene. Depletion of platelets and clotting factors ultimately results in plasmin activation and seepage of blood into skin. Minor hemorrhages in skin cause small (petechiae) or large red or purple (purpura) spots on the lower extremities.

Activation of the Complement Cascade. LOS also activates the alternative complement pathway. Complement fragment C5a is an anaphylatoxin, which releases histamine and preformed mediators from mast cells and basophils. Other complement fragments attract neutrophils in the infection nidus. Vasodilatation and neutrophil chemotaxis are major contributors to septic shock induced by *N. meningitidis*.

Meningococcal Septic Shock

Meningococcal septic shock is a consequence of a fulminating meningococcal bacteremia. Systemic manifestations of hypotension, shock, adrenal hemorrhage, and multiple-organ failure are also common. Meningococcal bacteremia carries a mortality rate of 40%.

Incidence and Frequency. The incidence of meningococcal disease is highest in the late winter and early spring. Infants under 12 months of age, adolescents, and young adults between the ages of 18 and 23 years are highly susceptible to meningococcal infections. Populations with the highest risk for developing the disease are college freshman living in dormitories and military recruits.

Infection rates for each serotype are age dependent. In infants under 1 year of age, 65% of the cases are caused by serotype B, for which no licensed vaccine is available. In older individuals, 75% of meningococcal disease is caused by serogroups C, Y, or W-135.

Treatment. Bacterial meningitis runs a rapid clinical course and has a high mortality rate. Treatment is predicated on bacterial morphology and gram stain characteristics. Therapy regimens for gram-positive and gram-negative bacteria are provided in Table 25-8.

Vaccines

Three meningitis vaccines are licensed in the United States: Menomune, which is also called the *Meningococcal Polysaccharide Vaccine 4 (MPSV4)*, Menactra (MCV), and Menveo.

Menomune

Menomune is a quadrivalent vaccine, which contains (A, C, Y, and W-135) capsular polysaccharides. Because Menomune contains T cell–independent antigens, it has poor

Table 25-8 Therapeutic Agents Used to Treat Meningitis Caused by Gram-Positive and Gram-Negative Bacteria

Gram-positive cocci	Vancomycin plus ceftriaxone or cefotaxime
Gram-negative cocci	Penicillin G
Gram-positive bacilli	Ampicillin plus an aminoglycoside
Gram-negative bacilli	Broad-spectrum cephalosporin plus an aminoglycoside

Modified from Razonable RR, Keating MR: Meningitis: Treatment and medication, Emedicine. emedicine.medscape.com/article/232915-overview. Accessed 11/01/10.

immunogenicity in children under 5 years of age and does not generate memory cells. The vaccine is recommended for individuals 2 to 55 years of age and for unvaccinated individuals in high-risk groups. High-risk groups include children entering high school, college freshman living in dormitories, military recruits, and individuals with complement deficiencies or a dysfunctional spleen.

Menactra

Menactra is a quadrivalent vaccine consisting of (A, C, Y, and W-135) capsular polysaccharides linked to the diphtheria toxoid. The toxoid evokes a T cell–dependent response to both the polysaccharides and the toxoid. Because of its capability to evoke a memory response, the vaccine has a long duration of protection and reduces the carrier state. Menactra is licensed for use among persons 11 to 55 years of age. Young adolescents 11 to 12 years of age are usually vaccinated during a preadolescent health care visit.

Menveo

Menveo is composed of meningococcal (A, C, Y, and W-135) oligosaccharides conjugated to the diphtheria CRM197 protein. It is indicated for immunization to prevent invasive meningococcal disease and approved for use in individuals 11 to 55 years of age. It does not protect against infection with serotype B bacteria.

POLIO

Poliovirus is an enterovirus, which is a genus within the picornavirus family. By definition, picornaviruses are small, icosahedral, non-enveloped, double-stranded ribonucleic acid (RNA) viruses. The three polio serotypes (P1, P2, and P3) have little antigenic cross-reactivity and immunity to one serotype does not confer immunity to other serotypes.

Humans are the only natural hosts for polioviruses. The virus is transmitted via the fecal–oral route and quickly infects the lymph tissue in the gastrointestinal tract. Following rapid replication, the virus enters the bloodstream and produces several different clinical outcomes.

Subclinical Infections

The majority of polio infections are asymptomatic. These individuals have no clinical symptoms but continue to shed the virus in saliva and feces for extended periods.

Abortive Infections

Some individuals infected with poliovirus develop a minor, nonspecific illness with symptoms similar to influenza infections. Most people recover within 1 week.

Nonparalytic Aseptic Meningitis

The virus infects the meninges, or tissue layers, covering the brain. Meningitis is characterized by stiffness of the neck, back, and legs. Usually, a complete recovery occurs within 10 days, often without supportive therapy.

Paralytic Polio

Over 85% of paralytic infections are caused by the P1 virus strain, which unilaterally infects motor neurons in the anterior horn of the spinal cord and the brain stem. Destruction of infected neurons disrupts the transmission of nerve impulses to select muscle groups, causing a flaccid paralysis.

Types of Paralytic Polio

Three types of paralytic polio exist: (1) The most common form is *spinal polio* (79%), with asymmetrical paralysis of the lower limbs. (2) *Bulbar polio* is associated with weakness in muscles innervated by the trigeminal (V), glosso-pharyngeal (IV), and accessory nerves (VI). These nerves control the muscles in the neck and tongue and the muscles used for swallowing. (3) *Bulbospinal polio* affects the spinal cord at the C3-5 level, which inhibits the function of the diaphragm and results in death.

Treatment

Currently, no antiviral treatment for polio is available. Most therapies are only supportive.

Post-Polio Syndrome

Between 20% and 40% of persons with a history of paralytic polio completely recover from the initial infection but experience new muscle weakness and paralysis 30 to 40 years after the initial event. The etiology of the post-polio syndrome (PPS) is unclear. One possible cause of PPS is reactivation of a latent polio virus. A second possible cause of PPS is the loss of slow-firing motor neurons in the anterior horn. To replace the rapid-firing neurons destroyed in the initial infection, a compensatory hypertrophy of small, slow twitch neurons occurs, restoring motor function. Over time, these neurons become fatigued and dysfunctional, and motor function is lost.

Vaccines

Two polio vaccines are licensed for use in the United States. The original inactivated poliovirus (IPV) vaccine developed by Jonas Salk consists of the three (P1–P3) formalin-inactivated polio strains. Over 95% of vaccinated individuals develop high levels of antibodies, which are protective against paralytic disease. The duration of immunity is unknown. A major disadvantage of the vaccine is that it does not stimulate the mucosal immune system, and individuals can be infected and transmit wild-type viruses. The vaccine was used extensively from 1955 to 1963 to eradicate polio in the United States.

The Sabin oral poliovirus vaccine (OPV) contains attenuated P1–P3 polio strains, which can replicate in the intestine. The OPV induces mucosal immunity and the synthesis of surface immunoglobulin A (sIgA), which prevents infection by the wild-type virus. Continued shedding of the virus also contributes to the natural vaccination of unprotected individuals.

Until 2000, a person was considered protected against polio following an IVP and OPV vaccination series. However, the risk of vaccine-associated paralytic poliomyelitis (VAPP) now outweighs the benefit of OPV. OPV is no longer recommended for routine vaccination in the United States. In other parts of the world, OPV is widely used in polio eradication programs.

Oral Polio Vaccine-Associated Paralytic Poliomyelitis

Since the OPV attenuated virus is able to replicate in the body, it has the ability to mutate or revert to a neurotropic form. From 1980 to 1995, VAPP accounted for 95% of all polio cases in the United States. The rate of VAPP is 1 case per 2.4 million vaccinations. A majority of these cases occurred in healthy vaccine recipients or household contacts of vaccine recipients.

MEASLES (RUBEOLA)

Rubeola is an enveloped, single-stranded RNA paramyxovirus that is closely related to the animal distemper, mumps, and respiratory syncytial viruses. It causes an acute viral disease that infects children and young adults. Classic rubeola begins with infection of the nasopharynx. Macrophages also transport the virus to the local lymph nodes. Replication of the virus in the lymph nodes allows the virus to enter the bloodstream and spreads the virus to multiple organs and to the skin.

The rubeola rash begins at the hairline, face, and upper neck. Over several days, the rash moves downward to the hands and feet. Early in the disease course, characteristic white spots, called *Koplik spots*, are found on the cheeks inside the mouth.

Complications

Because the rubeola virus localizes in multiple organs, major and minor sequelae are not unexpected. Minor complications include diarrhea and otitis media. More serious sequelae are immune suppression, encephalitis, and subacute sclerosing panencephalitis (SSPE).

Immune Suppression

Rubeola infections cause a prolonged immunosuppression in infected individuals. Measles-infected lymphocytes undergo apoptosis. As a consequence, increased susceptibility to secondary intestinal and respiratory infections occurs.

Encephalitis

Encephalitis occurs in 0.1% of measles infections and is fatal in 25% of cases. Survivors often have moderate to severe brain damage that results in intellectual disabilities.

Subacute Sclerosing Panencephalitis

SSPE is a rare, progressive deterioration of the central nervous system associated with a slow or persistent measles infection. Progressive deterioration of brain function results in ataxia, myoclonic seizures, dementia, and death. Onset is generally 7 to 10 years after the initial measles infection. It is considered rare in the developed countries. Fewer than 10 cases per year are reported in the United States.

Atypical Rubeola

Atypical measles is a hypersensitivity reaction in individuals who received the killed measles vaccine (KMV) between 1963 and 1967. This vaccine sensitized an estimated 600,000 to 900,000 persons to measles antigens. A second exposure to measles vaccines elicits delayed hypersensitivity reactions in the skin and inflammation of the serous membranes lining the pericardial, pleural, and peritoneal cavities.

Modified Measles

Modified measles is a mild illness that occurs in infants who have maternal antibodies to measles and in adults who have received IgG prophylaxis for measles infections. It is characterized by small, discrete measles rashes of short duration.

Treatment

Treatment for measles is supportive. Antibiotics may be indicated when the individual is diagnosed with secondary bacterial infections.

Table 25-9 Adverse Reactions of the Measles–Mumps–Pertussis Vaccine

Symptom	Percentage or Frequency
Fever	5–15
Rash	5
Joint symptoms	25
Thrombocytopenia	≤1/30,000
Encephalopathy	≤1/1,000,000

Modified from Centers for Disease Control and Prevention. Atkinson W, Hamborsky J, McIntyre S, editors: Epidemiology and prevention of vaccine preventable diseases, ed 10, Washington, DC, 2007, Public Health Foundation.

Vaccines

In 1963, the Edmonstron-Enders B strain measles vaccine, in both killed and attenuated forms, was licensed in the United States. Further attenuation of the Edmonstron-Enders measles strain produced the virus used in the current vaccine, which was licensed in 1968. The attenuated vaccine is available as a stand-alone product or in combination with rubella or mumps and rubella (MMR). Vaccination produces a mild, noncommunicable infection. Ninety-five percent of children vaccinated at 12 to 15 months of age produce antibodies and are protected from subsequent infection. If a second dose of vaccine is given at 4 to 6 years of age, 99% of children develop high titers of antibody, an anamnestic response, and lifelong immunity. Side effects of the vaccine range from fever to encephalopathy (Table 25-9).

MUMPS

Mumps is an acute viral illness caused by a single-stranded RNA paramyxovirus. Person-to-person transmission occurs by the respiratory route. The virus initially localizes in the nasopharynx and regional lymph nodes. Following several replication cycles in the lymph node, the virus enters the bloodstream and infects multiple organs, including the meninges, pancreas, testes, ovaries, and salivary glands. The most common symptom is unilateral or bilateral parotitis, which is an inflammation of the parotid salivary glands located on either side of the face.

Complications of Mumps

Complications of mumps infections include encephalitis, aseptic meningitis, and inflammation of the ovaries (oophoritis), breasts (mastitis), or testes. Inflammation of the testes (orchitis) is common in postpubescent males. The inflammation is bilateral in 30% of males and is characterized by testicular swelling and tenderness. Orchitis results in testicular atrophy in 30% of affected males, but sterility is rare. The mumps virus also causes unilateral deafness in approximately 1 per 20,000 infected individuals.

Vaccine

The current vaccine, licensed in 1967, is a live attenuated strain of mumps grown in chick embryo fibroblasts. Efficacy is estimated to be 75% to 91% after a single dose and 85% after two doses; immunity is believed to last 25 years or more.

The vaccine is available as a single-antigen preparation or in combination with measles and rubella (MMR), and additionally in combination with varicella (MMRV). Following vaccine licensure, the incidence of mumps decreased rapidly in the United States. Only 258 cases of mumps were reported in 2004.

Recent data suggest that the mumps virus may be evolving or a high rate of vaccine failure is present. In 2006, a multiple-state outbreak of mumps with 6500 cases was documented. The majority of infections occurred in college students (median age 22 years) who had been vaccinated with one or two doses of the MMR vaccine.

RUBELLA (GERMAN MEASLES)

The rubella virus is an enveloped, single-stranded RNA virus closely related to the eastern and western encephalitis viruses. German physicians were the first to describe the illness in the scientific literature, and thus the common name for the infection came to be *German measles*. The scientific name *rubella* is derived from the Latin word, meaning "little red," to denote that the lesions were smaller than those of rubeola.

The virus is transmitted by the respiratory route, and initial replication occurs in the nasopharynx and lymph nodes in the head and neck. After 5 to 7 days, the virus enters the bloodstream and infects the distal lymph nodes. Viral replication in tissue and nodes produces a second viremia. Infection of skin cells causes a maculopapular rash that appears 14 to 17 days after the initial infection. The rash begins on the face and progresses downward to the hands and feet.

Complications
Congenital Rubella Syndrome

Congenital rubella syndrome (CRS) is the major complication associated with rubella infections. Measles infection of the mother during the first trimester of pregnancy is associated with encephalitis, hearing loss, and blindness in the newborn infant, and, later, intellectual disabilities. Between 1964 and 1965, a rubella epidemic resulted in 12.5 million cases of rubella infection. CRS occurred in 20,000 newborns and resulted in 15,000 neonates being either deaf or blind, 2000 with encephalitis, and 1800 children with intellectual disabilities.

Rubella Infections in the Second and Third Trimesters

If the mother is infected with rubella during the fourth and fifth months of pregnancy, deafness is the most common complication in the offspring. Ocular, cardiac, and neurologic abnormalities have also been reported.

Arthritis

In 70% of women, rubella infection causes arthritis and arthralgia in the fingers, wrists, or knees. Symptoms may persist for 2 to 6 weeks.

Vaccine

The current licensed rubella vaccine is the RA27/3 live attenuated virus grown in human diploid fibroblasts. Individuals 1 year and older develop antibodies after a single dose. Antibodies protect against infection and viremia for 15 years or more.

The vaccine also is available as a single-antigen preparation, as MMR, or as MMR combined with varicella as MMRV. A mass vaccination program undertaken in 1969 eradicated rubella in the United States.

CHICKENPOX (VARICELLA ZOSTER VIRUS)

Varicella zoster virus (VZV), which causes chickenpox, is an enveloped deoxyribonucleic acid (DNA) virus and a member of the herpes virus family. It causes two diseases: (1) chickenpox (varicella) and (2) shingles (zoster), which is a reactivation of a latent varicella virus.

The virus enters the host through the respiratory route and the conjunctiva. Like other viruses, the initial replication occurs in the nasopharynx and in the lymph nodes. A second viremia infects multiple organs and skin cells. Some viruses infect sensory nerves and take up lifelong residence in the sensory dorsal root ganglia near the spinal cord.

In contrast to measles and rubella infections, the skin rash begins on the torso (centripetal distribution) and progresses outward to the arms, legs, and head. Lesions progress from red papules to generalized blisters (vesicular lesion) containing a clear fluid and infective virus. Successive crops of lesions may occur over several days. When all lesions have scabbed over, the individual is no longer infectious.

Treatment of Varicella Infections

Treatment is designed to reduce or manage symptoms and prevent secondary bacterial infections. Therapeutic agents used to treat chickenpox are listed in Table 25-10.

Complications of Varicella Infection
Disseminated Varicella Neonatorum

Disseminated varicella neonatorum is observed in infants born to women who develop active varicella infections 5 days before or after delivery. Because the neonate is often without the benefit of maternal antibodies and cannot generate an immune response, infants have overwhelming hemorrhagic infections of the lungs and liver. Mortality rate in these infants is over 30%.

Reye Syndrome

Reye syndrome is associated with aspirin use during an active varicella zoster virus (VZV) infection. In the infected cells in the brain, liver, and kidney, aspirin inhibits mitochondrial function and the generation of ATP. Without ATP, cells cannot synthesize the proteins necessary for survival. As a consequence, a loss of neurons in the brain, degeneration of the proximal tubules in the kidney, and hepatocyte destruction occur.

Congenital Infections

Infection of the fetus during the first 20 weeks of gestation is associated with congenital varicella syndrome, which includes low birth weight, skin scarring, muscular atrophy in the arms and legs, encephalitis, and microencephaly. After 20 weeks of gestation, VZV infection causes a latent infection that is associated with reactivation varicella, or shingles.

Table 25-10 Agents Used to Treat Chickenpox

Diphenhydramine	First-generation antihistamine
Hydroxyzine	H1 receptors agonist
Acyclovir	Synthetic purine nucleoside that inhibits the replication of viral deoxyribonucleic acid (DNA)
Varicella zoster immunoglobulin, human	Provides passive immunity and binds free virus
Acetaminophen	Reduces fever by acting directly on hypothalamic heat-regulating centers

Table 25-11	Agents Used to Treat Herpes Zoster
Acyclovir	Synthetic purine nucleoside analog that inhibits the replication of viral deoxyribonucleic acid (DNA)
Famciclovir	Active metabolite, penciclovir, inhibits viral DNA synthesis/replication
Valacyclovir	L-valyl ester of acyclovir, which is converted to acyclovir
Varicella zoster vaccine	Boosts immunity against herpes zoster virus (shingles) in older patients

VARICELLA ZOSTER (SHINGLES)

In young individuals, varicella reactivation in nerve tracts is prevented by a vigorous cellular immune response. As the immune system wanes with age, the risk of varicella reactivation increases. Shingles or varicella zoster results from a reactivation and eruption of the latent varicella virus in the dorsal root ganglia and supporting cells. The virus moves down the nerve tact and localizes in the skin, where it causes a unilateral, painful skin rash. Eruptions usually occur in the sensory ganglia of the face, head, or torso.

Complications of Herpes Zoster
Post-Herpetic Neuralgia
After resolution of the zoster lesions, persistent pain, or post-herpetic neuralgia (PHN), may persist for a year. Although the pathology is unclear, PHN is believed to involve neuronal atrophy, scarring of the dorsal root ganglia, and loss of epidermal nerve innervations. Sensory loss is often surrounded by areas where normal stimuli (e.g., light touching) cause intense pain.

Ramsay Hunt Syndrome
In Ramsay Hunt syndrome, varicella infection of the seventh cranial nerve (CNVII) gives rise to ulceration of the ears, tongue, and soft palate. It begins with lesions on the external ear canal, with or without facial paralysis.

Treatment of Herpes Zoster
Treatment is directed at inhibiting viral replication and prevention of PHN. Nucleoside analogs are often effective in reducing the duration of zoster infections and the severity of PHN. Therapeutic agents used to treat zoster are listed in Table 25-11.

Vaccines
Varicella Vaccine
The varicella vaccine (Varivax) was licensed in 1995 and is indicated for the vaccination of individuals 1 year of age and older. The vaccine comprises an attenuated strain of VZV that has been passed sequentially through human embryonic lung cells, embryonic guinea pig fibroblasts, WI-38, and MRC-5 human diploid cells. After two doses of the vaccine, over 99% of individuals develop protective antibodies, and the risk of varicella infection is reduced by 80% to 90%. Efficacy studies have shown that protection lasts 10 years or longer. Breakthrough infections in vaccinated individuals are rare and usually milder than the infections in unvaccinated individuals.

Varicella Zoster Vaccine
In 2006, a varicella zoster vaccine (Zostavax) was approved for use in persons 60 years of age and older. Zostavax contains a 14-fold higher concentration of the attenuated strain used in the Viravax vaccine. The vaccine reduces the incidence of shingles by 51.3% and PHN by 61.3%. The vaccine efficacy, however, declines with age. In persons 80 years of age and older, the efficacy is only 18%. With the scheduled use of Viravax, this vaccine will become unnecessary.

HEPATITIS
Viral hepatitis is a generic term for liver inflammation caused by six hepatitis viruses (A, B, C, D, E, and G). Types A, B, and E are more prevalent and cause acute hepatitis, chronic hepatitis, or both, in humans. Because of the occult and chronic nature of hepatitis C virus infection, it is viewed as the most serious form of hepatitis. The pathophysiology of hepatitis has not been fully delineated. However, cellular injury is not apparent until cytotoxic T cells accumulate in the portal and periportal areas of the liver. This suggests that the immune response to the virus-infected cells causes tissue destruction and hepatitis.

Hepatitis A
The hepatitis A virus (HAV) is a non-enveloped, single-stranded RNA enterovirus that is a member of the picornavirus family. The virus is transmitted via the fecal–oral route and occasionally by the parenteral route. The incidence of symptomatic illness varies with age. Children younger than 6 years of age usually have asymptomatic infections. In adolescents and adults, infection is symptomatic, with nausea, abdominal discomfort, dark urine, and jaundice (yellowing of the skin and eyes). Symptoms usually last less than 2 months but may persist for as long as 6 months.

Hepatitis B
The hepatitis B virus (HBV) is a member of the Hepadnaviridae family and is closely related to animal hepatitis viruses. Unlike other viruses, HBV can persist outside the body for extended periods and is highly resistant to extreme temperatures. The viral DNA is circular but only partially double-stranded.

The presence of hepatitis B surface antigen (HBsAg), which is an envelope protein, is considered evidence for acute HBV infections. Another antigen called *HBeAg* is only found when free virus is present in blood. It is used as a marker for infectivity and the ability to spread the virus to others.

HBV is transmitted through mucosal exposure to the blood or other bodily fluids of the infected person. Although rare, it is also possible to transmit HBV through percutaneous exposure, such as with tattooing, ear piercing, or needle sticks. HBV can also be transmitted perinatally from mother to infant.

Several populations are at high risk for developing hepatitis B. Intravenous drug users are a high-risk group because of needle sharing. Other high-risk populations are household contacts of individuals with hepatitis, residents and staff of facilities for developmentally disabled persons, and health care workers who have possibly been exposed to the blood, blood products, or bodily fluids of patients.

Acute Hepatitis B
After a nonspecific stage, which is characterized by malaise, nausea, and vomiting that last for 3 to 10 days, jaundice emerges and lasts for 1 to 3 weeks. In addition to jaundice, hepatic tenderness and hepatomegaly are often present.

Table 25-12	Agents Used to Treat Hepatitis Infections
Interferon alpha 2b (IFN-α2b)	Prevents the spread of virus to uninfected cells
Amantadine	Prevents penetration of virus into host by inhibiting uncoating of virus
Famciclovir	Active metabolite, penciclovir, inhibits viral deoxyribonucleic acid (DNA) synthesis
Entecavir	Guanosine nucleoside analogue which inhibits hepatitis B virus (HBV) polymerase
Prednisone	Anti-inflammatory agent

Chronic Hepatitis

Chronic active infection is responsible for most HBV morbidity and mortality. Fifteen to twenty percent of infected individuals develop cirrhosis of the liver within 5 years. When compared with the general population, persons with chronic HBV disease also have a 12- to 300-fold higher risk of developing liver cancer. If cirrhosis is present, the risk of hepatocellular carcinoma is further increased.

Treatment

Therapeutic agents are available for treatment of HBV with the goals of reducing inflammation, fibrosis, and progression to cirrhosis. Therapeutic agents are listed in Table 25-12.

Vaccines

Hepatitis A Vaccine

Havrix and VAQTA are two killed or inactivated virus vaccines licensed in the United States for use in children and adults. The vaccine is prepared from tissue culture–adapted virus is grown in diploid human fibroblasts, purified, and formalin treated. Viral fragments are adsorbed to aluminum adjuvants.

Both vaccines are efficacious. After a single dose of either vaccine, protective antibody develops in 97% of children and adults within 4 weeks. The incidence of clinical hepatitis is reduced by 94% in children receiving two doses of the vaccine. Data from computer-based kinetic models suggest that antibodies may persist for 20 years or longer. The duration of cell-mediated immunity to the virus is unclear.

Hepatitis B Vaccines

Recombivax and Engerix–B are licensed for both adult and pediatric populations. Both are recombinant subunit vaccines containing HBsAg protein. The vaccines differ only in the concentration of the HBsAg antigen and the nature of aluminum adjuvants. Recombivax contains aluminum hydrophosphate sulphate. Engerix-B uses aluminum hydroxide as an adjuvant and trace amounts of thimerosal from the manufacturing process.

In addition to single-antigen vaccines, two combination vaccines have been licensed in the United States. Comvax is HBV combined with *Haemophilus influenzae* type B vaccine. It can be administered to infants aged 12 to 15 months when the mother's HBV status is unknown. Pediatrix is the first licensed multiple-component vaccine. It contains diphtheria–tetanus–acellular pertussis (DTaP Infantrix), hepatitis B virus (Engerix), and the three-strain inactivated polio virus (IPV). This vaccine can be used interchangeably with other HBV vaccines.

INFLUENZA

The influenza virus is a helical-shaped, single-stranded RNA virus within the Orthomyxoviridae family. The viral RNA is unique in that it is composed of eight separate genomic segments. Extending from the protein capsid are hemagglutinins and neuraminidase molecules. Hemagglutinins are spikes that facilitate viral binding to sialic acid residues in mammalian cell membranes. Neuraminidase is a mushroom-shaped glycoprotein enzyme, which contributes to the infectivity of the virus. As the virus exits the cell, it coats itself with host cell membrane containing sialic acid residues. Sialic acids are the target molecules for hemagglutinins. As a consequence, the hemagglutinins on one virion bind to sialic residues on another virion, creating large, noninfectious aggregates. Neuraminidase destroys sialic acid residues and frees the individual viruses to infect other cells. On the basis of the types of nuclear material, three basic influenza types exist: A, B, and C.

Type A Influenza

The natural hosts for type A viruses are wild aquatic birds. Influenza type A viruses from wild birds can infect multiple species, including humans, birds, and swine. When transmitted to humans, type A influenza causes moderate to severe disease. Type A influenza is usually associated with worldwide epidemics known as *pandemics*.

Type B Influenza

Influenza type B has no animal reservoir and causes only mild disease in humans. However, it is responsible for geographically localized epidemics that appear every 3 to 5 years.

Type C Influenza

Type C influenza can infect humans and pigs. In humans, it causes a mild respiratory disease or an asymptomatic infection. It does not have an impact on public health, as do types A and B, because it rarely causes epidemics.

Influenza Strains or Subtypes

Hemagglutinins and neuraminidase are the major influenza virulence factors. Sixteen hemagglutinins and 9 different neuraminidase molecules exist. An influenza strain expresses only one hemagglutinin and one neuraminidase serotype. Both molecules are antigenic and are not cross-reactive. Current serotypes of influenza A viruses are the H1N1 and H3N2 viruses.

Antigenic Drift

From year to year, genetic and epidemiologic pressures on influenza types A and B cause point mutations in genes coding for the antigenic epitopes in hemagglutinins (H) and often neuraminidase (N). Less than a 1% change in the hemagglutinin or neuraminidase structure creates novel epitopes that are not recognized by pre-existing antibodies or memory cells. The phenomenon is known as *antigenic drift*. An example of antigenic drift occurred in 1997–1998. Early in 1997, the type A/Wuhan/H3N2 was the dominant influenza strain included in the 1997 vaccine. Late in the same year, a drift variant called *type A/Sydney/H3N2* became the predominant virus. Although only a small difference in hemagglutinin structure was present, the two strains were antigenically dissimilar. The 1997 vaccine failed to protect against infection with the type

Table 25-13 Influenza Pandemics of the Twentieth Century

Year	Serotype	Origin	Antigenic Shift Type
1899	H3N2	Russia	Unknown
1918	H1N1	United States	Direct jump
1957	H2N2	Singapore	Reassortment
1968	H3N2	Hong Kong	Reassortment
1976	H1N1	New Jersey	Reassortment
2008	H5N3	China	Direct jump
2009	H3N1	Mexico	Reassortment

A/Sydney/H3N2 strain, which caused epidemics in late 1997 and early 1998.

Antigenic Shift

Antigenic shift occurs when a radical and abrupt change in influenza type A virus hemagglutinins occurs. In some cases, a 50% change occurs in the hemagglutinin structure. Antigenic shift can be the result of a direct jump from an unknown animal strain to humans or a reassortment of two or more influenza viruses within the same cell.

Evidence suggests that the 1918 influenza pandemic was the result of a direct jump from pigs to humans. The type A H1N1 pandemic flu killed 500,000 people in the United States. Worldwide, the death toll was estimated at 50 million.

Viral reassortment is a more complex form of antigenic shift. It occurs when two viruses simultaneously infect the same animal. For example, pigs carry an endemic strain of influenza and can be infected with both human and avian influenza strains. Within an infected porcine cell, reassortment of genetic material from both viruses creates a new, hybrid virus. The virus that caused the 2009 pandemic influenza (type A H1N1) is a *quadruple reassortment virus*. It contains genes from pigs normally found in Europe and Asia, avian–swine influenza genes, and human influenza genes.

Seven reassortments or antigenic shifts in type A influenza have been documented in the last 115 years. Influenza pandemics are listed in Table 25-13.

Transmission and Temporal Patterns

Person-to-person transmission of influenza virus is facilitated via large (5-micron diameter) droplets generated by sneezing or coughing. In adults, transmission can occur 1 day before symptoms occur to 5 days after symptoms begin. Transmission also occurs by touching virus-contaminated inanimate objects. Influenza virus remains viable for 24 to 28 hours on hard, nonporous materials.

Types of Influenza

Seasonal Influenza

In seasonal or yearly influenza, infections are localized in the lung because hemagglutinins can only bind to the epithelial cells in the respiratory tract. The incubation period is 2 to 4 days followed by fever, myalgia, sore throat, nonproductive cough, and headache. Influenza complications include secondary bacterial pneumonia, Reye syndrome, and myocarditis. During an average influenza season, 36,000 persons die from influenza infections in the United States. If the predominate type A strain expresses the genetically unstable H3 hemagglutinin, mortality increases significantly. Over 90% of deaths occur in persons 65 years of age and older.

Pandemic Influenza Mortality

Pandemic influenza strains usually cause a severe infection that is often fatal. Unlike the seasonal flu viruses, pandemic strains can infect multiple organs. An aberrant immune response known as a *cytokine storm* is responsible the pathophysiology of pandemic influenza.

Infection of macrophages and monocytes by a pandemic avian influenza strain (H5N1) causes an exaggerated and prolonged production of proinflammatory cytokines and chemokines. T cells activated following interactions with macrophages also produce proinflammatory cytokines. The cytokine storm causes pulmonary edema, alveolar hemorrhage, and acute respiratory distress syndrome (Figure 25-3). The major cytokine contributors to the pathophysiology are tumor necrosis factor alpha (TNF-α), IL-6, and interferon gamma (IFN-γ).

Treatment

Treatment for influenza is designed to prevent the spread of the virus and boost immunity with the administration of influenza vaccines. Therapeutic agents are listed in Table 25-14.

Vaccines

Two vaccines are licensed by the FDA. A trivalent inactivated vaccine (TIV) was licensed in 1940, and the live attenuated influenza vaccine (LAIV) became commercially available in 2003. The composition of these vaccines changes every year but usually contains both type A and B strains.

Preparation of Trivalent Inactivated Vaccine (TVI)

The epidemic strains of the vaccine are propagated in the embryonic fluid of fertilized chicken eggs, harvested by centrifugation, purified, inactivated by betapropiolactone, and disrupted by detergent treatment. Subunit hemagglutinin and neuraminidase proteins are purified and prepared for inclusion into the vaccine. Only subunit vaccines are licensed in the United States. TIV is 70% to 90% effective in adults under 65 years of age. In older adults, the vaccine is only 30% to 40% effective in preventing clinical illness. It does, however, reduce hospitalization and prevent influenza-induced deaths by 50% to 80%.

Live Attenuated Influenza Vaccine (LAIV)

LAIV uses influenza strains adapted to replicate at 25°C by the passage of the virus through primary chicken kidney cells at progressively lower temperatures. When administered by the intranasal route, the vaccine strains infect the nasal pharynx and the throat, which are usually at 25°C, but cannot infect the lung that has a temperature of 37°C. In the nasal pharynx and the throat, the virus produces hemagglutinins and neuraminidase, which stimulate mucosal immunity. It is 87% effective against infection with the vaccine strains. In vaccinated adults, 20% to 27% fewer febrile and upper respiratory illnesses occur.

ROTAVIRUS

Rotavirus is a double-stranded RNA virus that consists of three concentric protein shells. This virus is found in every part of the world and is the major cause of severe diarrhea in children.

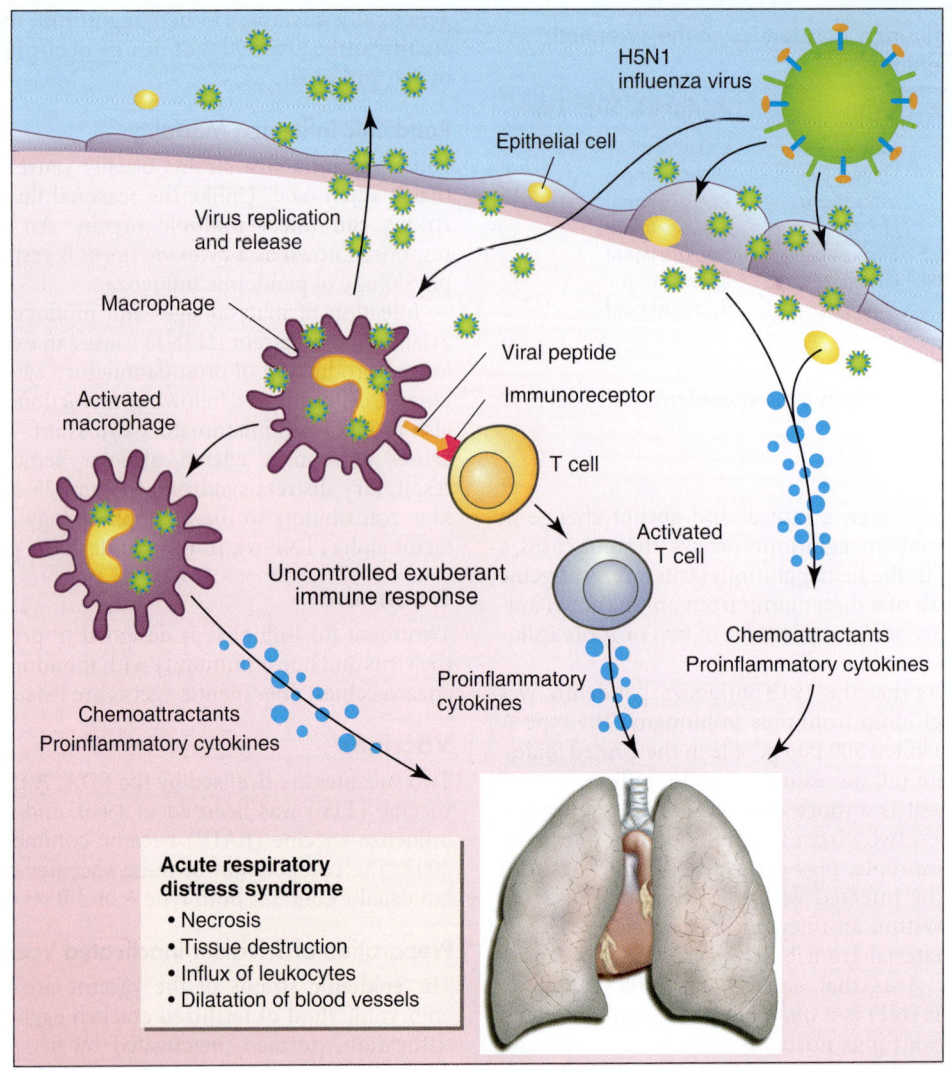

Figure 25-3

The proposed mechanism of the cytokine storm evoked by influenza virus. (Osterholm, MT: Preparing for the next pandemic, N Engl J Med 352:1839-1842, 2005.)

Table 25-14 Agents Used to Treat or Prevent Influenza Infections

Amantadine	Inhibits fusion between viral and target cell membrane
Remantadine	Same as above
Zanamivir	Neuraminidase inhibitor
Oseltamivir	Same as above
Peramivir	Same as above

Groups at risk for rotavirus infection are children in daycare centers, hospitalized children (nosocomial infection), and parents of infected children. Each year in the United States, 55,000 children between 4 and 36 months require hospitalization for rotavirus infections.

The virus enters the body by the oral route and infects the villous epithelium in the upper two thirds of the small intestine. Viral replication causes damage to the intestinal mucosa which results in the malabsorption of sodium and glucose and decreased levels of lactase, phosphatase, and sucrase. This leads to isotonic diarrhea, dehydration, electrolyte imbalance, and metabolic acidosis.

The major groups, subgroups, and serotypes are determined by the differences in viral capsid proteins. Seven major groups of rotavirus (A–G) have been described, but most human infections are caused by group A. Two structural viral proteins (VP4 and VP7) are the major virulence factors and determine the serotype. Eight different VP4 protein isoforms (P1–P8) have been described. These isoforms act as viral enterotoxins that cause diarrhea. The VP7 structural protein is a cased glycoprotein, also known as the *G protein*. Nine different allelic forms of the G protein (G1–G9) are known to exist. A rotavirus strain expresses only one P and one G isoform. Over 80% of diarrheal disease in the United States is caused by the P8G1 serotype.

Treatment

In most cases, the individual recovers without medications. Medications such as antidiarrheals and antiemetics should be used with extreme caution.

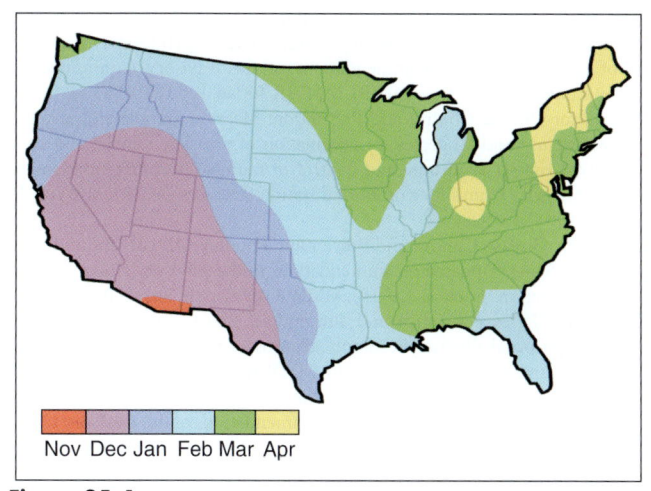

Figure 25-4
Seasonal infections with rotaviruses. (From Parashar U, Bresee S, Gentsch J, et al: Rotavirus, Emerg Infect Dis 4(4):1998.)

Table 25-15	Agents Used to Treat Human Papilloma Virus Infections
Imiquimod	Induces secretion of interferon alpha (IFN-α), tumor necrosis factor (TNF), interleukin 1 (IL-1), IL-6, and IL-8
IFN-α n3 and IFN-α2b	Prevents the spread of virus to uninfected cells
Podofilox	Topical anti-mitotic
Podophyllin	Cytotoxic agent that arrests mitosis in metaphase
Fluorouracil	Interferes with the synthesis of deoxyribonucleic acid (DNA) and ribonucleic acid (RNA), which creates thymine deficiency
Trichloroacetic acid and bichloroacetic acid	Keratolytic agents that chemically cauterize skin and keratins
Salicylic acid	Desquamation of the horny layer of skin
Papillomavirus vaccine, quadrivalent (Gardasil)	Vaccine containing serotypes 9, 11, 16, and 18
Papillomavirus vaccine, bivalent (Cervarix)	Vaccine containing serotypes 16 and 18

Vaccine

In 1998, the FDA licensed Rotashield (RRV-TV), a rhesus-based reassortment vaccine for administration to infants. The vaccine was withdrawn within a year because it caused bowel obstructions as a consequence of the intestine wrapping around itself (intussusceptions).

The FDA subsequently licensed Rotarix and RotaTeq for the prevention of rotavirus infections. RotaTeq is a reassortment vaccine developed from human and bovine rotavirus strains. The vaccine is composed of four reassortment human viruses (G1–G4), a bovine G6 virus, and attachment proteins P1A (human) and P7 (bovine). The duration of RotaTeq protection lasts, at least, throughout the rotavirus season. In the United States, the rotavirus season begins on the west coast between November and January. It moves quickly to the southern states, and then to the northern and the midwestern states (Figure 25-4).

Rotarix is indicated for the prevention of rotavirus gastroenteritis caused by G1 and non-G1 types (G3, G4, and G9), which are the four predominant strains in the United States. The vaccine contains a live attenuated virus associated with the P8G1 serotype. After two doses of the vaccine, 77% to 86% of the recipients develop high antibody titers. The vaccine is efficient in reducing both gastroenteritis and hospitalizations for rotavirus infections over 2 years.

PAPILLOMA VIRUS

Papilloma virus is a small DNA virus. On the basis of antigenic differences in viral capsid L1 proteins, 100 different human papilloma virus serotypes have been classified. Sixty serotypes cause warts on hands and feet. The remaining 40 serotypes infect the mucosa or the genital area. Two serotypes (6 and 11) cause 99% of genital warts and 80% of laryngeal papillomas. Twenty-three other serotypes are oncogenic and cause cervical changes that can transition into cervical intraepithelial neoplasia (CIN) and cancers of the anus, penis, vulva, and vagina. Serotypes 16 and 18 cause 70% of cervical cancers in women and 90% of anal cancers in men.

Papilloma virus infection is the most common sexually transmitted disease in the United States and, perhaps, the world. New infections are estimated at 6.2 million annually. Over 70% of new infections are being reported in the 15- to 24-year age group, and the infection rate among adolescent girls may be as high as 64% and among boys may be greater than 20%. Recent computer-based models also estimate that 80% of sexually active women will be infected with the papilloma virus by age 50.

Infection estimates are both alarming and deceiving. Estimates are based on infection with any one of the 23 genital strains. Only four of these strains pose a high risk of adverse health effects, and 91% of infections resolve within 2 years and cause no further health effects. The incidence of infections with vaccine strains causing genital warts or cervical cancer may be relatively low in the United States.

Human papilloma virus (HPV) has a two-stage reproductive cycle. Basal cells are infected with the virus when the epithelial layer is disturbed during sexual intercourse. The virus targets keratinocyte stem cells and remains dormant in these cells until HPV genes are activated as the keratinocytes leave the basal layer. Replication of the virus occurs in highly differentiated keratinocytes at the epithelial surface. Desquamation of epithelial cells releases the virus into the environment.

Treatment

Biologic modifiers are used to reduce symptoms and external lesions. Infected cells can also be destroyed by cytotoxic agents. Therapeutic agents used to treat HPV infections are listed in Table 25-15.

Vaccines

Gardasil and Cervarix are FDA-licensed HPV vaccines. The quadrivalent HPV recombinant vaccine (Gardasil) contains L proteins that reassemble to form an empty viral shell called a *viral-like protein (VLP)*. Gardasil contains VLPs from serotypes 6, 11, 16, and 18. Cervarix is a bivalent vaccine that contains only serotypes 16 and 18. To sustain the immune response, VLPs are adsorbed to an aluminum adjuvant and stabilized with sodium chloride, L-histidine, polysorbate 30, and sodium borate.

Both vaccines have advantages and disadvantages. Since VLPs do not contain DNA or other genetic material, they cannot infect cells, reproduce, or induce neoplastic changes. A major disadvantage of both vaccines is that they are only effective against papilloma strains used in the vaccine. They do not protect against 21 other strains that may cause cervical cancers in women and penile cancers in men.

Gardasil

Within 1 month of completing the three-dose series, 99.5% of subjects develop high levels of IgG antibody to all four L1 serotypes. This suggests that the vaccine is highly immunogenic and that memory cells have been created. The vaccine is also highly efficacious. Double-blind studies showed that the vaccine reduced the incidence of advanced stage CIN2/3 and carcinoma in situ (CIS). CIS is synonymous with high-grade dysplasia in the cervix. The vaccine is also 99% effective against genital warts. The duration of protection is believed to be 3 to 5 years.

Cervarix

Cervarix is a bivalent (types 16 and 18) HPV vaccine prepared from L1 proteins produced in bioreactors by using a baculovirus expression system. The vaccine is indicated in girls and women (aged 10–25 years) for the prevention of diseases caused by oncogenic HPV types 16 and 18. These diseases include cervical cancer, cervical intraepithelial neoplasia grades 1 and 2, and adenocarcinoma in situ. The vaccine is 93% effective in preventing diseases caused by serotypes 16 and 18.

SUMMARY

- Herd immunity forms the theoretical basis for mass vaccination programs.
- In the twentieth century, mass vaccination programs were highly successful in eradicating childhood diseases such as diphtheria, pertussis, and tetanus.
- Vaccines administered by the subcutaneous or intramuscular route prevent dissemination of bacteria or viruses to multiple organs but may not prevent infection.
- Vaccines that are administered by the intranasal route prevent both infection and dissemination of bacteria or viruses.
- Bacterial antigens used in vaccines are usually stable.
- Viral antigens often change as a consequence of antigenic drift, antigenic shift, or genetic reassortment.

REFERENCES

Atkinson W, Hambrosky J, McIntyre L, et al: Centers for Disease Control and Prevention. Epidemiology and prevention of vaccine preventable diseases, ed 10, Washington, DC, 2007, Public Health Foundation.

Bellini WJ, Rota JS, Lowe LE, et al: Subacute sclerosing panencephalitis: More cases of this fatal disease are prevented by measles immunization than was previously recognized, J Infect Dis 192(10):686, 2005.

Belshe RB, Mendelman PM, Treanor J, et al: The efficacy of live attenuated, cold-adapted, trivalent, intranasal influenza virus vaccine in children, N Engl J Med 338(20):1405, 1998.

Centers for Disease Control and Prevention: A comprehensive immunization strategy to eliminate transmission of hepatitis infections in the United States: Recommendations of the Advisory Committee on Immunization Practices (ACIP), MMWR 54(No. RR-16):1, 2005.

Centers for Disease Control and Prevention: Haemophilus type b conjugate vaccine for prevention of Haemophilus type b among children two months of age and older: Recommendations of the Advisory Committee on Immunization Practices (ACIP), MMWR 40(No. RR-1):1, 1991.

Centers for Disease Control and Prevention: Measles, mumps and rubella-vaccine use and strategies for elimination of measles, rubella, and congenital rubella syndrome and control of mumps: Recommendations of the Advisory Committee on Immunization Practices (ACIP), MMWR 47 (No. RR-8):1, 1998.

Centers for Disease Control and Prevention: Poliomyelitis prevention in the United States: Updated recommendations of the Advisory Committee on Immunization Practices (ACIP), MMWR 49(No. RR-5):1, 2000.

Centers for Disease Control and Prevention: Prevention and control of meningococcal disease: Recommendations of the Advisory Committee on Immunization Practices (ACIP), MMWR 54(No. RR-7):1, 2005.

Centers for Disease Control and Prevention: Prevention of hepatitis A through active or passive immunization: Recommendations of the Advisory Committee on Immunization Practices (ACIP), MMWR 52(No. RR-x):1155, 2006.

Centers for Disease Control and Prevention: Preventing tetanus, diphtheria and pertussis among adolescents: Recommendations of the Advisory Committee on Immunization Practices (ACIP), MMWR 55(No. RR-3):1, 2006.

Centers for Disease Control and Prevention: Prevention of rotavirus gastroenteritis among infants and children: Recommendations of the Advisory Committee on Immunization Practices (ACIP), MMWR 55(No. RR-12):1, 2006.

Centers for Disease Control and Prevention: Prevention of varicella: Recommendations of the Advisory Committee on Immunization Practices (ACIP), MMWR 45(No RR-6):1, 1996.

Freed GL, Konrad TR, DeFriese GH, Lohr JA: Adoption of a new Haemophilus influenzae type b vaccine recommendation, Am J Dis Child 147(2):124, 1993.

Halperin SA: Recommendation for an adolescent dose of tetanus and diphtheria toxoids and acellular pertussis vaccine: Reassurance for the future, J Pediatr 149(5):589, 2006.

Juskewitch JE, Tapia CJ, Windebank AJ: Lessons from the Salk polio vaccine: Methods for and risks of rapid translation, Clin Transl Sci 3(4):182, 2010.

Koopman JS, Monto AS: The Tecumseh Study. XV: Rotavirus infection and pathogenicity, Am J Epidemiol 130(4):750, 1989.

Kretsinger K, Broder KR, Cortese MM, et al: Preventing tetanus, diphtheria, and pertussis among adults: Use of tetanus toxoid, reduced diphtheria toxoid and acellular pertussis vaccine recommendations of the Advisory Committee on Immunization Practices (ACIP) and recommendation of ACIP, supported by the Healthcare Infection Control Practices Advisory Committee (HICPAC), for use of DTaP among health-care personnel, MMWR Recomm Rep 55(RR-17):1, 2006.

Mellinger AK, Cragan JD, Atkinson WL, et al: High incidence of congenital rubella syndrome after a rubella outbreak, Pediatr Infect Dis J 14(7):573, 1995.

Moxon ER, Vaughn KA: The type b capsular polysaccharide as a virulence determinant of Haemophilus influenzae: Studies using clinical isolates and laboratory transformants, J Infect Dis 143(4):517, 1981.

Murphy TV, Gargiullo PM, Massoudi MS, et al: Intussusception among infants given an oral rotavirus vaccine, N Engl J Med 344(8):564, 2001.

Poland GA, Jacobson RM: Clinical practice: Prevention of hepatitis B with the hepatitis B vaccine, N Engl J Med 351(27):2832, 2004.

Rosenstein NE, Perkins BA, Stephens DS, et al: Meningococcal disease, N Engl J Med 344(18):1378, 2001.

Seward JF, Watson BM, Peterson CL, et al: Varicella disease after introduction of varicella vaccine in the United States, 1995-2000, JAMA 287(5):606, 2002.

Smith DR, Leggat PA: Pioneering figures in medicine: Albert Bruce Sabin—inventor of the oral polio vaccine, Kurume Med J 52(3):111, 2005.

Sukupolvi-Petty S, Grass S, St Geme JW III: The Haemophilus influenzae type b hcsA and hcsB gene products facilitate transport of capsular polysaccharide across the outer membrane and are essential for virulence, J Bacteriol 188(11):3870, 2006.

Whitney CG: Preventing pneumococcal disease. ACIP recommends pneumococcal polysaccharide vaccine for all adults ages, Geriatrics 58(10):20, 2003.

ASSESSMENT QUESTIONS

1. The diphtheria toxin targets:
   A. Pertactin
   B. G protein
   C. Elongation factor 2
   D. Filamentous hemagglutinin

2. The tetanus toxin acts by:
   A. Preventing the release of gamma amino butyric acid
   B. Accelerating the release of acetylcholinesterase
   C. Preventing muscle contraction
   D. Increasing the concentration of cyclic adenosine monophosphate (cAMP)

3. In the whole-cell pertussis vaccine, which of the following is responsible for the adverse health effects induced by the vaccine?
   A. Hemaggutinins
   B. Neuraminidase
   C. Pertactin
   D. Endotoxin

4. The major virulence factor for *Haemophilus influenzae* type B is a/an:
   A. Capsular polysaccharide
   B. Hemagglutinin
   C. Outer membrane protein
   D. Endotoxin

5. Which of the following is the *least* effective vaccine for *Streptococcus pneumoniae*?
   A. Pneumovax
   B. Prevnar
   C. Prevnar 13
   D. Prennar 12

6. In meningitis, the activation of the coagulation and complement pathways is caused by:
   A. Capsular polysaccharide
   B. Lipooligosaccharide (LOS)
   C. Outer membrane proteins
   D. Pertactins

7. Which of the following meningitis vaccines is recommended for administration to unvaccinated high-risk groups?
   A. Menveo
   B. Menomune
   C. Menactra
   D. Menoligo

8. Which of the following is a life-threatening form of polio?
   A. Spinal polio
   B. Nonparalytic aseptic meningitis
   C. Bulbar polio
   D. Bulbospinal polio

9. Which of the following is *not* a complication of rubeola?
   A. Immune suppression
   B. Encephalitis
   C. Deafness
   D. Subacute sclerosing panencephalitis (SSPE)

10. The most life-threatening form of hepatitis is:
    A. Hepatitis B
    B. Hepatitis A
    C. Hepatitis E
    D. Hepatitis C

11. Which of the following influenza types are associated with pandemics?
    A. Type B
    B. Type A
    C. Type C
    D. Type E

12. Antigenic shift in influenza hemagglutins is caused by:
    A. Mutations that change the hemagglutinin structure by 50%
    B. A direct jump of the virus from animals to humans
    C. Reassortment of genetic material from two or more influenza strains
    D. All of the above

13. Tissue damage in pandemic influenza infections is caused by:
    A. Viral replication
    B. Production of an enterotoxin
    C. Cytokine storm
    D. Production of anti-inflammatory cytokines

14. The major complication of rubella infections in women is:
    A. Congenital rubella syndrome
    B. Arthritis
    C. Subacute sclerosing panencephalitis
    D. Secondary bacterial infection

15. Which of the following is *not* caused by varicella zoster virus?
    A. Chickenpox
    B. Shingles
    C. Post-herpetic neuralgia
    D. Encephalitis

16. The major cancer-causing human papilloma virus strains are:
    A. 6 and 9
    B. 16 and 18
    C. 6 and 11
    D. 14 and 16

CHAPTER 26

Acquired Immune Deficiency Syndrome

LEARNING OBJECTIVES

- Recognize the origin of human immunodeficiency virus 1 (HIV-1) and HIV-2
- Define clade
- Identify the HIV-1 clade predominant in most of the world
- Describe the structure of HIV-1
- Compare the roles of structural, regulatory, and accessory genes in HIV-1 integration and replication
- Compare and contrast HIV-1 binding to lymphocytes and monocytes
- Explain the mechanisms involved in the fusion of HIV and the host cell membrane
- Explain the reverse transcription of HIV
- Understand the two-step process used to integrate viral deoxyribonucleic acid (DNA)
- Identify the process by which HIV exits host cells
- Discuss the roles of follicular dendritic cells in the pathogenesis of HIV
- List the possible mechanisms in the killing of CD4 cells
- Identify the possible mechanisms involved in CD8 dysfunction
- Identify HIV target cells in the brain
- Differentiate between the three states of HIV infection
- Compare and contrast HIV infection and acquired immune deficiency syndrome (AIDS)
- List the AIDS-defining medical conditions
- Understand the rationale for using highly active antiretroviral therapy (HAART)
- Explain the mechanism of action of fusion inhibitors
- Compare and contrast nucleoside and non-nucleoside reverse transcriptase inhibitors
- Explain the mechanism of action of integrase inhibitors
- Identify the biologic role of protease inhibitors

KEY TERMS

Acquired immune deficiency syndrome (AIDS)
Capsid
Chemokine
Clade
Env
Follicular dendritic cells
Gag
Gp120/gp41
Iccosomes
Integrase
Matrix
Nef
Pol
Protease
Rev
Reverse transcriptase
Simian immunodeficiency virus (SIV)
Syncytia
Tat
Vif
Vpr
Vpu

INTRODUCTION

Human immunodeficiency virus (HIV) is closely related to simian immunodeficiency viruses (SIVs), which are found in equatorial Africa. SIVs are found in nine classes of monkeys and chimpanzees. Genetic sequencing strongly suggests that an SIV endemic to a chimpanzee subspecies (*Pan troglodytes troglodytes*) first crossed the species barrier in 1930. This virus is the ancestral HIV-1. In Gabon and Cameroon, the Sooty Mangabey monkey population is infected with a different SIV. Sometime between 1955 and 1972, the monkey SIV crossed the species barrier in several direct jumps to humans. The genome of this virus differs from HIV-1 by 30% to 40% and is designated HIV-2.

Subsequent studies linked HIV with the destruction of the immune system and acquired immune deficiency syndrome (AIDS). The syndrome is characterized by infections with unusual opportunistic pathogens (e.g., *Pneumocystis jiroveci*) and the development of aggressive sarcomas.

HIV-1 causes over 90% of human infections in the world. In the United States, 1.1 million individuals are infected with HIV-1, and 56,000 new cases are reported each year. HIV-2 is responsible for at least six epidemics in Africa. The World Health Organization (WHO) estimates that 4.3 million individuals are newly infected with HIV each year. Over 95% of

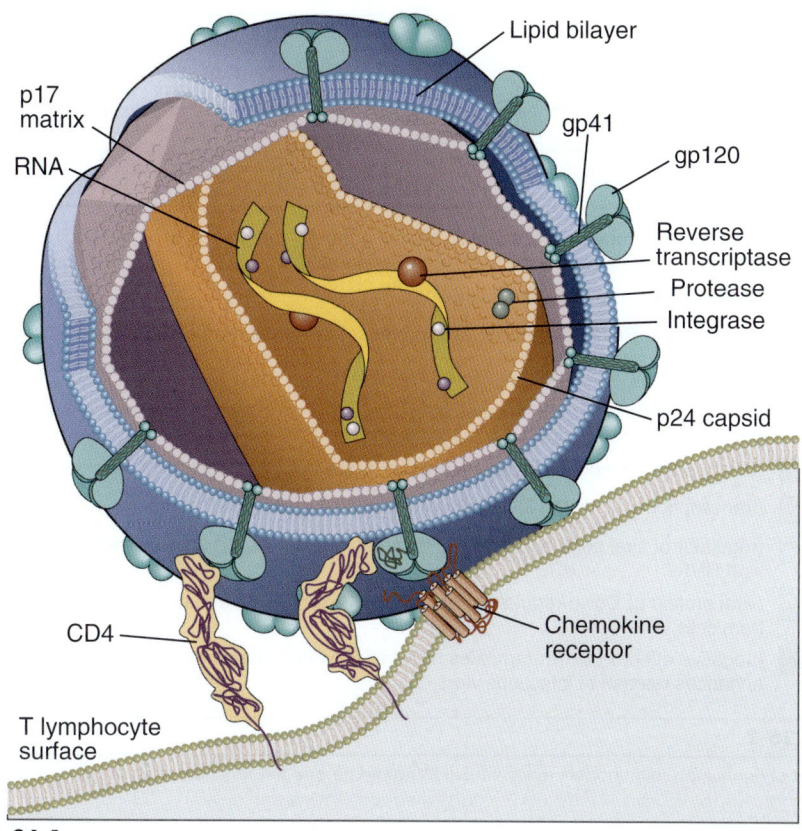

Figure 26-1

Structural features of human immunodeficiency virus (HIV). (From Abbas AK, Lichtman AH: Basic immunology, ed 3 [updated edition], Philadelphia, 2010, Saunders.)

these infections are occurring in the developing countries and Sub-Saharan Africa.

HUMAN IMMUNODEFICIENCY VIRUS GROUPS AND CLADES

According to the frequency of infections and the genetic diversity, HIV-1 is subdivided into groups and clades. HIV-1 is initially grouped into M (major), O (outlying), and N (new) groups. The HIV-1 M group has spread throughout the world. Groups N and O are restricted to West Equatorial Africa. Mutations within the M group, environmental pressure, and therapeutic selection have given rise to HIV clades. By definition, a *clade* is a virus subgroup that arose from a single common ancestor. The HIV-1 M group has nine major genetically diverse clades (A, B, C, D, F, G, H, J, and K). In the Western world, the B clade is the predominant virus. Transmission of HIV-1 B is rapid and associated with sex between men, intravenous drug use, and transmission of the virus from mothers to babies. HIV-1 A and C clades are found in southern and eastern Africa. Recombinant A-G and A-E clades also are emerging as infectious agents in Africa and Asia. In areas where subtypes C or A-E are common, heterosexual transmission is more frequent. Heterosexual transmission occurs because these clades replicate more efficiently in the Langerhans and dendritic cells of the vagina, and the virus is then shed into vaginal fluids. In the United States, the emerging trend in heterosexual HIV transmission has occurred because of the introduction of the A-E or C clade into North America.

STRUCTURE OF THE HUMAN IMMUNODEFICIENCY VIRUS

HIV virus comprises an inner core, a capsid, a matrix shell, and a host cell–derived outer membrane. The inner core contains two single strands of ribonucleic acid (RNA). One RNA strand, called the *plus* (+) or *coding strand*, contains viral genes that are transcribed. A second strand, the *negative* (−) *strand*, is complementary to the plus strand. The RNA and several proteins necessary for viral replication are encased in a cone-shaped capsid (Figure 26-1).

Additional protection for the capsid core is provided by an icosahedral shell or matrix. The shell anchors a lipid membrane to the outer surface of the virus. Protruding from the HIV membrane is the gp120 viral protein, which is anchored by a transmembrane gp41 protein. Three molecules of the gp120–gp41 aggregate to form a trimolecular structure necessary for docking to HIV target cells.

HUMAN IMMUNODEFICIENCY VIRUS GENES

The HIV-1 genome codes for all the gene products necessary for viral replication. The genome is divided into structural genes (*gag*, *pol*, and *env*), regulatory genes (*tat* and *rev*) and accessory genes (*vpr*, *nef*, *vpu*, and *vif*). The organization of the HIV genome and the function of individual genes are shown in Figure 26-2.

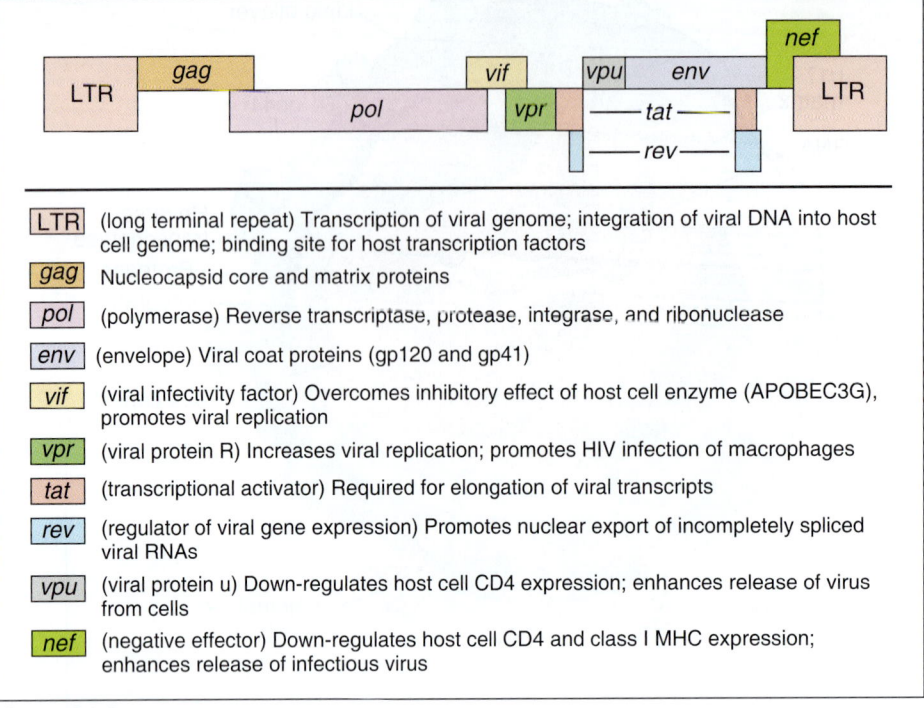

Figure 26-2

LTR	(long terminal repeat) Transcription of viral genome; integration of viral DNA into host cell genome; binding site for host transcription factors
gag	Nucleocapsid core and matrix proteins
pol	(polymerase) Reverse transcriptase, protease, integrase, and ribonuclease
env	(envelope) Viral coat proteins (gp120 and gp41)
vif	(viral infectivity factor) Overcomes inhibitory effect of host cell enzyme (APOBEC3G), promotes viral replication
vpr	(viral protein R) Increases viral replication; promotes HIV infection of macrophages
tat	(transcriptional activator) Required for elongation of viral transcripts
rev	(regulator of viral gene expression) Promotes nuclear export of incompletely spliced viral RNAs
vpu	(viral protein u) Down-regulates host cell CD4 expression; enhances release of virus from cells
nef	(negative effector) Down-regulates host cell CD4 and class I MHC expression; enhances release of infectious virus

Figure 26-2
Structure of the human immunodeficiency virus (HIV) genome and the function of each gene. (From Abbas AK, Lichtman AH: *Basic immunology*, ed 3 [updated edition], Philadelphia, 2010, Saunders.)

LIFE CYCLE OF THE HUMAN IMMUNODEFICIENCY VIRUS

The life cycle of HIV is divided into several stages, which include attachment, membrane fusion, uncoating, reverse transcription of viral RNA into DNA, and integration into the host cell genome. When HIV is integrated into the host cell DNA, it is called a *latent provirus*. Latency is characterized by the lack of viral gene expression. At some point in time, intracellular *tat* levels increase, and viral RNA is transcribed. After synthesis of multiple copies, the double-stranded RNA is packaged and exported from the cell.

Attachment

Different receptors are used to attach the virus gp120–gp41 to lymphocytes or monocytes. Attachment to T cells requires both CD4 and the chemokine receptor (CXCR4). Monocyte attachment points for HIV gp120–gp41 are a cell surface heparin molecule and a macrophage-specific chemokine (CCR5) receptor. Interaction with two receptors is necessary for the fusion of HIV with the host cell membrane (Figure 26-3).

Membrane Fusion

After interaction with gp120, the membrane attachment component (gp41) disassociates itself and undergoes a conformational change to become a long, cylindrical fusion protein, which bridges the divide between the virus and the cell membrane. After inserting itself into the host cell membrane, the gp41 fusion protein refolds itself using two specialized molecular H-1 and H-2 sequences called *heptadrepeats*. The H-1 and H-2 regions fold and form a six-helix fusion protein bundle, which brings the virus and host cell membrane into close contact (see Figure 26-3). Several six-helix fusion proteins form a narrow fusion pore in the membrane, which expands to allow viral entry into the cell.

After uncoating of the virus in the host cell cytoplasm, the *nef* gene is translated; it accelerates the endocytosis of the CD4 virus complex and downregulates the expression of class I molecules, which decreases the risk of the CD8-mediated destruction of infected cells.

Reverse Transcription (RT)

Pol gene products are critical for the synthesis and integration of viral DNA into the host genome and the generation of capsid proteins. *Pol* gene products include the HIV-1 reverse transcriptase, an integrase, and the late-phase protease. The *pol* gene proteins complex with RNase and *vpr* in the cell membrane to form the viral reverse transcription complex. The complex docks with the actin microfilaments in the cell and begins the RT process. After degradation of the negative RNA strand, the plus, or coding, strand is prepared for transcription. The plus RNA stand consists of the following: (1) R regions, which are direct repeats at both ends of the genome, (2) a U5 noncoding region, which is initially transcribed and forms the 3′ end of new DNA; (3) a leucine transfer RNA (tRNA) primer binding site (PBS), which is used to initiate reverse transcription; (4) a leader sequence, which is located downstream of the transcription start site and upstream of the structural genes; (5) structural, regulatory, and accessory genes; (6) a polypurine tract (PPT), which is responsible for initiating plus strand synthesis; and (7) a U3 noncoding region, which contains the promoter elements of the single-stranded DNA and a noncoding 5′ end of the genome (Figure 26-4).

Reverse transcription begins from the 5′ terminus and proceeds to the 3′ terminus. In the initial stages of reverse transcription, the leucine tRNA binds to the PBS near the 5′ end of the viral RNA. Complementary DNA binds to the U5

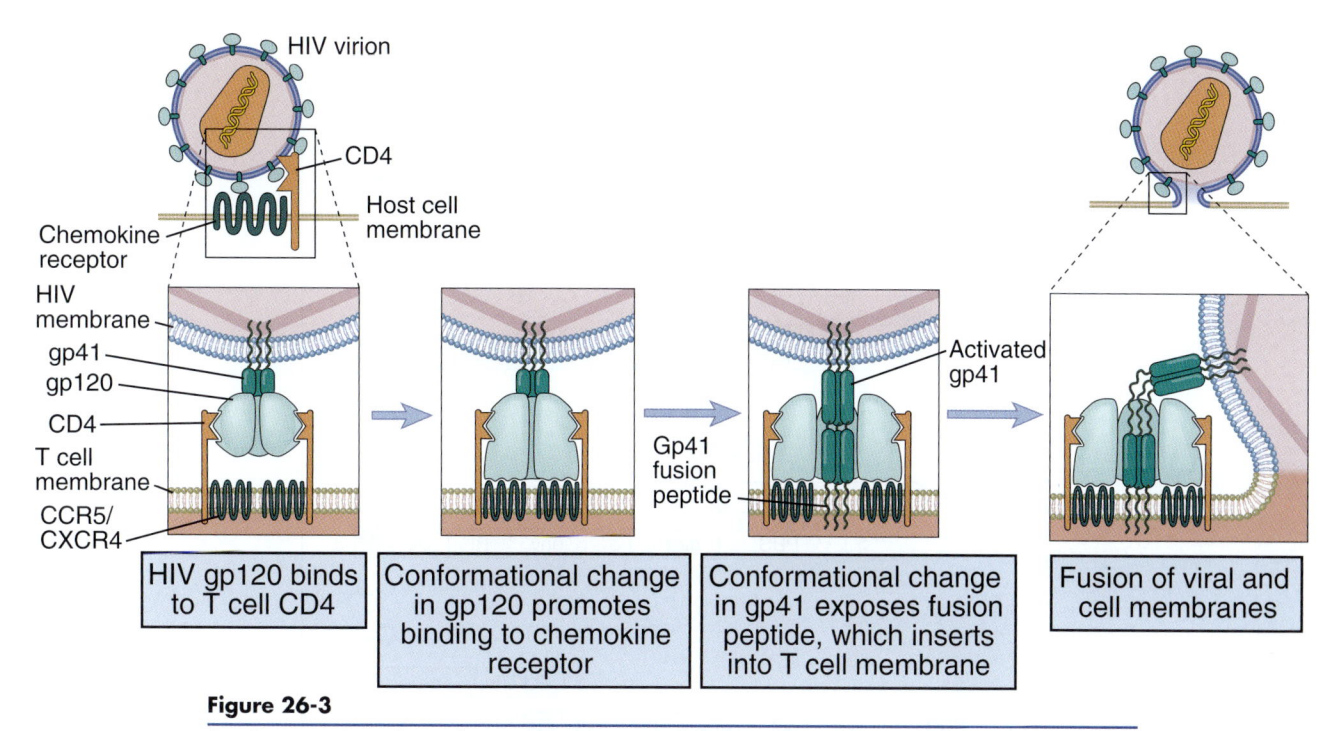

Figure 26-3

Attachment and membrane fusion of human immunodeficiency virus (HIV). (From Abbas AK, Lichtman AH: Basic immunology, ed 3 [updated edition], Philadelphia, 2010, Saunders.)

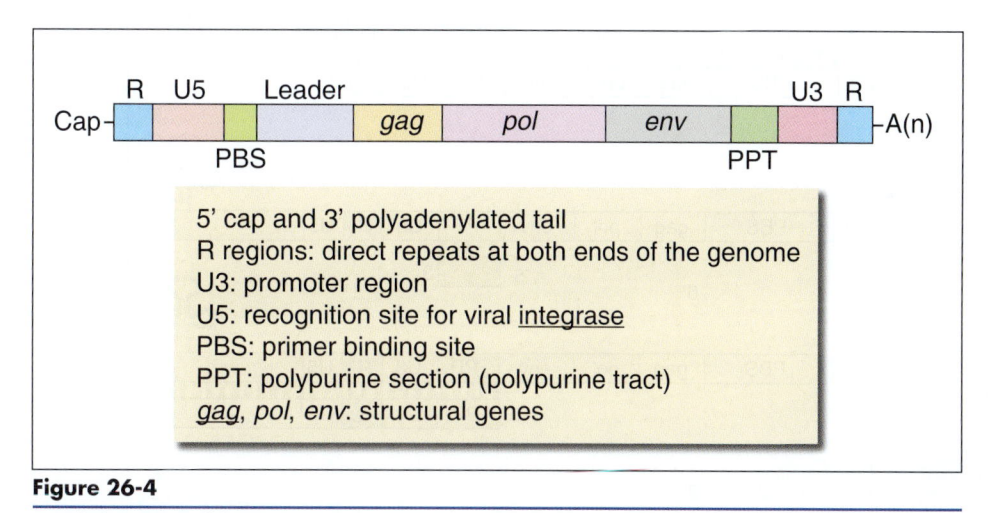

5' cap and 3' polyadenylated tail
R regions: direct repeats at both ends of the genome
U3: promoter region
U5: recognition site for viral integrase
PBS: primer binding site
PPT: polypurine section (polypurine tract)
gag, pol, env: structural genes

Figure 26-4

Detailed structure of the HIV genome.

and R sites and the tRNA, creating a complex consisting of a small fragment of DNA linked to the viral RNA. Subsequently, the 5' end of the viral RNA in the complex is degraded by the enzyme RNase to create a DNA primer. The primer consists of the tRNA and DNA complementary U5 and R regions (see Figure 26-4). Since the reverse transcriptase synthesizes DNA from the 5' end to the 3' prime end, the primer must jump to the other end of the viral DNA, where it binds to the R region. The reverse transcriptase is activated and elongates a plus, or sense, DNA strand.

Subsequently, most of the RNA is degraded by the RNase leaving only the PPT. Using a DNA polymerase and the polypurine primer, a small piece of negative, or antisense, DNA is synthesized in a 5' end to 3' end direction. The DNA fragment codes for the U3, R, and U5 segments. This fragment jumps to the 5' of the plus strand DNA and binds to the PBS tract. A DNA polymerase extends the plus strand and assists in the synthesis of double-stranded DNA (Figure 26-5).

Preintegration Complex

Following the synthesis of double-stranded viral DNA, a preintegration complex (PIC) forms for the transport of DNA to the nucleus. The PIC consists of DNA, viral protein R (*vpr*), and the integrase. The PIC switches attachment from actin microfilaments to microtubules, which actively transports HIV DNA to the nucleus. To increase the efficiency of viral DNA into the host chromosome, *vpr* arrests proliferating cells in the G2 phase of cell division.

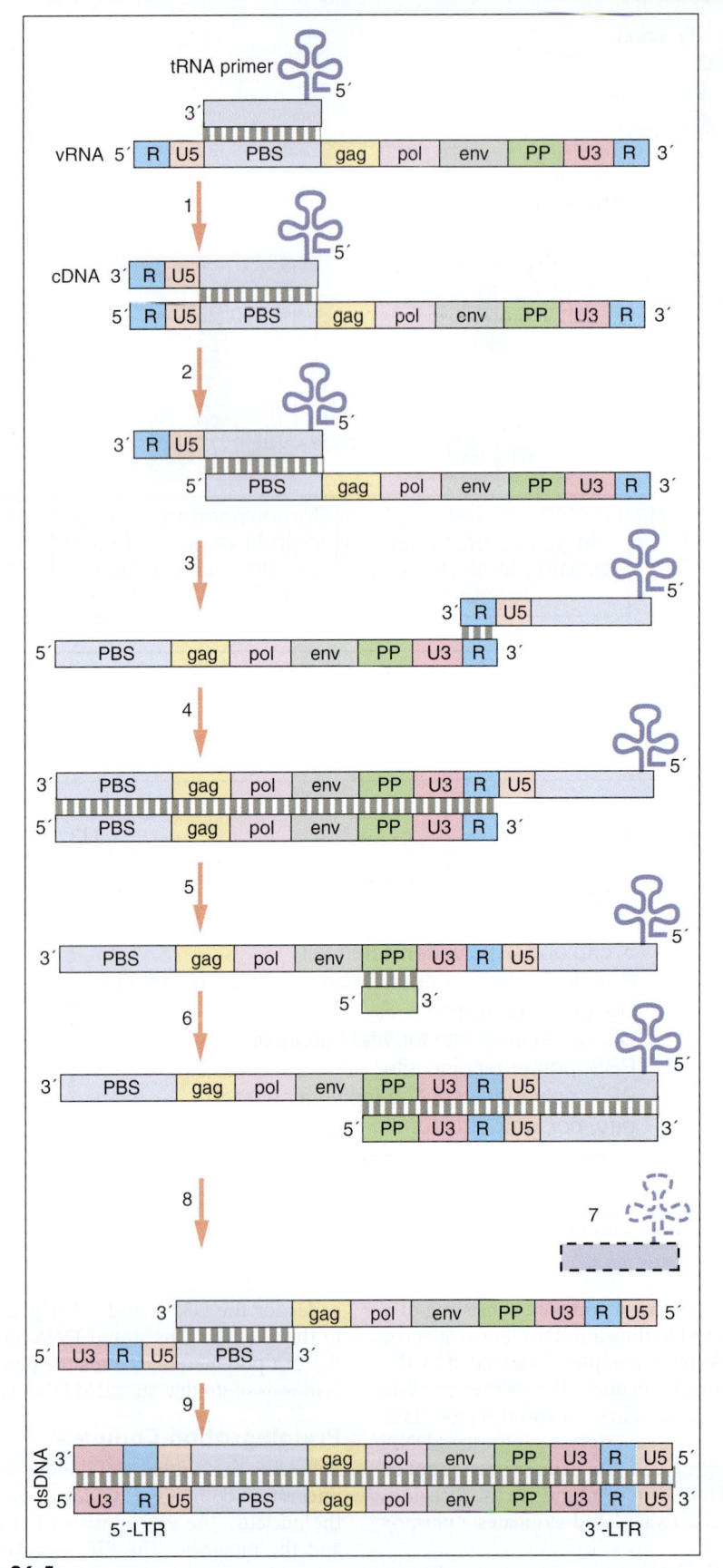

Figure 26-5

Synthesis of viral double-stranded deoxyribonucleic acid (DNA) from single-stranded ribonucleic acid (RNA). (From Wikimedia Commons. Licensed under the Creative Commons Attribution Unreported license. Image part of the Philip Greenspun Illustration Project.)

Integrase

Double-stranded viral DNA is integrated into the host genome by a two-step process that occurs in the cytoplasm and the nucleus. In the cytoplasm, the integrase binds to the blunt end of the DNA strands and removes two nucleotides from the 3′-OH end of each viral DNA strand in a process called *3′-end processing*. Processed viral DNA is transferred to the nucleus and the exposed 3′-OH ends ligated to the cellular DNA (3′ end joining). Host cell DNA repair enzymes fill in any gaps in DNA and remove unpaired nucleotides. Viral DNA is synthesized and inserted within 6 hours of infection.

Viral Assembly and Release

Tat gene translation is essential for viral replication. *Tat* promotes full length synthesis of viral RNA by stabilizing the RNA polymerase and preventing the termination of protein synthesis. Interactions between *Tat* and the polymerase increase the production of viral RNA and messenger RNA (mRNA) approximately 100-fold.

Rev binds to mRNA, which contains a *Rev* response element (RRE). This promotes stabilization and export of mRNA from the nucleus to the cytoplasm of unspliced and single-spliced RNA. Under normal circumstances, only unspliced RNA is exported. The ability to transport both types of genetic material is necessary for viral replication. Early in the replication process, unspliced RNA that codes for RNase, *nef*, *tat*, and *rev* exits the nucleus. As *rev* levels increase, single-spliced RNA coding for matrix and capsid proteins are exported from the nucleus. The vif protein protects RNA from degradation by cytoplasmic enzymes.

Translation of the *gag* and *env* genes is necessary for the formation of HIV capsid and matrix proteins. *Gag* gene transcription generates a large p55 precursor protein, which is cleaved by the protease into small p24 (capsid) and p17 (nucleocapsid) proteins (see Figure 26-1). The *env* gene complex codes for gp120–gp41, regulatory, and accessory proteins. With the assistance of specialized proteins, the assembled virus passes through the host cell lipid bi-layer membrane and exits the cell by a process called *budding*. As a consequence, the virus is coated with a cholesterol-rich membrane. Since the budding process does not kill the host cell, viral synthesis is continual.

HUMAN IMMUNODEFICIENCY VIRUS AND THE IMMUNE SYSTEM

Follicular Dendritic Cells and Human Immunodeficiency Virus

During the initial phases of infection, HIV is concentrated in lymph node germinal centers. Follicular dendritic cells (FDCs) use dendritic extensions called *iccosomes* to trap viable viruses. Some CD4 cells are infected by contact with the iccosomes. Within 6 weeks, FDCs express FasR molecules on the cell surface and are killed by CD8 cells.

FDC destruction has far-reaching effects on T cell development. Interleukin 12 (IL-12) produced by dendritic cells is necessary for the differentiation of CD4Th1 cells and maintenance of CD4 memory cells. As a consequence of FDC destruction and a lack of IL-12, CD4Th1 inflammatory responses cannot be implemented, thus increasing the risk of infection with intracellular pathogens such as mycobacteria, *Histoplasma*, and *Pneumocystis*. In addition, the dysfunctional memory cells cannot facilitate isotypic switching required for an anamnestic response to extracellular pathogens such as *Staphylococcus aureus*, *Haemophilus influenzae*, and *Streptococcus pneumoniae*.

Destruction of CD4 Cells

The mechanisms used by HIV to destroy CD4 cells are unclear. CD4 cells may be killed in an *innocent bystander* reaction. HIV synthesizes a truncated gp120, which is released into the cytoplasm. Some noninfected CD4 cells bind the soluble gp120 and are killed by cytotoxic T cells. Infected CD4 cells also form syncytia with monocytes or other T cells and undergo rapid apoptosis. Evidence also indicates that HIV acts as a super-antigen that stimulates a massive polyclonal proliferation of CD4 cells. Proliferation and activation are followed by HIV infection and apoptosis of large numbers of CD4 cells. The destruction of CD4 cells results in an inversion in the normal C4–CD8 ratio in peripheral blood.

The ultimate collapse of the CD4 population is caused by stem cell exhaustion. Approximately 2.0×10^9 CD4 cells must be produced each day to match the number of dying cells. Over time, the number of stem cells able to produce CD4 cells is exhausted and the number of CD4 cells is permanently reduced.

Loss of CD8 Cell Function

Cytotoxic CD8 cells are important in containing HIV infections; individuals with normal CD8 numbers have longer survival rates. In children and adults, a loss of CD8 function correlates with increased viremia, spread of the virus within the host, and the onset of clinical symptoms. Decreased CD8 function, which can be restored by IL-2, is associated with reduced expression of T cell receptors and CD28.

HUMAN IMMUNODEFICIENCY VIRUS AND NEUROLOGIC EFFECTS

In 10% of patients with HIV, the virus crosses the blood–brain barrier and infects macrophages, microglial cells, and astrocytes. These cells produce proinflammatory cytokines, neurotoxins, and reactive oxygen species. Additional neurotoxins are produced by monocytes or macrophages recruited into the brain from peripheral blood. Toxin damage to neuronal cells is reflected in cognitive dysfunction and symptoms associated with the AIDS–dementia complex.

HUMAN IMMUNODEFICIENCY VIRUS INFECTION AND ACQUIRED IMMUNE DEFICIENCY SYNDROME

In 2008, the Centers for Disease Control and Prevention (CDC) revised its acquired immune deficiency syndrome (AIDS) classification system for adults and adolescents into a single case definition for HIV infection. The case definition is based on laboratory data and the presence of an AIDS-defining condition (Box 26-1).

Presumptive laboratory evidence of HIV infection includes a positive result in an HIV antibody screening test that is confirmed by an alternative HIV test (Western blot or immuno-fluorescence). The presence of HIV nucleic acids, p24 capsid antigen, or isolation of HIV from blood or bodily fluids is also considered evidence of HIV infection. If the patient meets the laboratory criteria for HIV infection and one of the three

BOX 26-1
Acquired Immune Deficiency Syndrome (AIDS)–Defining Conditions

Candidiasis of bronchi, trachea, or lungs
Candidiasis of esophagus
Cervical cancer, invasive
Coccidioidomycosis, disseminated or extrapulmonary
Cryptococcosis, extrapulmonary
Cryptosporidiosis, chronic intestinal (>1 month's duration)
Cytomegalovirus disease (other than liver, spleen, or nodes), onset at age >1 month
Cytomegalovirus retinitis (with loss of vision)
Encephalopathy, human immunodeficiency virus (HIV)–related
Herpes simplex: chronic ulcers (>1 month's duration) or bronchitis, pneumonitis, or esophagitis (onset at age >1 month)
Histoplasmosis, disseminated or extrapulmonary
Isosporiasis, chronic intestinal (>1 month's duration)
Kaposi's sarcoma
Lymphoma, Burkitt's (or equivalent term)
Lymphoma, immunoblastic (or equivalent term)
Lymphoma, primary, of brain
Mycobacterium avium complex or *Mycobacterium kansasii*, disseminated or extrapulmonary
Mycobacterium tuberculosis of any site, pulmonary, disseminated, or extrapulmonary
Mycobacterium, other species or unidentified species, disseminated or extrapulmonary
Pneumocystis jiroveci pneumonia
Pneumonia, recurrent
Progressive multifocal leukoencephalopathy
Salmonella septicemia, recurrent
Toxoplasmosis of brain, onset at age >1 month
Wasting syndrome attributed to HIV

Modified from CDC: Appendix A: AIDS-defining conditions, MMWR 57(RR10):9, 2008.

Table 26-1 Nucleoside or Nucleotide Reverse Transcriptase Inhibitors

Drug	Chemical Structure
Zidovudine	Thymidine analog, 3′ azido group (–N$_3$) replaces the 3′ hydroxyl group
Abacavir	Synthetic nucleoside, which lacks the 3′-OH group on sugar groups
Didanosine	Adenosine analog, which lacks the 3′-OH group on sugar groups
Emtricitabine	Synthetic cytidine analog, which has a fluorine in the 5′ position
Stavudine	Synthetic thymidine analog, which lacks hydroxyl radical at the 3′ position
Tenofovir	Analog of adenosine 5′ phosphate. Converted to an acrylic nucleoside phosphonate.

stages of HIV infection (stages 1–3), HIV infection is considered confirmed.
   HIV Infection Stage 1
   • No AIDS-defining condition and a CD4 lymphocyte count at or above 500 cell/μL or a CD4 lymphocyte percentage at or above 29%
   HIV Infection Stage 2
   • No AIDS-defining condition and a CD4 lymphocyte count of 200 to 499 cells/μL or a CD4 lymphocyte percentage between 14% and 28%
   HIV Infection Stage 3
   • CD4 lymphocyte count of at or below 200 cells/μL or a CD4 lymphocyte percentage at or below 14% and documentation of an AIDS-defining condition

TREATMENT OF HUMAN IMMUNODEFICIENCY VIRUS INFECTIONS

Highly active anti-retroviral therapy (HAART) is a treatment strategy that combines drugs that inhibit viral replication at different steps. These drugs are classified into five categories: (1) attachment and fusion inhibitors, (2) reverse transcriptase inhibitors (nucleoside and non-nucleoside inhibitors), (3) protease inhibitors, (4) integrase inhibitors, and (5) combination drugs. At the present time, over 30 drugs have been approved by the U.S. Food and Drug Administration (FDA) for the treatment of HIV infection.

Attachment and Fusion Inhibitors

Attachment and fusion inhibitors prevent the initial interactions between the virus and target cell membranes. At this point in time, two fusion inhibitors are licensed in the United States: (1) Maraviroc prevents the binding of gp120 to the CCR5 co-receptor for HIV. It is most effective when used to treat individuals infected with macrophage-tropic HIV strains and does not inhibit HIV attachment of CXCR4 lymphocyte-tropic HIV-1 strains. (2) Enfuvirtide is a synthetic 36-amino-acid segment of the HR2 region of gp41, which prevents the formation of a six-helix fusion protein necessary for membrane fusion.

Nucleoside Reverse Transcriptase Inhibitors

The reverse transcriptase (RT) is a major target in anti-retroviral therapy. RT inhibitors are classified as nucleoside reverse transcriptase inhibitors (NRTIs) or non-nucleoside reverse transcriptase inhibitors (NNRTIs). Nucleosides (adenine, cytosine, guanine, and thymidine) consist of a phosphate group and a sugar molecule, either deoxyribose (DNA) or ribose (RNA). In the synthesis of DNA, nucleosides are linked together using 5′-3′-hydroxyl linkages between sugars. In many of the NRTIs, the hydroxyl group at the 3′ position in the sugar is replaced by another molecule. The NRTIs can be inserted into new DNA, but chain synthesis is terminated (Table 26-1).

The most studied reverse transcriptase inhibitor is zidovudine or 3′-azido-2′,3′-dideoxythymidine (Figure 26-6).

The structure mimics thymidine. However, a 3′ azido group (N$_3$) replaces the 3′ hydroxyl group on the nucleotide. Other synthetic analogs are dehydroxylated forms of purines and pyrimidines. For example, didanosine is an adenosine analog, and zalcitabine is a cytosine analog (Figures 26-7 and 26-8).

Non-Nucleoside Reverse Transcriptase Inhibitors

Although the NNRTIs have different chemical structures, they are all highly specific to the HIV-1 RT. They bind to the RT and inhibit RNA and DNA polymerase activity. Delavirdine, etravirine, and nevirapine are NNTRIs that are currently licensed in the United States.

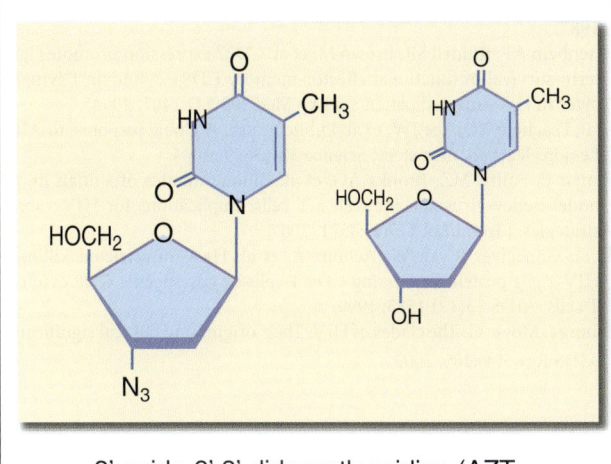

Figure 26-6
3'-azido-2',3'-dideoxythymidine (AZT, ziduovudine), analog to deoxythymidine

Deoxythymidine and the zidovudine nucleoside analogue.

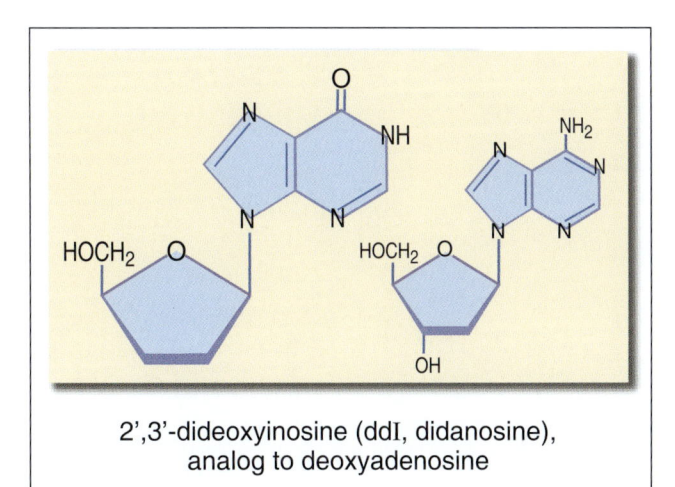

Figure 26-7
2',3'-dideoxyinosine (ddI, didanosine), analog to deoxyadenosine

Deoxyadenosine and the nucleoside analog didanosine.

Figure 26-8
2',3'-dideoxycytidine (ddC, zalcitabine), analog to deoxycytidine

Deoxycytidine and the nucleoside zalcitabine.

BOX 26-2
Non-Nucleoside Reverse Transcriptase Inhibitors

Amprenavir
Atazanavir
Darunavir
Fosamprenavir
Indinavir
Nelfinavir
Ritonavir
Saquinavir mesylate
Tipranavir

Protease Inhibitors

Protease inhibitors prevent the cleavage of the large *gag–pol* polyproteins into active proteins and enzymes. Protease inhibition results in disorganized capsid or matrix formation and the production of noninfectious viruses. Box 26-2 shows the currently licensed agents that are competitive inhibitors of the HIV protease.

Integrase Inhibitors

Integrase is an attractive drug target because integration of viral DNA into the host genome is critical to the infective process, and integrase has no functional analog in humans. Raltegravir is the only nontoxic, selective integrase inhibitor currently licensed by the FDA. This drug acts by inhibiting single-strand transfer of viral DNA to the host genome.

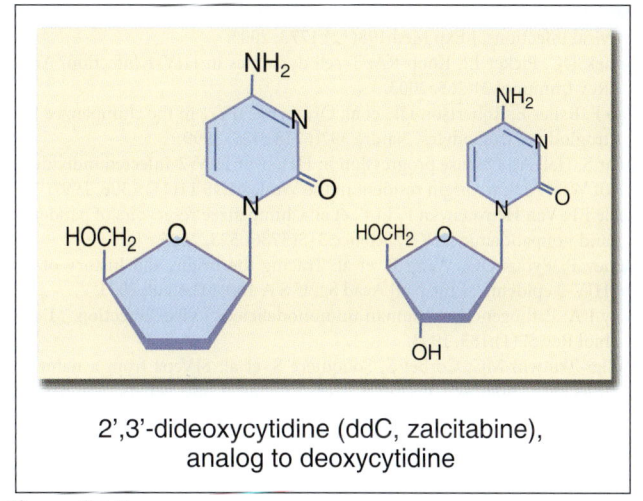

SUMMARY

- Human immunodeficiency virus 1 (HIV-1) and HIV-2 are chimpanzee and monkey immunodeficiency viruses that have crossed species barriers to infect humans.
- HIV-1 M is responsible for HIV infections in the developed countries.
- HIV-2 causes most infections in Africa.
- Genetic pressure and mutations have created HIV clades.
- Attachment to targets cells requires interaction between HIV and two cellular receptors.
- After membrane fusion, the virus integrates itself into host DNA by using a reverse transcriptase and an integrase.
- Over time, immune function is disrupted, and infected individuals become susceptible to opportunistic pathogens and tumor development.
- Therapeutic agents interrupt HIV membrane fusion, reverse transcriptase, integrase, and protease activity.

REFERENCES

Altfeld M, Allen TM, Yu XG, et al: HIV-1 superinfection despite broad CD8+ T-cell responses containing replication of the primary virus, Nature 420(6914):434, 2002.

Anonymous: Revised surveillance case definitions for HIV infections among adults and children ≤18 months and for HIV infection and AIDS among children aged 18 months to ≤13 years. Recommendations and Reports. Appendix A, MMWR 57(RR10):9, 2008.

Day CL, Walker BD: Progress in defining CD4 helper cell responses in chronic viral infections, J Exp Med 198(12):1773, 2003.

Douek DC, Picker LJ, Koup RA: T cell dynamics in HIV-1 infection, Annu Rev Immunol 21:265, 2003.

Gao F, Bailes E, Robertson DL, et al: Origin of HIV-1 in the chimpanzee Pan troglodytes troglodytes, Nature 397(6718):436, 1999.

Jaffar S, Hall AJ: Disease progression in HIV-1 or HIV-2-infected individuals of West African origin resident in the West, AIDS 11(11):1398, 1997.

Keele BF, Van Heuverswyn F, Li Y, et al: Chimpanzee reservoirs of pandemic and nonpandemic HIV-1, Science 313(5786):523, 2006.

Lemey P, Pybus OG, Wang B, et al: Tracing the origin and history of the HIV-2 epidemic, Proc Natl Acad Sci U S A 100(11):6588, 2003.

Levy J A: Pathogenesis of human immunodeficiency virus infection, Microbiol Rev 57(1):183, 1993.

Muller-Trutwin MC, Corbet S, Souquière S, et al: SIVcpz from a naturally infected Cameroonian chimpanzee: Biological and genetic comparison with HIV-1N, J Med Primatol 29(3-4):166, 2000.

Noireau F: HIV transmission from monkey to man, Lancet 1(8548):1498, 1987.

Ochsenbein AF, Riddell SR, Brown M, et al: CD27 expression promotes long-term survival of functional effector-memory CD8+ cytotoxic T lymphocytes in HIV-infected patients, J Exp Med 200(11):1407, 2004.

Piot P, Feachem RG, Lee JW, et al: Public health. A global response to AIDS: Lessons learned, next steps, Science 304(5679):2004.

Rollman E, Smith MZ, Brooks AG, et al: Killing kinetics of simian immunodeficiency virus-specific CD8+ T cells: Implications for HIV vaccine strategies, J Immunol 179(7):4571, 2007.

Salerno-Goncalves R, Lu W, Achour A, et al: HLA-unrestricted killing of HIV-1 *gag* protein-expressing CD4 T cells by *gag*-specific CD8 cytotoxic T cells, AIDS 13(12):1583, 1999.

Stebbing J, Moyle G: The clades of HIV. Their origins and clinical significance, AIDS Rev 5(4):205, 2003.

ASSESSMENT QUESTIONS

1. Which of the following human immunodeficiency virus (HIV) clades is responsible for most infections in developed countries?
   A. HIV-1B
   B. HIV-1C
   C. HIV-2M
   D. HIV-1A/C

2. Which of the following interactions are required for HIV attachment to monocytes?
   A. Gp120–gp41 binding to CD4
   B. Gp120–gp41 binding to CD4 and binding to the CXCR5 chemokine receptor
   C. Gp120–gp41 binding to the chemokine receptor CCR5
   D. Gp120–gp41 binding to the chemokine receptor CCR5 and sodium heparin in the cell membrane

3. In the synthesis of new HIV, which of the following promotes synthesis of ribonucleic acid (RNA)?
   A. *Tat*
   B. *Nef*
   C. *Vif*
   D. *Vpr*

4. HIV infection of follicular dendritic cells inhibits the synthesis of _____, which is necessary for the maturation of CD4Th1 and memory cells.
   A. Interleukin 2 (IL-2)
   B. IL-4
   C. IL-8
   D. IL-12

5. Which of the following is *not* a mechanism by which CD4 cells are killed during HIV infection?
   A. "Innocent bystander" reaction
   B. Syncytium formation
   C. Downregulation of the T cell receptor (TCR)
   D. Superantigen stimulation

6. Which of the following is an integrase inhibitor?
   A. Delavirdine
   B. Etravirine
   C. Nevirapine
   D. Raltegravir

7. Which of the following is *not* a true statement concerning non-nucleoside reverse transcriptase inhibitors?
   A. Inhibit RNA polymerase activity
   B. Prevent cleavage of the *gag* protein
   C. Inhibit DNA polymerase activity
   D. Bind to reverse transcriptase

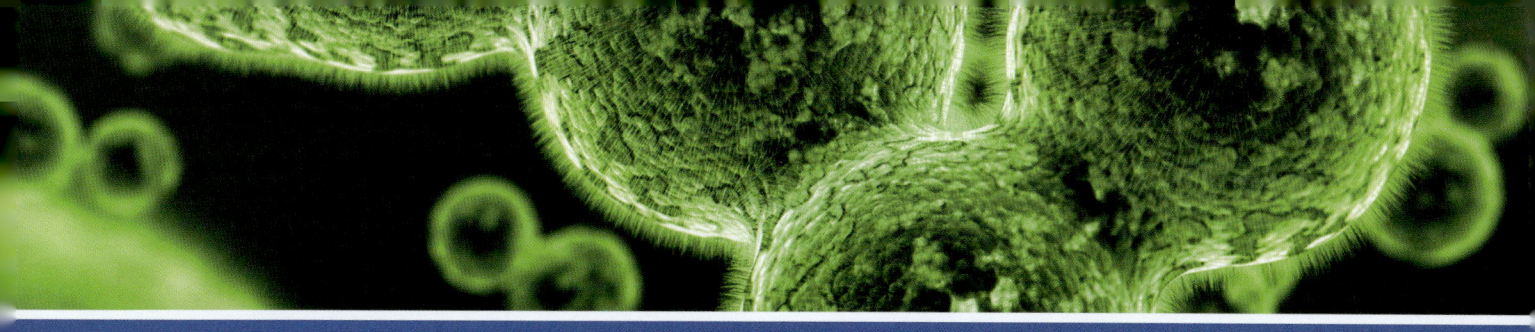

ANSWERS TO ASSESSMENT QUESTIONS

CHAPTER 1
Answers: 1-D, 2-A, 3-A, 4-C, 5-A, 6-B, 7-A, 8-A, 9-D

CHAPTER 2
Answers: 1-E, 2-B, 3-C, 4-E, 5-A, 6-D, 7-E, 8-C, 9-C

CHAPTER 3
Answers: 1-D, 2-C, 3-B, 4-E, 5-B, 6-C, 7-D, 8-C, 9-A

CHAPTER 4
Answers: 1-E, 2-C, 3-A, 4-B, 5-D, 6-B, 7-A, 8-B, 9-A

CHAPTER 5
Answers: 1-E, 2-A, 3-B, 4-A, 5-C, 6-A

CHAPTER 6
Answers: 1-E, 2-D, 3-E, 4-D, 5-A, 6-A

CHAPTER 7
Answers: 1-B, 2-D, 3-A, 4-A, 5-B, 6-B

CHAPTER 8
Answers: 1-D, 2-A, 3-C, 4-C, 5-E, 6-B

CHAPTER 9
Answers: 1-A, 2-C, 3-C, 4-A, 5-C, 6-A

CHAPTER 10
Answers: 1-A, 2-C, 3-B, 4-D, 5-C, 6-D

CHAPTER 11
Answers: 1-E, 2-B, 3-A, 4-C, 5-D, 6-A

CHAPTER 12
Answers: 1-D, 2-C, 3-C, 4-D, 5-E, 6-B

CHAPTER 13
Answers: 1-D, 2-B, 3-C, 4-D, 5-B, 6-C

CHAPTER 14
Answers: 1-D, 2-A, 3-C, 4-B, 5-D

CHAPTER 15
Answers: 1-D, 2-D, 3-E, 4-A, 5-E, 6-A

CHAPTER 16
Answers: 1-B, 2-D, 3-B, 4-E, 5-B, 6-C, 7-C, 8-D

CHAPTER 17
Answers: 1-C, 2-A, 3-B, 4-C, 5-C, 6-D

CHAPTER 18
Answers: 1-C, 2-D, 3-D, 4-A, 5-E, 6-D

CHAPTER 19
Answers: 1-C, 2-E, 3-B, 4-D, 5-C, 6-B

CHAPTER 20
Answers: 1-A, 2-D, 3-A, 4-D, 5-D, 6-D

CHAPTER 21
Answers: 1-A, 2-A, 3-C, 4-D, 5-A, 6-C

CHAPTER 22
Answers: 1-A, 2-C, 3-A, 4-D, 5-C, 6-B
199

CHAPTER 23
Answers: 1-C, 2-C, 3-A, 4-A, 5-C, 6-D

CHAPTER 24
Answers: 1-D, 2-B, 3-A, 4-C, 5-D, 6-C

CHAPTER 25
Answers: 1-C, 2-A, 3-D, 4-A, 5-A, 6-B, 7-B, 8-D, 9-C, 10-C, 11-B, 12-D, 13-C, 14-A, 15-D, 16-B

CHAPTER 26
Answers: 1-A, 2-D, 3-A, 4-D, 5-C, 6-D, 7-B

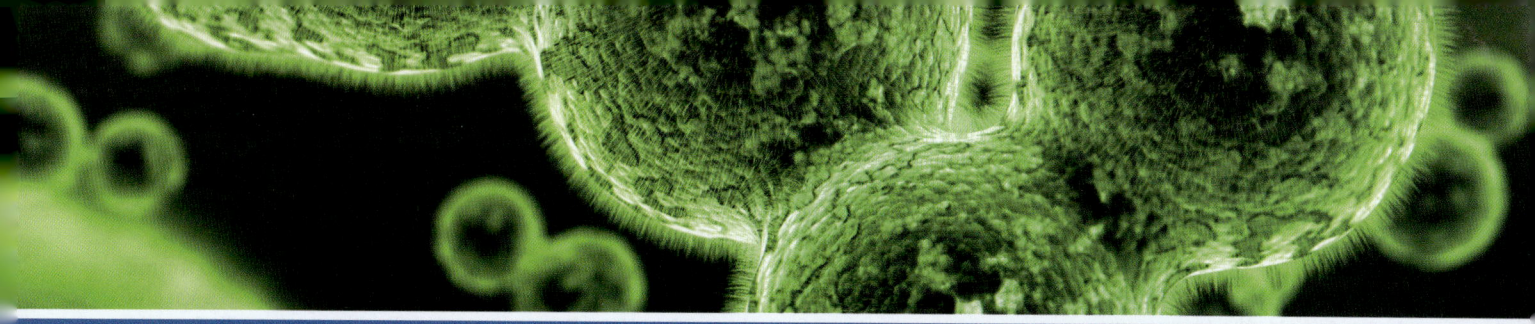

GLOSSARY

A

Abatacept: a co-stimulator inhibitor in a new class of drugs called *disease modifying antirheumatic drugs (DMARDs)*.

Acetylcholine: neurotransmitter causing muscle contraction.

Acetylcholinesterase: enzyme that destroys acetylcholine.

Acquired immunodeficiency disease: also known as *acquired immune deficiency syndrome (AIDS)* and characterized by infections with unusual opportunistic pathogens (e.g., Pneumocystis pneumoniae) and the development of aggressive sarcomas.

Activation complex: enzyme that cleaves protein molecules.

Active immunity: results from exposure to microbes such as streptococcus and pneumococcus or vaccination with dead or weakened microbes.

Acute-phase proteins: synthesized as part of the acute-phase response to tissue injury or infection to inhibit bacterial growth or activate the complement cascade.

Acute-phase response: mammalian response to tissue injury or infection characterized by fever, demargination of polymorphonuclear leukocytes (PMNs), the synthesis of acute-phase proteins by the liver, and white blood cell production of a wide variety of antimicrobial agents such as cathelicidins, defensins, and nitric oxide.

Acute rejection: begins within a week of transplantation and is mediated by alloreactive T cells that have been directly and indirectly stimulated. The response is initiated by the presence of donor dendritic cells (passenger leukocytes) expressing HLA and co-stimulatory molecules necessary to activate T cells.

Adaptive immune response: designed to protect the host against microbial antigens that constantly change and evolve. As the microbe changes its tactics for infection, the immune system adapts to counter the tactic and destroy the microbe. Adaptive immunity requires the stimulation of the immune system, the proliferation of effector cells, and the synthesis of cytokines and antibodies.

Adjuvant: compound that stimulates and directs the immune response by reducing antigen solubility and releasing small amounts of antigens over an extended period to augment systemic or mucosal immunity. When added to vaccines adjuvants enhance immune response to microbial and viral virulence factors.

Affinity: antibody binding strength resulting from the interaction between an antibody and a single antigenic determinant. Antibody affinity determines the rate at which an infection is terminated.

Affinity maturation: during an immune response cells are preferentially stimulated to produce high-affinity antibodies.

Alefacept: a fusion protein indicated for psoriasis vulgaris, an autoimmune skin disease.

Allele: each common variant of a polymorphic gene.

Allelic exclusion: antibody production from a single re-arranged set of parental genes.

Allelic polymorphism: several alternate forms of the same gene are present, providing additional genetic diversity critical to disease resistance.

Allergic contact dermatitis: a delayed type IV allergic reaction of the skin resulting from cutaneous contact with a specific allergen, with varying degrees of erythema, edema, and vesiculation.

Allergic rhinitis: immediate or delayed inflammation of the mucous membranes of the nose in response to an allergen to which a person has previously been exposed and has developed antibodies. Usually accompanied by swelling of the mucosa and a nasal discharge.

Alloantigens: glycoproteins expressed by white blood cells that are part of the body's self-recognition system.

Allogeneic graft: Allograft. Surgical transplantation of tissue between two genetically dissimilar individuals of the same species, such as between two humans who are not monozygotic twins.

Alpha/beta T cell receptor: α/β T cell receptor (TCR) recognizes a peptide–major histocompatibility complex (MHC) to fully activate the T cell.

Alternative complement pathway: a process of antigen-antibody interaction in which activation of the C3 step occurs without prior activation of C1, C4, and C2.

Anamnestic response: the proliferation and differentiation of memory B cells into IgG-producing plasma cells after a second antigenic challenge.

Anaphylactoid: pseudoallergic reaction not mediated by immunoglobulin E but the symptoms mimic severe anaphylaxis.

Anaphylatoxin: a molecule that induces the movement of eosinophils and phagocytic cells (chemotaxis) toward increasing concentrations of C3a. Fragment produced during the pathways of the complement system that mediates changes in mast cells leading to the release of histamine and other immunoreactive or inflammatory reactive substances. If the degranulation of mast cells is too strong, it can cause allergic reactions.

Anaphylaxis: an exaggerated, life-threatening hypersensitivity reaction to a previously encountered antigen. It is mediated by antibodies of the E or G class of immunoglobulins and results in the release of chemical mediators from mast cells.

Anergy: an immunodeficient condition characterized by a lack of or diminished reaction to an antigen or group of antigens. This state may be seen in advanced tuberculosis and other serious infections, acquired immunodeficiency syndrome, and some malignancies.

Ankylosing spondylitis: a chronic inflammatory disease of the spinal sacroiliac region, which connects spine to the pelvis. The disease appears to be mediated by CD8 cells. Constant inflammation causes fusion of the vertebrae, which results in chronic back pain and limited mobility.

Antibody-cross matching: a test for the presence in the serum of a prospective transplant recipient of cytotoxic antibodies against donor tissue antigens: donor lymphocytes are placed in serum of the recipient; the presence of cytolysis indicates incompatibility and the likelihood of hyperacute graft rejection.

Antigen: protein or carbohydrate molecule recognized as foreign by the host.

Antigen recognition complex: part of the cascade of the classic complement pathway, consists of antibody (Ab) and C1q.

Antigenic drift: over time, mutations result in slight changes in the protein structure and formation of new antigenic epitopes. Yearly influenza epidemics are a reflection of antigenic drift.

Antigenic shift: genetic recombination of animal and human influenza viruses to create major changes in hemagglutinins and neuraminidase. The "swine flu" pandemic of 1918 is an example of antigenic drift.

AP-1 complex: a nuclear transcription factor for the transcription of messenger ribonucleic acid (RNA) and the translation of IL-2 protein.

Artemis: enzyme that removes the hairpin curves in DNA in the recombination of light chain V and J regions.

Arthritis: any inflammatory condition of the joints, characterized by pain, swelling, heat, redness, and limitation of movement.

Arthroconidia: fungus with septate hyphae.

Aspirin induced asthma: attacks occur within 1 hour of aspirin ingestion and are often accompanied by rhinorrhea and conjunctival irritation. Aspirin-sensitive patients have a single nucleotide polymorphism in the LTC_4 synthetase gene that causes the overproduction of LTC4. The C4 leukotriene is converted to LTD_4 that causes airway narrowing, mucus secretion, and increased vascular permeability.

Asthma: a disease characterized by partial airway obstruction that is partially reversible either spontaneously or with treatment. Allergic response, chronic airway inflammation, airway injury, and airway repair (airway remodeling) also contribute to the pathogenesis of asthma and permanent abnormalities in lung function.

Atopic dermatitis: a chronic, eczematous skin disease that is characterized by itching, swelling, cracking, and weeping skin lesions. Unlike contact dermatitis, atopic dermatitis is an IgE-mediated allergic reaction.

Atopy: a familial genetic tendency to develop rhinitis, urticaria, and asthma. The condition is characterized by elevated IgE levels directed at common aero-allergens or food allergens.

Attenuation: reduces virulence while maintaining immunogenicity so that a live organism can be used in a vaccine.

Autocrine signaling: activated T cells produce IL-2, which binds to receptors on the same cell to initiate T cell growth and proliferation.

Autograft: A type of transplant where the same individual serves as the donor and the recipient of the transplanted tissue.

Avidity: the combined strength of multiple interactions between antibodies and epitopes, geometrically higher than the affinity.

B

B cell: small lymphocyte differentiated in the bone marrow.

B cell receptor (BCR): a monomeric form of an antibody called *immunoglobulin M* found on the surface of B lymphocytes.

B lymphocyte stimulator (BLyS): cytokine that engages with its ligands to promote B cell survival and differentiation into plasma cells.

B7 molecules: expressed on monocytes, macrophages, interstitial dendritic cells, and epithelial dendritic cells and activate or downregulate T cells to determine the nature of the immune response.

Bacillus Calmette-Guérin (BCG): an attenuated strain of *M. bovis* used in tuberculosis vaccine.

Bacteremia: the presence of bacteria in the blood.

Bacteriophage: a bacterial virus.

Bence Jones proteins: light chains excreted into urine.

Bruton's tyrosine kinase (BtK): a gene that is important in B cell maturation and intracellular signaling pathways.

C

C1 esterase inhibitor (C1INH): a soluble protein that inhibits C1 activation by disassociating C1r and C1s and preventing the activation of C4.

C3 convertase: catalyzes the cleavage of C3 into C3a and C3b. This is the most important step in the complement cascade and occurs in the classic, alternative, and MBL pathways. Also called *C4b2a complex.*

C4 Binding Protein (C4BP): a plasma protein that inhibits the classic and MBL complement pathways by blocking the interaction between C4b and C2a.

C5 convertase: an AbC4bC2aC3b complex on the cell surface containing most C3b in the classic complement pathway.

Calreticulin: a chaperone protein found in the sarcoplasmic reticulum and also in the endoplasmic reticulum of non-muscle cells; its many functions include roles in protein folding, calcium homeostasis, control of viral RNA replication, lymphocyte activation, and cytotoxicity.

Capsid: the layer of protein enveloping the genome of a virion. A capsid is composed of structural units called *capsomeres.* Its symmetry may be cubic or helical.

Catalase: a heme enzyme, found in almost all biologic cells, that catalyzes the decomposition of hydrogen peroxide to water and oxygen.

Cathepsin C: activates granzymes to kill infected or tumor cells.

CD1: a third lineage of antigen-presenting molecules (unrelated to class I and II molecules) that are expressed by B cells, monocytes, and dendritic cells.

CD11a: an α_1 integrin-subunit that associates with an integrin β_2-subunit (CD18) to form LFA-1.

CD2: a glycoprotein present on 90% to 95% of mature T cells and NK cells. Ligation with lymphocyte function-associated antigen (LFA-3 or CD58) on APCs results in the production of proteins that regulate the cellular response to IL-2.

CD28: interacts with a B7 molecule on the APC (antigen-presenting cell) in the final step of the T cell activation sequence.

CD3 complex: pan T cell maker composed of five subunit (α, β, ζ, ϵ, and γ) signalling proteins created by association with TCR.

CD4: molecule binds to class II molecules and stabilizes the TCR–class II complex as part of the T cell activation process. Expressed on CD4Th1 and CD4Th2 cells, macrophages, and dendritic cells

CD40L: CD40 ligand, a 261-amino-acid membrane glycoprotein expressed on activated CD4 lymphocytes shortly after T cell activation.

CD4Th1 cell: inflammatory cell. CD4 molecules are expressed on CD4Th1 and CD4Th2 cells.

CD4Th2 cell: T helper cells in antibody production. CD4 molecules are expressed on CD4Th1 and CD4Th2 cells.

CD59: a GPI-linked protein that binds to C8 and C9 and inhibits complement-mediated lysis of red blood cells, platelets, and leukocytes.

CD8: molecule on cytotoxic T cells that stabilizes the interaction between the TCR and the APCs expressing HLA molecules.

CD8Tc1: a principal effector of delayed-type hypersensitivity (DTH) reactions. CD8Tc1 cells provide defense against tumors and viral infections and secrete IL-2, interferon gamma (IFN-γ), and TNF-β.

CD8Tc2: not strongly cytotoxic and may play a role in neurologic and autoimmune diseases. CD8Tc2 cells secrete IL-4, IL-5, and IL-10.

Cell-mediated immunity: the mechanism of acquired immunity characterized by the dominant role of T cell lymphocytes. Cellular immunity is involved in resistance to infectious diseases caused by viruses and some bacteria and in delayed hypersensitivity reactions, some aspects of resistance to cancer, certain autoimmune diseases, graft rejection, and certain allergies. It does not involve the production of humoral antibody but instead involves the activation of Mo and natural killer cells.

Chemokine: any of a group of low-molecular-weight cytokines, such as interleukin-8, identified on the basis of their ability to induce chemotaxis or chemokinesis in leukocytes (or in particular populations of leukocytes) in inflammation. They function as regulators of the immune system and may also play roles in the circulatory system and CNS.

Chimeric antibodies: genetically engineered monoclonal antibodies with reduced immunogenicity, composed of murine V_H and V_L domains and constant domains from human IgG.

Chronic granulomatous disease (CGD): any of a group of immunodeficiencies of X-linked or autosomal recessive inheritance, caused by failure of the respiratory or metabolic burst, resulting in deficient microbicidal ability. The clinical picture consists of frequent, severe, prolonged bacterial and fungal infections of the skin, oral and intestinal mucosa, reticuloendothelial system, bones, lungs, and genitourinary tract. The course of the disease varies: symptoms may appear in the neonate, with death during the first decade, or a patient may survive into middle age. The X-linked types seem to be associated with higher morbidity and mortality than the autosomal recessive types.

Chronic rejection: occurs after 6 months to a year and involves both cell-mediated and antibody-mediated responses to transplanted tissue.

Clade: a virus subgroup that arose from a single common ancestor.

Class I molecules: found on all the nucleated cells in the body and present antigen to CD8 T cells. They consist of a single α-chain transmembrane protein that is stabilized by a second protein known as β_2-*microglobulin*.

Class I region: division of the HLA gene complex, further subdivided into three major loci (*HLA-A*, *HLA-B*, and *HLA-C*) and several minor loci.

Class II molecules: present antigens to CD4Th1 and CD4Th2 cells. Class II molecules consist of heavily glycosylated α- and β-chains and are much larger than class I molecules.

Class II region: division of the HLA gene complex, further subdivided into three loci (DP, DR, and DQ) involved in antigen presentation.

Class III region: division of the HLA gene complex with 62 genes. Gene products include three complement components and the tumor necrosis factor (TNF).

Classic complement pathway: cascade of nine proteins that results in the lysis of antibody-coated bacteria. (NOTE: I changed "classical" to "classic" to match text.)

Classic de nova nucleic acid synthesis pathway: a complex pathway in which folic acid donates single carbon aldehyde groups necessary for the synthesis of purines and prymidines.

CLIP: class II-associated invariant chain peptide, a 3-kDal peptide truncated from the invariant chain of an antigen-containing endosome or phagolysosome.

Cluster of differentiation (CD) markers: cell surface glycoproteins and glycolipids.

Colony-stimulating factor (CSF): a diverse group of glycoproteins that induce differentiation of white blood cells in bone marrow.

Combinatorial diversity: generates antibodies with a wide range of antigen specificities in gene recombination.

Complement: nine serum proteins produce proinflammatory factors that are chemotactic for phagocytic cells (resolve microbial infections).

Complement receptor 1 (CR1): is found on erythrocytes and inhibits the formation of the classic and alternative pathway C3 convertase. It often acts in concert with DAF.

Complementarity determining regions (CDRs): hypervariable regions in the α/β-chains that form a three-dimensional antigen pocket and contact antigens.

Conformational epitope: created when protein segments are folded into a tertiary structure.

Congenital rubella syndrome (CRS): the major complication associated with rubella infections. CRS is a collection of birth defects caused by transmission of the rubella virus from an infected mother to a fetus during the first trimester of pregnancy.

Conidia: asexual fungal spores that are deciduous (shed at maturity) and formed by budding or splitting off from the summit of a conidiophore.

Cord factor: lipoarabinomannan that inhibits the interferon (IFN)–induced activation of macrophages and stimulates the production of tumor necrosis factor alpha (TNF-α).

Cross-priming: a unique mechanism that allows the generation of an inflammatory response to endogenous antigens and a cytotoxic response to exogenous antigens. Dendritic and tumor cells are obtained from the patient and purified then mixed together and incubated for several days in the laboratory. DCs ingest intact tumor cells and process the appropriate antigens, increasing the immunogenicity of tumor cells for use in vaccines.

Cryopyrin-associated periodic syndrome (CAPS): a group of inherited diseases that are characterized by the overproduction of IL-1β. CAPS is characterized by short, intense inflammatory reactions with rashes, fever or chills, redness of eyes, joint pain, and adolescent deafness.

Cyclosporine A (CsA): therapeutic agent that inhibits T cell signaling and downregulates immune responses used as prophylaxis to prevent organ rejection or severe, active rheumatoid arthritis.

Cytokine storm: an aberrant immune response that is responsible for the pathophysiology of pandemic influenza.

Cytokines: one of a large group of low-molecular-weight proteins secreted by various cell types and involved in cell-to-cell communication, coordinating antibody and T cell immune interactions, and amplifying immune reactivity. Cytokines include colony-stimulating factors, interferons, interleukins, and lymphokines, which are secreted by lymphocytes.

Cytotoxic T cells: a type of T lymphocyte that has the ability to cause lysis of specific target cells, such as cells containing viral antigens or intracellular bacteria. Cytotoxic T cells are activated by dendritic cells that express antigen-loaded class I molecules.

D

Decay Accelerating Factor (DAF): a glycoprotein that is anchored in the membrane by a covalent linkage to glycosylphosphatidylinositol (GPI). It functions to disassociate the C3 convertases by releasing C2a from the AbC4bC2a complex in the classic pathway and C3b and Bb in the alternative pathway.

Dendritic cell: "professional" antigen-producing cell present in lymphoid and nonlymphoid tissues.

Dendritic cell cancer vaccine: intact tumor cells or tumor-specific antigens are reacted with mature dendritic cells isolated from peripheral blood. Tumor cells are ingested and processed and presented in context with class I and class II molecules. In vitro, dendritic cells are often stimulated with GM-CSF, IL-4, and interferon gamma (IFN-γ) that induce dendritic cell maturation. Antigen-pulsed dendritic cells are re-injected into the host to stimulate an immune response.

Deoxynucleotidyl transferase: enzyme that mediates the addition of P- nucleotides and N- nucleotides for junctional diversity during recombination.

Diabetes: a clinical condition characterized by the excessive excretion of urine. The excess may be caused by a deficiency of antidiuretic hormone, as in diabetes insipidus, or it may be the polyuria resulting from the hyperglycemia that occurs in diabetes mellitus.

Disseminated intravascular coagulopathy (DIC): caused by activation of the coagulation pathway. DIC is a coagulopathy resulting from the overstimulation of clotting and anticlotting processes in response to disease or injury, such as septicemia, acute hypotension, poisonous snakebites, neoplasms, obstetric emergencies, severe trauma, extensive surgery, and hemorrhage.

E

Early phase IgE response: occurs within 20 minutes of the second exposure to an allergen, involves IgE–antigen interactions, and is mediated by preformed pharmacologic mediators.

Elongation factor-2 (EF-2): protein that assists in joining amino acids during protein synthesis.

Endogenous antigen: generally large molecules that must be digested and fragmented before presentation to lymphocytes, e.g., intracellular microbes, viruses, and tumor cells. Endogenous antigens elicit a cellular response comprising lymphocytes, macrophages, and natural killer cells.

Endosome: vacuole formed by endocytosis in B cells.

Endotoxin: lipopolysaccharide component of the gram-negative cell wall. Unlike exotoxins, endotoxins are only released on the death of the bacteria.

Enterotoxin: secreted by *Staphylococcus aureus;* similar to exotoxin but usually only causes moderate to severe diarrhea.

Env: structural gene of the HIV-1 genome. Translation of the *env* gene is necessary for the formation of HIV capsid and matrix proteins.

Enzyme-linked immunosorbent test: a laboratory technique for detecting specific antigens or antibodies by using enzyme-labeled immunoreactants and a solid-phase binding support, such as a test tube. A primary test used in screening for HIV antibodies. Also *enzyme-linked immunosorbent assay (ELISA).*

Epitope: the molecular fragment of an antigen that interacts with effector cells or antibodies, also called an *antigenic determinant.*

Erythroblastosis fetalis: a type of hemolytic anemia in newborns that results from maternal-fetal blood group incompatibility, specifically involving the Rh factor and the ABO blood groups. The condition is caused by an antigen-antibody reaction in the bloodstream of the infant caused by placental transmission of maternally formed antibodies against the incompatible antigens of the fetal blood. In Rh factor incompatibility the hemolytic reaction occurs only when the mother is Rh negative and the infant is Rh positive.

Exogenous antigen: enter the body via the oral, respiratory, and parenteral routes. In general, exogenous antigens are immunogenic structures expressed on extracellular bacteria, fungi, viruses, and pollens.

Exotoxin: proteins synthesized and secreted by gram-positive bacteria that are immunogenic and toxic to mammalian tissue. Lipopolysaccharide endotoxins are an integral part of the gram-negative cell wall and are released into the circulation following bacterial death.

Extensively drug resistant tuberculosis (XDR-TB): resistant to isoniazid and rifampin as well as fluoroquinolones and any of the second-line drugs. When second-line drugs for tuberculosis are mismanaged or misused, extensively drug-resistant tuberculosis strains develop.

F

F(ab′)₂: two Fab linked together by heavy-chain disulfide bonds, can bind two antigens.
Fab: fragment antigen binding, binds a single antigen.
Factor H: downregulates the alternative pathway by inactivating soluble or bound C3b and amplifying the decay of the C3bBb complex.
Factor I: a serine protease that cleaves C3b and C4b and prevents further activation of complement in the alternative pathway.
FADD protein: Fas-associated protein with death domains (FADD). An adaptor protein that binds with death domains on target cells causing FADD domains to activate caspases 8 and 10.
Fas ligand (FasL): expressed on the surface of activated CD8 cells, also known as *CD95L*.
Fas receptor (FasR): activates death domains when ligated on target cells. Also known as *CD95*.
Fc: fraction crystallized portion of antibodies that binds to receptors (FcR) on immunocompetent cells.
Fimbriae: bacterial appendages that are used to adhere to one another and mammalian cells.
Flow cytometer (FCM): consists of four components: (1) a fluidics system, (2) single or dual lasers, (3) optical detectors, and (4) an on-board computer system that collects and analyzes data. FCM is used in clinical medicine to screen for immunodeficiencies, evaluate disease progress, support a tentative diagnosis, and provide prognostic information to the clinician.
Fluorescence-activated cell sorter (FACS): an automated instrument that separates cell populations labeled with fluorescent antibodies or other fluorescent labels. The sample stream is broken up into droplets which are electrostatically charged and deflected into different collecting tubes depending on the measured fluorescence of the droplets.
Follicular dendritic cell (FDC): a subset of dendritic cells derived from a myeloid stem cell migrated to the lymph node. FDCs use dendritic extensions called *iccosomes* to trap viable viruses.
Fos: protein that associates with Jun protein to create the AP-1 complex, an early transcriptional activator.
FOXp3: intracellular forehead helix or winged transcription factor.
Freund's adjuvant: Freund's complete adjuvant (FCA) is composed of killed *Mycobacterium tuberculosis* or *M. butyricum* suspended in mineral oil, water, and a surfactant called *mannide monoleate*. FCA cannot be used in humans because it causes inflammatory reactions, ulcerations, and granulomas at the injection site. Freund's incomplete adjuvant (FIA) comprises oil and water emulsions without killed mycobacteria. FIA stimulates only an antibody response and is occasionally used in vaccines.

G

Gag: structural gene of the HIV-1 genome. Translation of the *gag* gene is necessary for the formation of HIV capsid and matrix proteins.

Gamma amino butyric acid (GABA): an amino acid that functions as an inhibitory neurotransmitter in the brain and spinal cord. It is also found in the heart, lungs, and kidneys and in certain plants.
Gamma/delta T cell receptor: γ/δ T cell receptor is one of two forms of the unique antigen binding receptor on T cells. Rare in peripheral blood but are found in abundance in mucosal tissue.
Gaucher's disease: a deficiency in β-glucosidase or glucosylceramidase, which is necessary for the intracellular degradation of senescent red blood cells—a normal function of macrophages and monocytes. As a consequence, glucocerebroside (a membrane lipid component) accumulates in phagocytic cells in the liver, spleen, bone marrow, lymph nodes, and alveolar capillaries. The high lipid concentration inhibits protein kinase C that is necessary for macrophage activation and phagocytosis.
Gliadin: a fraction of the gluten protein that is found in wheat and rye and to a lesser extent in barley and oats. Its solubility in diluted alcohol distinguishes it from another grain protein, glutenin. Those with celiac disease are sensitive to this substance, and it must be excluded from their diet.
Goiter: an enlarged thyroid gland (glandular hyperplasia) usually evident as a pronounced swelling in the neck.
Goodpasture syndrome: characterized by pulmonary hemorrhage and a rapidly progressing glomerulonephritis. Patients present to the physicians with hemoptysis, dyspnea, and generalized weakness. The syndrome is characterized by antibodies directed at noncollagenous domains (NC1) of the α3-chains of type IV collagen in the basement membranes of the lungs and kidneys.
Gp120/gp41: protein that protrudes from the HIV membrane and is anchored by a transmembrane gp41 protein. Three molecules of the gp120/gp41 aggregate to form a trimolecular structure necessary for docking to HIV target cells.
Graft versus host disease (GVHD): occurs when allo-reactive T cells from the donor attack the recipient's tissue. The reaction develops when cells or tissue containing lymphocytes or lymphocyte progenitors are infused into immunosuppressed individuals.
Granuloma: an accumulation of macrophages, lymphocytes, and fibroblasts surrounding a lesion to contain infection.
Granulysin: alters membrane permeability and facilitates the insertion of perforin into target cell membranes or forms a complex to create pores in the endoplasmic membrane and insert into cytoplasm.
Granzyme: enzyme released by T lymphocyte (CTL) degranulates. Five different granzymes cause apoptosis in target cells.
Graves' disease: the most common cause of hyperthyroidism in children and young women. The disease is caused by IgG_1 antibodies reacting with thyrotropin or TSH receptors.

H

Haplotype: a set of HLAs (HLA-A, -B, -C, -DP, -DQ, and -DR) on the same chromosome.
Hapten: small-molecular-weight compounds that evoke an immune response only when they are attached to carrier proteins.

Hashimoto's thyroiditis: the most common form of hypothyroidism. Individuals mount both an antibody response and a cellular response to thyroid tissue. The disease is caused by a break in peripheral tolerance to thyroid tissue, the failure of regulatory cells to control auto-reactive T and B cells.

HAT selection: process in which aminopterin (a folic acid inhibitor) blocks the production of DNA by the classic de novo pathway and kills the myeloma cells.

Hemagglutinin: structure of a virus that agglutinates red cells

Herd immunity: when a high proportion of a population is vaccinated, person-to-person disease transmission is interrupted by surrounding the infected person with vaccinated individuals.

Hereditary angioneurotic edema (HANE): caused by failure to regulate complement activation, or by C1 INH deficiency. During a clinical episode, well-circumscribed edema is localized to the face, tongue, and larynx (restricts normal breathing).

Heterozygosity: the inheritance of duplicate genes at the same locus; ensures that some members of the species will survive microbial infections.

Homologous Restriction Factor (HRF): a 20,000–molecular-weight (MW) protein that inhibits the interaction of the C8 and C9 terminal complement components.

Human leukocyte antigen (HLA) complex: human version of the gene cluster on chromosome 17 that determines rejection or acceptance of grafts (called *major histocompatibility complex (MHC)* in animals).

Humanized monoclonal antibodies: derived from murine hybridomas. Genes coding for the six murine CDRs (three each on heavy and light chains) are amplified by PCR and inserted into a plasmid vector. Genes for human variable and constant regions also are inserted into the same vector. Transfected bacteria or transformed human B cells produce humanized monoclonal antibodies.

Hybridoma: a hybrid cell formed by the fusion of a myeloma cell and an antibody-producing cell. Hybridomas are used to produce monoclonal antibodies.

Hyper IgM syndrome (HIGM): commonly inherited as an X-linked recessive trait. Individuals with HIGM lack a functioning CD40 ligand (CD40L) on activated T cells, impacting immunity.

Hyperacute rejection: occurs within minutes when the recipient has pre-existing IgM antibodies to the donor's HLA antigens.

Hyposensitization therapy: a form of immunotherapy that can either reduce or eliminate hypersensitivity. Hyposensitization therapy induces the synthesis of IgG antibodies, which are called *blocking antibodies.*

I

Iccosomes: beaded, three-dimensional structures of processed and unprocessed antigens bound by follicular dendritic cells (FDCs).

Idiopathic thrombocytopenic purpura (ITP): an autoimmune pediatric disease that is associated with low platelet counts. In most cases, antibody-coated platelets bind to Fc receptors on macrophages in the spleen and liver.

Idiotope: an antigenic determinant on a variable region of an immunoglobulin molecule. Each complementarity-determining region (CDR) amino acid sequence is called an *idiotope.*

Idiotype: the portion of an immunoglobulin molecule that confers the molecule's unique character, most often including its antigen-binding site. Collectively, clusters of idiotopes in and around the CDR are called the *antibody idiotype.*

Idiotypic cancer vaccine: a therapeutic target for treatment of B cell malignancies. Since the malignant cells are derived from a single B cell clone, each B cell in the malignant population has a B cell receptor (a monomeric IgM) with a homogeneous idiotope. Isolation and purification of idiotypic molecules form the basis for the vaccine.

IgA: immunoglobulin A, one of five antibody isotypes and a dimeric antibody found in both serum and external secretions such as tears, saliva colostrums, and intestinal secretions.

IgD: immunoglobulin D, one of five antibody isotypes and bound to B cells via the Fc receptor or free in serum.

IgE: immunoglobulin E, one of five antibody isotypes and the major mediator of asthma, urticaria, and rhinitis (immediate allergic reactions).

IgG: immunoglobulin G, one of five antibody isotypes and able to penetrate extracellular and intracellular spaces.

IgM: immunoglobulin M, one of five antibody isotypes and the antibody formed during the initial response to an antigen or microbe.

Immunological synapse: structure that initiates T cell receptor (TCR)–mediated signalling, also known as *supramolecular activation cluster (SMAC).*

Immuno-receptor tyrosine-based activation motifs (ITAMs): chains of 44 to 81 amino acid sequences essential to TCR signal transduction.

Induction immunosuppression: used at the time of transplantation and is designed for short-term use when the risk of transplantation rejection is the highest.

Infectious asthma: caused by influenza, respiratory syncytial virus (RSV), or parainfluenza viruses. The replication of viruses often destroys the epithelial layers of the respiratory tract and exposes the sensory nerve endings. Stimulation of nerve endings by cold air or irritants causes a reflex bronchoconstriction. Asthma symptoms abate when the respiratory epithelium regenerates. Also called *nonallergic asthma.*

Innate immune response: phagocytic cells, antimicrobial proteins, and serum enzymes are activated by molecules common to most bacteria. The innate immune response functions to contain an infection until an adaptive response can be mounted against the infective agent.

Integrase: enzyme critical for the integration of viral DNA into the host genome.

Interferon (IFN): a natural glycoprotein formed by cells exposed to a virus or another foreign particle of nucleic acid. It induces the production of translation inhibitory protein (TIP) in noninfected cells. TIP blocks translation of viral RNA, thus giving other cells protection against both the original and other viruses.

Interferon-gamma (IFN-γ): a CD4Th1-produced cytokine that activates IFN-γ receptors expressed by other T cells, NK cells, and macrophages or monocytes. IFN increases bacterial killing by monocytes and alveolar macrophages. Individuals with an IFN-γ receptor deficiency are at risk for infection with *M. tuberculosis, M. africanum,* and *M. bovis.*

Interleukin 1 (IL-1): a protein with numerous immune system functions, including activation of resting T cells, endothelial cells, and macrophages; mediation of inflammation; and stimulation of the synthesis of lymphokines, collagen, and collagenases.

Interleukin 11 (IL-11): a cytokine produced by bone marrow stromal cells. It induces IL-6-dependent murine plasmacytoma cells to proliferate and plays an important role in early platelet hematopoiesis.

Interleukin 2 (IL-2): a protein with various immunologic functions, including the ability to initiate proliferation of activated T cells. IL-2 is used in the laboratory to grow T cell clones with specific helper, cytotoxic, and suppressor functions.

Interstitial dendritic cell: a subset of dendritic cells derived from a myeloid stem cell found in nonlymphoid tissue.

Intrinsic factor: a glycoprotein secreted by the gastric mucosa that is essential for the intestinal absorption of cyanocobalamin. Intrinsic factor forms a bond with molecules of cyanocobalamin, and this complex is transported across the ileal membrane. A deficiency of intrinsic factor, caused by gastrectomy, myxedema, or atrophy of the gastric mucosa, causes pernicious anemia.

Intussusceptions: intestinal obstruction as a result of the intestine wrapping around itself.

Invariant chain: polypeptide that associates with class II molecules for antigen presentation.

Isoantigen: Red blood cell antigens are water-soluble glycopeptides consisting of heterosaccharides attached by a glycosidic linkage at the reducing ends.

Isograft: tissue transplanted between genetically identical twins. Also called a *syngeneic transplant*.

Isotypes: differentiated by the chemical structure of the heavy chain. Antibody isotypes have different molecular structures, different affinity constants, appear at different times in an immune response, and have different functions.

J

Jun: protein that associates with Fos protein to create the AP-1 complex, an early transcriptional activator.

Junctional diversity: Adding six or more amino acids to the J domains to create more TCR diversity and allow the immune system to respond to all known antigens.

K

Kawasaki disease: a self-limiting, febrile disease that is characterized by vasculitis of peripheral and coronary vessels. Also called *mucocutaneous lymph node syndrome (MLNS)*.

Koplik spots: small red spots with bluish-white centers on the lingual and buccal mucosa, characteristic of measles. The rash of measles usually erupts a day or two after the appearance of Koplik spots.

L

Langerhans cell: skin interstitial dendritic cell that serves as a sentinel for detecting foreign or antigenic molecules.

Large granular lymphocyte (LGL): arises in bone marrow, has large nuclei, plentiful cytoplasm, and multiple azurophilic granules. LGLs function as NK cells, which nonspecifically lyse virus-infected cells and tumor cells.

Late-phase IgE response: occurs 4 to 8 hours following the second exposure to an allergen, does not involve antibodies, and is facilitated by the newly synthesized products of the arachidonic acid pathway.

Leukotrienes: a class of biologically active compounds that occur naturally in leukocytes and produce allergic and inflammatory reactions similar to those of histamine. They are thought to play a role in the development of allergic and autoallergic diseases such as asthma, rheumatoid arthritis, inflammatory bowel disease, and psoriasis.

Ligase: enzyme that catalyzes the formation of a bond between substrate molecules coupled with the breakdown of a pyrophosphate bond in ATP or a similar donor molecule.

Linear epitope: six to eight contiguous amino acids in the primary amino acid sequence of a polypeptide.

Lipo-oligosaccharide (LOS): specialized endotoxin that is a major neisserial virulence factor in meningitis.

Liposomes: small, spheric particles consisting of a bilayer of phospholipid molecules surrounding an aqueous solution.

Lysosomes: cytoplasmic, membrane-bound particles that contain hydrolytic enzymes that function in intracellular digestive processes. The organelles are found in most cells but are particularly prominent in leukocytes and the cells of the liver and kidney. If the hydrolytic enzymes are released into the cytoplasm, they cause self-digestion of the cell.

M

Macrophage: "professional" antigen-presenting cell resulting from circulating monocytes migrating into tissue where they digest foreign material.

Maintenance immunosuppression: usually consists of a corticosteroid, a calcineurin inhibitor, and a lymphocyte proliferation inhibitor to decrease chance of graft rejection. Uses less toxic therapeutic doses than induction immunosupression that can be administered for long periods.

Mantoux test: a tuberculin skin test that consists of intradermal injection of a purified protein derivative of the tubercle bacillus. A hardened, raised red area of 8 to 10 mm, appearing 24 to 72 hours after injection, is a positive reaction. This method is the most reliable means of testing tuberculin sensitivity. Also known as the *PPD (purified protein derivative of tuberculosis) skin test*.

Matrix: icosahedral shell that provides additional protection for the virus's capsid core. The shell anchors a lipid membrane to the outer surface of the virus.

Membrane attack complex: a cluster of complement components that creates a pore in the plasma membrane of a cell, leading to the lysis of a cell.

Membrane Cofactor Protein MCP: in combination with other proteins, inactivates C4b.

Messenger RNA splicing: process that removes introns between J and C genes during transcription of mRNA.

Metastable C3: covalently binds to highly conserved microbial polysaccharides (e.g., inulin, zymosan) and lipopolysaccharides in the alternative pathway or complement activation.

Molecular mimicry: an antigenic similarity between unrelated macromolecules, believed to play a role in the pathogenesis of rheumatic fever and other diseases.

Monoclonal antibody (MAB): an antibody produced in a laboratory from a single clone of B lymphocytes. All MABs produced from the same clone are identical and have the same antigenic specificity.

Monocyte: the largest white blood cell in peripheral blood, containing large, indented nuclei as well as abundant cytoplasm and azurophilic granules. A "professional" antigen-presenting cell that circulates in the blood and digests foreign material.

Multi-drug resistant tuberculosis (MDR-TB): a tuberculosis strain that is resistant to, at least, isoniazid and rifampin.

Multiple myeloma: a B cell malignancy that is characterized by destruction of skeletal bone and the production of monoclonal antibodies.

Myasthenia gravis: a rare disorder in which the patient exhibits progressive weakness of skeletal muscles. Individuals with the disease produce antibodies directed at postsynaptic acetylcholine receptors at the neuromuscular junctions of skeletal muscle. Surface receptors are destroyed as a result of complement activation or are internalized and destroyed by proteolytic enzymes.

Mycolic acids: comprise 50% of the dry weight of the mycobacterium cell wall and form a hydrophobic barrier that prevents the entry of drugs, disinfectants, and other harsh chemicals.

Myeloperoxidase (MPO): a peroxidase enzyme occurring in phagocytic cells that can oxidize halide ions, producing a bactericidal effect.

N

Natural resistance–associated macrophage protein (NRAMP): plays a role in the destruction of mycobacteria early in infection. NRAMP1 is localized in endosomal vesicles that fuse with phagosomes. NRAMP1 reduces the pH of the phagosome to levels that are toxic to the bacteria. NRAMP2 is an efflux pump that exports iron and other cations from the phagosome. Mutations in NRAMP1 and NRAMP2 genes influence the phagosomal function of alveolar macrophages.

Nef: accessory gene of the HIV-1 genome. Translation of the *nef* gene accelerates the endocytosis of the CD4 virus complex and downregulates the expression of class I molecules, which decreases the risk of the CD8-mediated destruction of infected cells.

Neoantigen: immunogenic protein created by mutating genes producing self-proteins, may stimulate an immune response.

Neuraminidase: a mushroom-shaped glycoprotein enzyme, which contributes to the infectivity of the influenza virus. Neuraminidase destroys sialic acid residues and frees the individual viruses to infect other cells.

NFAT: the second nuclear transcription factor necessary for synthesis of IL-2. A product of the calcium–PLC signaling pathway.

Nonhomologous end joining: process in light chain VJ recombination in which double strands are tied together using ligase IV (NHEJ).

Nosocomial infections: hospital-acquired diseases.

NTreg cell: natural Tregs, educated in the thymus during the negative selection process. Thymocytes binding to the HLA molecules with intermediate affinity are considered NTregs that exit the thymus and circulate in peripheral blood.

Nuclear factor-κB (NF-κB) paracrine: the third transcription factor necessary for synthesis of IL-2. A product of the calcium-independent PLC$_\gamma$1–DAG/PKC pathway.

Nucleic acid salvage pathway: provides a second conduit for DNA synthesis. In this pathway, thymidine and hypoxanthine are recycled into new nucleotides.

O

Oligonucleotide: a compound formed by linking a small number of nucleotides.

Omenn syndrome: an autosomal recessive form of severe combined immunodeficiency (SCID).

One turn-two turn rule: recombination restriction: genes can only recombine when they are located on the same side of the chromosome (12/23 rule). Only RSS 12 and RSS 23 segments can combine.

Opisthotonos: contractions in the long muscles of the back that arch the back in a characteristic form, which often results in fractures of the spine.

Opsonin: leukocyte surface molecules that attach to microbes and promote phagocytosis.

Orchitis: Inflammation of the testes.

Osteomyelitis: local or generalized infection of bone and bone marrow, usually caused by bacteria introduced by trauma or surgery, by direct extension from a nearby infection, or via the bloodstream. Staphylococci are the most common causative agents.

Otitis media: an inflammation or infection of the middle ear, common in early childhood.

Oxygen-dependent intracellular killing: dependent on the presence of oxygen, a respiratory burst, and the generation of reactive oxygen species.

Oxygen-independent intracellular killing: uses preformed granules containing proteolytic enzymes to kill microbes.

P

P and N nucleotides: alternately join with Dβ-chains and junctional flexibility to create additional TCR diversity.

P nucleotide additions: palindromic sequences of amino acids inserted at single strand breaks to create additional TCR diversity in somatic cells.

Paracrine: an endocrine function in which effects of a hormone are localized to adjacent or nearby cells.

Paroxysmal nocturnal hemoglobinuria (PNH): short, rapid episodes (paroxysmal) of red blood cell lysis caused by lack of membrane-bound complement inhibitors.

Passive immunity: the administration of antibodies to correct an immunodeficiency or provide short-term immunity against microbial infection.

Perforin: contributes to cytolysis through two mechanisms. It forms homopolymeric pores in cell membranes, through which granzymes are injected into the target cell. Or perforin acts as part of a complex to create pores in the endosomal membrane and release several granzymes into the cytoplasm of target cells.

Pernicious anemia (PA): a megaloblastic anemia characterized by the presence of immature, dysfunctional red blood cells (megaloblasts) in the blood. In PA, antibodies are directed at a glycoprotein known as *intrinsic factor*. These autoantibodies also neutralize any soluble intrinsic factor in the intestinal lumen, which prevents the transport of vitamin B$_{12}$ across the intestinal mucosa to portal blood. Without this essential vitamin, red blood cell precursors cannot divide.

Peroxidase: any of a group of iron-porphyrin enzymes that catalyze the oxidation of some organic substrates in the presence of hydrogen peroxide.

Pertactin: a virulence factor and adhesin that is a component of some of the acellular vaccines.

Phagocytosis: the process by which certain cells engulf and destroy microorganisms and cellular debris. Phagocytosis and intracellular killing comprise the final step in the resolution of extracellular microbial infections.

Phagosome: vacuole in monocytes and macrophages that ingests bacteria and antigens by phagocytosis.

Phosphokinase C (PKC): the initiating signal for the NF–κB activation.

Phospholipase C: adaptor protein that forms short-lived complexes with other proteins to transduce membrane activation signals to the major cytoplasmic signaling pathways.

Photocontact dermatitis: a cell-mediated response to drugs or drug metabolites that act as haptens. Quinolones, sulfonamides, tetracyclines, and trimethoprim are the major agents of photocontact dermatitis.

Pili: fine filamentous appendages found on certain bacteria and similar to flagellum except that they are shorter, straighter, and found in greater quantities in the organism. Pili consist solely of protein and are associated with antigenic properties of the cell surface.

Pinocytosis: the process by which extracellular fluid is taken into a cell. The plasma membrane develops a saccular indentation filled with extracellular fluid and then pinches off the indentation, forming a vesicle or vacuole of fluid within the cell.

Plasma cell: differentiated B cell lymphocyte that produces soluble protein antibodies.

Plasmacytoid dendritic cell: localized in the T cell compartment within the lymph node (also known as *lymphoid dendritic cell*). Captures and processes antigens.

Pol: structural gene of the HIV-1 genome. *Pol* gene products are critical for the synthesis and integration of viral DNA into the host genome and the generation of capsid proteins.

Polymerase chain reaction (PCR): used to amplify stretches of genomic DNA encoding HLA molecules.

Post-herpetic neuralgia (PHN): persistent pain that may persist for a year after resolution of zoster lesions.

Properdine: molecule that stabilizes a C3 convertase in the alternative pathway of complement activation.

Prostaglandins: potent unsaturated fatty acid products of the arachidonic acid pathway. Two prostaglandins (PGD$_2$ and PGE$_2$) play critical roles in late-phase reactions by increasing vascular permeability, contracting smooth muscle, and acting as an NCF (neutrophil chemotactic factor).

Protease: an enzyme that is a catalyst in the breakdown of peptide bonds that join the amino acids in a protein.

Proteasome: a large, cylindrical protease complex occurring in both the nucleoplasm and cytoplasm, consisting of a 20S core that in eukaryotes and Archaea is capped by a regulatory complex at one or both ends; it degrades intracellular proteins that have been marked by the attachment of ubiquitin.

Pyrogen: interleukins that can raise body temperature.

Q

Qa-1: a nonclassic HLA glycoprotein that presents a small hydrophobic peptide (AMAPRTLLL) derived from the leader sequences of other HLA class I molecules.

R

Radioallergosorbent test (RAST): a test in which a technique of radioimmunoassay is used to identify and quantify the presense of allergen-specific IgE. The test is an in vitro method of demonstrating allergic reactions.

RAG enzymes: facilitate the recombination of genes (part of a recombinase family).

Ramsay Hunt syndrome: varicella infection of the seventh cranial nerve (CNVII) gives rise to ulceration of the ears, tongue, and soft palate.

RANKL: receptor activator of nuclear factor kappa-B ligand. A fibroblast-produced factor that stimulates osteoclasts to destroy bone tissue.

Ras: protein that transduces signals from the surface receptor to the MAPK pathway.

Reactive arthritis: a unique arthritic condition characterized by skin plaques, conjunctivitis, urethritis, arthritis, and spondylitis. It usually occurs 1 month after infection with sexually transmitted microbes (*Chlamydia* or *Neisseria gonorrhoeae*) or select enteric organisms (*Yersinia*, *Salmonella*, *Shigella*, *Campylobacter*, and *Clostridium*). It is a classic example of a disease caused by molecular mimicry with the generation of antigen-specific CD8 cells.

Reactive oxygen species: toxic to microbes. Singlet oxygen disrupts bacterial cell walls. Hydrogen peroxide and hydroxyl radicals attack cell membranes and also cause damage to bacterial DNA.

Receptor-mediated endocytosis: used by B cells to ingest foreign material. Receptor binding activates membrane clathrin and facilitates an inward folding of the cell membrane to form a vesicle and then a membrane-bound vacuole.

Recognition signal sequences: a heptamer followed by either 12 or 23 bases and an AT-rich nonamer that aligns genes on the same side of the DNA for recombination. (RSS).

Regulator cells: play a role in downregulating auto-reactive lymphocytes, reducing inflammation, mediating tolerance to superantigens, and maintaining self-tolerance.

Rescue immunosuppression: used during an episode of graft rejection. It uses intense, short-term therapy that varies according to the nature of the transplant.

Respiratory burst: rapid production of singlet oxygen (O$_2$-) and hydrogen peroxide (H$_2$O$_2$) and energy in the form of adenosine triphosphate (ATP) following the ingestion of microbes.

Rev: regulatory gene of the HIV-1 genome. *Rev* binds to mRNA, which contains a *Rev* response element (RRE). This promotes stabilization and export of mRNA from the nucleus to the cytoplasm of unspliced and single-spliced RNA.

Reverse transcriptase: an enzyme of RNA viruses that catalyzes the transcription of RNA to DNA, which is then incorporated into the genome of the host cell. This is the reverse of the usual mechanism for replication of genetic information; in the presence of this enzyme, it is the RNA that serves as the template for DNA copies.

Reye syndrome: associated with aspirin use during an active varicella zoster virus (VZV) infection. In the infected cells in the brain, liver, and kidney, aspirin inhibits mitochondrial function and the generation of ATP. Without ATP, cells cannot synthesize the proteins necessary for survival. As a consequence, a loss of neurons in the brain, degeneration of the proximal tubules in the kidney, and hepatocyte destruction occur.

Rheumatic fever (RF): a systemic inflammatory disease that may develop as a delayed reaction to an inadequately treated infection of the upper respiratory tract by group A beta-hemolytic streptococci. The disease usually occurs in young school-age children and may affect the brain, heart, joints, skin, or subcutaneous tissues.

Rheumatoid factor (RF): Immune complexes found in both the serum and synovial fluids of patients with rheumatoid arthritis (RA). RF is an autoantibody against the Fc portion of another antibody.

S

Sabin vaccine: oral poliovirus vaccine (OPV) that contains attenuated P1–P3 polio strains, which can replicate in the intestine. The OPV induces mucosal immunity, and the synthesis of surface immunoglobulin A (sIgA), which prevents infection by the wild-type virus. Continued shedding of the virus also contributes to the natural vaccination of unprotected individuals.

Salk vaccine: the original inactivated poliovirus (IPV) vaccine consists of the three (P1–P3) formalin-inactivated polio strains. A major disadvantage of the vaccine is that it does not stimulate the mucosal immune system, and individuals can be infected and transmit wild-type viruses.

Sequence-specific oligonucleotides (SSO): used to identify allelic polymorphism within each loci in tissue cross-matching. The PCR-SSO is a low-cost, high-volume assay that can screen a large number of potential donors with low or intermediate HLA resolution. Each probe is complementary to different motifs within an allelic hypervariable region of HLA molecules. Thus, the technique can identify heterozygous or homozygous combinations.

Sequence-based typing (SBT): used to identify allelic polymorphism within each loci in tissue cross-matching. PCR-SBT has the highest resolution for determining allelic polymorphisms. In the assay, the coding region of the entire HLA sequence on chromosome 6 is amplified by PCR. Coding sequences in exons 2 and 3 (HLA-A, HLA-B, and HLA-C) and exon 2 (DR, DQ, and DP) are then sequenced to determine HLA alleles. Employing different formats, SBT can be used to determine heterozygous sequences at each loci, haploid sequences, or a combination of heterozygous and homozygous sequences.

Sequence-specific primers (SSP): used to identify allelic polymorphism within each loci in tissue cross-matching. PCR-SSP has intermediate resolution for HLA-A, HLA-B, HLA-C, DR, and DQ and can be performed rapidly, usually within 3 to 4 hours. It is especially useful in typing cadaver organs that are used for transplantation or identifying closely related HLA alleles.

Serglycin: a protein that assembles a complex of granulysin, perforin, and granzymes in the small gap between effector and target cells. The complex is ingested by target cells by using receptor-mediated endocytosis and is placed into a cytoplasmic endosome.

Serum sickness: caused by the administration of large amounts of any foreign protein. Within 7 to 10 days after administration, an immunoglobulin M (IgM) antibody response to the foreign protein develops.

Signal joints: large loops containing introns between coding genes in recombination.

Simian immunodeficiency virus (SIV): a lentivirus that produces an acquired immunodeficiency syndrome-like disease in nonhuman primates. The cytopathologic changes caused by SIV are similar to those caused by the human immunodeficiency virus (HIV). SIV also shares with HIV a group of genes lacking in other retroviruses, and animals infected with either virus experience a similar decrease in the number of $CD4^+$ lymphocytes.

Single chain Fab variable (scFv) protein: antibody-variable regions (antigen-combining sites) that can be expressed in the protein coat of bacterial viruses, or bacteriophages, and are used in the construction of genetic libraries.

Single nucleotide polymorphism: single base pair changes in genes coding for each HLA allele, providing additional genetic diversity critical to disease resistance.

Singlet oxygen: metabolite of oxygen that disrupts bacterial cell walls and is toxic to microbes.

Sirolimus: blocks the signaling from the high-affinity IL-2 receptor.

Skin test: a test to determine the reaction of the body to a substance by observing the results of injecting the substance intradermally or of applying it topically to the skin. Skin tests are used to detect allergens, to determine immunity, and to diagnose disease.

Small lymphocyte: has a large, dark-staining nucleus, little cytoplasm, and no granules. Most small lymphocytes are localized in secondary lymphoid tissue (e.g., spleen or lymph nodes).

Sodium dodecyl sulfate (SDS): the more usual name for sodium lauryl sulfate when used as an anionic detergent to solubilize proteins. Denatures proteins during Western blotting.

Somatic cell recombination: a process of rearranging genes in somatic cells to create a repertoire of antigen-specific TCRs.

Somatic mutation: theory proposes that a limited number of inherited genes undergo mutations to general antibody repertoires. A sudden change in the chromosomal material in somatic cell nuclei affecting derived cells but not offspring.

S-Protein (vitronectin): a plasma protein that associates C5bC6C7 with C8 as an inhibitor of complement activation in the classic complement pathway.

Squalene: a naturally occurring molecule found in plants and some foods. Squalene is a weak adjuvant and other immunogenic molecules are usually added to increase immunogenicity for use in vaccines.

Superantigen: molecules that indiscriminately stimulate up to 20% of all T lymphocytes to release massive amounts of proinflammatory cytokines, possibly causing life-threatening hypovolemic shock and organ failure.

Superoxide dismutase: enzyme that converts singlet oxygen to oxygen (O_2) and H_2O_2.

Syncytia: a group of cells in which the cytoplasm of one cell is continuous with that of adjoining cells, resulting in a multinucleate unit.

Systemic lupus erythematosus (SLE): a multiple-organ disease occurring primarily in women of child-bearing age. It is characterized by multiple-organ inflammation. Almost any organ system can be involved, but the central nervous system (CNS), the renal system, and the pulmonary organs are common targets.

T

T cell: small lymphocyte differentiated in the thymus.

T cell receptor: gene found on the surface of T lymphocytes.

Tacrolimus: an anti-rejection agent that binds to a cytoplasmic protein called *FK506-binding protein 12 (FKBP-12)* and blocks the activity of calcineurin in the calcium–PKC signaling pathway.

TAP: transporter-associated antigen processing proteins used to move antigenic fragments from the cytoplasm into the endoplasmic reticulum. TAP is actually a heterodimer of TAP1 and TAP2. Both isoforms are required for antigen transport and for the stabilization of class I molecules.

Tapasin: a transmembrane-associated protein, called the *TAP-binding protein.*

Tat: regulatory gene of the HIV-1 genome. *Tat* gene translation is essential for viral replication. *Tat* promotes full-length synthesis of viral RNA by stabilizing the RNA polymerase and preventing the termination of protein synthesis.

Tetanospasmin: protein exotoxin released by vegetative bacteria. Tetanospasmin is a 150-kiloDalton (kDal) A+B toxin that is responsible for the recognized pathophysiology of tetanus.

TH3 cell: a subpopulation of CD4 Tregs. TH3 is found in the intestinal mucosa and is important in establishing oral tolerance or in downregulating the immune response to ingested antigens.

Thymus-dependent (TD) antigens: require the help of T cells for the stimulation of B cells to produce antibodies.

Thymus-independent (TI) antigens: can initiate antibody production without antigen processing or the help of T cells.

Thyroid releasing hormone (TRH): produced by the hypothalamus, travels through blood to the anterior pituitary gland as part of the process to control synthesis of T3 and T4.

Thyroid stimulating hormone (TSH): released by the anterior pituitary gland, the hormone interacts with thyrotropin receptors and stimulates iodine uptake and the production of T3 and T4.

Toll receptor: ligates pathogen-associated microbial patterns (PAMPs) to accelerate the phagocytosis of microbes.

Toll-like receptor: present on lymphocytes, macrophages, and dendritic cells and plays an important role in innate immunity. The 11 different TLRs in mammals each usually recognize only one type of pathogen-associated microbial pattern (PAMP).

Toxoids: modified bacterial exotoxins used in vaccines. Toxoids are treated with iodine, pepsin, ascorbic acid, or formalin to reduce toxicity while retaining the ability to stimulate an immune response.

TRADD protein: tumor necrosis factor receptor–associated protein with death domains (TRADD). TRADD complexes with proteins known as *RIP* and *RAIDD* and activate caspase 2 of the apoptotic pathway. In the TNF-related apoptosis-inducing ligand (TRAIL) pathway, TRADD complexes with FADD and activates caspases 8 and 10 that are critical to the induction of apoptosis.

Treg1 cell: T regulatory cells type 1. These cells have variable expression of FOXp3, require antigen stimulation, and do not need IL-2 stimulation or cell-cell contact for activation. Treg1 cells lyse effector cells using the classical perforin-granzyme lytic pathway.

Trismus: lockjaw, the first sign of generalized tetanus.

Tumor-associated antigen: an antigen produced by a particular type of tumor that also appears on normal cells of the tissue in which the tumor developed.

Tumor infiltrating lymphocyte (TIL): often found in melanomas and solid tumors of the kidney, colon, and lung. TILs comprise CD8 cells and a small population of cytotoxic CD4 cells and are the result of antigen-driven recruitment and proliferation of oligoclonal T cells within the tumor.

Tumor necrosis factor (TNF): a natural body protein, also produced synthetically, with anticancer effects. The body produces it in response to the presence of toxic substances, such as bacterial toxins. Adverse effects are toxic shock and cachexia.

Tumor necrosis factor-beta: produced by activated T and B cells and belongs to the TNF superfamily that also includes TNF-α. It has many of the proinflammatory properties of TNF-α, but it also is involved in biologic processes that include cell proliferation and apoptosis. Also known as *lymphotoxin.*

Tumor-specific antigen (TSA): an antigen produced by a particular type of tumor that does not appear on normal cells of the tissue in which the tumor developed.

Type I thymus-independent antigens: require interaction with a BCR and a second signal to activate B cells (e.g., bacterial endotoxins, glycolipids, and nucleic acids).

Type II thymus-independent antigens: polysaccharide antigens with repeating epitopes that cross-link multiple BCRs to stimulate B cell activation.

U

Ubiquitination: a process by which antigens are marked for enzymatic degradation involving the small polypeptide ubiquitin.

Urticaria: a rash characterized by raised, flat-topped areas with associated red edematous welts. Uticaria is an immunoglobulin E–mediated allergic reaction.

Urushiol: a toxic resin in the sap of certain plants of the genus *Rhus,* such as poison ivy, poison oak, and poison sumac, that produces allergic contact dermatitis in many people.

V

Vaccine: a suspension of attenuated or killed microorganisms administered intradermally, intramuscularly, orally, or subcutaneously to induce active immunity to infectious disease.

Vaccine-associated paralytic poliomyelitis (VAPP): the Sabin oral poliovirus vaccine (OPV) attenuated virus is able to replicate in the body so it has the ability to mutate or revert to a neurotropic form. The rate of VAPP is 1 case per 2.4 million vaccinations. A majority of these cases occurred in healthy vaccine recipients or household contacts of vaccine recipients.

Vif: accessory gene of the HIV-1 genome. The Vif protein protects RNA from degradation by cytoplasmic enzymes.

Vitamin D receptor (VDR): when associated with vitamin D, initiates transcription and translation of gene products that activate macrophages and Th1 cells while suppressing the activity of Th2 cells.

Vpr: accessory gene of the HIV-1 genome. Viral protein R (*Vpr*) acts as part of a complex to transport viral DNA into the nucleus.

Vpu: accessory gene of the HIV-1 genome. *Vpu* helps in virus release.

W

Waldenström's macroglobulinemia: a rare non-Hodgkin's lymphoma, which causes an overproduction of monoclonal IgM.

Western blotting: a laboratory blood test to detect the presence of antibodies to specific antigens. It is regarded as more precise than the enzyme-linked immunosorbent assay (ELISA) and is sometimes used to check the validity of ELISA tests. Conformational epitopes are irreversibly denatured by SDS in Western blotting and cannot be detected.

Whole-cell cancer vaccine: prepared using irradiated autologous or allogeneic tumor cells. To increase immunogenicity, whole-cell vaccines are genetically modified to express co-stimulatory molecules or combined with an adjuvant. Adjuvants create an insoluble depot of antigens, which are slowly released over time and continually stimulate the immune system.

X

Xenograft: when organs are transplanted across species barriers from animals to humans.

X-linked agammaglobulinemia: immunologic defect mapped to the Bruton's tyrosine kinase gene (*BtK*). Also known as *early onset agammaglobulinemia* or *Bruton's agammaglobulinemia*.

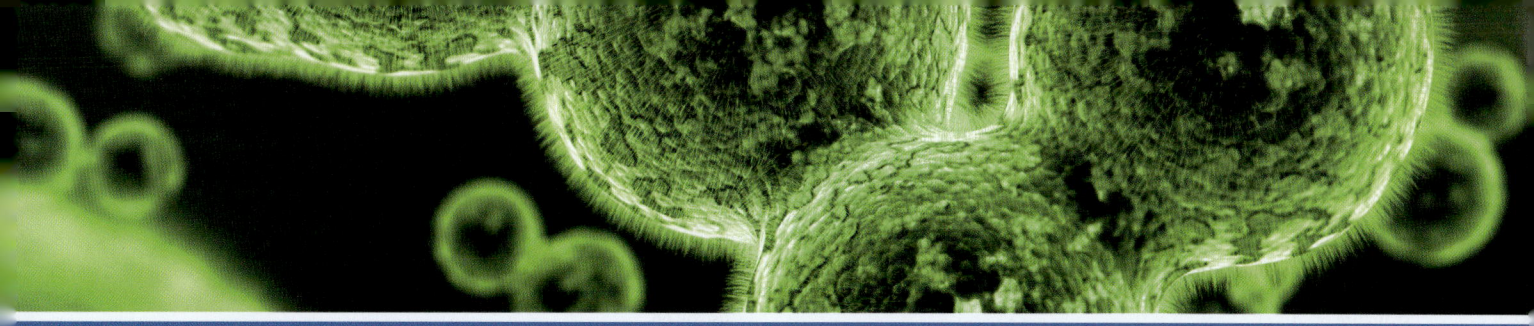

INDEX

A
A antigen, 24–25, 26f
Abatacept, 50
ABO isoantigen, 25
Abortive infection, 204
Acellular pertussis vaccine, 200t
N-acetylglucosamine, 24–25
Acid-fast organism, 153
Acquired immune deficiency syndrome (AIDS), 214
    characteristics of, 214
    defining conditions of, 220b
    diagnosis of, 114
    human immunodeficiency virus (HIV) and, 219–220
Activation complex, 88–89
    control of, 88
Activation-induced cell death, 178
Active immunity, 102
Acute B cell leukemia (ABCL), 110
Acute graft-versus-host disease, 144
Acute hepatitis B, 207
Acute phase protein
    inflammatory response, produced during, 20t
    types of, 19
Acute phase response, 18–20
Acute rejection, 141
    of graft, 142f–143f
Acute rheumatic fever
    group A *Streptococcus* species and, 135
    treatment of, 135
Adaptor protein, 56
Adenosine deaminase (ADA), 13
Adenosine diphosphate (ADP)-ribosylating toxin, 199f
Adjuvant, 20
    mucosal immunity and
        bacterial enterotoxins, 193
        monophosphoryl lipid A, 192–193
        oligodeoxynucleotide, 193
    systemic immunity and
        aluminum salts, 192
        Freund's complete, 192
        liposomes, 192
        muramyl peptides, 192
        squalene, 192
    vaccines and, 192
Affinity, 71
Affinity maturation, 84
Age, immunogenicity and, 24
Agrobacterium tumefaciens, 192
AIDS. *See* Acquired immune deficiency syndrome (AIDS)
Alefacept, 50
Allele, 33
Allelic exclusion, 84
Allelic polymorphism, 33–34
    of human leukocyte antigen, 34

Allergen
    cockroach-related, 124
    exposure to, 119
        early-phase reaction/preformed mediators, 119
        late-phase reaction/synthesized mediators, 119–120
    in food products, 122t
    latex, 124
    mite, 124
Allergic conjunctivitis
    characteristics of, 121
    treatment of, 121
Allergic reaction. *See also* Immediate allergic reaction
    agents causing, 122
    anaphylactoid reaction as, 124
    anaphylaxis as, 122
    occurrence/signs of, 118
Allergic rhinitis
    cause of, 120
    complications of, 120
    treatment of, 120
Alloantigen, WBC expressing, 24
Allogeneic graft
    antigen presentation in, 140
    tissue compatibility for, 139–140
Allogeneic transplant, 139
    diseases treated by, 143b
Allograft, 139f
Allo-reactive T cell, high frequency of, 141
Allorecognition, 140f
    direct versus indirect, 141f
Alpha/beta T cell receptor, 46–47
    V regions of, 46
        complementary determining region (CDR), 46
Alpha-defensin, 19
Alpha fetal protein (AFP), 184
Aluminum salt, 192
Amplification, of B cell signaling, 64
Anamnestic response, 74–76
Anaphylactoid reaction, 124
Anaphylaxis, 27–28, 122
    prevention of, 122
Anesthetic, 28
Ankylosing spondylitis (AS), 134
    pathophysiology of, 134
    treatment of, 134
Anthrax, 190–191
Antibiotic
    for chronic sinus/respiratory infections, 70
    as excipient, 193
    hapten as, 27–28
Antibiotics, antibody therapy and, 102
Antibody, 70
    anti-idiotype serum containing, 179f
    characteristics/location of, 70

Page numbers followed by *b*, indicate box; *f*, figure, *t*, table.

Antibody *(Continued)*
  encoding of, 79
  flexibility of, 71f
  gene coding in light/heavy chains, 80t
  molecular weight of, 70
  non-self blood group antigens and, 25
  passive immunity and, 102
  structure of, 70–71
Antibody binding, affinity/avidity of, 71
Antibody blocking, 176f
Antibody cross-matching, 139–140
Antibody-dependent cell-mediated cytotoxicity (ADCC), 171, 171f
Antibody diversity, 79
  generation of, 79, 84, 84b
Antibody fragment, 71–72
Antibody idiotype, 178
Antibody isotype
  differences in, 72–74
  immunoglobulin M isotype, 72–74
Antibody specificity, 71
Antibody therapy
  antibiotics and, 102
  side effects of, 103
Antigen
  B cell and, 39
  binding in pockets/grooves/extended surfaces, 71f
  class II MHC pathway and, 42f
  concentration of, 176, 176f
  dendritic cell and, 41
  exogenous and endogenous, 26–27
  form of/administration route for, 175–176
  immunocompetent macrophages and, 7–8
  ingestion of, 98
  microfold (M) cell and, 10
  presentation of, 46f
    CD1 protein and, 148–149
    cross-priming and, 149–150
    drugs and, 150
  thymus-independent, 63
  types of
    RBC isoantigen, 24–25
    TRALI, 24
    WBC alloantigen, 24
  yeast expression system and, 192
Antigen-antibody complex, precipitation of, 97
Antigenic determinant, 24, 25f
Antigenic drift, 208–209
Antigenicity, 23
  size and, 23
Antigenic shift, 165, 209
Antigen-presenting cell, 37, 51f
  bone-marrow derived, 40f
  heat shock protein and, 185f
  maturity of, 176
  T cell and, 50t
  T cell receptor (TCR) and, 49–50
  types of
    dendritic cells as, 37–39
    monocytes and macrophages as, 37
Antigen-presenting molecule, 31
  immunodeficiency and, 35
Anti-HLA antibody, 139
Anti-idiotype serum, 179f
Antimicrobial agent, 19–20
AP-1 complex, 56
Apolactoferrin, role of, 2
Apoptosis
  Granzyme A mediated, 165f
  of plasma cell, 6f
Artemis, 80
Arthritis, 206
Artificial passive immunity, 102
Aspirin-induced asthma, 124

Asthma
  characteristics of, 120
  chromosomal location/genes associated with, 119t
  latex allergen and, 124
  treatment of, 120
Atacicept
  B cell differentiation, inhibition of, 68t
  use of, 66
Atopic dermatitis
  characteristics of, 121
  pathogenesis of, 121
  treatment of, 121
Atopic eczema, 121f
Atopy
  characteristics of, 118–119
  chromosomal location/genes associated with, 119t
Attachment
  HIV and, 216, 217f
    inhibitors of, 220
Atypical measles, 205
Autoantibody, lymphocyte producing, 75–76
Autoantigen, 27
Autocrine interleukin 2 signaling, agents blocking, 59
Autograft, 139, 139f
Autoimmune disease
  of thyroid, 128–129
    Graves' disease, 128
    Hashimoto's thyroiditis, 128
Autoimmune hemolytic anemia
  complement receptor deficiency and, 100
  drugs inducing, 136
  treatment of, 136
Autoimmune lymphoproliferative syndrome type 2 (APLS2)
  characteristics of, 166
  treatment of, 166
Autoimmunity, 127
  infection, role of, 133f
  toll-like receptors and, 17
Autologous graft, 139
Autologous transplant, diseases treated by, 143b
Avidity, 71
Azathioprine, 142–143
Azurophilic granule(s), 2

B
B-1 lymphocyte, 75–76
Bacille Calmette-Guérin (BCG), 155–156
  for Tuberculosis, 191
  use of, 190–191
Bacteremia, 202
  fatality rate of, 203
Bacteria
  flow cytometry identifying, 112
  growth range and temperature, 19
  intracellular killing of, 98
    prevention of, 99
  meningitis and, 203
  pathogen-associated microbial patterns in, 16t
  skin as barrier to, 15
  toxins produced by, 190
Bacterial enterotoxin, 193
Bacterial meningitis. *See* Meningitis
B antigen, 26f
Bare lymphocyte syndrome
  effects of, 35
  treatment of, 35, 35t
Basiliximab, 59
  inhibiting IL-2 binding to receptors, 61t
Basophil, 3
B cell
  activation of, 89–90
  ADA deficiency and, 13
  antigens and, 39
  epitopes and, 24
  identification of, 5

B cell (Continued)
  lamina propria lymphocyte (LPL) as, 10
  maturation of, 6–7
  PALS and, 9
  plasma cells and, 5
  role of, 5
  T cells and, 67f
  vacuoles in, 40
  V genes, somatic hypermutation of, 84
B cell activation, 63
  complement role in, 66f
  initial stage of, 63
  occurrence of, 64
B cell differentiation, 65
  fusion protein/monoclonal antibodies inhibiting, 68t
  into plasma cells, agents blocking, 66
B cell maturation antigen (BCMA), 65
B cell-myeloma cell hybrid, 104
B cell priming, 176f
B cell proliferation, 65
B cell receptor, 7
B cell receptor complex, 63, 64f
  signal transduction by, 65f
B cell receptor signaling, 63
B cell signaling, 63
  amplification of, 64
Belimumab
  B cell differentiation, inhibition of, 68t
  use of, 66
Beta-defensin, 19
Bi-functional antibody, 107
Biologic response modifier
  colony-stimulating factor (CSF) as, 184
  cytokine and, 181
  interferon and, 183
  interleukin 11 as, 182
  interleukin 1 as, 182
  interleukin 2 as, 182
  role of, 181
  tumor necrosis factor (TNF) as, 183
Bi-specific antibody, 107
Blocking antibody, 122
Blood, 2
  PMNs in, 2–3
  white cells of
    basophils as, 3
    definition of, 2
    eosinophils as, 3
    lymphocytes as, 4–6
    macrophages as, 4
    mast cells as, 3–4
    monocytes as, 4
Blood transfusion, disease transmission from, 104
B lymphocyte stimulator (BLyS), 65–66
  interaction of, 67f
Bone marrow
  cell lineage in, 2
  location/composition of, 1–2
  Peyer's patches and, 7
  as primary lymphoid organ, 1
Bone-marrow derived antigen-presenting cell, 40f
Bone marrow stem cell, 144
Bone marrow transplantation, 144
  for Chediak-Higashi syndrome, 172t
Bordetella pertussis, 199
  virulence factors for, 199
BR3-Fc, B cell differentiation, inhibition of, 68t
Bronchial-associated lymphoid tissue (BALT), 190
Bronchiole-associated lymphoid tissue (BALT), 1
Bronchiolitis obliterans, 142
Bruton, Colonel Ogden, 66–67
Bruton agammaglobulinemia, effects of, 66–67
Budding, 219
Burnet, MacFarland, 45–46

C
C1
  activity of, regulation of, 91f
  proteins of, 88
  structure of, 88–89
C1 inhibitor, 95f
C3 convertase, 88
  inhibition of formation of, 94f
Calcineurin inhibitor, 142
Calcium-PKC signaling pathway, 59
Calcium-PLC signaling pathway, 56
Calcium release activated channel (CRAC), 56, 59f
Calreticulin, 147–148
Campylobacter, diarrhea from, 66–67
Canale-Smith syndrome
  characteristics of, 166
  treatment of, 166
Cancer, rapid cell division and, 99
Cancer vaccine. See also Vaccine
  dendritic cells and, 41
  dendritic cells vaccine as, 186
  idiotypic antigen vaccine as, 186
  purpose of, 185–186
  tumor antigens and, 184
  viral vector vaccine as, 186
  whole-cell vaccine as, 185–186
Capsular polysaccharide vaccine, 202
Carbohydrate, immunogenicity of, 23
Carbohydrate side chain, 73f
Carcinoembryonic antigen, 184
Cardiolipin, 23
Cathelicidin, 19
Caveolin, 12
CD1 protein, 148
  antigen presentation and, 148–149
CD28/B7 interaction, pathway for, 55
CD28/B7 signaling pathway, 56
CD3-T cell receptor protein complex, 48
CD4 cytotoxic cell
  destruction of, 219
  role of, 163
CD4 regulator cell, 176–177
  similarities/differences in, 178f
CD8 cytotoxic cell
  activation of, 162–163
  loss of function, 219
  subpopulation of, 163
CD8 regulator cell, 177–178
CD94-NKG2 receptor, 169
Celiac sprue, 159
  genetic component of, 159
  treatment of, 159–160
Cell
  antigen-presenting, 37
  antimicrobial agents produced by
    cathelicidins, 19
    defensins, 19–20
    nitric oxide, 20
  in thymus, 6f
Cell adhesion factor, 11t
Cell death, 178
Cell lineage, 1–2
Cephalic tetanus, 201
Cephalosporin, 28
Ceruloplasmin
  biologic effects of, 20t
  role of, 19
Cervarix, 211–212
Chediak-Higashi syndrome
  effects of, 172
  treatment of, 172, 172t
Chemokine, 10–11
Chicken pox (varicella zoster virus), 206
  treatment of, 206t

Chimeric antibody, 106
    generation of, 106f
    for immunotherapy, 107t
Chinese restaurant syndrome, 193
Cholera toxin, 193
Chronic asthma, 120
Chronic graft-versus-host disease, 144
Chronic granulomatous disease (CGD)
    effects of, 100
    treatment of, 100
Chronic hepatitis B, 208
Chronic lymphocytic leukemia (CLL), 110
Chronic rejection, 142
Chronic sinus infection, antibiotics for, 68
C-Jun N terminal kinase (JNK), 56
Class I major histocompatibility complex (MHC), 148f
Class I molecule
    antigen presentation and, 147–148
    location of, 147
Clathrin-dependent endocytosis, 39–40
    mechanism of, 41f
Clonal selection theory, tenets of, 45–46
Clostridium tetani, 200
    disease and, 200–201
Cluster of differentiation (CD) marker, 5
Coagulation pathway, meningitis and, 203
Coccidioides immitis, 158, 158f
Coccidioidomycosis (Valley Fever), 158
    pathophysiology of, 158
    treatment of, 158, 158t
Cockroach-related allergen, 124
Collagenase, role of, 2
Collectin, 16–17
    as oligomer, 17f
Colony-stimulating factor (CSF)
    as biologic response modifier, 184
    commercially available, 184t
    types of, 183–184
Colostrum, passive immunity and, 102
Combinatorial diversity, 80
Common variable immunodeficiency, 76
Community-acquired pneumonia (CAP), 201–202
Complement, 87
    activation of, 16, 90f
        alternative pathway of, 88–89, 93f
        molecules/receptors inhibiting, 91t
    alternative pathway for, 89
    B cell activation and, 66f
    cascades for, 87
        control of, 88
    cellular receptors for
        CR1, 97
        CR2, 98
        CR3, 98
    classic pathway for, 87–88, 89f
    Fc receptors for IgG, 98
    genetic defects for, 92–93
    mammalian cell inactivation of, 89
    mannose-binding lectin, 16–17
    pathways of, 18f
    schematic overview of, 17f
    serum proteins of, 16
Complementarity-determining region (CDR), 46, 71
    as amino acid sequences, 106
Complement deficiency
    hereditary angioneurotic edema, 90
    paroxysmal nocturnal hemoglobinuria, 90–92
    treatment of, 93
Complement pathway, meningitis and, 203
Complement receptor 1 (CR1), 89
Complement receptor deficiency, 100
    treatment of, 100
Concentration, immunogenicity and, 24
Congenital infection, from varicella zoster virus, 206
Congenital rubella syndrome, 206

Conjugate vaccine, 191
    licensed by U.S. FDA, 202t
    pneumococcal, 202–203
    Prevnar, 202–203
Constant region, 71, 79
    gene coding in light/heavy chains, 80t
Contact dermatitis, 159
    Toxicodendron and, 159
    treatment of, 159, 159t
Cortex, 8
Corticosteroid, 142
Corynebacterium diphtheriae,
    strains of, 198
Co-stimulatory molecule
    blockade of, 50
    CD11a/CD18/CD54, 49
    CD28/B7 interaction, 49
    CD2/CD58, 49
    CD40 ligand/CD40, 49
CR1 complement receptor, 97
CR2 complement receptor, 98
CR3 complement receptor, 98
C-reactive protein (CRP)
    biologic effects of, 20t
    role of, 19
Cross-presentation, models of, 149f
Cross-priming, antigen presentation and, 149–150
Cryopyrin-associated periodic syndrome (CAPS)
    characteristics of, 182
    gene abnormalities in, 182t
    treatment for, 182t
Crypticidin, 19
Cyclophilin, 56–59
Cyclosporine A (CsA), 56–59
    side effects of, 59
    T cell activation/signaling, blocking of, 60t
Cytochrome, 2
Cytochrome b588, 100
Cytokine, 10–11
    biologic modifiers and, 181
    interleukins and, 181–182
Cytokine storm, 200f, 209
Cytolysis
    FasL-FasR, 164
    Perforin-granzyme, 163–164
    TNF-β–TNFR-1, 164
Cytoplasm
    granules in
        primary, 2
Cytoplasmic granule(s), 2
    ultrastructural analysis of, 3f
Cytotoxicity, 139
Cytotoxic T cell, 162
    activation of, 162–163
Cytotoxic T lymphocyte
    killing tumor/virus-infected cells, 165f
    perforin and, 164f
    targets and, 163f
Cytotoxic T lymphocyte protein 4 (CTLA-4), 49
    mechanism of action of, 50f

D

Daclizumab, 59
    inhibiting IL-2 binding to receptors, 61t
Dalton, 70–71
Dausset, Jean, 138
Death
    from meningitis, 203
    from *Neisseria meningitidis*, 203
    from pandemic influenza, 209
    toxic shock syndrome and, 52
Decay accelerating factor (DAF), 89
Defensin, 19–20, 98
    gram-positive/negative bacteria and, 19
    influenza and, 20

Delayed-type hypersensitivity reaction, 152
  in intestine, 159
  in lungs, 153–158
  in skin, 158–159
    contact dermatitis, 159
    photo contact dermatitis, 158
Dendritic cell, 37–39
  cancer vaccines and, 41
  cytotoxic T cells and, 162–163
  disease and, 41
  follicular, 38
  human immunodeficiency virus (HIV) and, 41, 219
  interstitial, 38–39
  lymphoid, 37–38
  pathway for, 38f
  plasmacytoid, 39
Dendritic cell vaccine, 186
Deoxyadenosine, 221f
Deoxycytidine, 221f
Deoxyribonucleic acid (DNA)
  double-stranded viral, 217
    integration of, 219
    synthesis of, 218f
  exchange of, 33
  HAT selection process and, 104
  immunogenicity of, 23
  V(D)J recombination and, 81f
    sequential events during, 82f
Deoxythymidine, 221f
Dermonecrotic lethal toxin
  effects of, 200
  treatment of, 200
  vaccine for, 200
Desensitization, 123f
Diabetes (type 1a), 133–134
  characteristics of, 134
  molecular mimicry and, 133
  pathophysiology of, 134
  treatment of, 134
Diapedesis, 10–12
  of neutrophil, 12f
Diarrhea, *Giardia/Campylobacter* causing, 66–67
Didanosine nucleoside transcriptase, 221f
DiGeorge syndrome, 12–13
Diphtheria
  cause of, 198
  pathophysiology of, 199
  treatment of, 199
    therapeutic agents for, 199t
  vaccine for, 199
Diphtheria exotoxin, 198–199
Diphtheria toxoid, 199
Direct allorecognition, 141f
Disease
  Clostridium tetani and, 200–201
  herd immunity thresholds for, 198t
  human leukocyte antigen, 34
  interleukin 1 and, 182
  natural killer T cell in, 172
  tumor necrosis factor (TNF) and, 183
  vaccinations reducing, 198
  vaccine-preventable, 197
Disease modifying antirheumatic drug (DMARD), 50
Disseminated varicella neonatorum, 206
Disulfide bond, 70–71
Diversity gene, 79
Diversity segment, gene coding in light/heavy chains, 80t
DNA vaccine, 186
Double-stranded viral DNA, 217
  integration of, 219
  synthesis of, 218f
Double-stranded viral RNA, 216
Drug
  antigen presentation and, 150
  autoimmune hemolytic disease and, 136

Drug (Continued)
  immediate allergic reaction and, 124–125
  neoantigens and, 28
  RBC/serum protein reaction to, 29b
Drug-induced "lupus-like" disease, 132
  drugs causing, 132b
Dtox gene, 198

E
Early endosome, 40
Early-onset agammaglobulinemia
  effects of, 66–67
  treatment of, 67–68
Edible vaccine, 192
Efalizumab, 50
Effector cell, types of, 1
Effector T cell, regulation of, 177f
Egg albumin, in vaccines, 193, 194t
Egg allergen, 122t
Egg protein, as excipient, 193
ELK, 56
Encephalitis, 205
Endocytosis, 98
Endogenous antigen, 27
Endogenous pyrogen, 19
Endothelial cell, chemokine and, 10–11
Endotoxin
  domains for, 64–65
  effects of, 190
Endotoxin-induced B cell stimulation, 65
Enterotoxin
  bacterial, 193
  effects of, 190
  exotoxins versus, 51
Env gene, 219
Enzyme-linked immunosorbent assay (ELISA)
  alternative formats for
    indirect assay, 112
    sandwich assay, 112
  diseases diagnosed with, 115t
  plate preparation for, 114f
  use of, 112
Enzyme replacement therapy (ERT), 100
Eosinophil
  characteristics of, 3
  role of, 3
  structure of, 3f
Epithelioid cell, 154
  of granulomatous hypersensitivity, 154f
Epitope, 24
  T cell/B cell recognition of, 24
Epratuzumab
  B cell differentiation, inhibition of, 68t
  use of, 66
Equine antiserum therapy, 102
ERK, 56
Erythroblastosis fetalis
  cause of, 26
  effects of, 26
  prevention of, 104
Erythrocyte, 2
Escherichia coli
  effects of, 190
  Oprelvekin and, 182
  plasmids and, 192
E-selectin, 11
Excipient
  antibiotics as, 193
  egg protein as, 193
  gelatin as, 193–194
  monosodium glutamate as, 193
  purpose of, 193
Exercise-induced asthma, 123
Exogenous antigen, 26–27
  presentation of, 39–41

Exophthalmos, 128
Exotoxin
  dermonecrotic lethal toxin as, 200
  enterotoxins versus, 51
  role of, 190
Extensively drug-resistant tuberculosis (XDR-TB), 156
Extruded granule(s), role of, 3

F

Fab fragment
  construction of, 107
  usefulness of, 72
Factor H, 89
Familial erythrophagocytic lymphohistiocytosis type 2 (FHLH2)
  cause of, 165–166
  treatment of, 166
Fas-associated protein with death domain (FADD), 164
FasL-FasR, engagement and disease, 178
FasL-FasR cytolysis, 164
Fc receptors for IgG, 98
Feedback loop, 129f
Fernandez reaction, 155f
Ferritin
  biologic effects of, 20t
  role of, 19
FK506-binding protein 12 (FKBP-12), 59
Flow cytometer, 111–112
Flow cytometry (FCM)
  bacteria/virus identification by, 112
  components of, 110
  leukemia and, 110
  of peripheral blood cells, 111f
  principle of, 113f
  use of, 110
Fluorescence-activated cell sorter (FACS)
  flow cytometer as, 111–112
  principle of, 113f
Fluorescence isothiocyanate (FITC), 111
Follicle-associated epithelium, microfold (M) cell and, 10f
Follicular dendritic cell, 38
  human immunodeficiency virus (HIV) and, 219
  view of, 39f
Food allergy, 122
  allergens causing, 122t
  treatment of, 122
Forehead helix (FOX), 177
N-formyl-1-methionyl-1-leucyl-1-phenylalamine (FMLP), Polymorphonuclear leukocyte (PMN) and, 2
Forward scatter, 110
FOXp3
  deficiency of, 177
  role of, 177f
Fraction antigen binding (Fab), 71–72
Fraction crystallized (Fc), 71–72
Freund's adjuvant, 192
Fucosyltransferase enzyme, 24–25
Fulminating bacteremia, 203
  meningococcal septic shock and, 203
Fungal immunosuppressive agent, T cell activation/signaling, blocking of, 60t
Fungus, pathogen-associated microbial patterns in, 16t
Fusion protein
  B cell differentiation, inhibition of, 68t
  creation of, 50

G

Gag gene, 219
Gamma/delta T cell receptor, 47
Gammaglobulin, 70
Gardasil, 211–212
Gaucher's disease, 99–100
  treatment of, 100
Gelatin, as excipient, 193–194
Gelatinase, 2

Gene, immune receptors encoded by, 170t
Gene conversion, 33
Generalized tetanus, 200–201
Genetic information coding, 107
Genetics
  immune response and, 175
  immunogenicity and, 24
  Mycobacterium infection and, 154–155
  rheumatoid arthritis and, 135
Gentamicin, in vaccines, 194t
German measles. *See* Rubella
Germ line theory, 79
Gestation, hematopoiesis and, 1–2
Giant papillary conjunctivitis, 121
Giardia, diarrhea from, 66–67
Glandular hyperplasia, 128
Gliadin, 159
Gluten-sensitive enteropathy, 159
Goodpasture syndrome
  characteristics of, 132
  treatment of, 132–133
Graft-versus-host disease
  acute, 144
  chronic, 144
  occurrence of, 144
  treatment for
    acute rejection, 144–145
    chronic rejection, 145
Gram-negative bacteria
  defensins and, 19
  meningitis and, 203t
Gram-positive bacteria
  defensins and, 19
  meningitis and, 203t
Granule
  in cytoplasm, 2
    primary, 2
  phagosome, fusing with, 98
  proteins in, 3
  role of, 3t
Granulocyte, 2
Granulocyte-colony-stimulating factor, 184
Granulocyte macrophage-colony-stimulating factor, 184
Granuloma, 154
Granulomatous hypersensitivity, characteristic cell of, 154f
Granulysin, 163–164
Granzyme, 164
  familial erythrophagocytic lymphohistiocytosis type 2 and, 165
Granzyme A mediated apoptosis, 165f
Graves' disease
  effects of, 130f
  hyperthyroidism and, 128
  thyroid storm and, 128
  treatment of, 128
Graves' ophthalmopathy, 128
Group A streptococcus, cathelicidins and, 19
Group I CD I molecule, tissue distribution of, 35t
Guanosine diphosphate (GDP), 56
Guanosine triphosphate (GTP), 56
Guanosine triphosphate-guanosine diphosphate (GTP-GDP) exchange protein, 63–64
Gut-associated lymphoid tissue (GALT), 1, 190

H

Haemophilus infection, treatment of, 201t
Haemophilus influenzae, 208
  early-onset agammaglobulinemia and, 66–67
  as etiologic agent, 201
  vaccine for, 74
  virulence factor for, 201
Haemophilus influenzae type B (Hib)
  prevalence of, 201
  treatment of, 201
  vaccine for, 201
Hairpin, 80

Hairy cell leukemia
 flow cytometry and, 110
 treatment of, 110
Halothane, 28
Hansen's bacillus, 153
H antigen, 24–25, 26f
Haplotype, 33
Hapten, 27–29
 anesthetics as, 28
 cell-mediated reactions and, 29
 ovalbumin, conjugation to, 27f
 pharmaceuticals as, 27–28
  antibiotics, 27–28
Haptoglobin
 biologic effects of, 20t
 role of, 19
Hashimoto's thyroiditis, 128–129, 130f
 symptoms of, 129
 treatment of, 129
Heat labile *E. coli*, 193
Heat shock protein (HSP), 184
 peptides and, 185f
Heat shock protein, antigen-presenting cell and, 185f
Heavy chain
 example of, 73f
 gene recombination/expression, 83f
 light chain attachment to, 71
 molecular weight of, 70–71
 number of genes coding for, 80t
Heavy-chain constant domain, 71
Heavy chain VDJ recombination, 82–84
Helicobacter pylori, 16
Helper T cell, B cells and, 67f
Hemagglutins, 208
Hematopoiesis, definition of, 1–2
Hematopoietic stem cell transplantation, 143–144
Hemodynamic focusing, 110
Hemolytic transfusion reaction
 cause of, 25
 treatment of, 25, 26t
Hepatitis
 treatment of, 208, 208t
 types/effects of, 207
 vaccines for, 208
Hepatitis A, 207
 vaccine for, 208
Hepatitis B, 207–208
 as acute, 207
 as chronic, 208
 risk groups for, 207
 transmission of, 207
 treatment of, 208
 vaccine for, 208
Hepatitis B vaccine, 192
Heptadrepeat, 216
Herd immunity, 198
 for disease, 198t
Hereditary angioneurotic edema (HANE), 90
 cause of, 90
 clinical appearance of, 95f
 emergency intervention for, 90
 inherited versus acquired forms of, 90
 treatment of, 90
Herpes virus, 206
Herpes zoster
 complications of
  post-herpetic neuralgia, 207
  Ramsay Hunt syndrome, 207
 treatment of, 207, 207t
Heterologous antisera
 immunogenicity and, 102
 passive immunity and, 102–103
Heterologous recombinant protein, 192
Heterozygosity, 33
Hevein (amine), 124

Hevin, 12
High determinant model, 141
Histamine, 119
 in food products, 124
Histoplasma capsulatum, 157f, 158
 methenamine silver stain of, 157f
 prevalence of, 156–157
Histoplasmin, 157f
Histoplasmosis
 frequency of reactors to, 157f
 pathophysiology of, 157–158
 prevalence of, 156–157
 treatment of, 158, 158t
HIV-1. See Human immunodeficiency virus (HIV)
Homologous restriction factor (HRF), 89
Hormone, T cell maturation and, 7
Human immunodeficiency virus (HIV)
 AIDS and, 219–220
 dendritic cells and, 41
 diagnosis of, 114, 219–220
 follicular dendritic cells and, 219
 groups and clades of, 215
 immune system and, 219
 integrase and, 219
 neurologic effects and, 219
 preintegration complex and, 217
 prevalence of, 214–215
 sirian immunodeficiency virus versus, 214
 stages of, 216–220
  attachment, 216, 217f
  membrane fusion, 216, 217f
  reverse transcription, 216–217
 structure of, 215, 215f–216f
 treatment of, 220–221
  attachment/fusion inhibitors, 220
  integrase inhibitor, 221
  non-nucleoside reverse transcriptase inhibitor, 220, 221b
  nucleoside reverse transcriptase inhibitor, 220, 220t
  nucleotide reverse transcriptase inhibitor, 220t
  protease inhibitor, 221
 viral assembly and release, 219
Human immunodeficiency virus (HIV) genome, 215, 217f
Human immunoglobulin locus, germ-line organization of, 80f
Humanized antibody, 106
 generation of, 106f
 for immunotherapy, 107t
Human leukocyte antigen
 allelic polymorphism of, 34t
 inheritance of, 33
 polymorphic residues of, 34
 single nucleotide polymorphism and disease, 34
Human leukocyte antigen complex
 antigen-presenting molecules outside of, 34
 class III region, 32–33
  structure of, 33f
 class II region, 32
  molecules of, 32–33
 class I region, 31
  molecules of, 32
  structure of, 33f
 map of, 32f
 pseudogenes and, 31
Human leukocyte antigen glycoprotein, immune response and, 175
Human leukocyte antigen marker, transplantation and, 139
Human leukocyte-specific antigen (HLA-A2), 138
Human monoclonal antibody, 106
 for immunotherapy, 107t
Human papilloma virus (HPV).. See Papilloma virus
Human stem cell, characteristics of, 144
Hybridoma, 104
Hydrogen peroxide, 2
Hyperacute rejection, 141, 141f
Hyperimmunoglobulinemia E (Job syndrome)
 composition of, 77
 treatment of, 77

Hyper-immunoglobulin M syndrome
  treatment of, 52
  X-linked immunodeficiency with, 52
Hyperosmolar radiocontrast media, 124
Hypersensitivity. See also Delayed-type hypersensitivity
  nickel and, 159
  plants and, 159
    poison ivy, 159
Hyperthyroidism, 128
Hypochlorous acid, 2
  formation of, 98
Hyposensitization therapy, 122
Hypothyroidism, Hashimoto's thyroiditis as, 128
Hypoxanthine-aminopterin-thymidine (HAT) selection, 104–105
  DNA and, 104
Hypoxanthine-guanine phosphorylribosyl transferase (HPRT+), 104

I
Iccosome, 38, 219
Idiopathic thrombocytopenic purpura
  characteristics of, 103
  platelet count and, 103
  treatment of, 103
Idiotype network theory, 178–179
Idiotypic antigen vaccine, 186
Immediate allergic reaction. See also Allergic reaction
  drugs and, 124–125
  evolution of, 119
  mediation of, 118
Immune polyendocrinology, enteropathy, and X-linked disorder (IPEX)
  symptoms of, 177
  treatment of, 177
Immune receptor, 170t
Immune response, 75f
  evasion by virus, 164–165
  factors influencing, 175
  genetics and, 175
  human leukocyte antigen glycoprotein and, 175
  physical/biologic factors influencing, 175–176
Immune suppression, rubeola infection and, 205
Immune system
  human immunodeficiency virus (HIV) and, 219
  parts of, 1
Immunoblotting, 116f
Immunochromatographic testing, 112
Immunocompetent macrophage, antigen and, 7–8
Immunodeficiency
  antigen-presenting molecule and, 35
  Bruton agammaglobulinemia as, 66–67
  Chediak-Higashi syndrome as, 172
  DiGeorge syndrome as, 12–13
  effects of, 66–67
  innate immunity and, 20–21
  leukocyte adhesion deficiency as, 13
  Nezelof syndrome as, 13
  phagocytosis, associated with
    chronic granulomatous disease (CGD), 100
    complement receptor deficiency, 100
    Gaucher's disease, 99–100
    myeloperoxidase (MPO) deficiency, 100
  primary
    common variable immunodeficiency, 76
    hyperimmunoglobulinemia E (Job syndrome), 77
    immunoglobulin A (IgA) deficiency, treatment of, 77
    selective immunoglobulin A deficiency, 76–77
    transient hypogammaglobulinemia of infancy, 76
  T killer cell and, 165–166
  X-linked
    characteristics of, 60–61
    with hyper-immunoglobulin M, 52
Immunogen
  degradability of, 24
  foreignness of, 23
  internal rigidity/tertiary structure of, 23

Immunogenicity, 23
  ancillary factors influencing, 24
  biologic factors influencing
    age, 24
    genetics, 24
  heterologous antisera and, 102
  monoclonal antibodies and, 105–106
Immunoglobulin, 176
Immunoglobulin A (IgA)
  epithelium, transportation to, 76f
  secretory, production of, 74–75
Immunoglobulin A (IgA) antibody, 74
Immunoglobulin A (IgA) chain, 73f
Immunoglobulin A (IgA) deficiency, treatment of, 77
Immunoglobulin A (IgA) isotope, 74
Immunoglobulin D (IgD), 75
Immunoglobulin D (IgD) chain, 73f
Immunoglobulin E (IgE), 76
  immediate allergic reaction and, 118
  pseudoallergic reactions not mediated by nonallergic asthma, 123–124
Immunoglobulin E (IgE) chain, 73f
Immunoglobulin E (IgE)-mediated allergic reaction
  allergic conjunctivitis
    characteristics of, 121
    treatment of, 121
  allergic rhinitis as
    cause of, 120
    complications of, 120
    treatment of, 120
  asthma as
    characteristics of, 120
    treatment of, 120
  atopic dermatitis as
    characteristics of, 121
    pathogenesis of, 121
    treatment of, 121
  urticaria as
    as acute or chronic, 121
    characteristics of, 121
    photo of, 121f
    treatment of, 121
    types of, 121
Immunoglobulin G (IgG)
  clinical implications of, 74
  fragments of, 72f
  N terminal characteristics of, 71f
  subclasses of, 74
  systemic lupus erythematosus and, 132f
Immunoglobulin G (IgG) antibody, 74
Immunoglobulin G (IgG) chain, 73f
Immunoglobulin G isotope, 74
Immunoglobulin heavy-chain/light-chain gene recombination/expression, 83f
Immunoglobulin immunodeficiency, 76
Immunoglobulin M (IgM), 63
  antibody response to, 102–103
  formation of, 72–74
  monomeric, location/function of, 74
  secretory, production of, 74
  structure of, 74
Immunoglobulin M (IgM) chain, 73f
Immunoglobulin M isotope, 72–74
Immunologic synapse, 55–56, 57f
Immuno-receptor tyrosine-based inhibitory motif (ITIM), 170
  inhibitory receptors and, 171f
Immunostimulatory sequence (ISS), 193
  classes of, 193t
Immunosuppressive agent, T cell activation/signaling, blocking of, 60t
Immunotherapy, 123f
  monoclonal antibody for, 107t
Inactivated vaccine, 191
Indirect allorecognition, 141f

Infection
　acute phase response to, 18–20
　diapedesis and, 10–11
　PMNs and, 2–3
Infectious asthma, 123
Inflammation
　acute phase proteins and, 20t
　diapedesis and, 10–11
　eosinophils and, 3
　PMNs and, 2–3
　tissue, causing damage to, 99
Influenza virus
　antigenic drift and, 208–209
　antigenic shift and, 209
　cytokine storm and, 200f
　defensin and, 20
　pandemics of, 209t
　strains/subtypes of, 208
　transmission/temporal patterns of, 209
　treatment/prevention of, 209, 210t
　types of, 208
　　pandemic, 209
　　seasonal, 209
　　type A, 208
　　type B, 208
　　type C, 208
　vaccine for, 209
　　live attenuated, 209
　　trivalent inactivated, 209
Inhibitory receptor, 170f
　phosphatases and, 171f
Injury, acute phase response to, 18–20
Innate immunity, 15
　immunodeficiency and, 20–21
　injury and infection, 18–20
　toll-like receptor and, 16–17
Innocent bystander, 219
Integrase, 219
Integrase inhibitor, 221
Integrin, location of, 11t
Intercellular adhesion molecule (ICAM), leukocyte tethering and, 11–12
Intercellular signaling, 55
Interferon
　commercially available, 183t
　synthetic and natural, 183
　types/role of, 183
　viral infections and, 183
Interferon gamma receptor deficiency, 155
Interleukin, cytokine and, 181–182
Interleukin 1
　as biologic response modifier, 182
　disease and, 182
　overview of, 182
Interleukin 11, 182
　as biologic response modifier, 182
Interleukin 2
　as biologic response modifier, 182
　monoclonal antibodies inhibiting binding, 61t
　synthesis of, 182
　　AP-1 complex and, 56
　　signaling pathways for, 55
Interleukin 2 receptor, 59
Interleukin 3, role of, 183–184
Interleukin 7, 6–7
Interstitial dendritic cell, 37–39
Intestine
　delayed-type hypersensitivity in, 159
　stomach acid and, 16
Intracellular bacteria, destruction of, 2
Intracellular killing, 97
　of bacteria, 98
　microbial evasion of, 99
　by natural killer cells, 170
　oxygen-dependent, 98
Intracellular signaling, 17–18

Intraepithelial lymphocyte (IEL), location of, 10
Intravenous immunoglobulin, T cell-mediated autoimmune disease, 104
Intravenous preparations of human immunoglobulin (IVIG), 103
　safety concerns with, 104
　use of, 103
Intrinsic factor, 129
In vitro radioallergosorbent test, 122
In vitro test for tuberculosis, 156
Isoantigen, in RBCs, 24–25
Isograft, 139, 139f
ITAM, ZAP proteins and, 61

J

Janus tyrosine kinase-signal transducer activator of transcription (JAK-STAT), 56
J chain, 73f
Jenner, Edward, 189
Job syndrome (Hyperimmunoglobulinemia E)
　composition of, 77
　treatment of, 77
Joining segment, gene coding in light/heavy chains, 80t
Junctional diversity, 82–84, 84f
Juvenile rheumatoid arthritis, complement receptor deficiency and, 100

K

Kappa light chain, number of genes coding for, 80t
Kawasaki disease, 103–104
　treatment of, 104
Killer cell immunoglobulin-like receptor, 169, 170f
Koplick spots, 205

L

Lambda light chain, number of genes coding for, 80t
Lamina propria lymphocyte (LPL), 10
Large granular lymphocyte (LGL), 2
　characteristics of, 4
Latent provirus, 216
Latex allergen, 124
　diagnosis of, 124
　natural rubber and, 194
　products containing, 124b
Leader peptide, from class 1 MHC, 171f
Left shift, 2–3
Leprosy bacillus, 155f
Leukemia, flow cytometry and, 110
Leukocyte adhesion deficiency (LAD), 13
Leukocyte receptor complex region, 170t
Leukocyte. See also White blood cell
　movement of, 11
　tethering of, 11–12
Ligand, for toll-like receptors, 20t
Light chain
　example of, 73f
　gene recombination/expression, 83f
　heavy chains, attachment to, 71
　molecular weight of, 70–71
　number of genes coding for, 80t
　types of, 80
Light chain VJ recombination, 80–82
Lingual tonsils, 10
Linker for activation of T cells (LAT), 56
　function of, 56
Lipid, immunogenicity of, 23
Lipooligosaccharide (LOS), 203
　complement pathway, activation of, 203
　lipid-binding protein and, 203
Lipopolysaccharide endotoxin, 17–18
　release of, 64–65
Liposome, 192
Live attenuated *Bacillus anthracis* Sterne strain, 190–191
Live attenuated influenza vaccine (LAIV), 209
Live attenuated vaccine, 190–191
　advantages/disadvantages of, 191
Localized tetanus, 201

"Lupus-like" disease, drugs and, 132
Lymph node
   characteristics of, 8–9, 8f
   location/role of, 8f
   morphology of, 8f
   as secondary lymphoid organ, 1
Lymphocyte
   circulation of, 11f
   location of, 10
   population of, verifying, 111
   secretory IgA, production of, 74–75
   tumor-infiltrating, 164
Lymphocyte diapedesis, 10–12
Lymphocyte function-associated antigen (LFA-3), 49
Lymphocyte phenotyping, purpose of, 110
Lymphocyte. See also Small lymphocyte
   characteristics of, 4–6
   as effector cell, 1
   large granular, 2
   marker expression by, 5t
   production of, 2
Lymphocyte subset enumeration, 110, 112t
Lymphocyte VLA-4, 11
Lymphocytotoxicity, 139
Lymphoid dendritic cell, 37–38
   pathway for, 38f
Lymphoid organ. See Primary lymphoid organ. See also Secondary lymphoid organ
Lymphoid tissue
   bronchial-associated, 190
   composition of, 1
   gut-associated, 1, 190
   mucosal-associated, 9–10, 190
   nasal-associated, 190
   organization of, 9–10
Lymphokine-activated killer cell, 172
Lymph system, role of, 7
Lysozyme, 2

M

Macrophage
   as effector cell, 1
   as immunocompetent, 7–8
   location of, 4
   nomenclature for, 4t
   PAMPs, recognition of, 19f
   role of, 37
   types of, 4
   vacuoles in, 40
Macrophage-colony-stimulating factor, 184
MAGE-A3, 184
Maintenance dose, 122
Major histocompatibility complex (MHC)
   class I, 148f
      leader peptides from, 171f
   class II, 47f
      functions of, 42f
      pathway for, 42f
   thymocyte and, 7
   transplantation and, 139
Mannose-binding lectin complement activation pathway, 16–17
Mantle cell leukemia
   flow cytometry and, 110
   treatment of, 110
Mantoux skin test, for tuberculosis, 155
   interpretation of, 155–156
Mast cell
   mediators, releasing of, 120f
   overview of, 3–4
   in rat peritoneum, 4f
Matrilysin, 178
M cell. See Microfold (M) cell
Measles (rubeola)
   cause/effects of, 205
   complications of, 205

Measles (Continued)
   atypical measles, 205
   encephalitis, 205
   immune suppression, 205
   modified measles, 205
   subacute sclerosing panecephalitis (SSPE), 205
   rash from, 205
   treatment of, 205
   vaccine for, 205
Measles-mumps-pertussis-vaccine (MMR), 205t
Medulla, 6, 8
Melanin, 184
Melanoma, 184
Melanoma antigen, T cells and, 184–185
Membrane attack complex, 88
   control of, 88
   formation of, regulation of, 94f
   structure of, 91f
Membrane cofactor protein (MCP), 89
Membrane fusion, 216, 217f
   inhibitors of, 220
Memory cell, 74
Menactra, 204
Meningitis, 202
   bacterial growth and, 203
   coagulation pathway, 203
   complement pathway, 203
   mortality rate of, 203
   Neisseria meningitidis as agent for, 203
   nonparalytic aseptic, 204
   treatment of, 203, 203t
   vaccine for, 203–204
      Menactra, 204
      Menomune, 203–204
      Menveo, 204
Meningococcal bacteremia, 203
Meningococcal disease, Neisseria meningitidis as agent for, 203
Meningococcal septic shock
   fulminating bacteremia and, 203
   incidence/frequency of, 203
   treatment of, 203, 203t
Meningococcal vaccine, 74
Menomune, 203–204
Menveo, 204
Microbe
   ingestion of, 98
      oxygen-dependent respiratory burst, 98
   intracellular killing of, 20f
Microfold (M) cell
   antigens and, 10
   follicle-associated epithelium and, 10f
Migratory cup, 12
Miliary tuberculosis, 154
Milk allergen, 122t
"Missing self" hypothesis, 170
Mite allergen, 124
Mitogen-activated protein (MAP) kinase, 63–64
Modified measles, 205
Molecular clustering, purpose of, 56
Molecular mimicry, 133–136
   diabetes (type 1a) and, 133–134
   disease, role in, 133
Molecule
   antigen-presenting, 31, 34
   of class 1 region of HLA complex, 32
   of class 2 region of HLA complex, 32–33
   stabilization of, 48–49
   virulence factors for, 189–190
Monoclonal antibody, 50
   Basiliximab as, 59
   B cell differentiation and
      inhibition of, 68t
      prevention of, 66
   for immunotherapy, 107t
   inhibiting IL-2 binding to receptors, 61t

Monoclonal antibody *(Continued)*
  nomenclature for, 106–107
    source, 106t
    target, 106t
  with reduced immunogenicity, 105–106
  role of, 59
  in tissue culture, 104–105
  transplantation rejection and, 143
Monocyte
  overview of, 4
  role of, 37
  ultrastructure of, 4f
Monomeric IgM, location/function of, 74
Monophosphoryl lipid A, 192–193
Monosodium glutamate (MSG)
  as excipient, 193
  in vaccines, 194t
Montagu, Lady Mary Wortley, 189
mRNA splicing, 82
MSG symptom complex, 193
Mucin, 185
Mucociliary escalator
  dysfunction of, 15
  factors affecting, 15–16
  mechanism of, 15
Mucosal-associated lymphoid tissue (MALT), 9–10, 10f, 190
Mucosal immunity
  adjuvants and, 192
    bacterial enterotoxins, 193
    monophosphoryl lipid A, 192–193
    oligodeoxynucleotide, 193
  administration of, 190
Multidrug-resistant tuberculosis (MDR-TB), 156
Multiple-colony-stimulating factor, 183–184
Multiple determinant model, 141
Multiple myeloma, 77
  treatment of, 77
Mumps
  cause/symptoms of, 205
  complications of, 205
  vaccine for, 205–206
Muramyl dipeptide, 20
Muramyl peptide, 192
Murine monoclonal antibody
  generation of, 105f
  for immunotherapy, 107t
  production of, 105
Myasthenia gravis
  effects of, 129
  ptosis and, 131f
  treatment of, 130–131
Mycobacterial cell wall, 153f
Mycobacterium africanum, 153, 153t
Mycobacterium avium, 153, 153t
Mycobacterium avium complex (MAC),
    infections caused by, 156
Mycobacterium bovis, 153, 153t
  Bacille Calmette-Guérin (BCG) and, 155–156
Mycobacterium genus/species, 153
  laboratory identification of, 153
Mycobacterium infection, genetics and, 154–155
Mycobacterium leprae, 153, 153t
Mycobacterium tuberculosis, 153, 153t
Mycophenolate mofetil, 142
Myeloid cell, production of, 2
Myeloid dendritic cell, pathway for, 38f
Myeloperoxidase (MPO), 98
  role of, 2
Myeloperoxidase (MPO) deficiency, 100
  treatment of, 100

N

Nasal-associated lymphoid tissue (NALT), 190
Natural antibody, 65
Natural CD4 Treg, 176

Natural interferon
  biologic modifiers and, 183
  commercially available, 183t
Natural killer cell, 169
  ADA deficiency and, 13
  function of, 171–172
  intracellular killing by, 170
  lymphokine-activated, 172
  marker expression by, 6
  phosphatases and, 171f
  role of, 6, 170
  subpopulations of, 171
Natural killer cell receptor
  CD94-NKG2 receptors as, 169
  killer cell immunoglobulin-like receptor as, 169, 170f
Natural killer T cell, 172
  in disease, 172
Natural passive immunity, 102
Natural resistance-associated macrophage protein (NRAMP)
  defect in production of, 154–155
  role of, 155
Negative selection, auto-reactive cell removal and, 6–7
Neisseria, vaccine for, 74
Neisseria meningitidis
  carrier for, 203
  fatality rate from, 203
  serotypes for, 203
Neoantigen, pharmaceuticals and, 28
Neomycin, in vaccines, 194t
Neonatal Fc receptor (FcRn)
  pooled IVIG and, 103
  role of, 103f
Neonatal tetanus, 201
Nerve impulse, 131f
Neuraminidase, 208
Neutrophil, diapedesis of, 12f
Neutrophilic band, 2–3
Nezelof syndrome, 13
Nickel hypersensitivity, 159
Nitric oxide, 20
  tumor necrosis factor (TNF) and, 183
N-nucleotide, 82
Nonallergic asthma
  aspirin-induced, 124
  exercise-induced, 123
  infectious, 123
Nonallergic food reaction, histamine in food, 124
Nongranulocyte, 2
Nonhomologous end joining (NHEJ), 80
Non-inhibitory receptor, 170f
Non-nucleoside reverse transcriptase inhibitor, 220, 221b
Nonparalytic aseptic meningitis, 204
Non-self blood group antigen, 25
Novel antibody configuration
  bi-functional antibody and, 107
  bi-specific antibody and, 107
  Fab fragments and, 107
Nuclear Factor-$_\kappa$B (NF-$_\kappa$B), 56
Nuclear transcription factor (NFAT), 56
Nucleic acid vaccine, 186
Nucleoside reverse transcriptase inhibitor, 220, 220t
Nucleotide, J gene, removal from, 82
Nucleotide reverse transcriptase inhibitor, 220t
Nucleus, ultrastructural analysis of, 3f
NY-ESO-1, 185

O

O antigen, 24–25
Oligodeoxynucleotide, 193
Oligomer, collectin as, 17f
Omenn syndrome, 52
Opisthotonos, 200, 210f
O-polysaccharide, 64–65
Oprelvekin, 182
Oral allergy syndrome, pollen and, 121–122

Oral polio vaccine-associated poliomyelitis, 204
Original inactivated poliovirus (IPV), 204
Orthomyxoviridae family, 208
Otitis media, 202
Ovalbumin, hapten conjugation to, 27f
Oxygen-dependent intracellular killing, 98
Oxygen-dependent killing by phagocytic cells, 99f
Oxygen-dependent respiratory burst, 98

P

Palatine tonsils, 10
Pandemic influenza
    mortality rate of, 209
    in twentieth century, 209t
Paneth cell defensin, 19
Papain, 71–72
Papilloma virus
    prevalence of, 211
    serotypes for, 211
    strains of, 211
    treatment of, 211, 211t
    vaccine for, 211–212
        Cervarix, 212
        Gardasil, 212
Papillon-Lefèvre syndrome
    characteristics of, 166
    treatment of, 166
Paracortex, 8
Paralytic polio
    cause of, 204
    types of, 204
Paroxysmal nocturnal hemoglobinuria (PNH), 90–92
    treatment of, 92
Passive immunity
    definition of, 102
    heterologous antisera and, 102–103
Pasteur, Louis, 189
Pathogen-associated molecular pattern (PAMP), 16
    lipopolysaccharide endotoxin as, 17–18
    macrophages recognizing, 19f
    receptor recognition of, 16–17
    serum complement components and, 16–17
    toll-like receptors and, 17
    types of, 16t
    vaccines and, 20
Pathogenic bacteria, growth range and temperature, 19
Peanut allergy, 122t
Penicillin
    composition of, 27–28
    metabolites for, 28, 28f
Pepsin, 71–72
Perforin
    cytotoxic T lymphocyte and, 164f
    familial erythrophagocytic lymphohistiocytosis type 2 and, 165
    role of, 165f
    synthesis of, 163f
Perforin-granzyme cytolysis, 163–164, 164f
Periarteriolar lymphoid sheath (PALS), 9
Peripheral blood stem cell, 144
Pernicious anemia
    bone marrow aspirate smear for, 130f
    intrinsic factor and, 129
    treatment of, 129
Pertussis (whooping cough)
    coughing pattern for, 199
    etiologic agent of, 199
    treatment of, 200t
    vaccine for, 200t
Pertussis (whooping cough) toxin, 199
Peyer's patches, 10f
    Bone marrow and, 7
    location/composition of, 9–10
pH, of skin, 15
Phagocyte, adhesion of, 11f
Phagocytic cell, oxygen-dependent killing by, 99f

Phagocytosis, 97–98
    antigen-antibody complex and, 97
    immunodeficiencies associated with
        chronic granulomatous disease (CGD), 100
        complement receptor deficiency, 100
        Gaucher's disease, 99–100
        myeloperoxidase (MPO) deficiency, 100
    microbe killing and, 20f
    toll-like receptor and, 17
Phagolysosome, 17, 40
Phagosome, 17, 40, 98
    granules fusing with, 98
Pharmaceutical, neoantigens and, 28
Pharyngeal tonsils, 10
Phosphokinase C (PKC) pathway, 56
Photo contact dermatitis, 158
    treatment of, 159
Phycoerythrin (PE), 111
Picornavirus, 204
Pig, for transplants, 139
Pinocytosis, 98
Plant
    hypersensitivity reactions to, 159
        poison ivy, 159
Plant vaccine, 192
Plasma cell
    apoptosis of, 6f
    B cell differentiation into, agents blocking, 66
    B cells and, 5–6
    characteristics of, 5f
    longevity of, 65–66
Plasma cell differentiation, 65
Plasma cell dyscrasias
    multiple myeloma as, 77
        treatment of, 77
    Waldenström's macroglobulinemia as
        effects of, 77
        treatment of, 77
Plasmacytoid dendritic cell, 39
Plasmid, 186
    Escherichia coli and, 192
Plasmid vaccine, 186
Platelet
    hematopoiesis and, 1–2
    idiopathic thrombocytopenic purpura and, 103
    production of, 2
$PLC_{GAMMA}1$, T cell signaling downstream of, 59f
$PLC_{GAMMA}1$-DAG/PKC pathway, 56
PLC signaling pathway, calcium and, 56
Pneumococcal conjugate vaccine, 202–203
    Prevnar as, 202–203
Pneumococcal disease, 202
    treatment of, 202
    types of
        bacteremia as, 202
        meningitis as, 202
        otitis media as, 202
        pneumonia as, 202
    vaccines for, 202–203
        capsular polysaccharide, 202
Pneumococcus, 201–203
    active immunity and, 102
    polysaccharide capsule and, 189–190
    serotyping for, 202
    vaccine for, 74
    virulence factors for, 202
Pneumonia, 202
    Neisseria meningitidis as agent for, 203
Poison ivy dermatitis, 159, 159t
Pol gene, 216
Polio, 198
    abortive infection form, 204
    host for, 204
    post-polio syndrome, 204
    serotypes for, 203

Polio *(Continued)*
  subclinical infections from, 204
  treatment of, 204
  vaccines for, 204
Poliomyelitis, oral polio vaccine-associated, 204
Pollen
  cross-reactive agents and, 122t
  oral allergy syndrome and, 121–122
Polymerase chain reaction-sequence-based typing (PCR-SBT), 140
Polymerase chain reaction-sequence-specific oligonucleotide (PCR-SSO), 140
Polymerase chain reaction-sequence-specific primer (PCR-SSP), 140
Polymeric beta 1-4 linkage, 2
Polymorphic, 33
Polymorphonuclear neutrophils (PMN)
  composition/function of, 2
  cytoplasm, granules in, 2
  demargination of, 2
  N-formyl-1-methionyl-1-leucyl-1-phenylalamine (FMLP) and, 2
  half-life of, 2
  mobility, increasing, 2
  production of, 2
  structural/histological features of, 2f
Polymyxin B, in vaccines, 194t
Polypeptide chain, 73f
Polyribosyl phosphate (PRP), 201
Polysaccharide capsule, 189–190
Pooled human immunoglobulin
  administration of, 103
  bacterial/viral pathogens and, 176
  diseases treated with, 103b
    erythroblastosis fetalis, 104
    idiopathic thrombocytopenic purpura, 103
    Kawasaki disease, 103–104
  limitations of, 104
  preparation of, 103
Porcine gelatin, in vaccines, 195t
Positive selection, auto-reactive cell removal and, 6
Post-herpetic neuralgia, 207
Post-polio syndrome, 204
Preformed mediator, 119
Pregnancy, measles infection and, 206
Pregnancy testing
  as immunochromatographic testing, 112
  reaction, test and control zones of, 114f
Preintegration complex (PIC), formation of, 217
Prevnar, 202–203
Prevnar 13, 203
Primary ciliary dysfunction (PCD), 15
Primary granule(s), 2
Primary immune response, 75f
Primary immunodeficiency
  common variable immunodeficiency as, 76
  hyperimmunoglobulinemia E (Job syndrome) as, 77
  immunoglobulin A (IgA) deficiency, treatment of, 77
  selective immunoglobulin A deficiency as, 76–77
  transient hypogammaglobulinemia of infancy as, 76
Primary lymphoid organ, 1, 6–7
Professional antigen-presenting cell. *See* Antigen-presenting cell
Proliferation-inducing ligand (APRIL), 65
  interaction of, 67f
Properidin, 89
Propionibacter acnes, 15
Protease inhibitor, 221
Protein
  alpha fetal, 184
  CD1, 148
  epitopes and, 24
  in granules, 3
    role of, 3t
  heat shock, 184, 185f
  immunogens as, 23
  transporter-associated with antigen processing (TAP), 147
Proteolysis, 25f
P-selectin, 11

Pseudogene, 31
Pseudomonas, 189–190
Pseudomonas aeruginosa, 20
Pseudopodia, 39–40
Psoriasis, dendritic cells and, 41
Ptosis, 131f
Puberty, thymus and, 6
Purified protein derivative of tuberculosis, 155
Purine nucleoside phosphorylase (PNP), 13

Q
QuantiFERON Gold test (GFT-G), 156

R
Rac-JNK pathway, 56
Rac protein kinase, 56
Radioallergosorbent test (RAST), in vitro, 122
Radioimmunoassay (RIA), 115f
Radioimmunotherapy, 108
Ramsay Hunt syndrome, 207
Rapamycin-associated protein (RAP), 59
Ras-MAPK pathway, 56
  in T cell activation, 58f
Rationale attenuation, 190–191
Rat sarcoma protein (Ras), 56
  mode of action for, 58f
Reactive arthritis, 134
Reassortment vaccine, 191–192
  recombinant bacterial vaccine as, 191
  recombinant viral vaccine as, 191–192
Recognition complex, 88
  control of, 88
Recognition signal sequence (RSS), 80
Recombinant bacterial vaccine, 191
Recombinant viral vaccine, 191–192
Recombination activating gene (RAG), 47, 48f
Red blood cell
  drugs reacting to, 29b
  hematopoiesis and, 1–2
Red blood cell isoantigen, 24–25
  hemolytic transfusion reaction and
    cause of, 25
    treatment of, 25, 26t
Red pulp
  composition of, 9
  location of, 1–2
  stem cells from, 2
Regulator cell
  CD4 as, 176–177
  CD8 as, 177–178
  role of, 176
  TH3 as, 177
Regulator factor X (RFX), 35
Respiratory burst
  as defective, 100
  oxygen-dependent, 98
Respiratory infection, 68
Respiratory syncytial virus (RSV), 67–68
Respiratory tract, barriers for, 15
Rev gene, 219
Reye syndrome, 206
Rhesus antigen, 26
  role of, 26
Rhesus factor isoantigen, 26
Rheumatic fever
  group A *Streptococcus* species and, 135
  treatment of, 135
Rheumatoid arthritis
  characteristics of, 135
  effects of, 135f
  genetics and, 135
  treatment of, 66, 136
  triggers for, 135
  tumor necrosis factor (TNF) and, 183
Rheumatoid factor (RF), 135

INDEX

Rh factor incompatibility, 104
Rotarix, 211
Rotashield (RRV-TV), 211
RotaTeg, 211
Rotavirus
    groups, subgroups, serotypes for, 210
    risk groups for, 209–210
    seasonal infections with, 211f
    transmission of, 210
    treatment of, 210
    vaccine for, 211
Rotavirus vaccine, 191
Rubella (German measles)
    complications of
        arthritis, 206
        congenital rubella syndrome, 206
    history of, 206
    transmission/effects of, 206
    vaccine for, 206
Rubeola. *See* Measles

S

Sabin oral poliovirus vaccine (OPV), 204
Sandwich enzyme-linked immunosorbent assay (ELISA), 112, 115f
Sclerosing panecephalitis (SSPE), 205
Seasonal influenza, 209
Sebaceous gland, 15
Sebum, 15
Secondary granule(s), 2
Secondary immune response, 75f
Secondary lymphoid organ, 1, 8–9
Secretory (sIgM), production of, 74
Secretory granule(s), 2
Secretory IgA
    clinical importance of, 74–75
    production of, 74–75
Sedimentation rate (Svedberg unit), 70
Selectin, 2
    location of, 11t
Selection
    of B cell-myeloma cell hybrid, 104
    necessity of, 104
    tissue culture-based system and, 104
Selective immunoglobulin A deficiency, 76–77
Self-peptide
    allorecognition and, 140
    T cell activation and, 140
Serial summation, 141
Seroglycin, 163–164
Serum amyloid protein
    biologic effects of, 20t
    drugs reacting to, 29b
    role of, 19
Serum sickness, cause of, 102–103
Severe combined immunodeficiency (SCID), 35
    Omenn syndrome and, 52
    treatment of, 61
    X-linked, 60–61
Shingles (varicella zoster)
    cause of, 207
    complications of
        post-herpetic neuralgia, 207
        Ramsay Hunt syndrome, 207
    treatment of, 207, 207t
Sialyl-Lewis[x], 11
Sialyl Tn antigen (sTn), 185
Sider scatter, 110
Signal joint, 80
Signal transducer activator of transcription (STAT), 56
Single-chain Fab variable fragment (scFv), 107–108
    advantages/disadvantages of, 108
    expression of, 108, 108f
    generation of, 107–108
Single nucleotide polymorphism (SNP), 33

Sinus, role of, 9
Sirian immunodeficiency virus (SIV), human immunodeficiency virus (HIV) versus, 214
Sirolimus, 59
    T cell activation/signaling, blocking of, 60t
Sjögren syndrome, complement receptor deficiency and, 100
Skin
    as barrier, 15
    delayed-type hypersensitivity in, 158–159
        contact dermatitis, 159
        photo contact dermatitis, 158
Small lymphocyte
    characteristics of, 4
    subdivision of, 5
Small nuclear riboprotein (snRAP), 82
Solid organ rejection
    acute, 141, 142f–143f
    chronic, 142
    hyperacute, 141
    prevention of, 142–143
Somatic cell recombination, 47
Somatic mutation theory, 79
Son of sevenless (SOS), 63–64
Soybean allergen, 122t
Spina bifida, 124
Spleen
    characteristics of, 9f
    hematopoiesis and, 1–2
    location of, 9
    morphology of, 9f
    as secondary lymphoid organ, 1
Squalene adjuvant, 192
Staphylococcal superantigen, 51, 52t
Staphylococcal toxic shock syndrome, 52
Staphylococcus, toll-like receptors and, 16–17
Staphylococcus aureus, enterotoxins and, 51
Staphylococcus aureus protein A, 193
Stem cell
    maturation of, 1–2
    from red pulp, 2
Stoma, 1–2
Stomach, barriers for, 16
Stomach acid, 16
Stratum corneum, 15
Streptococcal superantigen, 51, 52t
Streptococcal toxic shock syndrome, 51
    risk for, 52
    symptoms/effects of, 52
Streptococcus, 10
    active immunity and, 102
    cathelicidins and, 19
    toll-like receptors and, 16–17
Streptococcus pneumoniae
    early-onset agammaglobulinemia and, 66–67
    prevalence/effects of, 201–202
Streptomycin, in vaccines, 194t
Subacute sclerosing panecephalitis (SSPE), 205
Subclinical infection, 204
Subunit vaccine, 191
Superantigen, 50–51, 51f
Superoxide dismutase, 98
Suppressor cell, 176
Supramolecular activation cluster (SMAC), 55–56
Survival rate, for transplantation, 142–143, 143f
Syk, docking sites for, 63
Synergic transplant, 139
Syngeneic graft, tissue compatibility for, 139–140
Synthesized mediator, 119
Synthetic interferon
    biologic modifiers and, 183
    commercially available, 183t
Systemic immunity, adjuvants and, 192
    aluminum salts, 192
    Freund's complete, 192
    liposomes, 192

Systemic immunity (Continued)
   muramyl peptides, 192
   squalene, 192
Systemic lupus erythematosus (SLE)
   characteristics of, 131
   complement receptor deficiency and, 100
   effects of, 133f
   facial rash and, 132f
   immunoglobulin G, deposition of, 132f
   treatment of, 66, 131–132

T

Tacrolimus (FK506), 59
   T cell activation/signaling, blocking of, 60t
Tampon use, 51
Target cell, 170
   lysis of, 163–164, 171
Target of rapamycin (TOR), 59
Tat gene translation, 219
T cell, 7f
   ADA deficiency and, 13
   antigen-presenting cells and, reagents blocking interactions, 50t
   B cells and, 67f
   classification of, 5
   epitopes and, 24
   identification of, 5
   lamina propria lymphocyte (LPL) as, 10
   maturation of, 6–7
      hormones and, 7
   melanoma antigen recognizing, 184–185
   natural killer cell and, 6
   role of, 5
   subpopulation of, 5
T cell activation, 55
   FasR and ligand, expression of, 178f
   fungal immunosuppressive agent blocking, 60t
   ras-MAPK pathway in, 58f
   self-peptide and, 140
   of transcription factors, 60f
T cell-derived cytokine, 67f
T cell-mediated autoimmune disease, intravenous immunoglobulin, 104
T cell receptor (TCR)
   as alpha/beta, 46–47
      V regions of, 46
   antigen-presenting cells and
      agents blocking interactions, 49–50
      blocking interactions, 50
   CD3-T cell receptor protein complex, 48
   as gamma/delta, 47
   genetic rearrangement of, 6, 7f, 48f
   somatic cell recombination and, 47
   structure of, 46f
T cell receptor (TCR) complex, components of, 49f
T cell receptor (TCR) diversity, 47–48
T cell receptor (TCR)-mediated signaling, 55–56
T cell receptor (TCR) signaling, agents inhibiting, 56–59
T cell receptor (TCR) V_β isoform, 52
T cell receptor-human leukocyte antigen (TCR-HLA) interaction, pathways activated by, 55
T cell receptor-human leukocyte antigen (TCR-HLA) molecule, engagement of, 55
T cell signaling
   as defective, 60–61
   fungal immunosuppressive agent blocking, 60t
   PLC$_{GAMMA}$1, downstream of, 59f
Temperature, bacteria growth range and, 19
Terminal deoxyribonucleotidyl transferase, 82
Tertiary granule(s), 2
Tetanospasmin, 200
Tetanus
   forms of, 200
      cephalic, 201
      generalized, 200–201
      localized, 201
      neonatal, 201

Tetanus (Continued)
   in humans, 200
   prevalence of, 200
   treatment of, 201
      agents used in, 201t
   vaccine for, 201
Tetanus immune globulin (TIG), 201
Tetanus toxin, 190
   treatment of, 201
TH3 regulator cell, 177
Three'-end processing, 219
Thymocyte, 6
   major histocompatibility complex (MHC) and, 7
Thymus
   cell types in, 6f
   location/composition of, 6
   as primary lymphoid organ, 1
   puberty and, 6
   role of, 6
   T cells maturation in, 6–7
Thymus-dependent (TD) antibody production, 63
Thymus-dependent (TD) antigen, 64
Thymus-independent (TI) antigen, 63–65
   type I, 64–65
   type II, 65
Thyroid
   autoimmune diseases of, 128–129
      Graves' disease, 128
      Hashimoto's thyroiditis, 128
   function of, 128
Thyroid-releasing hormone (TRH), 128
Thyroid storm, 128
Thyrotoxicosis. See Graves' disease
Tissue
   antimicrobial agents produced by
      cathelicidins, 19
      defensins, 19–20
      nitric oxide, 20
   compatibility for grafts, 139–140
   inflammation causing damage to, 99
Tissue cross-matching, 140
Tissue culture-based system
   homogeneous antibody production by, 104
   selection and, 104
T killer cell
   evasion by tumor cells, 164
   immunodeficiency and, 165–166
TNFR-associated proteins with death domains (TRADD), 164
TNF-related apoptosis-inducing ligand (TRAIL) pathway, 164
Toll-like receptor
   autoimmunity and, 17
   innate immunity and, 16–17
   ligands for, 20t
   pathogen-associated molecular pattern (PAMP) and, 17
   phagocytosis and, 17
Tonsils
   composition of, 10
   location of, 10
   as secondary lymphoid organ, 1
   secretory antibodies and, 10
Toxicodendron, contact dermatitis and, 159
Toxic shock syndrome (TSS)
   staphylococcal, 52
   streptococcal, 51–52
   tampon use and, 51
   treatment of
      antibiotics, 52t
      pharmacotherapy for, 52
Toxin, bacteria producing, 190
Toxoid vaccine, 191
Tracheal antimicrobial peptide (TAP), 20
Tracheal cytotoxin, 199–200
Transfusion, disease transmission from, 104
Transfusion-related acute lung injury (TRALI), 24
Transient hypogammaglobulinemia of infancy, 76

Transplantation, 138
  bone marrow for, 144
  diseases treated with, 143b
  hematopoietic stem cell, 143–144
  human leukocyte antigen marker and, 139
  rejection of, 139f
Transplantation (Continued)
    monoclonal antibodies, 143
    types of, 141–142
  solid organ rejection, 141–142
  survival rates for, 142–143, 143f
    rejection prevention, 142–143
  tissue compatibility and, 139–140
  types of, 139
Transplantation protocol, 144
Transporter-associated with antigen processing (TAP) protein, 147
Treg (T regulator), 176
Treg 1 cell, 177
T regulator (Treg), 176
T-SPOT.TB test, 156
TSST-1 receptor, 51
Tuberculin, cellular movements after, 155f
Tuberculosis
  Bacille Calmette-Guérin (BCG) for, 191
  characteristics of, 154f
  diagnosis of, 156
  extensively drug-resistant, 156
  genetics and, 154–155
  Mantoux skin test for, 155
  multidrug-resistant strains of, 156
  natural resistance-associated macrophage protein and, 154–155
  pathophysiology of, 153–154
  treatment of, 156
    first-line drugs for, 156t
    second-line drugs for, 156t
  types of, 153, 153t
  virulence factors for, 153
  in vitro test for, 156
  in vivo tuberculin skin test and, 155–156
Tumor antigen, cancer vaccines and, 184
Tumor cell
  cytotoxic T lymphocyte killing, 165f
  T killer cell, evasion of, 164
Tumor-infiltrating lymphocyte, 164
Tumor necrosis factor (TNF), 4, 183
  as biologic response modifier, 183
  disease and, 183
  effects of, 183
  nitric oxide and, 183
Tumor necrosis factor (TNF) beta, 164
Tumor necrosis factor (TNF) receptor 1, 166f
Tumor necrosis factor (TNF) receptor 1 cytolysis, 164
Tumor-specific transportation antigen (TSTA)
  expression of, 184
  tyrosinase as, 184
Type A influenza, 208
Type B influenza, 208
Type C influenza, 208
Type II thymus-independent antigen, 65
Type I thymus-independent antigen, 64–65
Tyrosinase, 184

U
Ubiquitination, 147
Ultra-centrifugation, 70
Umbilical cord blood stem cell, 144
Urogenital tract, 16
Urticaria
  as acute or chronic, 121
  characteristics of, 121
  photo of, 121f
  treatment of, 121
  types of, 121
Urushiol, 159

V
Vaccination, 189
  disease reduction, 198
  routes of, 190f
Vaccine-preventable disease, 197
Vaccine. See also Cancer vaccine
  conjugate, 202t
    pneumococcal, 202–203
  dendritic cells and, 41
  for dermonecrotic lethal toxin, 200
  for diphtheria, 199
  DNA, 186
  as edible, 192
  egg albumin in, 193, 194t
  excipients in, 193–194
  for Haemophilus influenzae type B (Hib), 201
  for hepatitis, 208
  for influenza virus, 209
    live attenuated, 209
    trivalent inactivated, 209
  for measles (rubeola), 205
  measles-mumps-pertussis (MMR), 205t
  for meningitis, 203–204
    Menactra, 204
    Menomune, 203–204
    Menveo, 204
  monosodium glutamate in, 194t
  for mumps, 205–206
  neomycin in, 194t
  PAMPs and, 20
  for papilloma virus, 211–212
  plant, 192
  for pneumococcal disease, 202–203
  for polio, 204
  polymyxin B, gentamicin, streptomycin in, 194t
  porcine gelatin in, 195t
  reassortment, 191–192
  for rotavirus, 211
  for rubella (German measles), 206
  for tetanus, 201
  in theory and practice, 189
  types of, 190–192
    conjugate, 191
    inactivated, 191
    live attenuated, 190–191
    subunit, 191
    toxoid, 191
  for varicella zoster, 207
Vacuole, 40
Valley Fever. See Coccidioidomycosis
Vanishing bile duct syndrome, 142
Variable segment, gene coding in light/heavy chains, 80t
Varicella vaccine, 207
Varicella zoster vaccine, 207
Varicella zoster virus
  complications of
    congenital infection, 206
    disseminated varicella neonatorum, 206
    Reye syndrome, 206
  diseases of, 206
  rash from, 206
  reactivation as shingles, 207
  replication of, 206
  treatment of, 206
  vaccine for, 207
Variola, 189
V(D)J recombination, 81f
  sequential events during, 82f
Vernal conjunctivitis, 121
Vesicle, 98
V genes, somatic hypermutation of, 84
Viral hepatitis, 207
Viral-like protein (VLP), 211–212
Viral RNA, 216
Viral vector vaccine, 186

Virulent organism, 189
Virus
  cytotoxic T lymphocyte killing, 165f
  flow cytometry identifying, 112
  immune response, evasion of, 164–165
  interferon and, 183
  pathogen-associated microbial patterns in, 16t
Vitamin D receptor deficiency, 155
von Behring, Emil, 102

W

Waldenström's macroglobulinemia
  effects of, 77
  treatment of, 77
Western blotting
  limitations of, 114
  use of, 114
Wheal-and-flare skin reaction
  allergen causing, 122
  view of, 123f
White blood cell
  basophils as, 3
  definition of, 2
  eosinophils as, 3
  hematopoiesis and, 1–2
  lymphocytes as, 4–6
  macrophages as, 4
  mast cells as, 3–4
  monocyte as, 4
  PMNs as, 2

White blood cell alloantigen, 24
White pulp, composition of, 9
Whole-cell vaccine, 185–186
Whooping cough. *See* Pertussis

X

Xenograft, 139, 139f
Xenotransplantation, 139
X-linked agammaglobulinemia (XLA), effects of, 66–67
X-linked disorder
  symptoms of, 177
  treatment of, 177
X-linked immunodeficiency, 52
X-linked severe combined immunodeficiency (SCID), 60–61

Y

Yeast expression system, 192
Yellow pulp, 1–2

Z

Zalcitabine nucleoside analog, 221f
ZAP-70, 56
ZAP-70 immunodeficiency, 61
ZAP proteins, ITAMs and, 61
Zeta-chain-associated protein kinase (ZAP), 170
Zidovudine nucleoside analog, 221f
Ziehl Neelsen stain, 153